Designing Resistance Training Programs

Third Edition

Designing Resistance Training Programs

Third Edition

Steven J. Fleck

The Colorado College

William J. Kraemer

University of Connecticut

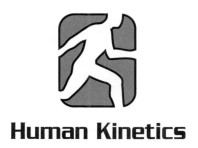

Human Kinetics

Library of Congress Cataloging-in-Publication Data

Fleck, Steven J., 1951-
  Designing resistance training programs / Steven J. Fleck, William J.
Kraemer.-- 3rd ed.
      p. cm.
Includes bibliographical references and index.
  ISBN 0-7360-4257-1 (Hard Cover)
  1. Isometric exercise. I. Kraemer, William J., 1953- II. Title.
  GV505.F58 2004
  613.7'1--dc21

                                        2004008524

ISBN: 0-7360-4257-1

Acquisitions Editor: Michael S. Bahrke, PhD
Developmental Editor: Anne Rogers
Assistant Editor: Amanda S. Ewing
Copyeditor: Patsy Fortney
Proofreader: Pam Johnson
Indexer: Schroeder Indexing Services
Permission Manager: Dalene Reeder
Graphic Designer: Fred Starbird
Graphic Artist: Angela K. Snyder
Photo Manager: Kareema McLendon
Cover Designer: Keith Blomberg
Photographer (cover): Dan Wendt
Photos on pages xiv, 129, and 151 © Kristiane Vey/JUMP; photo on page 3 © Marco Grundt/JUMP; photo on page 13 courtesy of Strive Enterprises; photos on pages 53 and 303 © CORBIS; photos on pages 148 and 187 courtesy of FreeMotion; photo on page 209 courtesy of Kytec; photo on page 241 © Empics; photo on page 260 © Creatas; photo on page 263 © Getty Images; photo on page 287 courtesy of William J. Kraemer.
Art Manager: Kelly Hendren
Illustrators: Mic Greenberg and Jennifer Delmotte
Printer: Transcontinental Printing
Printed in Canada   10   9   8   7   6   5   4   3   2   1

Human Kinetics
Web site: www.HumanKinetics.com

United States: Human Kinetics
P.O. Box 5076
Champaign, IL 61825-5076
800-747-4457
e-mail: humank@hkusa.com

Canada: Human Kinetics
475 Devonshire Road Unit 100
Windsor, ON N8Y 2L5
800-465-7301 (in Canada only)
e-mail: orders@hkcanada.com

Europe: Human Kinetics
107 Bradford Road
Stanningley
Leeds LS28 6AT, United Kingdom
+44 (0) 113 255 5665
e-mail: hk@hkeurope.com

Australia: Human Kinetics
57A Price Avenue
Lower Mitcham, South Australia 5062
08 8277 1555
e-mail: liahka@senet.com.au

New Zealand: Human Kinetics
P.O. Box 105-231, Auckland Central
09-523-3462
e-mail: hkp@ihug.co.nz

Contents

Preface

We welcome you to our third edition of *Designing Resistance Training Programs,* which over the years has been a solid resource in the field of exercise and sport science. This textbook has been used by a wide variety of readers seriously interested in resistance training—from undergraduate students in resistance training theory courses to sport scientists wanting to further their understanding of the theoretical approaches of resistance training. Because the concept of individualization is so important in designing a resistance training program, this text has also been highly individualized for many different needs and settings. Ultimately, this book will provide you with the tools to understand and design resistance training programs for almost any situation or need. It also offers a comprehensive background in resistance training program design from both scientific and practical perspectives. We hope you will gain an understanding of the dynamic nature of the program design process and will pick up on the many subtleties needed to bring the science of resistance training into practice. The third edition was written as the field moves forward quickly and the knowledge of the past combines with the dramatic amount of new information that has been produced over the past several years. Thus, readers of our previous editions will also find the important updates needed to fill in the blanks of the past and enjoy the resulting paradigms that have been created.

In the early 1980s we were both struck with the importance of understanding how to design a resistance training program. We sought to develop a theoretical paradigm to meet this need, and it resulted in the identification of two important variables related to program design—acute program variables and chronic program variables. These structures have provided the theoretical framework for both practical applications and the scientific study of resistance training. Our own work with athletes and in the laboratory has benefited from this more quantitative approach to resistance training, and we have been overwhelmed through the years at its acceptance and use by a multitude of readers. It was also our intention to create a book "beyond the exercises" that were vintage at the time

we put together our first edition and focused on the various aspects of science and practice needed to develop an effective exercise prescription. Because we both understand that the process of program design is related to the art of using science, each edition has attempted to fill in the blanks of our understanding of the science of resistance training. Thus, a literature-based book resulted and was a relatively novel approach to this area of study and for textbooks on this topic. Over the years students, instructors, and even those just interested in what they are doing in the weight room have found this book to be a valuable reference and a "good read." We continue in this tradition. This new edition brings to bear the many new perspectives in the field and updates both student and professional on this topic of program design.

Since our last edition, more than 10,000 manuscripts in the broad scientific literature of resistance training have been published with a wide variety of applications and in many areas of study. Although this textbook can no longer be a comprehensive source for such a dramatic amount of new data, we have used this large database to continue to mature and develop the concepts we put forth in our previous editions. The field is clearly moving forward at what might be called "warp speed," with the interest in resistance training as great as ever. This textbook will give you some tools to help you evaluate resistance training programs and better understand the context and efficacy of the host of information coming at you from sources beyond the scientific literature, such as the Internet, magazines, television, radio, videos, and infomercials. More than ever we need a paradigm for understanding the information now available in the growing field of resistance training.

We have reorganized this book by starting in chapter 1 with the basic principles of resistance training and exercise prescription. This chapter is vital to lay the foundation for each subsequent chapter. For example, one of the hallmarks of resistance training is the concept of training specificity, which affects everything from the cellular-level events in the muscle to the performance of athletic skills. We then take you through a detailed examination of the different types of strength training (chapter 2) from isometrics to isokinetics and make some unique comparisons among types of resistance training to help you understand how muscle action type influences adaptations and performance changes.

From here is it vital that you have a fundamental understanding of the basic physiology and adaptations to resistance training to be able to utilize new information in the future and put into context expectations for resistance training. For example, Is there such a concept as aerobic weight training? What might be the expectations for muscle hypertrophy in the first 6 weeks of a program? A fundamental understanding of basic physiology will help you distinguish fact from fiction when assessing the physical changes that occur with resistance training. Chapter 3 provides this comprehensive and important view of physiology from the perspective of resistance training influences. This chapter is one of the few in the literature to take on such a perspective and offers a new look at some basic concepts in physiological science. This chapter also provides undergraduate students studying kinesiology, exercise and sport sciences, and physical education a chance to integrate into understanding resistance training what they have learned from their other basic courses in anatomy, physiology, and exercise physiology.

Because resistance training is only one component of the "total conditioning" program, we felt that it was very important to show you how resistance training programs interact with the other conditioning components such as aerobic endurance training, interval training, and flexibility training. Chapter 4 offers an overview of these other important conditioning components and how they interact with resistance training.

In chapter 5 the design of a single workout session is addressed. Proper design of each session is important as individual sessions are the building blocks of long-term training programs. Here the acute program variables come into play and we continue in the tradition of using a specific paradigm to understand what you are asking someone to do in the weight room and why. From starting with a needs analysis to developing sound rationales for the various acute program variables and setting reasonable goals, this chapter discusses one of the individual sessions and one of the pillars of success in resistance training. Chapter 6 presents an overview of the many resistance training systems that have historically been around in both the popular and scientific literature from the perspec-

tive of the understanding of workout design offered in chapter 5. You get the chance to use what you learned about program variables in chapter 5 to see different resistance training systems in a new light. This skill of evaluating programs based on an analysis of the variable structure used is important in helping you to evaluate the many new programs that come out each year. This process allows you to predict potential physiological stress and extrapolate realistic training adaptations for programs that may not have been studied scientifically.

In chapter 7 we have newly structured our overview of the chronic program variables by including important concepts of how one progresses in a resistance training program over time. Principles such as periodization are important to this process. Work from laboratories around the world, including our own, has shown that without variation in training, adaptations and gains can plateau well before one's potential has been reached. We also cover the popular topic of plyometrics, which has now gained more importance in power development and is a part of many training strategies used in conditioning today. With the obvious need for rest in any resistance training program as a fundamental principle of periodization comes the question of detraining, which occurs when training is stopped or significantly reduced. How does this affect the average person or athlete? What about training in-season? How long can one go without working out? These are some of the questions addressed in chapter 8 to help those in resistance training complete the continuum of progression and prevent loss of training adaptations.

In the final section of the book we take a careful look at resistance training exercise prescription in different populations, because our understanding has been based on the "normative college-age man" for too long. Chapter 9 begins this section with a discussion of women and resistance training. Although women undertaking resistance training are similar to men in many respects, some true gender differences do exist. The exercise prescription process must take these factors into account and adjust in order to offer optimal gains. This theme continues in chapter 10, which addresses resistance training in children, who have been subjected to adult programs for too long. With the benefits of resistance training now being established for children of all ages, you must be able to prescribe programs that are safe and effective for this unique population. Given the epidemics of obesity and inactivity in children today, resistance training appears to be one fun way to attract more children to an active lifestyle. Furthermore, this chapter helps create the proper mind-set for working with young children and young adults while discarding the idea that children are just "little adults."

We end the book by addressing the other end of the aging continuum, that of older adults. This area of study has exploded over the past 20 years as a host of new information has come to light. We now know that resistance training can be effective in older adults and positively affect their health and functional abilities. However, program design concerns with this population are as important as ever, as improper program design may limit tissue activation and needed adaptations. In addition, joint compression and pain are problems that must be addressed with this group to facilitate the successful use of and adherence to resistance training programs.

We feel that this book will provide a cornerstone in your understanding of resistance training and continue to be a literature-based book on this topic. We understand that the ideas, philosophies, and approaches to resistance training change by the day, but ultimately the factual basis of what we know creates the stability needed to design effective programs in resistance training. We have provided extensive literature citations and selected readings to give you context and a historical feel for the field. This book will be an important component in your preparation for designing resistance training programs. We wish you good reading and good training!

Acknowledgments

I would like to acknowledge my many friends and colleagues who have influenced me throughout my career. In particular, I would like to acknowledge Wayne Batchelder for his support and guidance while I was a student at the University of Wisconsin at La Crosse and for helping me obtain a graduate fellowship at Ohio State University. I am also grateful to Robert Bartels for his support and guidance during my graduate career at Ohio State University.

Steve Fleck

At this point in my career, writing acknowledgments to so many who have helped to shape, support, and guide me in my career is beyond the scope of a typical acknowledgment section. This edition has come full circle from the first, which was published when I was here at the University of Connecticut in the late 1980s, and the second, published while I was at Penn State. Scientists, coaches, friends, and family have all helped to mold the creative process of putting this book together, from coaching to science.

I would like to thank all of the people at Human Kinetics who have been involved in the production process of this book from start to finish for their patience, professional skills, and support of our efforts. I am also grateful to Bruce Noble for his mentorship and belief in me during my graduate career. I thank my friend of over 30 years, Steve Fleck, for his patience with the whole process of book writing together over the years, as it has always been a process filled with joy and satisfaction. I also want to thank all of my fellow colleagues in the field for their inspirational work and excellence. I have been truly blessed to have a superb group of scientific collaborators and friends to work with in the process of undertaking scientific studies, many of which are referenced in this text. My deepest gratitude to each of you for your understanding and friendship (as the saying goes, "you know who you are").

I have been privileged to work with an outstanding and dedicated group of graduate students now and over the years who have all kept me on the cutting edge each day. I thank you all for your help, support, and loyalty to our vision.

Finally, thanks to Carl Maresh, who has supported this process as a friend of 30 years and the chair of the department of kinesiology here at the University of Connecticut. My career started on his desk in the laboratory long ago. I am truly humbled by all, and in a time when the world is filled with so many more dramatic and important challenges and life struggles, writing this book was truly a luxury and privilege. May God bless.

William J. Kraemer

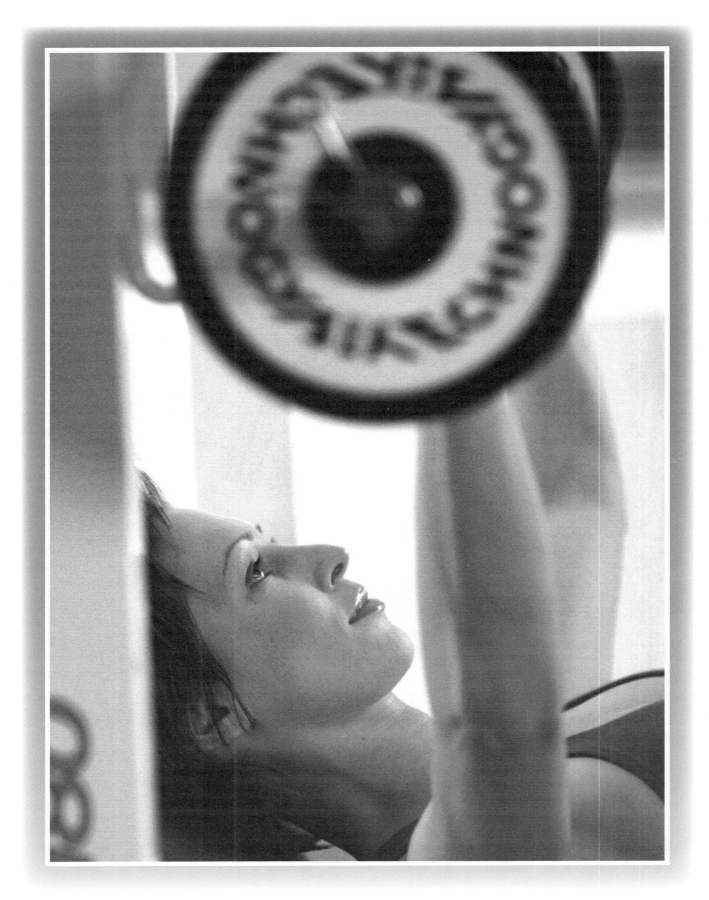

PART I

Foundations of Resistance Training

Like all fields of study, resistance training is based on underlying principles, concepts, and definitions. The information presented in the first four chapters is necessary to understand and successfully design any resistance training program. Chapter 1 presents the principles and definitions needed to effectively design and perform all resistance training programs in a safe manner. The characteristics of various types of resistance training are detailed in chapter 2. Different types of resistance training programs are desirable for different populations and for people seeking different physiological adaptations. Chapter 3 describes how muscles function and how they are controlled and adapt to resistance training. This chapter also describes how the cardiovascular system adapts to resistance training. This information will help you design resistance training programs to meet the goals and needs of a particular individual or population. Resistance training should be a part of a total fitness program, and how it fits into a total training program is discussed in chapter 4.

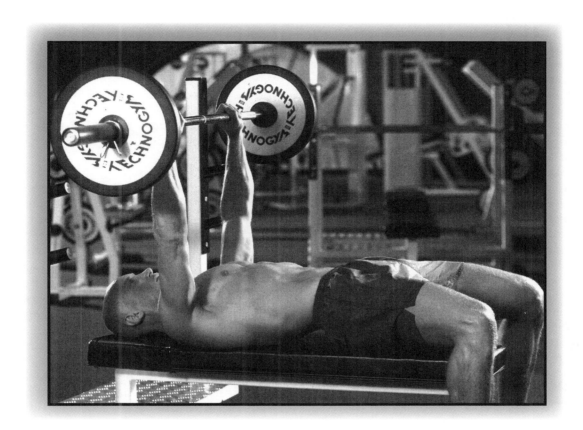

CHAPTER 1

Basic Principles of Resistance Training and Exercise Prescription

Resistance training, also known as strength or weight training, has become one of the most popular forms of exercise for enhancing an individual's physical fitness as well as for conditioning athletes. The terms *strength training, weight training,* and *resistance training* have all been used to describe a type of exercise that requires the body's musculature to move (or attempt to move) against an opposing force, usually presented by some type of equipment. The terms *resistance training* and *strength training* encompass a wide range of training modalities, including plyometrics and hill running. *Weight training* typically refers only to normal resistance training using free weights or some type of weight training machine.

The increasing number of health club, high school, and college resistance training facilities attests to the popularity of this form of physical conditioning. Individuals who participate in a resistance training program expect the program to produce certain health and fitness benefits, such as increased strength, increased fat-free mass, decreased body fat, and improved physical performance in either a sporting activity or daily life activities. A well-designed and consistently performed resistance training program can produce all of these benefits.

The fitness enthusiast, recreational weight trainer, and athlete all expect gains in strength or muscle size (muscular hypertrophy) from a resistance training program. Many different types of resistance training modalities (e.g., isokinetic, variable resistance, isometric, plyometric) can be used to accomplish these goals. In addition, many different training systems or programs (e.g., combinations of sets, repetitions, and resistances) can produce significant increases in strength or muscular hypertrophy as long as an effective training stimulus is presented to the muscle. Fitness gains will continue as long as the training stimulus remains effective. The effectiveness of a specific type of resistance training modality, training system, or training program depends on its proper use in the total exercise prescription.

Most athletes and fitness enthusiasts expect the gains in strength and power produced by a resistance training program to result in improved sport or daily life activity performance. Resistance training can improve motor performance (e.g., the ability to sprint, throw an object, or climb stairs), which can lead to better performance in various games, sports, and daily life activities. The amount of carryover from a resistance training program to a specific physical task depends on the transfer specificity or transfer carryover between the training program and the task. For example, multijoint exercises, such as clean pulls from the knees, would have greater transfer carryover to vertical jump ability than would isolated single-joint exercises, such as knee extensions or leg curls. Both multijoint and single-joint exercises increase the strength of the quadriceps and hamstring muscle groups. However, a greater similarity of biomechanical movements and muscle fiber recruitment patterns between a multijoint exercise and most sporting or daily life activities results in greater transfer specificity. Thus, in general, multijoint exercises have a greater transfer specificity than single-joint exercises.

Body compositional change is also a goal of many fitness enthusiasts and athletes engaged in resistance training programs. Normally the changes desired are a decrease in the amount of body fat and an increase in fat-free mass. However, some individuals also desire a gain or loss in total body weight. All of these changes can be achieved by a properly designed and performed resistance training program. The success of any program in bringing about a specific adaptation depends on the effectiveness of the exercise prescription, which ultimately produces the training stimulus.

Resistance training can produce the changes in body composition, strength, muscular hypertrophy, and motor performance that many individuals desire. To achieve optimal changes in these areas, individuals must adhere to some basic principles. These principles apply regardless of the resistance modality or the type of system or program the individual uses.

Basic Definitions

Before discussing the basic principles of resistance training, we will define some basic terms commonly used in describing resistance training programs or principles.

■ When a weight is being lifted, the muscles involved normally are shortening or performing a **concentric muscle action** (see figure 1.1a). During a concentric muscle action, shortening of the muscle occurs, and therefore the word *contraction* is also appropriate for this type of muscle action.

■ When a weight is being lowered in a controlled manner, the muscles involved are normally lengthening in a controlled manner, which is termed an **eccentric muscle action** (see figure 1.1b). Muscles can only shorten or lengthen in a controlled manner; they cannot push against the bones to which they are attached. In most exercises, gravity will pull the weight back to the starting position of an exercise. To control the weight as it returns to the starting position, the muscles must lengthen in a controlled manner, or the weight will fall abruptly.

■ When a muscle is activated and develops force, but no visible movement at the joint occurs, an **isometric muscle action** takes place (see figure 1.1c). This can occur when a weight is held stationary or when a weight is too heavy to lift any farther. Maximal isometric action force is greater than maximal concentric force at any velocity of movement, but less than maximal eccentric force at any movement velocity.

■ A **repetition** is one complete movement of an exercise. It normally consists of two phases: the concentric muscle action, or lifting of the resistance, and the eccentric muscle action, or lowering of the resistance.

■ A **set** is a group of repetitions performed continuously without stopping or resting. Although a set can consist of any number of repetitions, sets typically range from 1 to 15 repetitions.

▪ A **repetition maximum** or **RM** is the maximal number of repetitions per set that can be performed with proper lifting technique using a given resistance. Thus, a set at a certain RM implies that the set is performed to momentary voluntary fatigue. The heaviest resistance that can be used for 1 complete repetition of an exercise is 1RM. A lighter resistance that allows completion of 10, but not 11, repetitions with proper exercise technique is 10RM.

▪ **Power** is the rate of performing work. Power during a repetition is defined as the weight lifted multiplied by the vertical distance the weight is lifted divided by the time to complete the repetition. If 100 lb (45 kg or 445 N) are lifted vertically 3 ft (0.9 m) in 1 second, the power is 100 lb multiplied by 3 ft and divided by 1 second, or 300 ft lb s^{-1} (or about 400 W). Power during a repetition can be increased by lifting the same weight the same vertical distance in a shorter period of time. Power can also be increased by lifting a heavier resistance the same vertical distance in the same period of time as a lighter resistance. Normally, factors such as arm and leg length limit increasing power by moving a weight a greater distance. Thus, the only ways to increase power are to increase movement speed or lift a heavier resistance with the same or greater movement speed than a lighter resistance.

▪ **Strength** is the maximal amount of force a muscle or muscle group can generate in a specified movement pattern at a specified velocity of movement (Knuttgen and Kraemer 1987). In an exercise such as a bench press, 1RM is a measure of strength at a relatively slow speed. The classic concentric strength–velocity curve indicates that as the velocity increases, maximal strength decreases. On the other hand, as eccentric velocity increases, maximal strength increases and then plateaus.

Voluntary Maximal Muscular Actions

Voluntary maximal muscular actions appear to be an effective way to increase muscular strength (see the discussion of dynamic constant external resistance training in chapter 2). This does not mean that the maximal resistance possible for one complete repetition (1RM) must be lifted. Performing **voluntary maximal muscular actions** means that the muscle must move with as much resistance as its present fatigue level will allow. The force a partially fatigued muscle can generate during a voluntary maximal muscular action is not as great as that of a nonfatigued muscle. The last repetition in a set to momentary concentric failure is thus a voluntary maximal muscular action, even though the force produced is not the absolute maximum because the muscle is partially fatigued. Many resistance training systems use momentary concentric failure or RM resistance as a way to ensure the performance of voluntary maximal muscular actions. This ensures that the desired increases in strength, power, or local muscular endurance will occur (see chapter 2). Performing voluntary maximal muscular actions in resistance training is often referred to as overloading the muscle. The muscle must act against a resistance that it normally does not encounter for physiological changes resulting in the desired training effects to occur.

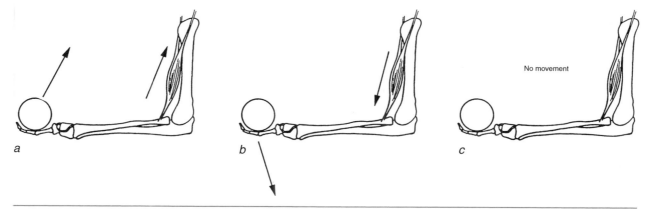

Figure 1.1 Major types of muscle actions. *(a)* During a concentric muscle action, a muscle shortens. *(b)* During an eccentric muscle action, the muscle lengthens in a controlled manner. *(c)* During an isometric muscle action, no movement of the joint occurs, and no shortening or lengthening of the total muscle takes place.

However, maximal increases in strength can occur, at least in some populations (i.e., seniors) without the performance of voluntary maximal muscular actions during each training session per week (Hunter et al. 2001). In this study equivalent strength and fat-free mass gains were demonstrated in a group performing maximal voluntary muscular actions during all of three training sessions per week and in a group performing maximal voluntary muscular actions in only one of three training sessions per week. However, it is important to note that maximal voluntary muscular actions were performed at least once per week.

In some exercises, performance of maximal voluntary muscular actions does not necessarily mean that the last repetition in a set is not completed. For example, when some muscle fibers become fatigued during power cleans, the velocity of the bar decreases and the weight is not pulled as high as it could be during the first repetition of a set even though the trainee is exerting maximal effort. Because the trainee developed maximal force in a partially fatigued state, by definition this is a maximal voluntary muscle action.

Some resistance training machines have been specifically designed to force the muscle to perform voluntary maximal muscular actions either through a greater range of motion or for more repetitions in a set. Developments in equipment such as variable resistance and isokinetic equipment (see chapter 2) attest to a belief in the necessity for voluntary maximal actions. All competitive Olympic weightlifters, power lifters, and bodybuilders use voluntary maximal muscular actions at some point in their training programs. This indicates that competitive lifters realize the need for voluntary maximal actions at some point in the training process to bring about optimal gains in strength or muscular hypertrophy.

Intensity

Closely related to voluntary maximal muscular actions is the intensity and power output of training. Power can be increased by using a heavier resistance and performing repetitions at the same speed of movement in some exercises or by lifting or moving a given resistance at a faster velocity in other exercises. The closer the concentric velocity is to maximal, the greater the power. This is true for both single-joint and multijoint exercises (Komi 1979). Increasing the power of an exercise by increasing the velocity of movement is important when a major goal is to increase the power

output of the muscle and not just its ability to develop maximal force (1RM ability).

Intensity of an exercise can be estimated as a percentage of the 1RM or any RM resistance for the exercise. The minimal intensity that can be used to perform a set to momentary voluntary fatigue in young, healthy individuals to result in increased strength is 60 to 65% of the 1RM (McDonagh and Davies 1984; Rhea et al. 2003). However, progression with resistances in the 50 to 60% of 1RM range may be effective and may result in greater 1RM increases than the use of heavier resistances in some populations (e.g., in senior women; see chapter 11). Additionally, approximately 80% of 1RM results in maximal strength gains in weight trained individuals (Rhea et al. 2003). Performing a large number of repetitions with a very light resistance will result in no or minimal strength gain. However, the maximal number of repetitions per set of an exercise that will result in increased strength will vary from exercise to exercise and from muscle group to muscle group. For example, the maximal number of repetitions possible at 60% of 1RM for the leg press is 34 and for the knee curl is 11 (Hoeger et al. 1987).

Unlike the intensity of endurance exercise, the intensity of resistance training cannot be estimated by heart rate during the exercise. Heart rate during resistance exercise does not consistently vary with the exercise intensity (see figure 1.2). Heart rate

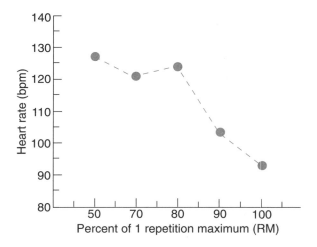

Figure 1.2 Maximal heart rate of a moderately trained group of males during knee-extension sets to momentary voluntary fatigue at various percentages of the 1RM. The heart rate does not reflect the intensity (% of 1RM) of the exercise.

Adapted, by permission, from S.J. Fleck and L.S. Dean, 1987, "Previous resistance-training experience and the pressor response during resistance exercise," *Journal of Applied Physiology* 63 (1): 118.

attained during sets to momentary voluntary fatigue at 50 to 80% of 1RM can be higher than the heart rate attained during sets with 1RM or sets performed to momentary voluntary fatigue at higher percentages of 1RM (Fleck and Dean 1987).

Training Volume

Training volume is a measure of the total amount of work (joules) performed in a training session, in a week of training, in a month of training, or in some other period of time. Frequency (number of training sessions per week, month, or year), training session duration, number of sets performed, number of repetitions per set, and number of exercises performed per training session all have a direct impact on training volume. The simplest method to estimate volume is to sum the number of repetitions performed in a specific time period, such as a week or a month of training. Volume can also be estimated by the total amount of weight lifted. For example, if 100 lb (45 kg) are used to perform 10 repetitions, the volume of training is 1,000 lb (450 kg) (10 repetitions multiplied by 100 lb or 45 kg).

Training volume is more precisely determined by calculating the work performed. Total work in a repetition is the resistance multiplied by the vertical distance the weight is lifted. Thus, if 100 lb (45 kg or 445 N) is lifted vertically 3 ft (0.9 m) in a repetition, the volume or total work is 100 lb multiplied by 3 ft or 300 ft · lb (445 N × 0.9 m = 400 J). Training volume for a set of 10 repetitions in this example is 300 ft · lb (400 J) per repetition multiplied by 10 repetitions, which equals 3,000 ft lb (4,000 J). The calculation of training volume is useful in determining the total training stress.

A relationship exists between training volume and training outcomes, such as muscular hypertrophy, decreased percentage of body fat, increased fat-free mass, and even motor performance. Larger training volumes may also result in a slower loss of strength gains after cessation of training (Hather et al. 1992). Thus, training volume is a consideration when designing a resistance training program.

Periodization

Planned variation in the training volume and intensity (periodization) is extremely important for continued optimal gains in strength, as well as other training outcomes. Additionally, changes in other training variables, such as exercise choice, can also be made on a regular basis or in a periodized fashion.

Variations in the position of the foot, hand, and other body parts that do not affect the safety of the lifter can also be used as a training variation and do affect muscle fiber recruitment patterns. The use of several exercises to vary the conditioning stimulus of a particular muscle group is also a valuable means by which muscle fiber recruitment patterns can be changed in an attempt to produce continued increases in strength and muscle fiber hypertrophy (see the discussion of motor unit activation in chapter 3). Periodization is needed to achieve optimal gains in strength and power as training progresses (American College of Sports Medicine 2002).

Progressive Overload

Progressive resistance exercise or progressive overload refers to the practice of continually increasing the stress placed on the muscle as it becomes capable of producing greater force or has more endurance. At the start of a training program the 5RM for arm curls might be 50 lb (23 kg), which may be a sufficient stimulus to produce an increase in strength. As the program progresses, 5 repetitions with 50 lb (23 kg) would not be a sufficient stimulus to produce further gains in strength because the trainee can now easily perform 5 repetitions with 50 lb (23 kg); consequently, this resistance is no longer a 5RM. If the training stimulus is not increased at this point, no further gains in strength will occur.

There are several methods to progressively overload the muscle (American College of Sports Medicine 2002). The most common method is to increase the resistance to perform a certain number of repetitions. The use of RMs or RM training zones (i.e., weight that allows between 6 and 8 repetitions per set) automatically provides progressive overload because as a muscle's strength increases, the resistance necessary to perform an RM or stay within an RM training zone increases. For example, a 5RM may increase from 50 lb (23 kg) to 60 lb (27 kg) after several weeks of training.

Other methods to progressively overload the muscle include increasing the total training volume by increasing the number of repetitions or sets performed; increasing repetition speed with submaximal resistances; changing rest period length between exercises (i.e., shortening rest period length for endurance improvements or lengthening rest period length for maximal strength and power training); and changing total training volume by changing repetitions, sets, and the number of exercises performed. In order to allow sufficient time for adaptations, progressive overload of any kind should be gradually introduced into the training program and sufficient time allowed for the trainee to become accustomed to and make physiological adaptations. Because of these factors and the possibility of overtraining, changes in total training volume should be made in small increments of 2.5 to 5% (American College of Sports Medicine 2002).

Rest Periods

Rest periods between sets of an exercise, between exercises, and between training sessions allow recovery and are important for the success of any program. The rest periods allowed between sets and between exercises during a training session are in large part determined by the goals of the training program. Rest period length affects the recovery between sets and exercises and the hormonal responses to a training session (see chapter 3). The rest periods between sets and exercises, the resistance used, and the number of repetitions performed per set all affect the design and goals of the program (see chapter 5). In general, if the goal is to increase the ability to exhibit maximal strength, relatively long rest periods (several minutes), heavy resistances, and 3 to 6 repetitions per set are suggested. When the goal is to increase the ability to perform high-intensity exercise for a period of several seconds, rest periods between sets should be less than 1 minute. Repetitions and resistance can range from 5RM to 15RM, depending on the exact type of high-intensity ability one wishes to enhance. If enhancement of long-term endurance (aerobic power) is the goal, then circuit-type resistance training with short rest periods (less than 30 seconds), relatively light resistances, and 10 to 15 repetitions per set is one training prescription.

Many fitness enthusiasts and some athletes allow one day of recovery between resistance training sessions for a particular muscle group. This is a good general rule, although some evidence indicates that other patterns of training sessions and recovery periods are equally or even more beneficial (see the discussion of rest periods between workouts in chapter 5 and the discussion of two training sessions per day in chapter 7). A practical indication of rest periods between training sessions is residual muscular soreness. When it interferes with performance of the following training session, the rest between training sessions was probably insufficient.

Velocity Specificity

Many coaches and athletes maintain that some resistance training should be performed at the velocity required during the actual sporting event. For many sporting events this means a high velocity of moment. Velocity specificity is the concept that resistance training produces its greatest strength gains at the velocity at which the training is performed. Closely associated with movement speed is power development (see chapter 7). There is velocity specificity; however, if the training goal is to increase strength at all velocities of movement, an intermediate velocity is the best choice. Thus, for an individual interested in general strength, an intermediate training velocity might be recommended. However, training at a fast velocity against light resistance and training at a slower velocity against heavy resistance both demonstrate velocity-specific strength gains. Thus, velocity-specific training to maximize strength and power gains is appropriate for athletes and fitness enthusiasts at some point in their total training program.

Muscle Action Specificity

If an individual trains isometrically and evaluates progress with a static muscle action, a large increase in strength may be apparent. However, if this same individual determines progress using concentric or eccentric muscle actions, little or no increase in strength may be demonstrated. This is termed muscle action or testing specificity. This muscle action or testing specificity indicates that gains in strength are in part specific to the type of muscle action used in training (e.g., isometric, variable resistance, isokinetic). This specificity of strength gains is caused by neural adaptations resulting in the ability to recruit the muscles to perform a particular type of muscle action (see the discussion of nervous system adaptations in chapter 3). Therefore, the training program or a specific sport or activity should include the types of muscle actions encountered in that sport or activity. For example, isometric muscle actions are frequently performed while wrestling, so it is beneficial to incorporate some isometric training into the resistance training program of wrestlers.

Muscle-Group Specificity

Muscle-group specificity simply means that each muscle group requiring strength gains or other adaptations to the training program must be trained. If an increase in strength is desired in the flexors (biceps group) and extensors (triceps) of the elbow, exercises for both muscle groups need to be included in the program. Exercises in a training program must be specifically chosen for each muscle group in which a training adaptation is desired, such as increased strength, local muscle endurance, or hypertrophy.

Energy-Source Specificity

Energy-source specificity refers to the concept that any physical training may bring about adaptations of the metabolic systems predominately used to supply the energy needed by muscles to perform a given physical activity. There are two anaerobic sources and one aerobic source of energy for muscle actions. The anaerobic sources of energy supply the majority of energy for high-power, short-duration events such as sprinting 100 m, whereas the aerobic energy source supplies the majority of energy for longer-duration, lower-power events, such as running 5,000 m. If an increase in the ability of a muscle to perform anaerobic exercise is desired, the bouts of exercise should be of short duration and high intensity. To increase aerobic capability, training bouts should be of longer duration and lower intensity. Resistance training is most commonly used to bring about adaptations of the anaerobic energy sources. The number of sets and repetitions, and the number and length of rest periods between sets and exercises, need to be appropriate for the energy source in which training adaptations are desired (see chapter 5).

Safety Aspects

Successful resistance training programs have one prominent feature in common—safety. Resistance training has some inherent risk, as do all physical activities. The chance of injury can be greatly reduced or completely removed by using correct lifting techniques, spotting, and proper breathing; by maintaining equipment in good working condition; and by wearing appropriate clothing.

The chance of being injured while performing resistance training is very slight. In college football players (Zemper 1990) the weight room injury rate was very low (0.35 per 100 players per season). Weight room injuries accounted for only 0.74% of the total reported time-lost injuries during the football season. This injury rate may be reduced to even lower levels through more rigorous attention to proper procedures in the weight room (Zemper 1990), such as proper exercise technique and use of collars with free weight bars. Injury rates in a supervised health and fitness facility that included resistance training as part of the total training program were also very low (0.048 per 1,000 participant-hours) (Morrey and Hensrud 1999). A review of the U.S. Consumer Product Safety Commission National Electronic Injury Surveillance System indicates that 42% of resistance training injuries occur at home (Lombardi and Troxel 1999), and 29% and 16% of resistance training injuries occur at sports facilities and schools, respectively. These results indicate that lack of supervision is a contributor to injury. So, although resistance training is a very safe activity, all proper safety precautions should be taken with special attention to all factors related to safety when performing resistance training in an unsupervised setting.

Spotting

Proper spotting is necessary to ensure the safety of the participants in a resistance training program. Spotting refers to the activities of individuals other than the lifter that help ensure the safety of the lifter. Spotters serve three major functions: to assist the trainee with completion of a repetition if needed, to critique the trainee's exercise technique, and to summon help if an accident does occur. Briefly, the following factors should be considered when spotting:

- Spotters must be strong enough to assist the trainee if needed.
- During the performance of certain exercises (e.g., back squats) more than one spotter may be necessary to ensure the safety of the lifter.
- Spotters should know proper spotting technique and the proper exercise technique for each lift for which they are spotting.
- Spotters should know how many repetitions the trainee is going to attempt.
- Spotters should be attentive at all times to the lifter and to his or her exercise technique.
- Spotters should summon help if an accident or injury occurs.

Following these simple guidelines will aid in the avoidance of weight room injuries. A detailed description of spotting techniques for all exercises is beyond the scope of this text, but spotting techniques for a wide variety of individual resistance training exercises have been presented elsewhere (Fleck 1998; Kraemer and Fleck 1993).

Breathing

Excessively holding one's breath with a closed glotis (Valsalva maneuver) during resistance training exercises is not recommended since blood pressure rises substantially (see the discussion of acute cardiovascular responses in chapter 3). Figure 1.3 depicts the intra-arterial blood pressure response to maximal isometric muscle actions during one-legged knee extensions. The blood pressure response during an isometric muscle action in which breathing was allowed is lower than the response observed during either an isometric action performed simultaneously with a Valsalva maneuver or a Valsalva maneuver in the absence of an isometric muscle action. This demonstrates that the elevation of blood pressure

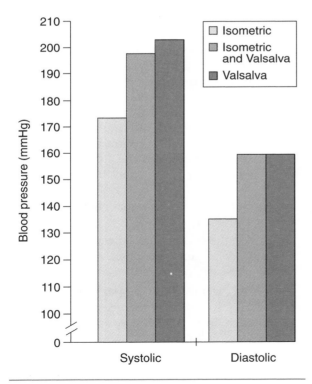

Figure 1.3 Systolic and diastolic blood pressure during an isometric action only, simultaneous isometric action and Valsalva maneuver, and Valsalva maneuver only.

Unpublished data of authors. $n = 6$.

during resistance training is lower if breathing occurs during the muscle action compared to if a Valsalva maneuver is performed during the muscle action. Elevated blood pressure increases the afterload on the heart; this requires the heart to develop more pressure to eject blood, which makes the work of the heart more difficult.

Exhaling during the lifting of the resistance and inhaling during the lowering of the resistance are normally recommended, although little difference in the heart rate and blood pressure response during resistance training is observed if exhaling occurs during lowering and inhaling during lifting of the resistance, respectively or vice versa (Linsenbardt, Thomas, and Madsen 1992). During an exercise using 1RM or during the last few repetitions of a set performed to momentary voluntary fatigue, performance of a Valsalva maneuver will occur. However, excessive breath holding should be discouraged.

Proper Exercise Technique

Proper technique for resistance training exercises is partially determined by the specific muscle groups being trained. Altering the proper form of an exercise causes other muscle groups to assist in performance of the exercise movement. This decreases the training stimulus on the muscles normally associated with a particular exercise. Proper technique is altered in several advanced resistance training techniques (e.g., the burn technique, the forced repetition technique), but these techniques are not recommended for beginning resistance trainers (see chapter 6).

Proper technique is also necessary to prevent injury, especially in some exercises in which improper technique exposes the low back to additional stress (e.g., squat, deadlift) or in which the resistance can be "bounced" off a body part (e.g., free weight bench press). Improper form often occurs when the lifter performs an exercise with resistances that exceed his or her present strength capabilities for a certain number of repetitions. If exercise technique deteriorates, the set should be terminated. Proper exercise technique for a large variety of exercises has been described elsewhere (Fleck 1998; Kraemer and Fleck 1993).

Full Range of Motion

Full range of motion refers to performing an exercise with the greatest possible range of movement. Exercises are normally performed with the full range of motion allowed by the body's position and the joints involved. Although no definitive studies are available, it is assumed that to develop strength throughout the joint's full range of motion, training must be performed throughout the joint's full range of motion. Studies demonstrating joint-angle specificity with isometric training indicate that if training is performed only at a specific joint angle, strength gains will be realized in a narrow range around that specific joint angle and not throughout the joint's full range of motion. Thus, performing exercises throughout a full range of motion ensures strength gains throughout the full range of motion and is important to proper exercise technique. Some specific training techniques (e.g., partial repetitions) intentionally limit the range of motion. These techniques are normally not recommended for beginning lifters, and their efficacy remains to be demonstrated.

Equipment Maintenance

Maintaining equipment in proper operating condition is of utmost importance for a safe resistance training program. Pulleys and cables or belts should be checked frequently for wear and replaced as needed. Equipment should be lubricated as indicated by the manufacturer. Cracked or broken free weight plates, dumbbells, or plates in a machine's weight stack should be retired or replaced. Upholstery should be disinfected daily. The sleeves on Olympic bars and other free weight bars should revolve freely to avoid tearing the skin off a lifter's hands. An injury resulting from improper equipment maintenance should never happen in a well-run resistance training facility or program.

Resistance Training Shoes

A safe shoe for resistance training does not have to be specifically designed for Olympic-style or power lifting, but should have good arch support, a nonslip sole, proper fit, and little shock-absorbing capability of the sole. The first three of these factors are for safety reasons. The last factor is important for a simple reason: Force produced by the leg muscles to lift the weight should not be wasted in compressing the shoe's sole. Additionally, if the heel area is very compressible, such as in a running shoe, in some exercises, such as back squats, compression of the heel area during the lift may cause the lifter to lose his or her balance. Shoes designed for cross-training offer all of these characteristics and are appropriate for all but the most advanced or competitive Olympic-style lifter or power lifter.

Resistance Training Gloves

Gloves for resistance training are designed without fingers, so the glove covers only the palm area. This design protects the palms from catching or scraping on barbell and machine handles, but still allows a good grip of the bar or handle. Gloves help prevent blisters and the ripping of calluses on the hand. However, they are not mandatory for safe resistance training.

Training Belts

Training belts have a wide back portion that supposedly helps support the lumbar area or low back. Training belts do help support the low back, but not because of the wide back area. Instead, the belt gives the abdominal muscles an object to push against. This helps to raise intra-abdominal pressure, which supports the lumbar vertebrae from the anterior (Harman et al. 1989; Lander, Hundley, and Simonton 1992; Lander, Simonton, and Giacobbe 1990). Increased intra-abdominal pressure prevents flexion of the lumbar vertebrae, which aids in maintaining an upright posture. Strong abdominal musculature helps to maintain intra-abdominal pressure. When intra-abdominal pressure increases, weak abdominal musculature will protrude anteriorly. This results in decreased intraabdominal pressure and so less support for the lumbar vertebrae. A training belt can be used for exercises that place significant stress on the lumbar area, such as squats and deadlifts. However, the belt is not necessary for safe performance of these exercises. A belt should not be used to alleviate technique problems caused by weak abdominal or low back musculature. If exercises placing a great deal of stress on the low back are to be performed, exercises to strengthen the low back and abdominal regions need to be included in the training program.

Wearing a tightly cinched belt during an activity increases blood pressure (Hunter et al. 1989), which can result in increased cardiovascular stress. Thus, a training belt should not be worn during activities such as riding a stationary bike or during exercises in which the lumbar area is not significantly stressed. Furthermore, belts should normally not be worn when performing exercises that do not require back support or that use moderate to light resistances (i.e., greater than 6RM).

Summary

Understandable and clear definitions of terminology are important to any field of study. Clear definitions of weight training terminology are necessary for accurate communication and exchange of ideas among fitness enthusiasts and strength and conditioning professionals. Proper safety precautions, such as spotting and proper exercise technique, are a necessity of all properly designed and implemented resistance training programs. An understanding of the basic terminology and safety aspects of weight training is important when examining the topic of the next chapter, different types of strength training.

Key Terms

concentric muscle action
eccentric muscle action
energy-source specificity
full range of motion
intensity
isometric muscle action
muscle action or testing specificity
muscle-group specificity
periodization
power
progressive overload
progressive resistance exercise
repetition
repetition maximum (RM)
rest periods
set
spotting
strength
training volume
Valsalva maneuver
velocity specificity
voluntary maximal muscular actions

Selected Readings

Fleck, S.J. 1998. *Successful long-term weight training.* Chicago: NTP/Contemporary Publishing Group.

Fleck, S.J. 1999. Periodized strength training: A critical review. *Journal of Strength and Conditioning Research* 13: 82-89.

Kraemer, W.J., and Fleck, S.J. 1993. *Strength training for young athletes.* Champaign, IL: Human Kinetics.

McDonagh, M.J.N., and Davies, C.T.M. 1984. Adaptive responses of mammalian skeletal muscle to exercise with high loads. *European Journal of Applied Physiology* 52: 139-155.

Willoughby, D.S. 1993. The effects of mesocycle-length training programs involving periodization and partially equated volumes on upper and lower body strength. *Journal of Strength and Conditioning Research* 7: 2-8.

CHAPTER 2

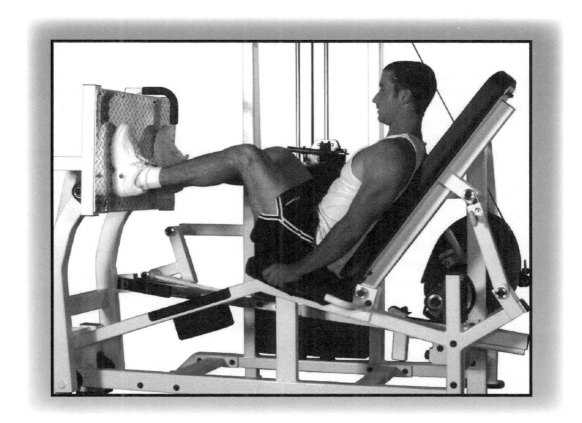

Types of Strength Training

Most athletes and many fitness enthusiasts perform strength training as a portion of their overall training programs. The main interest for athletes is not how much weight they can lift, but whether increased strength and power and changes in body composition brought about by weight training result in better performances in their sports. Fitness enthusiasts are interested in the health benefits associated with changes in body composition and the lean, fit appearance brought about by weight training.

There are several factors to consider when examining a type of strength training. Does this type of training increase motor performance? Vertical jump tests, a 40-yd or 30-m sprint, and throwing a ball for distance are common motor performance tests. Is strength increased throughout the range of motion and at all velocities of movement? Most sports and daily life activities require strength and power throughout a large portion (or the entire range of motion) of a joint. If strength and power are not increased throughout the entire range of motion, performance may not be enhanced as much as possible by a particular type of training. The majority of athletic events require strength and power at a variety of movement speeds, particularly at fast velocities. If strength and power are not increased over a wide variety of movement velocities, once again, improvements in performance may not be optimal.

Other questions to consider when examining types of strength training include the following: To what extent does the type of training cause changes in body composition, such as percentage of body fat or fat-free mass? How much of an increase in strength and power can be expected over a specified training period with this type of training? How does this type of training compare with other training types in the preceding factors?

A considerable amount of research concerns types of resistance training. The emergence of conclusions from this research, however, is hampered by several factors. The vast majority of studies have been of short-term duration (8 to 12 weeks) and used untrained or moderately trained individuals as subjects. This makes direct application of the studies' results to long-term training (years) and highly trained fitness enthusiasts or athletes questionable.

As an example, elite Olympic-style weightlifters during 1 year of training show an increase in 1RM snatch ability of 1.5% and in 1RM clean and jerk ability of 2%, and show an increase in fat-free mass of 1% or less and a decrease in percentage body fat up to 1.7% (Häkkinen, Komi et al. 1987; Häkkinen, Pakarinen et al. 1987). Over 2 years of training, elite Olympic-style weightlifters show an increase in lifting total (total = 1RM snatch + 1RM clean and jerk) of 2.7% and an increase in fat-free mass of 1% and a decrease in percentage body fat of 1.7% (Häkkinen, Pakarinen et al. 1988b). These changes

are much smaller than those shown by untrained or moderately trained individuals in strength and body composition (see table 3.3 on page 92) over much shorter training periods. This indicates that highly fit individuals such as athletes may have a harder time attaining changes in strength and body composition than untrained or moderately trained individuals. The idea that it is more difficult to increase strength in highly trained individuals compared to untrained individuals is supported by analysis (meta-analysis) of research studies (Rhea et al. 2003) and is clearly shown in figure 2.1.

Other factors that can affect gains in strength are the number of muscle actions (sets and repetitions) performed and the resistance used in training. These factors vary considerably from study to study and make interpretation of the results difficult. Another factor making interpretation and comparisons of studies difficult is the fact that different muscle groups do not necessarily respond at the same rate or to the same magnitude when performing the identical training program (Willoughby 1993). Ultimately, the outcome of any comparison of strength training types depends on the efficacy of the training programs used in the comparison. A comparison of the optimal dynamic constant external resistance training program to a very ineffective isokinetic program will favor dynamic constant external resistance training. Conversely, a comparison of the optimal isokinetic program to a very ineffective dynamic constant external resistance training program will favor the isokinetic program. Ideally, any comparison of strength training types would use the optimal program for the strength training types being compared and be of long duration. Unfortunately, strength training type comparisons of this nature do not exist. Enough research has been conducted, however, to reach some tentative conclusions concerning types of strength training and how to use them in a training program. This chapter addresses the major research concerning types of strength training and conclusions warranted.

Isometrics

Isometrics, or static resistance training, refers to a muscular action during which no change in the length of the total muscle takes place. This means that no visible movement at a joint (or joints) takes place. Isometric actions can take place voluntarily against less than 100% of maximal voluntary action, such as voluntarily holding a light dumbbell at a certain point in the range of motion of an

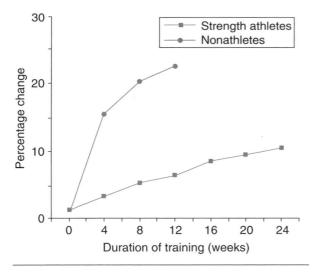

Figure 2.1 The percentage change in maximal squat ability from the pretraining value depends on the pretraining status of the trainees and the duration of training.

Adapted, by permission, from K. Häkkinen, 1985, "Factors influencing trainability of muscular strength during short-term and prolonged training," *National Strength and Conditioning Association Journal* 7: 33.

exercise or voluntarily generating less than maximal force against an object. An isometric action can also be performed at 100% of maximal voluntary action against an immovable object. Isometric training is most commonly performed against an immovable object such as a wall or a weight machine loaded beyond an individual's maximal concentric strength. Isometrics can also be performed by having a weak muscle group act against a strong muscle group, for example, activating the left elbow flexors maximally to try to flex the left elbow while simultaneously resisting movement by pushing down on the left hand with the right hand with just enough force to stop any movement at the left elbow. If the left elbow flexors are weaker than the right elbow extensors, the left elbow flexors would perform an isometric action at 100% of maximal voluntary action. Isometric actions can also be performed after a brief dynamic action in some exercises (see the discussion of functional isometrics in chapter 6). Thus, the cost of isometrics can range from minimal, when using a common object such as a wall as the immovable object, to quite extensive, when using a loaded weight machine as the immovable object.

Isometrics came to the attention of the American public in the early 1950s when Steinhaus (1954) introduced the work of two Germans, Hettinger and Muller (1953). Hettinger and Muller concluded that gains in isometric strength of 5% per week were produced by one daily 66% maximal isometric action 6 seconds in duration. Gains in strength of this magnitude with such little training time and effort seemed unbelievable. A review of subsequent studies demonstrated that isometric training leads to static strength gains, and that the gains can be substantial and variable over short-duration training periods (Fleck and Schutt 1985; see also table 2.1).

Table 2.1 Effects of 100% Maximal Voluntary Contractions on Isometric Strength

Reference	Duration of contractions	Contractions per day	Duration × contractions per day	Number of training days	MVIC increase (%)	MVIC increase % per day	Muscle
Bonde-Peterson 1960	5	1	5	36	0	0	Elbow flexors
Ikai and Fukunaga 1970	10	3	30	100	92	0.9	Elbow flexors
Komi and Karlsson 1978	3-5	5	15-25	48	20	0.4	Quadriceps
Bonde-Peterson 1960	5	10	50	36	15	0.4	Elbow flexors
Maffiuletti and Martin 2001	4	12	48	21	16	0.7	Quadriceps
Alway et al. 1989	10	5-15	50-150	48	44	0.9	Triceps surae
McDonagh et al. 1983	3	30	90	28	20	0.71	Elbow flexors
Grimby et al. 1973	3	30	90	30	32	1.1	Triceps
Davies and Young 1983	3	42	126	35	30	0.86	Triceps surae
Carolyn and Cafarelli 1992	3-4	30	90-120	24	32	1.3	Quadriceps
Garfinkel and Cafarelli 1992	3-5	30	90-150	24	28	1.2	Quadriceps

MVIC = maximal voluntary isometric contraction.

Adapted, by permission, from M.J.N. McDonagh and C.T. M. Davies, 1989, "Adaptive responses of mammalian skeletal muscle to exercise with high loads," *European Journal of Applied Physiology* 52: 140. © Springer-Verlag.

Increases in strength from isometric training are related to the number of muscle actions performed, the duration of the muscle actions, whether the muscle action is maximal, and the frequency of training. Because most studies involving isometric training manipulate several of these factors simultaneously, it is difficult to evaluate the importance of any one factor. Enough research has been conducted, however, to allow recommendations and tentative conclusions concerning isometric training.

Maximal Voluntary Muscle Actions

Increases in isometric strength can be achieved with submaximal isometric muscle actions (Alway, Sale, and MacDougall 1990; Davies et al. 1988; Davies and Young 1983; Hettinger and Muller 1953; Kubo et al. 2001; Lyle and Rutherford 1998; Macaluso et al. 2000). However, some research indicates that maximal voluntary muscle actions (MVMAs) are superior to submaximal voluntary isometric muscle actions in causing increases in strength (Rasch and Morehouse 1957; Ward and Fisk 1964). Additionally, there may also be adaptational differences depending on how a maximal voluntary isometric action is performed (Maffiuletti and Martin 2001). In this comparison of contraction training types, isometric actions were performed in a manner so that maximal force was developed as quickly as possible or such that maximal force was reached in 4 seconds during which force was voluntarily progressively increased. Both types of training resulted in significant and similar increases in maximal isokinetic and isometric force capabilities. However, electromyographic (EMG) and electrically evoked twitch contractile properties indicated that training in which maximal force was developed in 4 seconds resulted in modifications of the nervous system at the peripheral level (i.e., muscle membrane electrical activity). Training by developing maximal force as quickly as possible resulted in adaptations in contractile muscle properties (i.e., excitation-contraction coupling). As with other types of resistance training, the effect of the "quality" of the muscle action needs to be investigated further. Strength and conditioning coaches generally use MVMAs in training with healthy individuals, and submaximal isometric actions in rehabilitation programs or remedial strength training programs in which maximal muscular actions are contraindicated.

Number of Muscle Actions and Duration

Hettinger and Muller (1953) proposed that only one 6-second muscle action per day was necessary to produce maximal gains in strength. As shown in table 2.1, many combinations in the number and duration of MVMAs can result in significant strength gains. The majority of studies have used MVMAs of 3 to 10 seconds in duration, with 3 being the least number of muscle actions resulting in a significant strength gain. Similarly, many combinations in the number and duration of submaximal isometric actions can result in increased isometric strength. For example, four sets of 6 repetitions each of 2 seconds duration at 50% MVMA (adductor pollicus) and four muscle actions of 30 seconds in duration each at 70% MVMA (quadriceps) have both resulted in significant increases of isometric strength (Lyle and Rutherford 1998; Schott, McCully, and Rutherford 1995). It is important to note that generally these studies used healthy but non-weight-trained individuals as subjects.

The duration of the muscle action and the number of training muscle actions per day individually show weaker correlations to increases in strength than do duration and number combined (McDonagh and Davies 1984). This means that the total time spent in an isometric action (duration of each muscle action multiplied by the number of muscle actions) is directly related to increased strength. It also indicates that optimal gains in strength are the result of either a small number of long-duration muscle actions or a large number of short-duration muscle actions. As an example, seven daily 1-minute muscle actions at 30% of MVMA or 42 three-second MVMAs per training day over a 6-week training period both result in about a 30% increase in isometric MVMA (Davies and Young 1983).

However, some information indicates that longer-duration isometric actions may be superior to short-duration actions in causing strength gains (Schott, McCully, and Rutherford 1995). Training the quadriceps at 70% of MVMA with four 30-second actions and four sets of 10 repetitions each 3 seconds in duration both resulted in significant isometric strength gains. Even though total duration of the isometric muscle actions (120 seconds per training session) was identical between the two groups, the longer-duration isometric actions resulted in a significantly greater increase in isometric strength (median 55% vs. 32% increase).

The longer-duration isometric actions resulted in a significant increase in isometric strength after 2 weeks of training, whereas 8 weeks of training was necessary before a significant increase in strength was achieved with the short-duration isometric actions. This indicates that longer-duration submaximal isometric actions may be more appropriate when a quick increase in strength is desired.

Several intramuscular metabolite concentrations and acidity were higher, but not significantly so, immediately after the long-duration isometric action training compared to the short-duration training, which indicates that these factors may influence strength gains. During isometric actions, blood flow occlusion does occur and may be responsible in part for the increased metabolite concentrations and acidity due to the long-duration isometric actions. The possible role of occlusion resulting in increased metabolite concentrations and acidity affecting strength gains is supported by a comparison of training with either 30 to 50% of 1RM with blood flow occlusion or 50 to 80% of 1RM without blood flow occlusion (Takarada et al. 2000). Training with blood flow occlusion resulted in a significantly higher blood lactate concentration compared to training without occlusion, indicating greater concentrations of intramuscular metabolites. Over 16 weeks of training both programs resulted in significant increases in strength with no significant difference between groups shown. Thus, blood flow occlusion and the resulting increase in intramuscular metabolites appears to be a factor affecting strength increases.

Many studies using isometrics allow the trainee several seconds during which to increase the force of the muscle action until the desired percent of the MVMA is reached. Some information, however, indicates that rapid increase in the isometric force results in significantly greater increases in strength at the training joint angle (Maffiuletti and Martin 2001). During 7 weeks of training, a group performing isometric actions of the knee extensors with as rapid as possible an increase in muscle force (action lasting approximately 1 second) showed an increase in MVMA of 28%. A group performing more traditional isometric training during which force was increased to MVMA over 4 seconds showed an increase in MVMA of 16%. Similar and comparable increases in strength are shown at knee angles different from the training angle, and during eccentric and concentric isokinetic testing. Thus, the protocol involving increasing force as quickly as possible during training only showed a significantly greater increase in strength at the training joint angle.

Collectively, this information indicates that many combinations of maximal and submaximal isometric muscle action duration and number can bring about isometric strength gains. However, in typical training settings with healthy individuals, perhaps the most efficient use of training time when using isometrics is to perform a minimum of 15 to 20 MVMAs or near MVMAs of 3 to 5 seconds in duration for three sessions per week.

Frequency of Training

Three training sessions per week using either maximal or submaximal isometric actions results in a significant increase in isometric MVMA (Alway, MacDougall, and Sale 1989; Alway, Sale, and MacDougall 1990; Carolyn and Cafarelli 1992; Davies et al. 1988; Garfinkel and Cafarelli 1992; Lyle and Rutherford 1998; Macaluso et al. 2000; Maffiuletti and Martin 2001; Schott, McCully, and Rutherford 1995; Weir, Housh, and Weir 1994; Weir et al. 1995). Increases in isometric MVMA over 6 to 16 weeks of training ranged from 8% to 79% in these studies. However, whether three training sessions per week cause maximal increases in strength is not fully substantiated. Hettinger (1961) calculated that alternate-day isometric training is 80% as effective as daily training sessions and that once-a-week training is 40% as effective. Hettinger also concluded that training once every 2 weeks does not cause increases in strength, although it does serve to maintain strength. Daily training with isometrics is superior to less frequent training (Atha 1981), although the exact percentage of strength superiority is controversial and may vary by muscle group and other training variables (i.e., muscle action duration, number of muscle actions). To increase maximal strength, the optimal isometric program should consist of daily training; however, three training sessions per week will bring about significant increases in maximal strength.

Muscular Hypertrophy

Increases in limb circumferences from training are usually associated with muscular hypertrophy. Significant increases in strength accompanied by increased limb circumferences have been reported due to isometric training (Kanehisa and Miyashita 1983a; Kitai and Sale 1989; Meyers 1967; Rarick and Larson 1958). However, changes in limb circumferences do not necessarily accompany increased strength (Ward and Fisk 1964). Neural adaptations also play a role in increased strength due to isometric training.

Computerized tomography and magnetic resonance imaging (MRI) have been used to more directly determine muscle cross-sectional area changes due to isometric training. Six weeks of isometric training has resulted in elbow-flexor cross-sectional area increases of 5.4% and isometric strength increases of 14.5%. Nevertheless, no significant correlation between the increased strength and cross-sectional area was shown (Davies et al. 1988). Eight weeks of knee-extensor isometric training resulted in a 28% increase in isometric strength and a 14.6% increase in the cross-sectional area with a significant correlation shown between the increased strength and increased cross-sectional area (Garfinkel and Cafarelli 1992). Twelve weeks of training resulted in a significant increase of 8% in knee-extensor cross-sectional area and a 41% increase in isometric strength (Kubo et al. 2001).

Whether hypertrophy occurs and the extent to which it occurs may vary from muscle to muscle, as shown by the following studies. Type I and II muscle fiber diameters in the vastus lateralis did not change after 9 weeks of isometric training at 100% of MVMA (Lewis et al. 1984). Type I and II fiber areas increased in the soleus approximately 30% after 16 weeks of isometric training with either 30% or 100% of MVMA (Alway, MacDougall, and Sale 1989; Alway, Sale, and MacDougall 1990), whereas only the type II fibers of the lateral gastrocnemius increased in area 30 to 40% after the identical training program (Alway, MacDougall, and Sale 1989; Alway, Sale, and MacDougall 1990).

Some data indicate that longer-duration muscle actions result in greater gains in cross-sectional area than shorter-duration muscle actions (Schott, McCully, and Rutherford 1995). Muscle cross-sectional area (computerized tomography) was determined before and after training with four 30-second actions and four sets of 10 repetitions each 3 seconds in duration. Even though total duration of the isometric muscle actions (120 seconds per training session) were identical between the two groups, the longer-duration isometric actions resulted in a significant increase in quadriceps cross-sectional area (10-11%), whereas the shorter-duration muscular actions resulted in nonsignificant increases (4-7%) in quadriceps cross-sectional area. Similar

to increases in isometric strength, the blood flow occlusion and resulting increase in intramuscular metabolite concentrations may be related to the greater increase in muscle cross-sectional area with the longer-duration isometric actions.

Another study indicates 100% MVMAs results in significantly greater hypertrophy than 60% MVMAs (Kanehisa et al. 2002). In this study, training lasted 10 weeks and consisted of either 12 muscle actions at 100% MVMA with each action lasting 6 seconds or 4 actions at 60% MVMA with each action lasting 30 seconds. Muscle size changes were measured using magnetic resonance imaging. Collectively, these results indicate hypertrophy is dependent on both isometric muscle action duration and intensity (percent of MVMA used in training).

Muscle protein synthesis in the soleus after an isometric action at 40% of MVMA to fatigue (approximately 27 minutes) increases significantly by 49% (Fowles et al. 2000). This finding supports the efficacy of isometric actions inducing muscle hypertrophy. Collectively, this information indicates that muscular hypertrophy of both the type I and type II muscle fibers can occur from isometric training with submaximal and maximal muscle actions. Increases in strength may also occur due to neural adaptations (see chapter 3). Isometric training can bring about increases in hypertrophy and neural adaptations, both of which can increase strength.

Joint-Angle Specificity

Gains in strength occur predominantly at or near the joint angle at which the isometric training is performed; this is termed joint-angle specificity. The majority of research indicates that static strength increases from isometric training are joint-angle specific (Bender and Kaplan 1963; Gardner 1963; Kitai and Sale 1989; Lindh 1979; Meyers 1967; Thepaut-Mathieu, Van Hoeke, and Martin 1988; Weir, Housh, and Weir 1994; Weir et al. 1995; Williams and Stutzman 1959), although lack of joint-angle specificity gains in strength have also been shown (Knapik, Mawdsley, and Ramos 1983; Rasch and Pierson 1964; Rasch, Preston, and Logan 1961). Many factors may affect the degree to which joint-angle specificity occurs, including the muscle group(s) trained, the joint angle at which the training is performed, and the intensity and duration of the isometric actions. Joint-angle specificity is normally attributed to neural adaptations, such as increased muscle fiber recruitment at the trained angle and the inhibition of the antagonistic muscles at the trained angle.

Isometric training of the elbow extensors at an elbow joint angle of 90 degrees results in increased isometric MVMA at an angle of 90 degrees (Knapik, Mawdsley, and Ramos 1983). There is, however, a smaller but significant strength increase at elbow angles at 20 degrees on either side of the training angle. Training of the elbow flexors at an elbow angle of 80 degrees results in a carryover of strength increases over a large range of elbow angles (Thepaut-Mathieu, Van Hoeke, and Martin 1988), whereas training of the elbow flexors at elbow angles of 25 degrees or 120 degrees results in a much smaller carryover to other joint angles (see figure 2.2). Isometric training of the plantar flexors with the ankle joint at 90 degrees results in increased strength at the training angle and significant carryover of strength increases at only 5 degrees on either side of the training angle (Kitai and Sale 1989). Training the knee extensors at a knee angle of 135 degrees results in a strength carryover at 30 degrees on either side of the training angle (Weir, Housh, and Weir 1994; Weir et al. 1995) and at 65 degrees results in significant strength increases at knee angles of 55 and 75 degrees (Maffiuletti and Martin 2001).

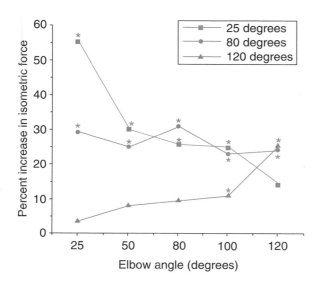

Figure 2.2 Percentage gain in isometric strength of elbow flexors due to isometric training at different elbow angles.

* = significant increase ($p < 0.05$).

Data from C. Thépaut-Mathieu et al., 1988.

Joint-angle specificity (see figure 2.2) is most marked when the training is performed with the muscle in a shortened position (25-degree angle) and occurs to a smaller extent when the training occurs with the muscle in a lengthened position (120-degree angle) (Gardner 1963; Thepaut-Mathieu, Van Hoeke, and Martin 1988). When training occurs at the midpoint of a joint's range of motion (80-degree angle), joint-angle specificity may occur throughout a greater range of motion (Kitai and Sale 1989; Knapik, Mawdsley, and Ramos 1983; Thepaut-Mathieu, Van Hoeke, and Martin 1988). In addition, twenty 6-second muscle actions result in greater carryover to other joint angles than six 6-second muscle actions (Meyers 1967). Thus, the longer the total duration of isometric training per training session (i.e., the number of muscle actions multiplied by the duration of each muscle action), the greater the carryover to other joint angles.

Some data indicate that isometric training at one joint angle may not result in dynamic power increases. Isometric training of the knee extensors at one joint angle results in inconsistent and for the most part nonsignificant changes in isokinetic torque across a wide range of movement velocities (Schott, McCully, and Rutherford 1995). This indicates that isometric training at a single joint angle is an inefficient means to train for increased dynamic strength and power. However, it has also been reported that isometric training at one joint angle does result in significant increases in dynamic (isokinetic) eccentric and concentric actions (Maffiuletti and Martin 2001), whereas isometric training of the elbow flexors at four different joint angles increases static strength at all four joint angles and significantly increases the dynamic power of the elbow flexors (Kanehisa and Miyashita 1983a). Thus, an individual wanting to increase dynamic power with isometric training should perform isometric actions at several points in the joint's range of motion.

This information from studies of joint-angle specificity offers some practical guidelines for increasing strength and power throughout the entire range of motion. First, the training should be performed at joint-angle increments of approximately 10 to 30 degrees. Second, the total duration of isometric training (the duration of each muscle action multiplied by the number of muscle actions) per session should be long (3- to 5-second actions, 15 to 20 actions per session). Third, if isometric actions cannot be performed throughout the entire range of motion, it is best to perform them with the muscle(s) in a lengthened position rather than a shortened position. It is also possible to use isometric training's joint-angle specificity to increase dynamic strength lifting ability by performing isometric actions at the sticking point of an exercise (see the section on functional isometrics in chapter 6).

Motor Performance

Maximal isometric strength has shown significant correlations to performance in sports such as basketball (Häkkinen 1987), rowing (Secher 1975), and sprinting (Mero et al. 1981), as well as to countermovement and static jump ability (Häkkinen 1987). However, a number of studies have shown nonsignificant correlations between maximal isometric strength and dynamic performance. An extensive review (Wilson and Murphy 1996) concluded that the relationship between maximal isometric strength and dynamic performance is questionable, even though some studies demonstrated significant correlations between the rate of force development during an isometric test and dynamic performance. Similarly, the majority of studies indicated that isometric tests are not sensitive to training adaptations induced by dynamic activity or consistently discriminate between athletes of differing caliber in the same sport or activity (Wilson and Murphy 1996). Thus, isometric testing is not the best modality to use when monitoring changes in dynamic motor performance. This information may also indicate that isometric training may not result in increases in dynamic motor performance such as sprinting or vertical jumping.

Isometric training at one joint angle does not increase dynamic motor performance (Clarke 1973; Fleck and Schutt 1985). This may be the result of several factors. Isometric training at one joint angle does not increase a limb's maximal velocity of movement with little or no resistance (DeKoning et al. 1982). Many motor performance tests and sport tasks (e.g., vertical jump, softball throw for distance) involve moving at maximal speed with little to moderate or no external resistance to movement. If the limb's maximal velocity of movement is not increased, improvement in many dynamic motor performance tasks will not occur. Other factors that may inhibit isometric strength gains from affecting dynamic motor performance include differences in muscle fiber recruitment patterns between isometric and dynamic actions and mechanical differences, such as little if any stretch-shortening cycle during an isometric action.

Maximal isometric force varies throughout the range of motion of a movement. The correlation between dynamic bench press ability and isometric strength varies drastically with the elbow angle at which the isometric test is performed (Murphy et al. 1995). This has led to the suggestion that isometric testing should be performed at the point within the range of motion at which maximal force is developed. However, the use of such an angle may not demonstrate the highest correlation between isometric strength and dynamic motor performance (Wilson and Murphy 1996). Thus, the exact angle at which isometric strength should be assessed remains unclear.

If isometric actions are to be used in an attempt to monitor dynamic motor performance or increase dynamic motor performance, several suggestions seem warranted. First, dynamic power can be increased with isometric training if the isometric actions are performed at several points within the range of motion (Kanehisa and Miyashita 1983a). Thus, performance of isometric actions at 10- to 20-degree intervals throughout the movement's range of motion may aid in carryover of isometric strength gains to dynamic actions. Second, most dynamic motor performance tasks are multijoint and multimuscle in nature. Thus, multijoint sport-specific isometric movements, such as a leg press movement for vertical jump ability, should be used to monitor or improve dynamic motor performance tasks. Third, if previous research indicates a point within the range of motion demonstrating a high significant correlation between isometric strength and a motor performance task, this point is where isometric strength should be assessed. If previous research does not indicate such a point within the range of motion, the strongest point within the range of motion can be used as the initial position for isometric strength testing.

Other Considerations

As with all resistance training, a Valsalva maneuver may occur resulting in an exaggerated blood pressure response during training. This should be discouraged during isometric training. Isometric knee extensions at 100% of MVMA with no breath holding result in systolic and diastolic blood pressures of 174 and 135 mmHg, respectively (see figure 1.3, page 10). The same isometric action with a Valsalva maneuver results in systolic and diastolic blood pressures of 198 and 158 mmHg, respectively. As duration, intensity (% MVMA), and muscle mass increase during an isometric action, the blood pressure response increases (Kjaer and Secher 1992; Seals 1993). The increased blood pressure response during high-intensity large-muscle-group isometric exercise can decrease left ventricular function (ejection fraction) (Vitcenda et al. 1990). These factors need to be considered when isometric actions are performed by individuals with compromised, or potentially compromised, cardiovascular function, such as older trainees.

Because they do not lift or move an actual weight, some trainees may experience motivational problems with isometric training. It is also difficult to evaluate whether the trainees are performing the isometric actions at the desired intensity without specialized equipment. Visual feedback of the force being developed, especially during unfamiliar movements, serves as positive feedback and encourages greater force production during isometric actions (Graves and James 1990). For such feedback, a force transducer and monitoring system are required. Such equipment may not be practical in many training situations. However, if isometric actions are to be used optimally in training, use of a feedback-monitoring system is warranted.

Dynamic Constant External Resistance Training

Isotonic is traditionally defined as a muscular action in which muscle exerts a constant tension. Free weight exercises and exercises on various weight training machines that are usually considered isotonic are not isotonic according to this definition. The force exerted by a muscle(s) in the performance of such exercises is not constant, but rather varies with the mechanical advantage of the joint(s) involved in the exercise. A better term for resistance training exercise in which the external resistance and weight does not change in both the lifting (concentric) and lowering (eccentric) phase is training. **Dynamic constant external resistance** (DCER) implies that the weight or resistance being lifted is constant and held constant and not that the force developed by a muscle(s) during the exercise is constant. When using free weights and many machines, the external resistance or weight lifted is held constant throughout the exercise movement. Thus, DCER better describes this type of resistance training than the old term *isotonic*.

Number of Sets and Repetitions

The optimal number of sets and repetitions for DCER exercises to achieve maximum gains in strength, power, and body compositional changes has received a great deal of attention from personal trainers, strength coaches, and sport scientists. The search for an optimal number of sets and repetitions assumes several factors: that an optimal number of sets and repetitions actually exists; that once found it will work for all individuals and exercises or muscle groups; that it will work equally well in untrained and trained individuals; and that it will promote maximal increases in strength, power, and body compositional changes for an indefinite period of time. These assumptions may not be correct.

The vast majority of research studies concerning DCER have used novice, college-age individuals as trainees and a relatively short duration of training (8 to 12 weeks, with several lasting 20 to 36 weeks). Pretraining status and the duration of the training will affect the results of any weight training project. Some studies do not report reliability of the tests, raising questions concerning the validity of the results. These factors make interpretation of the studies and drawing conclusions concerning long-term training effects difficult. Common to the vast majority of studies concerning DCER is the use of sets carried to volitional fatigue or the use of an RM resistance at some point in the training program.

Studies by Berger in the 1960s that focused on the bench press and back squat exercises indicated that optimal increases in 1RM in the bench press and back squat occurred with three sets using a resistance of 6RM (Berger 1962b, 1962c). In a later study, Berger concluded that significant but equivalent gains in 1RM strength occurred training with six sets at 2RM, three sets at 6RM, and three sets at 10RM (Berger 1963a). This demonstrated that various combinations of sets and repetitions cause similar gains in strength during an initial short period of training, especially in untrained individuals. The point that various combinations of sets and repetitions can bring about increased strength is well supported by research studies. Using nonperiodized training numbers of sets ranging from 1 to 6 and numbers of repetitions per set ranging from 1 to 20 have resulted in increased strength (see tables 2.2 and 2.3; Bemben et al. 2000; Calder et al. 1994; Dudley et al. 1991; Graves et al. 1988; Häkkinen 1985; Kraemer et al. 2000; Marx et al. 2001; Staron et al. 1989, 1994; Willoughby 1992, 1993).

Table 2.2 Changes in Bench Press Strength Due to Training

Reference	Gender of subjects	Type of training	Training duration (wk)	Training days/week	Sets and repetitions	% increase for equipment trained on	Comparative type of equipment	Comparative test % increase
Boyer 1990	F	DCER	12	3	3 wk = 3 × 10RM 3 wk = 3 × 6RM 6 wk = 3 × 8RM	24	VR	23
Brazell-Roberts and Thomas 1989	F	DCER	12	2	3 × 10 (75% 1RM)	37	—	—
Brazell-Roberts and Thomas 1989	F	DCER	12	3	3 × 10 (75% 1RM)	37	—	—
Brown and Wilmore 1974	F	DCER	24	3	8 wk = 1 × 10, 8, 7 6, 5, 4 16 wk = 1× 10, 6, 5, 4, 3	38	—	—
Calder et al. 1994	F	DCER	20	2	5 × 6-10RM	33	—	—
Hostler, Crill et al. 2001	F	DCER	16	2-3	4 wk = 2 × 7RM 4 wk = 3 × 7RM (10 days off) 8 wk = 3 × 7RM	47	—	—
Kraemer et al. 2000	F (college tennis)	DCER	36	3	1 × 8-10RM	8	—	—
Marx et al. 2001	F	DCER	24	3	1 × 8-10RM	12	—	—
Kraemer, Mazzetti et al. 2001	F	DCER	24	3	Periodized 3 × 3-8RM	37	—	—
Kraemer, Mazzetti et al. 2001	F	DCER	24	3	Periodized 3 × 8-12RM	23	—	—
Mayhew and Gross 1974	F	DCER	9	3	2 × 20	26	—	—
Wilmore 1974	F	DCER	10	2	2 × 7-16	29	—	—
Wilmore et al. 1978	F	DCER	10	3	40-55% 1RM for 30 s	20	—	—
Allen, Byrd, and Smith 1976	M	DCER	12	3	2 × 8, 1 × exhaustion	44	—	—

(continued)

Reference	Sex	Mode			Sets × reps			
Ariel 1977	M	DCER	20	5	4 × 3-8	14	—	—
Baker, Wilson, and Carlyon 1994b	M	DCER	12	3	3 × 6	13	—	—
Berger 1962b	M	DCER	12	3	3 × 6	30	—	—
Coleman 1977	M	DCER	10	3	2 × 8-10RM	12	—	—
Fahey and Brown 1973	M	DCER	9	3	5 × 5	12	—	—
Gettman et al. 1978	M	DCER	20	3	50% 1RM, 6 wk = 2 × 10-20, 14 wk = 2 × 15	32	IK (12 deg/s)	27
Hoffman et al. 1990	M (college football)	DCER	10	3	4 wk = 4 × 8RM, 4 wk = 5 × 6RM, 2 wk = 1 × 10, 8, 6, 4, 2RM	2	—	—
Hoffman et al. 1990	M (college football)	DCER	10	4	Same as 3/wk	4	—	—
Hoffman et al. 1990	M (college football)	DCER	10	5	Same as 3/wk	3	—	—
Hoffman et al. 1990	M (college football)	DCER	10	6	Same as 3/wk	4	—	—
Hostler, Crill et al. 2001	M	DCER	16	2-3	4 wk = 2 × 7RM, 4 wk = 3 × 7RM (10 days off), 8 wk = 3 × 7RM	29	—	—
Marcinik et al. 1991	M	DCER	12	3	1 × 8-12RM	20	—	—
Stone, Nelson et al. 1983	M	DCER	6	3	3 × 6RM	7	—	—
Wilmore 1974	M	DCER	10	2	2 × 7-16	16	—	—
Ariel 1977	M	VR	20	5	4 × 3-8	—	DCER	29
Boyer 1990	F	VR	12	3	3 wk = 3 × 10RM, 3 wk = 3 × 6RM, 6 wk = 3 × 8RM	47	DCER	15
Coleman 1977	M	VR	10	3	1 × 8-12RM	—	DCERa	12

Table 2.2 (continued)

Reference	Gender of subjects	Type of training	Training duration (wk)	Training days/ week	Sets and repetitions	% increase for equipment trained on	Comparative type of equipment	Comparative test % increase
Lee et al. 1990	M	VR	10	3	3 × 10RM	20	—	—
Stanforth, Painter, and Wilmore 1992	M and F	VR	12	3	3 × 8-12RM	11	IK (1.5 s/contraction)	17
Gettman and Ayres 1978	M	IK (60 deg/s)	10	3	3 × 10-15	—	DCER	11
Gettman and Ayres 1978	M	IK (120 deg/s)	10	3	3 × 10-15	—	DCER	9
Gettman et al. 1979	M	IK	8	3	4 wk = 1 × 10 at 60 deg/s 4 wk = 1 × 15 at 90 deg/s	22	DCER	11
Stanforth, Painter, and Wilmore 1992	M and F	IK (1.5 s/ contraction)	12	3	3 × 8-12RM	20	VR	11

DCER = dynamic constant external resistance; VR = variable resistance; IK = isokinetic; RM = repetition maximum; * = values for average training weights.

Table 2.3 Changes in Leg Press Strength Due to Training

Reference	Gender of subjects	Type of training	Training duration (wk)	Training days/week	Sets and repetitions	% increase for equipment trained on	Comparative type of equipment	Comparative test % increase
Brown and Wilmore 1974	F	DCER	24	3	8 wk = 1 × 10, 8, 7, 6, 5, 4 16 wk = 1 × 10, 6, 5, 4, 3	29	—	—
Calder et al. 1994	F	DCER	20	2	5 × 10-12RM	21	—	—
Cordova et al. 1995	F	DCER	5	3	1 × 10, 1 × 6, 2 × as many as possible normally up to 11	50	—	—
Kraemer et al. 2000	F (college tennis)	DCER	36	3	1 × 8-10RM	8	—	—
Marx et al. 2001	F	DCER	24	3	1 × 8-10RM	11	—	—
Mayhew and Gross 1974	F	DCER	9	3	2 × 10	48a	—	—
Staron et al. 1991	F	DCER (vertical leg press)	18 (8 wk, 1 wk off, 10 wk)	2	3 × 6-8RM	148	—	—
Wilmore et al. 1978	F	DCER	10	3	40-55% 1RM for 30 s	27	—	—
Allen, Byrd, and Smith 1976	M	DCER	12	3	2 × 8 1 × exhaustion	71b	—	—
Coleman 1977	M	DCER	10	3	2 × 8-10RM	17	—	—
Dudley et al. 1991	M	DCER	19	2	4-5 × 6-12RM	26	—	—
Gettman et al. 1978	M	DCER	20	3	50% 1RM, 6 wk = 2 × 10-20 14 wk = 2 × 15	—	IK	43
Pipes 1978	M	DCER	10	3	3 × 8	29	VR	8
Sale et al. 1990	M and F	DCER	11 (3 wk off) 11 more total 22	3	6 × 15-20RM (one-legged training)	30	—	—

(continued)

Table 2.3 (continued)

Reference	Gender of subjects	Type of training	Training duration (wk)	Training days/ week	Sets and repetitions	% increase for equipment trained on	Comparative type of equipment	Comparative test % increase
Tatro, Dudley, and Convertino 1992	M	DCER	19	2	7 wk = 4 × 10-12RM 6 wk = 5 × 8-10RM 6 wk = 5 × 6-8RM	25 (3RM)	—	—
Wilmore et al. 1978	M	DCER	10	3	40-55% 1RM for 30 s	7	—	—
Coleman 1977	M	VR	10	3	1 ×10-12RM	—	DCER	18
Gettman, Culter, and Strathman 1980	M	VR	20	3	3 × 8	18c	IK	17
Lee et al. 1990	M	VR	10	3	3 ×10RM	6	—	—
Pipes 1978	M	VR	10	3	3 × 8	27	DCER	8
Smith and Melton 1981	M	VR	6	4	3 × 10	—	VRd	11
Cordova et al. 1995	F	IK	5	3	2 × 10 at 60, 180, and 240 deg/s	64	—	—
Gettman et al. 1979	M	IK	8	3	4 wk = 1 × 10 at 60 deg/s 4 wk = 1 × 15 at 90 deg/s	38	DCER	18
Gettman, Culter, and Strathman 1980	M	IK	20	3	2 × 12 at 60 deg/s	42	VR	10
Smith and Melton 1981	M	IK	6	4	Sets to 50% exhaustion at 30, 60, and 90 deg/s	—	VR	10
Smith and Melton 1981	M	IK	6	4	Sets to 50% fatigue at 180, 240, and 300 deg/s	—	VR	7

DCER = dynamic constant external resistance; IK = isokinetic; RM = repetition maximum; a = values for 10RM; b = values for average training weights; c = values for number of weight plates; d = different type of VR equipment.

Other researchers' work substantiates the assertion that there is no one optimal combination of nonperiodized sets and repetitions for increasing strength. No significant difference in increases in 1RM were found when training consisted of five sets of three at 3RM, four sets of five at 5RM, or three sets of seven at 7RM (Withers 1970); three sets of two to three, five to six, or nine to ten at the same respective RM resistance (O'Shea 1966); or one, two, or four sets all at 7 to 12RM (Ostrowski et al. 1997).

Increases in maximal strength have been reported when doing one set of an exercise per training session (Alen et al. 1988; Berger 1962a; Graves et al. 1988; Kraemer et al. 2000; Luthi et al. 1986; Marcinik et al. 1991; Marx et al. 2001; Rasch and Morehouse 1957). The American College of Sports Medicine (1998) recommended that healthy adults interested in general fitness include a minimum of one set of 8 to 12 repetitions per set of at least one exercise for all major muscle groups in a weight training session. This recommendation is for healthy adults desiring fitness gains or maintenance of fitness. It is not for athletes or highly trained fitness enthusiasts, as multiple-set programs (American College of Sports Medicine 2002) as well as periodized multiple-set training programs do result in greater strength and fitness gains than single-set programs (Kraemer et al. 2000; Marx et al. 2001; McGee et al. 1992). Although one set per exercise per training session may be appropriate as a short-term in-season program for some athletes, it is not recommended as a long-term program for athletes desiring optimal fitness gains. Over the course of a training year or career, even small, superior gains in strength, power, or body composition from performing multiple sets in a periodized fashion as compared to one set can result in greater performance increases.

Maximal Voluntary Muscle Actions

The majority of training studies and training programs used by fitness enthusiasts and athletes incorporate maximal voluntary muscle actions (MVMAs) at some point in the training. This does not mean that a 1RM has to be performed; rather, it means that a set is performed to momentary concentric failure or sets are performed using RMs or close to RM resistances (see the discussion of exhaustion set technique in chapter 6).

Berger and Hardage (1967) demonstrated a need for MVMAs to bring about maximal gains in strength during 8 weeks of training. In this study, one group trained with one set of 10 repetitions at a 10RM resistance per training session. The first repetition for the other group was at a 1RM resistance. For the subsequent 9 repetitions the resistance was adjusted so that a maximal or near-maximal effort was required to complete each repetition. Both groups made significant gains in strength, but the group trained with the resistance adjusted so that a MVMA was performed during each repetition made significantly greater gains in strength. The results indicate that heavy resistances resulting in MVMAs need to be lifted multiple times per session to bring about optimal strength improvement.

Training Frequency

Training frequency, the numbers of sets and repetitions, and the number of exercises per training session determine total training volume. The optimal training frequency, therefore, may depend in part on total training volume per training session. The term *training frequency* is normally used to refer to the number of training sessions per week in which a certain muscle group is trained. It is possible to have daily training sessions and train a particular muscle group or body part from anywhere between not at all to seven sessions per week. Training frequency will be defined here as the number of training sessions per week in which a certain muscle group is trained or a particular exercise performed.

The importance of the definition of *training frequency* is made apparent by a comparison of an upper- and lower-body split program (see chapter 6) to a total-body weight training routine (Calder et al. 1994). Trainees in both the split routine and total-body programs performed the same exercises and numbers of set and repetitions per exercise. However, those in the total-body program performed all upper- and lower-body exercises in two training sessions per week, whereas those in the split program performed all of the upper-body exercises two days per week and the lower-body exercises on two other days per week resulting in four training sessions per week. Total training volume was not different between the split and total-body programs, yet training frequency was different between the two programs (unless it is defined as the number of sessions in which a certain body part or exercise is performed). Interestingly, the two training programs showed no difference in strength gains during the 10 weeks of training.

The optimal training frequency may also be different between muscle groups. A comparison of one, two, and three sessions per week training the bench press or squat concluded that three sessions were superior to one or two sessions in bringing about strength increases (Berger 1962a). Another comparison of training frequency for the bench press also concluded that three sessions were superior to one or two sessions (Faigenbaum and Pollock 1997). However, Graves and colleagues (1990) concluded that one session was equally as effective as two or three sessions per week when training for isolated lumbar extension strength. DeMichele and colleagues (1997) found that two sessions per week was equivalent to three and superior to one session per week when training for torso rotation. These studies indicate that three sessions per week are superior to one or two sessions per week when training arm and leg musculature, whereas when training spine muscles, one or two sessions per week result in equivalent gains compared to three sessions per week. The training frequency of three sessions per week when training the arms and legs results in a 20 to 30% greater strength gain than a frequency of two sessions per week (American College of Sports Medicine 1998).

Other factors may also affect optimal training frequency. In a comparison of varying self-selected training frequencies among collegiate football players using different body-part training programs over 10 weeks of training (see table 2.4), 1RM bench press ability significantly increased only in the five-sessions-per-week group (Hoffman et al. 1990), and 1RM squat ability significantly increased in the four-, five-, and six-sessions-per-week groups. All training frequencies did result in percentage gains in bench press (2-4%) and squat (5-8%) ability. Examining all of the tests (vertical jump, sum of skinfolds, 2-mi [1.61-km] run, 40-yd [36.6-m] sprint, thigh circumference, chest circumference) pre- and post-training, researchers concluded that a frequency of four or five sessions per week results in the greatest overall fitness gains. Note, however, that this means each muscle group was trained for only two or three times per week.

Table 2.5 presents two studies concerning training frequency. One study (Gillam 1981) compared from one to five training sessions per week. All subjects performed a large number of very intense sets (18 sets of 1RM) per training session. Five sessions were shown to be superior in causing increases in 1RM bench press ability compared to the other training frequencies. Additionally, five and three sessions per week showed significantly greater increases than two or one session per week. A study comparing training frequencies of four and three using male and female subjects reported significantly greater gains in both genders with more frequent training sessions (Hunter 1985). Both groups performed all exercises using a 7 to 10RM resistance with the three-sessions-per-week group performing three sets of each exercise per session and the four-sessions-per-week group performing two sets of each exercise 3 days per week and three sets 1 day per week. Thus, total training sets were equivalent between the two groups. Interestingly, the four-sessions-per-week subjects trained 2 consecutive days twice a week (i.e., Monday and Tuesday, and Thursday and Friday), while the three-sessions-per-week subjects trained in the traditional alternate-day

Table 2.4 Resistance Training Programs With Training Frequencies of Three to Six Sessions per Week

Frequency	Training days	Body parts trained
3	Mon., Wed., Fri.	Total body
4	Mon., Thurs. Tues., Fri.	Chest, shoulders, triceps, neck Legs, back, biceps, forearms
5	Mon., Wed., Fri. Tues., Thurs.	Chest, triceps, legs, neck Back, shoulders, biceps, forearms
6	Mon., Tues., Thurs., Fri. Wed., Sat.	Chest, triceps, legs, shoulders, neck Back, biceps, forearms

Adapted, by permission, from J.R. Hoffman et al., 1990, "The effects of self-selection for frequency of training in a winter conditioning program for football," *Journal of Applied Sport Science Research* 4: 76-82.

Table 2.5 Effect of Training Frequency on 1RM Bench Press		
Reference	Gender	Days per week of training and percent improvement
Gillam 1981	M	Days 1 2 3 4 5 % improvement 19 24 32 29 41
Hunter 1985	M	Days 3 4 % improvement 12 17
Hunter 1985	F	Days 3 4 % improvement 20 33

method (i.e., Monday, Wednesday, Friday). Results indicated that the necessity of the traditional 1 day of rest between weight training sessions may not apply to all muscle groups.

An extensive meta-analysis concluded that for untrained individuals a training frequency of 3 days per week per muscle group was optimal (Rhea et al. 2003), while a frequency of 2 days per week per muscle group was optimal for trained individuals. The difference in optimal training frequencies may be due to higher training volumes being used in the studies using trained individuals as subjects (Rhea et al. 2003). The results indicate optimal training frequency may vary with training status and training volume.

Periodization of weight training may allow more frequent training sessions and the use of a higher total training volume compared to nonvaried training programs. In comparisons of an undulating periodized program (see chapter 7) and a single-set nonvaried program over 6 and 9 months of training, the periodized program resulted in significantly greater strength and power, motor performance, and positive body composition changes than the nonvaried program (Kraemer et al. 2000; Marx et al. 2001). The periodized program used four training sessions per week with multiple sets of each exercise, and the nonvaried single-set program used three training sessions per week. Thus, the total training volume performed by those in the periodized program was substantially more than that performed by those in the nonvaried program.

Many of the aforementioned studies have design limitations: The majority of studies used beginning resistance exercisers (novice subjects); examined short training durations (up to 12 weeks); and some studies did not equate the total number of sets and repetitions performed by the different training groups. However, in general it appears that when using nonperiodized programs, two or three sessions per week result in near-optimal strength gains. Higher training frequencies, especially with periodized programs, may result in significantly greater strength and power, motor performance, and body compositional adaptations over long training periods.

Motor Performance

DCER exercise has been shown to increase motor performance. Many studies show significant increases in motor performance tests such as

- vertical jump ability (Adams et al. 1992; Campbell 1962; Kraemer et al. 2000; Kraemer, Mazzetti et al. 2001; Marx et al. 2001; Stone, Johnson, and Carter 1979; Stone, O'Bryant, and Garhammer 1981),
- the standing long jump (Capen 1950; Chu 1950),
- the shuttle run (Campbell 1962; Kusintz and Kenney 1958),
- a short sprint (Capen 1950; Marx et al. 2001; Schultz 1967),
- baseball throwing velocity (Thompson and Martin 1965), and
- the shot put (Chu 1950; Schultz 1967).

Statistically insignificant changes in short sprint time (Chu 1950; Hoffman et al. 1990; Marx et al. 2001) and in vertical jump ability (Hoffman et al. 1990; Marx et al. 2001; Newton, Kraemer, and Häkkinen 1999; Stone, Nelson, Nader, and Carter 1983) and standing long jump ability (Schultz 1967) have also been demonstrated. Training using over- and underweight balls increases overhand baseball throwing velocity (DeRenne, Ho, and Blitzblau 1990). However, overhand baseball throwing ability for speed and accuracy is not significantly affected by DCER training with weighted-ball or pulley-type exercises, according to two studies (Brose and Hanson 1967; Straub 1968). Significant changes in job-related motor performance tasks such as 1RM box lift and repetitive box lift have also been demonstrated (Kraemer, Mazzetti et al. 2001). Similar to strength increases, changes in motor performance tests will depend in part on the initial physical condition of the trainee, with smaller increases apparent with better initial physical fitness. The type of program employed can also influence whether a change occurs in a motor performance task. For example, in untrained women vertical jump power and 40-yd (36.6-m) sprint ability improved significantly more during 6 months of training with a multiple-set periodized program compared to a single set to momentary fatigue program (Marx et al. 2001). Similar results over 9 months of training of women collegiate tennis athletes have been shown, with vertical jump height and tennis serve velocity showing significant improvements with a multiple-set periodized program and no improvement with a single set to momentary fatigue program (Kraemer et al. 2000). These results indicate that higher-volume periodized programs can result in significantly greater gains in motor performance than nonvaried, low-volume programs. Although conflicting results concerning significant changes in motor performance can be found, as a whole research supports the assertion that DCER exercise can significantly improve motor performance ability.

Significant increases in vertical jump and shot put ability occurred in college-age individuals after training only the toe and finger flexors over a 12-week period (Kokkonen et al. 1988). Thus, the training of small-muscle groups involved in motor performance tasks is also important when an increase in performance is desired.

Many people assume that an increase in strength and power brought about by a training program can be usefully applied in a motor performance task. For this to occur, however, trainees must train all of the muscles involved in the motor performance task, especially the weakest muscles involved in the task, as they may limit the useful application of the strength and power from stronger muscle groups. Additionally, proper technique of the motor task must be trained, as technique may also limit the useful application of increased strength and power. This last point is supported by a project showing that direct practice, alone or combined with resistance training, increases standing long jump ability to a significantly greater extent than resistance training alone in previously untrained subjects (Schultz 1967).

Strength Changes

Strength increases in both women and men from DCER training in a large variety of muscle groups are well documented. Tables 2.2, 2.3, and 2.5 present changes in 1RM bench press and leg press ability in both genders after short-term DCER training. Women demonstrated substantial increases in 1RM bench press ability with increases ranging from 8% in college tennis athletes after 36 weeks of training (Kraemer et al. 2000) to 47% after 16 weeks of training (Hostler, Crill et al. 2001). Similarly, men experience strength increases ranging from 3% in college football players after 10 weeks of training (Hoffman et al. 1990) to 44% after 12 weeks of training (Allen, Byrd, and Smith 1976). Using 1RM as the testing criteria, women have demonstrated increases in leg press ability ranging from 8% in college tennis players after 36 weeks of training (Kraemer et al. 2000) to 148% after 18 weeks of training (Staron et al. 1991). Increases in men's leg press ability range from 7% after 10 weeks of training (Wilmore et al. 1978) to 71% after 10 weeks of training (Allen, Byrd, and Smith 1976). The wide ranges in strength increases are probably related to differences in pretraining status, familiarity with the exercise tests, the duration of training, and the type of program.

Body Composition Changes

The normal changes in body composition as a result of short-term DCER exercise in both genders are small increases in fat-free mass and small decreases in percent body fat (see table 3.3, page 92). The decrease in percent body fat is often due in large part to an increase in fat-free mass rather than a large decrease in fat weight. Normally these two changes occur simultaneously, resulting in little or no change in total body weight.

Safety Considerations

If DCER exercise is performed using free weights, appropriate spotting should be used. For machine DCER exercises, spotting is normally not needed. Because free weights must be controlled in three planes of movement, generally more time will be needed to learn proper lifting technique, especially of multijoint, multimuscle group exercises, compared to a similar exercise performed using a machine.

Variable Resistance Training

Variable resistance equipment has a lever arm, cam, or pulley arrangement that varies the resistance throughout the exercise's range of motion. One purpose of variable resistance equipment is to attempt to match the increases and decreases in strength (strength curve) throughout an exercise's range of motion. Proponents of variable resistance machines believe that by increasing and decreasing the resistance to match the exercise's strength curve, the muscle is forced to contract near maximally throughout the range of motion, resulting in maximal strength gains.

There are three major types of strength curves: ascending, descending, and bell-shaped (see figure 2.3). In an exercise with an ascending strength curve, it is possible to lift more weight if only the last half or last quarter of a repetition is performed than if the complete range of motion of a repetition is performed. For example, exercises with an ascending strength curve are the squat and bench press. If an exercise has a descending strength curve, it is possible to lift more weight if only the first half or first quarter of a repetition is performed. Such an exercise is upright rowing. An exercise in which it is possible to lift more resistance if only the middle portion of the range of motion is performed has a bell-shaped strength curve. Arm curls, like many single-joint exercises, have a bell-shaped strength curve. To match the three major types of strength curves, variable resistance machines must be able to vary the resistance in three major patterns. To date this has not been satisfactorily accomplished. Additionally, because of variations in limb length, the point of attachment of the muscle's tendons to the bones, and torso size, it is difficult to conceive of one mechanical arrangement that would successfully match all individuals' strength curves for a particular exercise.

Biomechanical research indicates that one type of variable resistance cam equipment does not match the strength curves of the elbow curl, multibiceps curl, chest fly, knee-extension, knee-flexion, and pullover exercises (Cabell and Zebras 1999; Harman 1983; Pizzimenti 1992). The equipment's ability to match the strength curve is especially ineffective at the extreme ranges of an exercise's range of motion (Cabell and Zebras 1999). A second type of cam equipment has been reported to match the strength curves

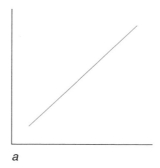

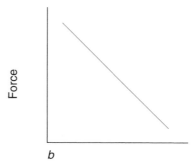

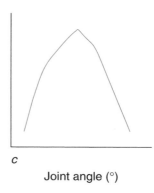

Figure 2.3 The three major types of strength curves are *(a)* ascending, *(b)* descending, and *(c)* bell shaped.

of females fairly well (Johnson, Colodny, and Jackson 1990). However, for females the cam resulted in too great a resistance near the end of the knee-extension exercise. The cam also provided too much resistance during the first half and too little during the second half of the elbow-flexion and -extension exercises. The knee-flexion machine matched the females' strength curves well throughout the range of motion. Thus, in general cam-type variable resistance equipment does not appear to successfully match the strength curve of exercises.

Sets and Repetitions

Significant strength gains from short-term (4 to 18 weeks) variable resistance training have been demonstrated in a large variety of muscle groups with various combinations of sets and repetitions. Significant increases in strength have been shown with the following protocols (sets × repetitions):

- 1 × 6 to 10RM (Jacobson 1986)
- 1 × 7 to 10RM (Braith et al. 1993; Graves et al. 1989)
- 1 × 8 to 12RM (Coleman 1977; Hurley, Seals, Ehsani et al. 1984; Keeler et al. 2001; Manning et al. 1990; Pollock et al. 1993; Silvester et al. 1984; Starkey et al. 1996; Westcott et al. 2001)
- 1 × 10 to 12RM (Peterson 1975)
- 1 × 12 to 15RM (Stone, Johnson, and Carter 1979)
- 2 × 10 to 12RM (Coleman 1977)
- 2 × 12 at 50% of 1RM (Gettman, Culter, and Strathman 1980)
- 2 to 3 × 8 to 10RM (LeMura et al. 2000)
- 3 × 6RM (Jacobson 1986; Silvester et al. 1984)
- 3 × 8 to 12RM (Starkey et al. 1996)
- 3 × 15RM (Hunter and Culpepper 1995)
- 6 × 15 to 20RM (Sale et al. 1990)
- 3 × 10RM for 3 weeks, 3 × 8RM for 3 weeks, and 3 × 6RM for 6 weeks (Boyer 1990)
- Four sets with increasing resistance and repetitions decreasing from 8 to 3 in a half-pyramid program (Ariel 1977)

Variable resistance training has been shown to increase maximal isometric strength throughout the full range of motion of an exercise (Hunter and Culpepper 1995). Thus, various combinations of sets and repetitions can cause significant increases in strength.

Strength Increases

Substantial increases in strength have been demonstrated with variable resistance training. For example, after 16 weeks of training males demonstrated an increase of 50% in upper-body exercises and 33% in lower-body exercises (Hurley et al. 1984a), and females demonstrated an increase of 29% in upper-body strength and 38% in lower-body strength (LeMura et al. 2000). Increases in bench press and leg press strength from variable resistance training are depicted in tables 2.2 and 2.3, respectively. This type of resistance training apparently can cause substantial increases in strength when tested using variable resistance equipment and other types of muscle actions.

Motor Performance

Several projects have examined changes in motor performance tasks as a result of variable resistance training. Peterson (1975) studied a group of American football players who participated in a combined program of in-season football training and total-body variable resistance strength training. The resistance training group demonstrated a small but greater mean decrease in the 40-yd (36.6-m) sprint and a small but greater mean increase in a vertical jump test than a control group performing only the in-season football training program. Whether the changes were statistically significant or whether a significant difference existed between the two groups was not addressed. Although this study showed a slightly greater increase in motor performance with variable resistance training, it offers little concrete evidence of a relationship between motor performance and variable resistance training.

Silvester and colleagues (1984) investigated strength increases in two groups that trained on different variable resistance equipment: One group trained on a cam-type variable resistance machine, and another group trained on an increasing lever arm–type variable resistance machine. The cam-type group trained 3 days per week for 6 weeks followed by 2 days per week for 5 weeks. This protocol was recommended by the manufacturer of the cam-type equipment. Participants did knee extensions immediately followed by the leg presses and performed each exercise for one set of 12 repetitions to failure. The increasing lever arm–type group trained 3 days per week for the entire 11-week training period performing the leg press for one set of 7 to 10 repetitions followed by one set to concentric failure. No difference in static leg strength gains was demonstrated between the two groups. The cam-type and lever arm–type groups increased their mean vertical jumps by 0.3 in. (0.69 cm) and 1.1 in. (2.91 cm), respectively. The increase in vertical jump shown by the lever arm–type group was significantly greater than the increase shown by the cam-type group. These results indicate that motor performance can increase as a result of variable resistance training and that the increase depends in part on the training protocol, equipment used, or both.

Body Composition

Significant increases in muscle thickness at some sites on the quadriceps and knee flexors (hamstrings) have been reported after variable resistance training (Starkey et al. 1996). Increases in fat-free mass and decreases in percent body fat also occur after variable resistance training. These changes in body composition are depicted in table 3.3 on page 92 and are of the same magnitude as the changes that occur from DCER training.

Safety Considerations

As with all types of weight training machines, safety is not a major concern when using variable resistance machines, and a spotter is not normally necessary. Similarly, as with all weight training machines, care must be taken to ensure that the variable resistance machine fits the trainee properly and that the trainee is properly positioned on the machine. Without proper fit and positioning, proper exercise technique is impossible and risk of injury increases. On some variable resistance machines jerky exercise movement may occur and may in part be caused by the strength curve of the individual not being closely matched. Such jerky exercise movement probably increases the possibility of injury such as muscle strain and joint discomfort.

Isokinetic

Isokinetic refers to a muscular action performed at constant angular limb velocity. Unlike other types of resistance training, there is no specified resistance to meet; rather, the velocity of movement is controlled. At the start of each movement, acceleration from 0 degrees per second takes place until the set velocity is achieved. After the set velocity is achieved, further acceleration is not possible and any force applied against the equipment results in an equal reaction force. The reaction force mirrors the force applied to the equipment throughout the range of movement of an exercise, until deceleration starts to occur at the end of the range of motion. It is theoretically possible for the muscle(s) to exert a continual, maximal force throughout the movement's range of motion except where acceleration at the start and deceleration at the end of the movement occurs.

The majority of isokinetic equipment found in resistance training facilities allows concentric-only actions. Thus, the effects of concentric-only isokinetic training will be reviewed here, although eccentric-only and coupled concentric-eccentric actions (the same exercise movement performed in a concentric followed by an eccentric action) are possible on some types of isokinetic equipment. After short-duration training (9 weeks), coupled concentric-eccentric isokinetic training has been shown to result in significant increases in concentric isokinetic, but not eccentric isokinetic strength (Caruso et al. 1997). Advantages of isokinetic training include the ability to exert maximal force throughout a large portion of an exercises' range of motion, the ability to train over a wide range of movement velocities, and minimal muscle and joint soreness. The major criticism of this type of training is that isokinetic muscle actions do not exist in the real world, making the application of isokinetic training to daily life and sport activity questionable.

Strength Changes

The vast majority of studies examining concentric-only isokinetic training have been of short duration (3 to 16 weeks) and have tested for strength gains using isometric, constant external resistance, and concentric-only isokinetic tests. Concentric-only isokinetic training has also been shown to increase eccentric isokinetic strength (Seger, Arvidsson, and Thorstensson 1998; Tomberline et al. 1991). As depicted in table 2.6, programs of 1 to 15 sets at various movement velocities and with various numbers of repetitions and sets cause significant increases in strength.

Significant gains in strength have also been achieved by performing as many repetitions as possible in a fixed period of time, as shown in the following studies:

- One set for 6 seconds at 180 degrees per second (Lesmes et al. 1978)
- One set for 30 seconds at 108 degrees per second (Lesmes et al. 1978)
- Two sets for 20 seconds at 180 degrees per second (Bell et al. 1992; Petersen et al. 1987)
- Two sets for 30 seconds at 60 degrees per second (Bell et al. 1991a)

Table 2.6 Isokinetic Training and Combinations of Sets and Repetitions Causing Significant Gains in Strength

Reference	Sets × reps at degrees per second
Bond et al. 1996	1 × 12 at 15
Jenkins, Thackaberry, and Killian 1984	1 × 15 at 60 1 × 15 at 240
Lacerte et al. 1992	1 × 20 at 60 1 × 20 at 180
Moffroid et al. 1969	1 × 30 at 22.5
Knapik, Mawdsley, and Ramos 1983	1 × 50 at 30
Pearson and Costill 1988	1 × 65 at 120
Gettman, Culter, and Strathman 1980	2 × 12 at 60
Gettman et al. 1979	2 × 10 at 60 followed by 2 × 15 at 90
Ewing et al. 1990	3 × 8 at 60 3 × 20 at 240
Tomberline et al. 1991	3 × 10 at 100
Morris, Tolfroy, and Coppack 2001	3 × 10 at 100
Gettman and Ayers 1978	3 × 15 at 90 3 × 15 at 60
Kanehisa and Miyashita 1983b	1 × 10 at 60 1 × 30 at 179 1 × 50 at 300
Seger, Arvidsson, and Thorstensson 1998	4 × 10 at 90
Colliander and Tesch 1990a	4-5 × 12 at 60
Coyle et al. 1981	5 × 6 at 60 5 × 12 at 300
Coyle et al. 1981	(6 sets total) 3 × 6 at 60 & 3 × 12 at 300
Cirello, Holden, and Evans 1983	5 × 5 at 60
Petersen et al. 1990	5 × 10 at 120
Mannion, Jakeman, and Willan 1992	6 × 25 at 240 5 × 15 at 60
Housh et al. 1992	6 × 10 at 120
Narici et al. 1989	6 × 10 at 120
Akima et al. 1999	10 × 5 at 120
Kovaleski et al. 1995	10 × 12 at 120 to 210
Cirello, Holden, and Evans 1983	5 × 5 at 60 15 × 10 at 60

- Two sets for 30 seconds at 120 degrees per seconds or at 300 degrees per second (Bell et al. 1989)

- One set for 60 seconds at 36 degrees per second or at 108 degrees per second (Seaborne and Taylor 1984)

Increases in strength have also been achieved by performing a set of voluntary maximal actions until a given percentage of peak force could no longer be generated. One set continued until at least 60%, 75%, or 90% of peak force could no longer be generated at each velocity of 30 degrees per second, 60 degrees per second, and 90 degrees per second (Fleck et al. 1982) and until 50% of peak force could no longer be maintained during slow-speed training (one set each at a velocity of 30 degrees per second, 60 degrees per second, and 90 degrees per second) or fast-speed training (one set each at a velocity of 180 degrees per second, 240 degrees per second, and 300 degrees per second) (Smith and Melton 1981).

Isokinetic velocity spectrum training has also resulted in significant strength gains. This type of isokinetic training involves performing several sets in succession at various movement velocities. Velocity spectrum training can be performed with either the faster velocities or the slower velocities being performed first. A typical fast-velocity spectrum exercise protocol is presented in table 2.7. A series of acute and short-duration (4-week) training studies (Kovaleski and Heitman 1993a, 1993b; Kovaleski et al. 1992) indicates that training protocols in which the fast-velocity sets are performed first result in greater power gains, especially at faster movement velocities, but not necessarily maximal torque gains across a range of movement velocities compared to protocols in which the slower movement velocities are performed first.

Tables 2.2 and 2.3 include changes in strength of the bench press and leg press, respectively, after isokinetic training. Apparently, many combinations of sets and repetitions of concentric-only training can cause significant increases in strength.

Number of Sets and Repetitions

Despite the vast quantity of research concerning the training effects of concentric-only isokinetic training, few studies have investigated the optimal training number of sets and repetitions. One study (Lesmes et al. 1978) showed no difference in peak torque gains between 10 sets of 6-second duration with as many repetitions as possible (approximately 3), and 2 sets of 30-second duration with as many repetitions as possible (approximately 10). Both groups trained at 180 degrees per second four times a week for 7 weeks. Another study compared all combinations of 5, 10, and 15 repetitions at slow, intermediate, and fast velocities of movement. After training 3 days a week for 9 weeks, groups showed no significant differences in strength (Davies 1977). Cirello, Holden, and Evans (1983) also compared 5 sets of 5 repetitions and 15 sets of 10 repetitions. In this study both groups trained at 60 degrees per second three times per week for 16 weeks. Both groups improved significantly at all concentric test velocities ranging from 0 to 300 degrees per second; only one significant difference existed between the two groups: At 30 degrees per second the 15-set group showed greater gains than the 5-set group. All three of these studies agree on at least one point: The number of repetitions performed appears to have little impact on increases in peak torque over short durations of training.

Training Velocity

Previously cited studies firmly support the contention that concentric-only isokinetic training can result in increased strength. One question inherent to isokinetic training is: What is the optimal training velocity—fast or slow? It is important to note that the optimal training velocity may depend on the task the training is meant to improve. If strength at a slow velocity of movement is necessary for success, the optimal training velocity may be different from that for a task in which strength at a fast velocity of movement is necessary for success.

Set	1	2	3	4	5	6	7	8	9	10
Velocity	180	210	240	270	300	300	270	240	210	180
Reps	10	10	10	10	10	10	10	10	10	10

Table 2.7 Typical Isokinetic Fast-Velocity Spectrum Training

The question of optimal training velocity is in part dependent on the velocity specificity of concentric-only isokinetic training. Velocity specificity refers to whether strength gains made training at one velocity are greatest at that training velocity and whether training at one velocity results in strength and power gains at movement velocities other than the training velocity. The majority of research indicates that isokinetic training does have velocity specificity (Behm and Sale 1993). This means that greater strength gains are made at or near the training velocity, indicating that if strength at a fast velocity of movement is necessary, training should be performed at a fast velocity, and likewise if strength at a slow velocity is necessary, training should be performed at a slow velocity. Neural mechanisms, such as selective activation of motor units, selective activation of muscles, and deactivation of co-contractions by antagonists, are generally believed to be the cause of velocity specificity (Behm and Sale 1993).

Other issues of optimal training velocity are to what extent velocity specificity exists and whether training at one velocity results in increased strength over a wide range of movement velocities. One of the first studies to investigate questions concerning optimal training velocity and velocity specificity was that of Moffroid and Whipple (1970). Their results indicated that both training velocities demonstrated some degree of velocity specificity (large strength gains at the training velocity). However, the faster training velocity demonstrated velocity specificity to a smaller extent and more consistent strength gains across the range of velocities at which strength was tested (see figure 2.4). It is important to note that both training velocities examined in this study were in reality relatively slow velocities of movement. Slow-speed training (4 seconds to complete one leg press repetition) has been shown to result in a greater strength increase than fast-speed training (2 seconds to complete one leg press repetition) (Oteghen 1975). Unfortunately, the velocity at which strength was tested is undefined.

Several studies do provide more insight into the fast-versus-slow optimal training velocity question. Kanehisa and Miyashita (1983b) trained groups at specified velocities of 60 degrees per second, 179 degrees per second, and 300 degrees per second six times per week for 8 weeks. The training consisted of 10, 30, and 50 voluntary maximal actions per session. All groups were tested for peak torque at a variety of velocities

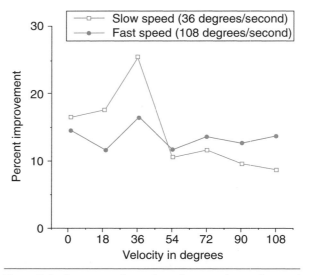

Figure 2.4 Percentage change in peak torque due to slow- and fast-speed, concentric-only isokinetic training.

Reprinted, by permission, from M.T. Moffroid and R.H. Whipple, 1970, "Specificity of speed of exercise," *Physical Therapy* 50: 1695.

ranging from 60 degrees per second to 300 degrees per second both before and after the training program. The varied number of repetitions at different training velocities limits general conclusions. However, the results indicate that an intermediate speed (179 degrees per second) may be the most advantageous for gains in average power across a range of movement velocities. Another study by Kanehisa and Miyashita (1983a) indicated velocity specific power gains after 6 weeks of training at either 73 degrees per second or 157 degrees per second.

Another study trained groups at 60 degrees per second and 240 degrees per second three times per week for 6 weeks (Jenkins, Thackaberry, and Killian 1984). Peak torque test results demonstrated that the 60-degrees-per-second group improved at all but the slowest and fastest velocities, whereas the 240-degree-per-second group improved significantly at all test velocities (see figure 2.5). No significant differences between improvement of the two training groups were shown. However, because of the nonsignificant improvement at the 30-degrees-per-second and 300-degrees-per-second test velocities by the 60-degrees-per-second group, it could be concluded that the 240-degrees-per-second training resulted in superior overall strength gains.

Another study examined three groups that trained at different velocities and with varying numbers of sets and repetitions (Coyle et al. 1981). A slow-speed group trained at 60 degrees per second with five sets of six maximal muscular

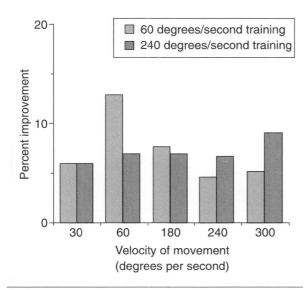

Figure 2.5 Percentage change in peak torque with training at 60 degrees per second and 240 degrees per second.

Adapted from W.L. Jenkins, M. Thackaberry, and C. Killian, "Speed-specific isokinetic training," *Journal of Orthopaedic and Sports Physical Therapy* 1984; 6: 182, with permission of the Orthopaedic and Sports Sections of the American Physical Therapy Association.

Table 2.8 Percent Increases in Peak Torque Due to Isokinetic Training at Specific Velocities			
Testing velocity	**Peak torque increases (in percentages)**		
PT/0	[Fast 23.6	Slow 20.3	Mixed] 18.9
PT/60	[Slow 31.8	Mixed 23.6	Fast] 15.1
PT/180	[Fast 16.8	Slow 9.2	Mixed] 7.9
PT/300	[Fast 18.5	Mixed] 16.1	Slow 0.9

PT/0-PT/300 = Peak torque at 0 to 300 degrees per second; Bracketed groups exhibit no statistically significant difference in peak torque.

Data from E.F. Coyle et al., 1981.

actions. A fast-speed group trained at 300 degrees per seconds with five sets of 12 maximal actions. A third group trained using a combination of slow and fast speeds, with two or three sets of 6 repetitions at 60 degrees per second and two or three sets of 12 repetitions at 300 degrees per second. Peak torque test results are presented in table 2.8. Each group showed its greatest gains at its specific training velocity, indicating that the velocity of training is in part dictated by the velocity at which peak torque increases are desired. However, substantial carryover to other velocities is also shown. This is especially apparent for velocities slower than the training velocity.

Some research suggests that there is little or no reason to favor a particular velocity when considering gains in strength. Training at 60 degrees per second or 180 degrees per second results in equal gains in peak torque at 60 degrees per second, 120 degrees per second, 180 degrees per second, and 240 degrees per second (Bell et al. 1989, Lacerte et al. 1992). Training at 60 degrees per second or 240 degrees per second results in equal isometric strength gains (Mannion, Jakeman, and Willan 1992). All of these projects used a short training duration of no more than 16 weeks, making conclusions concerning long-term training difficult.

Collectively, the studies indicate that if gains in strength over a wide range of velocities are desired, training should be at a velocity of some-

where between 180 degrees per second and 240 degrees per second. Additionally, if the training goal is to maximally increase strength at a specific velocity, training should be performed at that velocity. However, because the majority of the studies used relatively slow training velocities in general, any comparisons between slow and fast speeds is in reality a comparison of two or more relatively slow velocities. During many physical activities, angular limb velocities of greater than 300 degrees per second are easily achieved, making the application of conclusions to actual physical tasks tenuous.

Velocity Specificity and Strength Carryover

Closely associated with the concept of velocity specificity is the question, To what extent do increases in strength carry over to velocities other than the training velocity? The previously discussed Moffroid and Whipple study (1970) comparing training at 36 degrees per second and 108 degrees per second demonstrated that significant increases in peak torque carry over only at speeds of movement below the training velocity (see figure 2.4). A group trained at 90 degrees per second demonstrated significant increases in peak torque at 90 degrees per second and 30 degrees per second, but no significant increase in peak torque at 270 degrees per second (Seger, Arvidsson, and Thorstensson 1998). It is interesting to note that this same pattern of strength increases was noted when strength was tested eccentrically at 30 degrees per second and 270 degrees per second. The study illustrated in figure 2.5 indicates velocity specificity for slow (60 degrees per second) training and carryover below and above the training velocity, with less carryover as the velocity moves farther from the training velocity, while training at an intermediate velocity (240 degrees per second) results in carryover both below and above the training velocity. Another study testing strength gains at 60 degrees per second to 240 degrees per second (Ewing et al. 1990) suggests that there is carryover of peak torque gains at velocities above and below the training velocity. The carryover may be as great as 210 degrees per second below the training velocity and up to 180 degrees per second above the training velocity. Studies using training velocities of 60 degrees per second, 120 degrees per second, and 180 degrees per second indicate that significant gains in peak torque are made at all velocities from isometric to 240 degrees per second, but not necessarily at 300 degrees per second (Akima et al. 1999; Bell et al. 1989; Lacerte et al. 1992).

Collectively these studies indicate that significant gains in peak torque may occur above and below the training velocity except when the training velocity is very slow (30 degrees per second) and that generally the greatest gains in strength are made at the training velocity. These studies all determined peak torque irrespective of the joint angle at which peak torque occurred. It might be questioned whether the torque actually increased at a specific joint angle and therefore a specific muscle length, an indication that the mechanisms controlling muscle tension at that length have been altered.

Peak torque of the knee extensors irrespective of joint angle at velocities from 30 degrees per second to 300 degrees per second is slightly higher than joint-angle-specific torque at a knee angle 30 degrees from full extension (Yates and Kamon 1983). When subjects are grouped according to whether they have more or less than 50% type II muscle fibers, the two groups show no significant difference in the torque velocity curves for peak torque. For angle-specific torque, however, the torque velocity curves are significantly different between the two groups (Yates and Kamon 1983). This suggests that torque at a specific angle is influenced to a greater extent than peak torque by muscle fiber-type composition. Thus, comparisons of peak torque and angle-specific torque must be viewed with caution.

A study that determined torque at a specific joint angle trained groups at 96 degrees per second and 239 degrees per second (Caiozzo, Perrine, and Edgerton 1981). Figure 2.6 depicts the percentage improvement that occurred at the testing velocities. The results indicate that when the test criterion is angle-specific torque, training at a slow velocity (96 degrees per second) causes significant increases in torque at faster velocities as well as at slower velocities, whereas training at a faster velocity (239 degrees per second) results in significant increases only at slower velocities close to the training velocity.

The results of research concerning velocity specificity and carryover using peak torque and angle-specific torque as criterion measures are not necessarily contradictory (see figures 2.4, 2.5, and 2.6). All studies demonstrate that fast-velocity training (108 degrees per second up to 240 degrees per second) results in significant increases in torque below the training velocity and in some cases above the training velocity. Differences in the magnitude (significant or insignificant) of carryover to other velocities may in part be attributed to the velocities that were defined as fast (108 degrees per second up to 240 degrees per second). All studies also indicate that slow-velocity training (36 degrees per second up to 96 degrees per second) cause significant carryover in torque below and above the training velocity. Generally, whether fast- or slow-velocity training is performed, carryover at velocities substantially faster than the training velocity are the least evident.

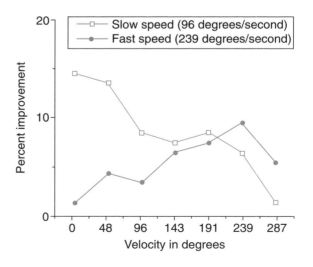

Figure 2.6 Percent changes in peak torque at a specific joint angle due to slow- and fast-speed, concentric-only isokinetic training.

Data from V.J. Caiozzo et al., 1988.

A previously cited study (Kanehisa and Miyashita 1983b) demonstrated that an intermediate training velocity (179 degrees per second) caused the greatest carryover of average power to a wider range of velocities both above and below the training velocity than at a slow (60 degrees per second) or fast (300 degrees per second) training velocity. The studies examining changes in peak torque previously discussed indicate that training velocities in the range of 180 degrees per second to 240 degrees per second result in carryover to velocities above and below the training velocity, but that the amount of carryover may decrease as the difference between the training and test velocity increases. The results of these studies indirectly support the contention that an intermediate training velocity offers the best possible carryover to velocities other than the training velocity.

Body Composition

Concentric-only isokinetic training has been reported to significantly increase mean muscle fiber area (Coyle et al. 1981; Ewing et al. 1990) and total muscle cross-sectional area (Bell et al. 1992; Housh et al. 1992; Narici et al. 1989). However, other studies demonstrate nonsignificant changes in muscle fiber area (Akima et al. 1999; Colliander and Tesch 1990a; Costill et al. 1979; Cote et al. 1988; Seger, Arvidsson, and Thorstensson 1998) and total muscle cross-sectional area (Akima et al. 1999; Seger, Arvidsson, and Thorstensson 1998). Increases of cross-sectional area in one muscle group (quadriceps) and not another (hamstrings) have also been reported after the same concentric-only isokinetic training program (Petersen et al. 1990). Thus, concentric-only isokinetic training can result in increased muscle fiber and muscle cross-sectional areas and increased fat-free mass. However, these increases are not necessarily an outcome of all isokinetic training programs.

Changes in body composition as a result of concentric-only isokinetic training are included in table 3.3 on page 92. These changes include increases in fat-free mass and decreases in percent fat and are of the same approximate magnitude as those induced by other types of training.

Motor Performance

Improved motor performance, specifically significant increases in vertical jump ability (Augustsson et al. 1998; Blattner and Noble 1979; Oteghen 1975; Smith and Melton 1981), standing broad jump ability (Smith and Melton 1981), and 40-yd (36.6-m) sprint ability (Smith and Melton 1981) have been shown after concentric-only isokinetic training. Ball velocity of a tennis serve has also improved with concentric-only isokinetic training (Ellenbecker, Davies, and Rowinski 1988). Power output during 6-second and 30-second maximal sprint cycling is also improved with isokinetic training (Bell et al. 1989; Mannion, Jakeman, and Willan 1992). Thus, concentric-only isokinetic training can improve motor performance.

Motor performance may be increased by fast-speed training more than by slow-speed training (Smith and Melton 1981). Training in this study consisted of one set to 50% fatigue in peak torque at each velocity of 180 degrees per second, 240 degrees per second, and 300 degrees per second for the fast-speed group and one set to 50% fatigue peak torque at each velocity of 30 degrees per second, 60 degrees per second, and 90 degrees per second for the slow-speed group. Each group trained three times weekly for 6 weeks. The fast-speed and slow-speed groups improved respectively, 5.4% and 3.9% in a vertical jump test, 9.1% and 0.4% in the standing long jump, and –10.1% and +4.1% in the 40-yd (36.6-m) sprint. However, increases in sprint cycling power output were shown not to be significantly different when isokinetic training was performed at 60 degrees per second, 180 degrees per second, or 240 degrees per second (Bell et al. 1989; Mannion, Jakeman, and Willan 1992). Thus, fast-speed isokinetic training may be more effective than slow-speed training for increasing some, but not all, motor performance tasks.

Other Considerations

There are other factors to consider with concentric-only isokinetic training. Training isokinetically has been reported to cause minimal muscular soreness (Atha 1981). Because neither a free weight nor a weight stack has to be lifted in this type of training, the possibility of injury is minimal, and no spotter is normally required.

It is difficult to judge an individual's effort unless the machine has an accurate feedback system of either force generated or work performed that is visible to the lifter while exercising. Furthermore, motivation may be a problem with some trainees because isokinetic equipment lacks visible movement of a weight or weight stack. Some equipment does have a monitor that displays such information as force for each repetition, but at present this type of equipment is not widely available in weight rooms or health clubs.

Eccentric Training

Eccentric training (also called negative resistance training) refers to a muscular action in which the muscle lengthens in a controlled manner. This type of muscle action occurs in many daily activities, such as walking. Walking down a flight of stairs requires the thigh muscles to perform eccentric muscle actions. During normal DCER training, when the weight is being lifted, the muscle shortens or performs a concentric action. When the weight is lowered, the same muscles that lifted the weight are active and lengthen in a controlled manner, or perform an eccentric action. If the muscles did not perform an eccentric action when the weight was lowered, the weight would fall due to the force of gravity.

Eccentric training can be achieved on many resistance training machines by lifting resistances greater than the 1RM of one arm or leg with both limbs and then lowering the resistance with only one limb. On some weight training machines it is also possible to perform the eccentric portion of repetitions with a resistance greater than that used in the concentric phase of repetitions. This type of training is termed accentuated eccentric training. Some isokinetic machines also have an eccentric mode. Resistances heavier than 1RM may also be achieved with free weights by having spotters add more weight after the weight is lifted, having spotters apply resistance during the eccentric phase of a repetition (forced negatives), or by having spotters help with the lifting of a heavier than 1RM resistance and then having the lifter perform the eccentric portion of the repetition without assistance. Weight release hooks are also available to achieve a heavier resistance than 1RM with free weights (Doan et al. 2002).

Whenever eccentric training is performed, proper safety precautions should always be used, especially when using free weights or nonisokinetic machines, because a lifter can attempt to use more weight than can be safely controlled during the eccentric portion of a repetition. Safety can be enhanced when performing eccentric training with some free weight exercises, such as the bench and squat, by setting the pins of a power rack so that they will catch the weight if needed at the lowest position of the exercise.

Strength Changes

Normal DCER training of the legs with both a concentric and an eccentric action causes greater concentric and eccentric strength increases than performing concentric-only resistance training for the same number of repetitions (Dudley et al. 1991). Performing 50% or 75% of the repetitions with an eccentric phase over 12 weeks of training results in greater increases in squat, but not bench press, ability than performing the same training program in a concentric-only manner (Häkkinen, Komi, and Tesch 1981). These results indicate that an eccentric component during DCER training appears to be important, especially for the leg musculature.

Eccentric-only DCER training has been shown to increase maximal strength. Maximal eccentric 1RM significantly increased (29%) after 8 weeks of training with three to five sets of 6 repetitions at 80% of the eccentric 1RM (Housh et al. 1996, 1998). Training in an eccentric-only manner with three sets of 120 to 180% of maximal isometric strength varied in a classic periodization style for 3 weeks significantly increased maximal isometric strength (Colduck and Abernathy 1997). Eccentric-only DCER training for 4 weeks with six sets of 5 repetitions at 100% of 1RM significantly increased isometric and isokinetic strength at all velocities tested ranging from 60 degrees per second to 360 degrees per second (Martin, Martin, and Morlon 1995).

Comparisons of DCER concentric-only and eccentric-only training indicated little difference between training modes. Two sets of 10 repetitions performed in a concentric-only manner at 80% of the normal 1RM or two sets of 6 repetitions performed in an eccentric-only fashion at 120% of the normal 1RM showed no difference in isometric or concentric-only 1RM increases (Johnson et al. 1976). Concentric-only and eccentric-only training for 20 weeks with four sets of 10 repetitions, at a contraction mode specific 10RM, demonstrated little advantage with either type of training (Smith and Rutherford 1995). No significant difference between groups was demonstrated for isometric strength at 10-degree intervals of knee extension; however, the concentric-only group did show significant increases in strength at a greater number of angles. Likewise, no significant differences between groups was demonstrated for concentric isokinetic strength at velocities of movement ranging from 30 degrees per second to 300 degrees per second; however, the eccentric-only group demonstrated significant increases in strength at a greater number of velocities. It is important to note that in neither of the previously mentioned studies was eccentric maximal strength tested. However, the results indicate that DCER eccentric-only training does significantly increase isometric and concentric strength.

Comparisons of concentric-only and eccentric-only isokinetic training demonstrate conflicting results. Training at 60 degrees per second for 12 weeks showed eccentric-only training to significantly increase isokinetic (60 degrees per second) eccentric strength to a greater extent than concentric-only training, with isometric and concentric isokinetic strength showing no significant difference between training modes (Hortobagyi et al. 1996). Training for 18 weeks at 60 degrees per second showed no significant difference in isokinetic (60 degrees per second) concentric or eccentric strength gains (Hawkins et al. 1999). Concentric-only training for 10 weeks at 90 degrees per second demonstrated a greater number of significant increases in concentric and eccentric isokinetic strength at velocities of 30 degrees per second, 90 degrees per second, and 270 degrees per second than eccentric-only training (Seger, Arvidsson, and Thorstensson 1998).

The aforementioned studies indicate that eccentric muscle actions are needed to optimally increase total muscle strength, especially when strength is measured in an eccentric manner. However, the majority of evidence indicates that eccentric-only training results in no greater gains in isometric, eccentric, and concentric strength than normal DCER training (Atha 1981; Clarke 1973; Fleck and Schutt 1985). It is now possible on some machines to perform **accentuated eccentric training**, which means using greater resistances in the eccentric phase of a repetition than is used during the concentric phase of a repetition. One practical question from a training perspective is, Does accentuated eccentric training result in greater strength gains than normal DCER training?

Unfortunately, only a few studies have compared accentuated eccentric training to a normal weight training protocol. Accentuated eccentric DCER training has been shown to have an acute effect on strength in moderately trained males (Doan et al. 2002). When accentuated eccentric DCER repetitions are performed with 105% of the normal 1RM immediately before 1RM bench press attempts, 1RM significantly increases on average from 214 lb (97.44 kg) to 221 lb (100.57 kg). Accentuated eccentric DCER training has been shown to increase strength to a greater extent than normal DCER training over 7 consecutive

days of training (Hortobagyi et al. 2001). Normal training consisted of five to six sets of 10 to 12 repetitions at approximately 60% of 1RM. Accentuated eccentric training used the same numbers of repetitions and sets; however, during the eccentric portion of each repetition the resistance was increased 40 to 50%. Concentric 3RM and isokinetic (90 degrees per second) concentric strength gains were not significantly different between the two types of training. However, accentuated eccentric training resulted in significantly greater gains in eccentric 3RM (27% vs. 11%), isokinetic (90 degrees per second), eccentric, and isometric strength than the normal training. Changes in electromyography (EMG) parameters paralleled the increases in strength, indicating that the majority of strength gains were related to neural adaptations as would be expected over such a short training period.

Accentuated eccentric isokinetic training for a moderately long time period of 10 weeks demonstrated gains in concentric-only isokinetic (30 degrees per second) strength to be not significantly different from isokinetic training with both a concentric and an eccentric repetition phase (Godard et al. 1998). Training for both groups consisted of one set of 8 to 12 repetitions at 30 degrees per second. Resistance for the isokinetic training with both a concentric and an eccentric repetition phase was initially set at 80% of maximal concentric isokinetic torque. The accentuated eccentric isokinetic training followed the same training protocol except that during the eccentric phase of each repetition, resistance was increased 40%. Unfortunately, no other strength measures were determined in this study. Nine weeks of training with eccentric accentuated DCER in moderately trained males demonstrated greater increases in concentric bilateral 1RM elbow extension, but not elbow flexion (preacher curl) than traditional DCER training (Brandonburg and Docherty 2002). In this study the DCER training consisted of four sets of 10 repetitions to concentric failure using approximately 75% of the concentric 1RM, whereas the accentuated eccentric DCER training consisted of three sets of 10 repetitions using the same resistance as the DCER for the concentric phase of repetitions, but 110 to 120% of the concentric 1RM for the eccentric phase of repetitions. This minimal information indicates that accentuated eccentric training with trained or moderately trained individuals does result in significant strength gains, especially when strength is determined in an eccentric manner, and may result in greater strength gains than normal resistance training. However, not all muscle groups may respond equally to accentuated eccentric DCER training.

Optimal Eccentric Training

Increases in strength have been reported after eccentric-only DCER training using the following:

- 120-180% of maximal isometric strength (Colduck and Abernathy 1997)
- 80% of the eccentric 1RM (Housh et al., 1996, 1998)
- 100% of normal 1RM (Martin, Martin, and Morlon 1995)
- 120% of normal 1RM (Johnson et al. 1976)
- 100% of 10RM (Smith and Rutherford 1995)

Increases in strength have also been shown using maximal isokinetic eccentric-only muscle actions (Hawkins et al. 1999; Hortobagyi et al. 1996; Seger, Arvidsson, and Thorstensson 1998). Accentuated eccentric DCER training using 40-50% more resistance than in the concentric phase of repetitions (Hortobagyi et al. 2001) and accentuated eccentric isokinetic training using 40% more resistance than in the concentric phase of repetitions (Godard et al. 1998) have also shown significant increases in strength. None of these studies, however, addressed what constitutes the optimal eccentric resistance to be used in eccentric training. Jones (1973) indicated the optimal resistance to be one that the trainee can lower slowly and stop at will. Using this definition, Johnson and colleagues (1976) claimed that a resistance of 120% of the DCER 1RM is the optimal eccentric resistance. Previous studies have shown significant strength increases using greater than and less than 120% of the DCER 1RM. For example, eccentric strength depending on velocity of movement is greater than or at least equal to maximal isometric strength and up to 180% of maximal isometric strength (Colduck and Abernathy 1997) has been used in eccentric-only DCER training. This may, however, be near the maximal resistance possible in eccentric training. If tension is applied rapidly or gradually to tetanized frog muscle, complete mechanical relaxation occurs at approximately 180% and 210%, respectively, of maximal voluntary contraction (Katz 1939).

Another practical question concerning eccentric training is, How many repetitions need to be performed in a heavy eccentric or accentuated eccentric manner? One study (see the section on negative system training in chapter 6) indicates that as few as 25% of the total number of DCER repetitions need to be performed in an accentuated eccentric manner to bring about greater strength increases than normal DCER training (Häkkinen and Komi 1981). It is important to note that this project was performed on highly trained competitive Olympic weightlifters. Thus, results are applicable to highly trained athletes.

Motor Performance and Body Composition

Eccentric training and accentuated eccentric training can increase strength across a number of contraction types (i.e., isometric, isokinetic). Thus, these types of training may increase motor performance ability. However, vertical jump ability has been shown to both increase (Bonde-Peterson and Knuttgen 1971) and remain unchanged (Stone, Johnson, and Carter 1979) with eccentric-only training. Tennis serve velocity has shown no change as a result of 6 weeks of shoulder and arm musculature isokinetic eccentric training (Ellenbecker, Davies, and Rowinski 1988) and has shown a significant increase with isokinetic eccentric training for 6 weeks, but the increase was not significantly different from isokinetic-concentric training (Mont et al. 1994). Thus, the potential impact of eccentric training on motor performance is unclear.

Net muscle protein synthesis is a balance of protein synthesis and protein breakdown. Both eccentric-only and concentric-only muscle actions have been shown to increase muscle protein synthesis and increase muscle protein breakdown, resulting in an increase in net muscle protein synthesis in untrained subjects with no difference by muscle action type (Phillips et al. 1997). Net protein synthesis rate has also been shown to significantly increase in both untrained and weight-trained individuals due to an eccentric exercise bout of eight sets of 10 repetitions at 120% of DCER 1RM (Phillips et al. 1999). These results indicate that eccentric training can increase fat-free mass over time.

Increases in limb circumference and muscle cross-sectional area are usually associated with muscular hypertrophy. Upper-arm circumference showed significant increases with eccentric-only training, but the increase did not differ significantly from the increase caused by concentric-only training (Komi and Buskirk 1972). Similarly, thigh circumference significantly increases with isokinetic training with both concentric and eccentric phases in a repetition, and with accentuated isokinetic eccentric training, but the increases are not significantly different (Godard et al. 1998). Eccentric-only DCER for 8 weeks has shown no significant change in muscle cross-sectional area (Housh et al. 1998), whereas isokinetic eccentric-only training has been shown to significantly increase muscle cross-sectional area, with concentric-only training showing no significant change in muscle cross-sectional area (Hawkins et al. 1999; Seger, Arvidsson, and Thorstensson 1998) and a significant increase in cross-sectional area, with the increase not being significantly different from concentric-only training (Jones and Rutherford 1987). Type I and type II muscle fiber cross-sectional area has shown no significant change after isokinetic eccentric-only training (Seger, Arvidsson, and Thorstensson 1998); and no significant change in type I, but a significant increase in type II cross-sectional area (Hortobagyi et al. 1996). Collectively, this information indicates that eccentric training can increase fat-free mass, but that the increase may not be different from that resulting from other types of muscle actions or training.

Postexercise Soreness

A possible disadvantage of eccentric training with greater than 1RM concentric strength or maximal eccentric actions is the development of greater postexercise soreness, also termed delayed-onset muscular soreness (DOMS), than that which accompanies isometric, DCER, or concentric-only isokinetic training (Fleck and Schutt 1985; Hamlin and Quigley 2001; Kellis and Baltzopoulos 1995). DOMS generally begins approximately 8 hours after exercise and peaks 2 to 3 days after the eccentric exercise bout and lasts 8 to 10 days (Clarkson, Nosaka, and Braun 1992; Hamlin and Quigley 2001; Kellis and Baltzopoulos 1995; Leiger and Milner 2001). Likewise, strength is decreased for up to 10 days after an eccentric exercise bout (Clarkson, Nosaka, and Braun 1992; Leiger and Milner 2001). However, one bout of eccentric exercise appears to result in protection from excessive soreness due to a successive eccentric exercise session for a period of up to 6 weeks in untrained or novice weight training individuals (Ebbling and Clarkson 1990; Clarkson, Nosaka, and Braun 1992; Golden and Dudley 1992; Hyatt and Clarkson 1998; Nosaka et

al. 1991). Protection from excessive soreness may occur as early as 13 days after the first eccentric bout (Mair et al. 1995) and appears to occur even with low-volume eccentric exercise bouts (one set of six maximal eccentric actions for two sessions) (Paddon-Jones and Abernathy 2001).

Some information indicates that for excessive soreness to develop, the eccentric actions must be performed with a resistance greater than the concentric 1RM (Donnelly, Clarkson, and Maughan 1992), which can be accomplished with maximal eccentric actions because more force can be developed during an eccentric action than during a concentric action. However, other data indicate little difference in the muscle damage immediately after exercise between maximal eccentric actions and eccentric actions performed with 50% of maximal isometric force (Nosaka and Newton 2002). However, markers (i.e., creatine kinase, force recovery) of muscle damage indicated that maximal eccentric actions resulted in greater muscle damage 2 to 3 days postexercise than the eccentric actions performed with 50% maximal isometric force. The performance of some eccentric actions before complete recovery from an eccentric exercise bout does not aid or hinder recovery from the initial eccentric exercise bout (Donnelly, Clarkson, and Maughan 1992; Nosaka and Clarkson 1995).

Although light concentric exercise for several days after an eccentric work bout may reduce muscle soreness slightly, it does not affect strength recovery (Saxton and Donnelly 1995). Stretching immediately before and immediately after an eccentric exercise bout does not affect muscle soreness or strength recovery (Lund et al. 1998). After 1 to 2 weeks of eccentric training, the soreness appears to be no greater than that which follows isometric training (Komi and Buskirk 1972) or DCER training (Colduck and Abernathy 1997).

Some individuals seem to be prone to excessive muscle soreness and muscle fiber necrosis due to eccentric muscle actions. As many as 21% of individuals exposed to an intense eccentric exercise bout (50 maximal eccentric actions) may not completely recover for 26 days, with some individuals requiring 89 days for complete recovery (Sayers and Clarkson 2001). Three percent of individuals may suffer from rhabdomyolysis after a strenuous eccentric exercise bout (Sayers, Clarkson et al. 1999). Rhabdomyolysis is degeneration of muscle cells resulting in myalgia, muscle tenderness, weakness, swelling, and myoglobinuria (dark-color urine). This condition results in a loss of the muscles' ability to generate force and may last as long as 6 to 7 weeks.

Why more soreness occurs after eccentric training than after normal DCER or concentric-only training is unclear. Electromyographic (EMG) activity can be less during an eccentric action than during a concentric action (Komi, Kaneko, and Aura 1987; Komi et al. 2000; Tesch et al. 1990). This indicates that fewer muscle fibers are active to develop force during an eccentric action than during a concentric action and that the force is distributed over fewer muscle fibers than during a concentric action. This could lead to muscle fiber damage. Evidence also shows that muscles performing eccentric actions rely more on type II muscle fibers than muscles performing concentric actions (Howell et al. 1995; McHugh et al. 2002; Nardone, Romano, and Schieppati 1989). Since type II muscle fibers are more susceptible to injury than type I muscle fibers during eccentric actions (Friden, Sjostrom, and Ekblom 1983), more reliance on type II muscle fibers could result in greater fiber necrosis and soreness.

A series of events within muscle fibers results in an attractive explanation of the soreness and strength loss after eccentric exercise. The eccentric exercise results in dilation of the sarcoplasmic reticulum, accompanied by slowing of calcium uptake (Byrd 1992; Hamlin and Quigley 2001). These changes are transient, lasting only about an hour, but they are related to decreased muscle fiber recruitment. This could account in part for the loss of strength immediately after an eccentric work bout and the increased EMG activity required to produce force as an eccentric work bout progresses. Extensive free calcium within muscle fibers may cause ever increasing damage to the sarcolemma. Sarcolemmal damage allows the influx of more calcium into muscle fibers. Calcium activates proteolytic enzymes, which degrade structures within muscle fibers (Z-disks, troponin, tropomyosin) and muscle fiber proteins by lysomal protease, increasing damage, edema, inflammation, and muscle soreness. Thus, muscle damage in itself may not be the cause of postexercise pain. Factors such as edema, swelling, and inflammation are more attractive explanations of the pain experienced several days after exercise (Clarkson, Nosaka, and Braun 1992; Stauber et al. 1990).

Repeated bouts of eccentric exercise may reduce sarcolemmal damage and hence the cascade of events resulting in muscle soreness. There are, however, other possible explanations of adaptations that reduce muscle damage and soreness due to repeated exercise bouts. Evidence indicates that repeated eccentric work bouts result in increased activation of type I muscle fibers and a concomitant decreased activation of type II fibers (Warren et al. 2000). Brockett, Morgan, and Proske (2001) also proposed that eccentric training results in a sustained increase in the length of muscle through the addition of sarcomeres, which protect the muscle from microdamage because they allow the muscle fibers to generally function at longer lengths, thus avoiding the descending limb of the length-tension diagram. The descending portion is the region of the length-tension diagram where damage to sarcomeres may be most likely to occur. Although the exact explanation of the adaptations that protect muscle from soreness after repeated exercise bouts is unclear, it is clear that some adaptation(s) do occur to protect muscle from soreness in successive exercise bouts.

Motivational Considerations

Some individuals derive great satisfaction from training with heavy resistances. Eccentric training for these individuals will be a positive motivational factor. However, the soreness that can accompany eccentric training, especially during the first week or two, can be a detriment to motivation.

Other Considerations

Because excessive soreness may accompany eccentric exercise, a program involving eccentric exercise should not be initiated immediately before a major competition. The soreness and loss of strength when beginning eccentric training will decrease physical performance. This may be especially true in rapid force development or power-type activities. In one study, one-legged vertical jump height significantly decreased after an eccentric exercise bout and remained decreased for 3 to 4 days (Mair et al. 1995). A successive eccentric exercise bout 4 days after the initial bout resulted in the same decrease in vertical jump height immediately after the eccentric bout as that experienced after the initial eccentric bout. Although jump height recovered more quickly after the second eccentric bout, it did not reach baseline values until 3 to 4 days after the eccentric exercise bout. However, 13 days after the initial eccentric bout a successive eccentric bout resulted in no significant decrease in vertical jump height. These results indicate that caution must be used concerning the time frame in which eccentric training is initiated before a competition or a point in time when optimal physical performance is desired.

The incorporation of eccentric training is appropriate when a goal of the training program is to increase 1RM and bench press and squat ability. One factor that separates great from good power lifters in the bench press and squat is the speed at which they perform the eccentric portion of the lift. Lifters who can lift heavier weights lower the resistance more slowly (Madsen and McLaughlin 1984; McLaughlin, Dillman, and Lardner 1977). This suggests that eccentric training may facilitate both the slowness of lowering the resistance and proper form while the resistance is being lowered.

Comparison of Training Types

Studies comparing the various types of resistance training are rare, and there are several difficulties in identifying the most beneficial type of training for a specific physiological adaptation. One issue is specificity of training and strength gains. When training and testing are performed using the same type of resistant equipment, a large increase in strength normally is demonstrated. If training and testing are performed on two different types of equipment, however, the increase in strength normally is substantially less and sometimes nonexistent. Ideally, strength should be tested using several types of muscular actions. This allows examination of training specificity as well as carry over to other types of muscular actions.

Problems in comparison also arise in equating total training volume (i.e., sets and repetitions), total work (i.e., total repetitions × resistance × distance the weight is moved), and duration of a training session. These discrepancies make it difficult to compare fairly and so prove the superiority of one resistance training type over another. Other study-design difficulties that hinder the generalization of results to different populations include the training status of the subjects, the fact that some studies train only one muscle group, and the length of the study. Many studies use untrained subjects, making generalization to highly trained individuals and to long-term training difficult. Application of results from training one muscle group or exercise to another muscle group or exercise can be difficult as muscle groups may not respond with the same magnitude or with the same time line of adapta-

tions. The typical length of many studies is 10 to 20 weeks, which makes the application of results to long-term training (i.e., years) tenuous.

Several of these difficulties are illustrated in one study (Leighton et al. 1967). Subjects trained twice a week for 8 weeks using several isometric and dynamic constant external resistance training (DCER) regimes (see table 6.1, page 190). Two particular regimes were an isometric program consisting of one 6-second maximal voluntary muscle action and a DCER program (Delorme system) using three sets of 10 repetitions progressing in resistance from 50% to 75% and finally to 100% of 10RM resistance. The isometric and DCER regimes resulted in a 0% and 9% increase in isometric elbow flexion, respectively, and a 35% and 16% increase in isometric elbow extension, respectively. Thus, depending on the muscle group tested, isometric and DCER training are both superior to the other training type for isometric strength gains. This same study also showed that a DCER cheat regime demonstrated a greater percentage of isometric strength gains in elbow flexion, elbow extension, and back and leg strength in a dead lift type movement than the isometric regime and the DCER regime. The overall results are therefore ambiguous: Isometric training is both inferior and superior to DCER training depending on the muscle group compared and the type of DCER regime. This study demonstrates that the result of comparing two types of training may vary by muscle group and by the training programs compared.

Perhaps the most important factor when comparing training types is the efficacy of the training programs. Is each training type program optimal in bringing about physiological adaptations? If the answer to this question is no, any conclusions based on the studies' results must be viewed with caution. Despite the interpretation difficulties, however, some conclusions concerning comparisons of training types can be made.

Isometric Versus Dynamic Constant External Resistance Training

Many comparisons of strength gains between isometric training and DCER training follow a pattern of test specificity. When isometric testing procedures are used, isometric training is superior (Amusa and Obajuluwa 1986; Berger 1962a, 1963b; Moffroid et al. 1969), and when DCER testing (1RM) is used, DCER training is superior (Berger 1962a, 1963c). However, it has also been shown that DCER training results in greater increases in isometric force than does isometric training (Rasch and Morehouse 1957). Isokinetic testing for increases in strength are inconclusive. When isokinetically tested at 20.5 degrees per second, both isometric and DCER training improved peak torque 3% (Moffroid et al. 1969). A second study demonstrated a 13% increase in peak torque for isometric training and a 28% increase for DCER training (the velocity of isokinetic testing was not reported) (Thistle et al. 1967). A review of the literature concludes that well-designed DCER programs are more effective than standard isometric programs for increasing strength (Atha 1981). Isometric training at one joint angle does not increase dynamic motor performance (Clarke 1973; Fleck and Schutt 1985), whereas DCER training can increase dynamic motor performance. It is not surprising, then, that motor performance is improved to a greater extent by DCER training than by isometric training at only one joint angle (Brown et al. 1988; Campbell 1962; Chu 1950). Thus, if an increase in motor performance is desired, DCER training would be a better choice than isometric training at one joint angle.

Isometric Versus Variable Resistance Training

The authors are aware of no studies that directly compare isometric and variable resistance training. However, it can be hypothesized that strength gains may follow a specificity of testing pattern similar to comparisons of isometric and DCER. It can also be hypothesized that because no improvement in motor performance has been reported from isometric training at one joint angle (Clarke 1973; Fleck and Schutt 1985), and because improvement in motor performance has been shown with variable resistance training (Peterson 1975; Silvester et al. 1984), variable resistance training may be superior to isometric training in this parameter. Thus, if an increase in motor performance is desired, variable resistance training would be a better choice than isometric training at one joint angle.

Isometric Versus Concentric Isokinetic Resistance Training

Comparisons of isometric and concentric isokinetic training for the most part follow a pattern of test specificity. However, direct comparisons

have used only relatively slow velocity isokinetic training (up to 30 degrees per second). Isometric is superior to isokinetic training at 22.5 degrees per second for increasing isometric strength (Moffroid et al. 1969). Isometric force of the knee extensors at knee angles of 90 degrees and 45 degrees increased 17% and 14%, respectively, with isometric training and 14% and 24%, respectively, with isokinetic training. Similarly, knee-flexor isometric strength at knee angles of 90 degrees and 45 degrees increased 26% and 24%, respectively, with isometric training and 11% and 19%, respectively, with isokinetic training. The isometrically trained group demonstrated superior isometric force improvements over the isokinetically trained group in three of these four tests. However, isokinetic training of the elbow extensors at 30 degrees per second resulted in greater increases in isometric force than isometric training (Knapik, Mawdsley, and Ramos 1983).

Isokinetic training is superior to isometric training in the development of isokinetic torque (Moffroid et al. 1969; Thistle et al. 1967). For example, knee-extensor strength for isokinetically and isometrically trained groups increased 47% and 13%, respectively (Thistle et al. 1967). Another study reported that isokinetically and isometrically trained groups increased 11% and 3%, respectively, in knee-extension peak torque at 22.5 degrees per second. For knee flexion the increases in peak torque were 15% and 3%, respectively, at 22.5 degrees per second (Moffroid et al. 1969). Thus, the phenomenon of test specificity is evident in the strength increases from both isometric and isokinetic training.

Training isometrically at one joint angle results in no improvement in motor performance (Clarke 1973; Fleck and Schutt 1985), whereas improvements in motor performance have been achieved with isokinetic training (Bell et al. 1989; Blattner and Noble 1979; Mannion, Jakeman, and Willan 1992). Thus, it can be hypothesized that isokinetic training is superior to isometric training for improving motor performance.

Isometric Versus Eccentric Resistance Training

The comparisons made in this section are between isometric training and eccentric training with free weights or normal resistance training machines, not isokinetic eccentric training. Measured isometrically, there is no difference in strength gains derived from isometric and eccentric training.

Bonde-Peterson (1960) trained the elbow flexors and knee extensors of both males and females for 36 training sessions in 60 days. The participants trained either only isometrically or only eccentrically. All trainees performed 10 maximal 5-second actions per day. The isometrically trained individuals experienced the following improvements in isometric strength: elbow flexion, 13.8% for males and 1% for females; knee extension, 10% for males and 8.3% for females. The eccentrically trained individuals exhibited the following improvements in isometric strength: elbow flexion, 8.5% for males and 5% for females; knee extension, 14.6% for males and 11.2% for females. Thus, there may be no significant difference between these two types of training with regard to increasing isometric strength.

Laycoe and Marteniuk (1971) reached the same conclusion after training subjects' knee extensors three times per week for 6 weeks. The isometric and eccentric groups improved 17.4% and 17%, respectively, in isometric knee-extension force. Other studies also reported no difference in strength gains between these two training methods (Atha 1981).

Reviews conclude that isometric training at one joint angle does not result in increased motor performance (Clarke 1973; Fleck and Schutt 1985), while the effect of eccentric training on motor performance is unclear, with increases (Bonde-Peterson and Knuttgen 1971) and no change (Ellenbecker, Davies, and Rowinski 1988; Stone, Johnson, and Carter 1979) in motor performance shown. Thus, the superiority of one of these training types over the other in terms of motor performance increases is unclear.

Dynamic Constant External Resistance Versus Variable Resistance Training

Comparisons of strength increases as a result of DCER and variable resistance training are equivocal. After 20 weeks of training, variable resistance training demonstrated a clear superiority over DCER training in 1RM free weight bench press ability (Ariel 1977). DCER and variable resistance training produced gains of 14% and 29.5%, respectively. In another bench press comparison after 12 weeks of training, a specificity of training phenomenon was demonstrated (Boyer 1990) with both training types showing significantly greater increases in 1RM than the other group when tested on the type of equipment on which training was performed. Further information concerning these studies is presented in table 2.2.

Leg press strength shows the phenomenon of test specificity for these two types of training. After 10 weeks of training, a variable resistance group increased 27% when tested with variable resistance equipment and 7.5% when tested with DCER methods (Pipes 1978). Conversely, a group trained with DCER improved 7.5% when tested on variable resistance equipment and 28.9% when tested with DCER methods. Three other exercises tested and trained for in the study demonstrated a similar test-specificity pattern. Likewise, after 12 weeks, DCER training significantly improved DCER and variable resistance leg press ability by 15.5% and 17.1%, respectively (Boyer 1990), whereas variable resistance training significantly improved DCER and variable resistance leg press ability by 11.2% and 28.2%, respectively. Both groups showed a significantly greater increase than the other group when tested on the type of equipment with which they trained. More information concerning these studies is presented in table 2.3.

In a 5-week program of three training sessions per week, DCER training was found to be superior to variable resistance training in producing strength gains determined by DCER testing (Stone, Johnson, and Carter 1979). No difference between the two types of training was shown when tested for variable resistance strength improvements.

After 10 weeks of training two to three times per week, variable resistance training and DCER training resulted in no significant difference in isometric knee-extension strength gains (Manning et al. 1990). Isometric force was tested throughout the range of motion starting at 9 degrees and ending at 110 degrees of full knee extension. Both types of training consisted of one set of 8 to 12 repetitions at 8 to 12RM. Another study (Silvester et al. 1984) supported the conclusion that these two training types result in the same gains in isometric strength. Collectively, this information indicates no clear superiority of either training type over the other in terms of strength gains.

Silvester and colleagues (1984) demonstrated that both DCER (free weight) and increasing lever-arm variable resistance training result in significantly greater increases in vertical jump ability than does cam-type variable resistance training. Thus, the superiority of either training type over the other may be explained in part by the type of variable resistance equipment or the training program used.

Table 3.3 (page 92) indicates that body composition changes from these two types of training are of the same magnitude. A 10-week (Pipes 1978) and a 12-week (Boyer 1990) comparative study demonstrated no significant difference between DCER and variable resistance training in changes of percent fat, fat-free mass, total body weight, and limb circumferences. Thus, body compositional changes with these two types of training are similar.

Concentric Versus Eccentric Resistance Training

Concentric and eccentric training can both be performed isokinetically or using DCER equipment. A review of comparative studies indicates that there is no significant difference in strength gains between concentric and eccentric training when the training is performed using DCER equipment (Atha 1981).

Strength gains tested with DCER elbow curls, arm presses, knee flexions, and knee extensions after 6 weeks of training three times per week are not significantly different between these two types of training (Johnson et al. 1976). Concentric training consisted of two sets of 10 repetitions at 80% of 1RM, and eccentric training consisted of two sets of 6 repetitions at 120% of 1RM. After 20 weeks of training little advantage was shown for either concentric or eccentric DCER training (Smith and Rutherford 1995). No significant difference in isometric strength or isokinetic strength gains between the two training methods was demonstrated (see the section on eccentric training for a more complete description of this study). It should be noted that maximal eccentric strength was not determined in either of the aforementioned studies.

Häkkinen and Komi (1981) compared three groups training with DCER methods for 12 weeks. All groups trained with the squat exercise. A concentric-only group performed the concentric phase of repetitions. A concentric-eccentric group performed primarily the concentric phase of repetitions with some eccentric phases of repetitions. An eccentric-concentric group trained primarily with the eccentric phase and some concentric phases of repetitions. The groups that trained with both eccentric and concentric actions made significantly greater gains in 1RM squat ability (approximately 29%) than the group that trained with concentric actions only (approximately 23%). This suggests that both eccentric and concentric

actions may be necessary to bring about maximal strength gains. This conclusion is supported by another 20-week training study in which normal DCER training was compared to concentric-only DCER training (O'Hagan et al. 1995a). However, a direct comparison of concentric-only and eccentric-only training cannot be made from these studies.

Concentric and eccentric resistance training have also been compared using isokinetic muscle actions. After 7 weeks of training, no significant difference in maximal isometric, eccentric, or concentric force was demonstrated between concentric and eccentric training (Komi and Buskirk 1972). Similarly, 18 weeks of training at 60 degrees per second showed no significant difference in isokinetic (60 degrees per second) concentric or eccentric strength gains between concentric-only or eccentric-only training (Hawkins et al. 1999). Testing specificity has also been shown when training with isokinetic concentric-only and eccentric-only actions. After 6 weeks of training at 100 degrees per second, concentric-only training increased concentric and eccentric isokinetic (100 degrees per second) torque (Tomberline et al. 1991). Eccentric-only training significantly increased eccentric, but not concentric, torque. The concentric-only training increased concentric strength significantly more than did the eccentric training. No significant difference between the two types of training in eccentric strength gains was demonstrated. Eccentric-only training (60 degrees per second) for 12 weeks demonstrated a significantly greater increase in eccentric isokinetic torque than concentric-only training, but no significant difference between training methods was demonstrated for isometric or concentric isokinetic torque (Hortobagyi et al. 1996). Conversely, concentric-only training for 10 weeks (90 degrees per second) demonstrated a greater number of significant increases in concentric and eccentric isokinetic torque at several velocities (30 degrees per second, 90 degrees per second, and 270 degrees per second) than did eccentric-only training (Serger, Arvidsson, and Thorstensson 1998). Thus, neither concentric-only nor eccentric-only isokinetic training shows a clear superiority over the other in terms of strength gains.

The effect isokinetic concentric-only and eccentric-only training of the shoulder internal and external rotators has on tennis serve velocity is also inconclusive. Six weeks of training with six sets of 10 repetitions at velocities ranging from 60 degrees per second to 210 degrees per second (velocity spectrum training) demonstrated eccentric but not concentric training to significantly increase serve velocity (Ellenbecker, Davies, and Rowinski 1988). Another comparison of 6-week training regimes of concentric-only and eccentric-only with eight sets of 10 repetitions at velocities ranging from 90 degrees per second to 180 degrees per second (velocity spectrum training) demonstrated that both eccentric and concentric training significantly increased serve velocity, but that there was no significant difference between training types (Mont et al. 1994). Neither of the studies demonstrated a clear superiority of either eccentric-only or concentric-only training in concentric or eccentric isokinetic strength gains.

As discussed in the section on eccentric training, although eccentric training does bring about increases in motor performance and changes in body composition, the changes appear not to be significantly different from those resulting from other types of muscle actions or training types. Postexercise soreness is a potential disadvantage of eccentric-only compared to concentric-only training, especially during the first several weeks of training. Thus, eccentric-only training should be incorporated slowly into a training program to minimize muscular soreness.

Dynamic Constant External Resistance Versus Isokinetic Resistance Training

Studies comparing DCER and concentric isokinetic resistance training indicate no clear superiority of either type over the other. After 8 weeks of training, the isokinetic torque of the knee extensors of an isokinetically trained group increased 47.2%, whereas that of a DCER group increased 28.6% (Thistle et al. 1967). Daily training of the knee extensors and flexors for 4 weeks demonstrated that isokinetic and isometric strength gains with isokinetic training (22.5 degrees per seconds) are superior to those with DCER training (Moffroid et al. 1969). The isokinetic and DCER groups exhibited increases of 24% and 13%, respectively, in isometric knee-extension force and 19% and 1%, respectively, in isometric knee-flexion force. Isokinetic peak torque at 22.5 degrees per seconds of the isokinetic and DCER groups increased 11% and 3%, respectively, in knee extension and 16% and 1%, respectively, in knee flexion.

In contrast to the previously mentioned studies, DCER training was demonstrated to be superior to isokinetic training in producing strength and power gains (Kovaleski et al. 1995). Both groups trained the knee extensors 3 days per week for 6 weeks with 12 sets of 10 repetitions. The isokinetic group trained using velocities of movement ranging from 120 degrees per second to 210 degrees per second in a velocity spectrum training protocol. The DCER group trained initially using 25% of peak isometric force during the first week with the resistance increased (5 Newton meters) weekly. The DCER training resulted in greater peak DCER power than the isokinetic training and greater peak isokinetic power at velocities of 120 degrees per second, 150 degrees per second, 180 degrees per second, and 210 degrees per second than the isokinetic training. DCER and isokinetic training have also shown testing specificity (Pearson and Costill 1988). After 8 weeks, DCER and isokinetic training demonstrated 32% and 4% increases, respectively, in 1RM strength tested in a DCER fashion. The isokinetic and DCER training resulted in 12% and 8% increases, respectively, in isokinetic force at 60 degrees per second and 10% and 1% increases, respectively, at 240 degrees per second, indicating testing specificity.

Lander and colleagues (1985) performed a biomechanical comparison of free weight and isokinetic bench pressing. Subjects performed a free weight bench press at 90% and 75% of their 1RM and maximal isokinetic bench presses at a velocity of movement corresponding to their individual movement velocities during their 90% and 75% free weight bench presses. No significant difference in maximal force existed between the isokinetic bench press and the 90% or the 75% of 1RM free weight bench press. This indicates that free weights may affect muscles in a manner similar to isokinetic devices, at least in the context of force production, during the major portion of an exercise movement.

Both DCER and isokinetic training can increase motor performance ability. A comparison of two-legged leg press training for 5 weeks with three training sessions per week demonstrated no significant difference in one-legged jumping ability (ground reaction force) (Cordova et al. 1995). These two training types appear to result in similar motor performance increases.

Body composition changes from DCER and isokinetic training are of the same magnitude. See table 3.3 on page 92 for information concerning comparative changes in percent fat, fat-free mass, and total body weight.

Isokinetic Versus Variable Resistance Training

Comparisons of isokinetic and variable resistance training demonstrate a test-specificity phenomenon. Smith and Melton (1981) compared slow- and fast-speed isokinetic training with variable resistance training. Slow-speed isokinetic training consisting of one set until peak torque declined to 50% at velocities of 30 degrees per second, 60 degrees per second, and 90 degrees per second. Fast-speed isokinetic training followed the same format as the slow-speed training, except that the training velocities were 180 degrees per second, 240 degrees per second, and 300 degrees per second. Variable resistance training initially consisted of three sets of 10 repetitions at 80% of 10RM; once all sets could be completed, the resistance was increased. All groups trained the knee extensors and flexors. Tables 2.9 and 2.10 present the results of this study. In measures of strength, the isokinetic groups demonstrated a relatively consistent pattern of test speed specificity. The

variable resistance group demonstrated consistent increases in knee flexion, irrelevant of the test criterion, but knee extension showed large increases in isometric force only. In leg press ability the variable resistance and slow-speed isokinetic groups showed similar and larger gains than the fast-speed isokinetic group. Another study involving changes in leg press strength also clearly illustrated a test-specificity phenomenon between these two types of training (Gettman, Culter, and Strathman 1980). See table 2.3 for information concerning this study.

Table 2.10 compares the motor performance benefits of isokinetic and variable resistance training. Fast-speed isokinetic training demonstrated greater increases in all three motor performance tests than the other two types of training, whereas the variable resistance and slow-speed isokinetic training groups showed similar changes in the motor performance tests. The training protocols used by all three groups were described previously (Smith and Melton 1981). These results indicate that fast-speed isokinetic training may be superior to slow-speed isokinetic and variable resistance training in the context of motor performance improvement.

Body compositional changes due to isokinetic and variable resistance training are presented in table 3.3 on page 92. Although minimal data is available, these two training types appear to bring about similar changes in body composition.

Table 2.9 Isokinetic Versus Variable Resistance Training: Strength Changes

Test and group	Test (% improvement)		
	Isometric	60 deg/s	240 deg/s
Knee extension			
VR	14.6	3.1	2.3
SIK	.5	21.3	24.7
FIK	6.7	3.4	60.9
Knee flexion			
VR	10.9	14.5	13.6
SIK	15.5	17.4	10.2
FIK	9.0	8.6	51.3

VR = variable resistance; SIK = slow-speed isokinetic; FIK = fast-speed isokinetic.

Adapted, by permission, from M.J. Smith and P. Melton, 1981, "Isokinetic versus isotonic variable resistance training," *American Journal of Sports Medicine* 9(4): 275-279.

Table 2.10 Isokinetic Versus Variable Resistance: Motor Performance Changes

Test	Group (% change)		
	VR	SIK	FIK
Leg press strength	10.5	9.8	6.7
Vertical jump	1.6	3.9	5.4
Standing long jump	.3	.4	9.1
40-yd dash	−1.4	+ 1.1	−10.1

VR = variable resistance; SIK = slow-speed isokinetic; FIK = fast-speed isokinetic.

Adapted by permission from M.J. Smith and P. Melton, 1981, "Isokinetic versus isotonic variable resistance training," *American Journal of Sports Medicine* 9(4): 276-277.

Summary

The information presented in this chapter concerning types of resistance training and changes in strength, body composition, motor performance, and test specificity should be considered in the design of all resistance training programs. The next chapter discusses the process of developing resistance training programs. Many decisions have to be made regarding the program design to satisfy the needs analysis and to meet the goals of individuals performing the program.

Key Terms

accentuated eccentric training
delayed-onset muscle soreness (DOMS)
dynamic constant external resistance (DCER)
eccentric
isokinetic
isometrics
joint-angle specificity
variable resistance

Selected Readings

Atha, J. 1981. Strengthening muscle. *Exercise and Sport Sciences Reviews* 9: 1-73.

Behm, D.G., and Sale, D.G. 1993. Velocity specificity of resistance training. *Sports Medicine* 15: 374-388.

Boyer, B.T. 1990. A comparison of the effects of three strength training programs on women. *Journal of Applied Sport Science Research* 4: 88-94.

Cabell, L., and Zebras, C.J. 1999. Resistive torque validation of the Nautilus multi-biceps machine. *Journal of Strength and Conditioning Research* 13: 20-23.

Clarke, D.H. 1973. Adaptations in strength and muscular endurance resulting from exercise. *Exercise and Sport Sciences Reviews* 1: 73-102.

Fleck, S.J., and Schutt, R.C. 1985. Types of strength training. *Clinics in Sports Medicine* 4: 150-169.

Golden, C.L., and Dudley, G.A. 1992. Strength after bouts of eccentric or concentric actions. *Medicine and Science in Sports and Exercise* 24: 926-933.

Häkkinen, K., and Komi, P. 1981. Effect of different combined concentric and eccentric muscle work on maximal strength development. *Journal of Human Movement Studies* 7: 33-44.

Hortobagyi, T., Devita, P., Money, J., and Barrier, J. 2001. Effects of standard and eccentric overload strength training in young women. *Medicine and Science in Sports and Exercise* 33: 1206-1212.

Kraemer, W.J., Mazzetti, S.A., Ratamess, N.A., and Fleck, S.J. 2000. Specificity of training molds. In *Isokinetics in the human performance*, edited by L.E. Brown. Champaign, IL: Human Kinetics.

Lacerte, M., deLateur, B.J., Alquist, A.D., and Questad, K.A. 1992. Concentric versus combined concentric-eccentric isokinetic training programs: Effect on peak torque of human quadriceps femoris muscle. *Archives of Physical Medicine and Rehabilitation* 73: 1059-1062.

Manning, R.J., Graves, J.E., Carpenter, D.M., Leggett, S.H., and Pollock, M.L. 1990. Constant vs. variable resistance knee extension training. *Medicine and Science in Sports and Exercise* 22: 397-401.

McDonagh, M.J.N., and Davies, C.T.M. 1984. Adaptive response of mammalian skeletal muscle to exercise with high loads. *European Journal of Applied Physiology* 52: 139-155.

CHAPTER **3**

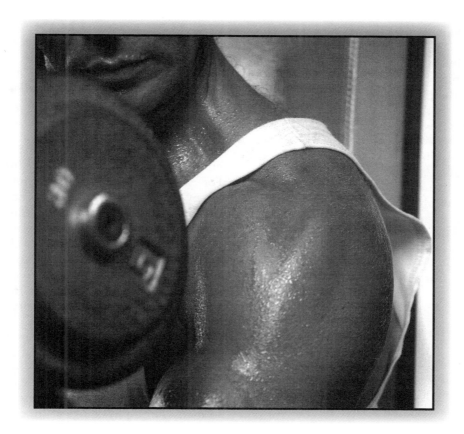

Neuromuscular Physiology and Adaptations to Resistance Training

With resistance exercise the body is challenged to produce force. Within a workout session this translates into a specific workout protocol, which is configured based on the choices made for each of the acute program variables (see chapter 5). Thus, muscle fibers are recruited to meet the demands of the force needed to lift a weight or perform a resistance exercise. With such exercise other physiological systems are engaged to support the acute demands of the workout (e.g., the cardiovascular system and the endocrine system) as well as help in the recovery process after the exercise has been completed (e.g., the endocrine system and the immune system).

Both acute and chronic physiological changes occur with exercise. An acute response to exercise usually results in an immediate change in the examined variable (e.g., an increase in heart rate), whereas a chronic change has to do with the body's response to repeated exercise stimulus exposure over the course of a training program. The physiological process by which the body responds to exercise is called an adaptation. Interestingly, each physiological variable will adapt on a different time line (e.g., nervous system versus protein accretion in muscle) and in a specific manner related to the exact type of exercise program performed, thus, the term exercise specificity. Adaptations can be observed after days of training to years of training (Häkkinen, Pakarinen et al. 1988c; Staron et al. 1994). Eventually, each physiological function or structure will express a maximum adaptation to the training program based on the trainee's genetics.

The specificity between the type of workout protocol performed and the resultant adaptation is a very important concept. It is important to be familiar with both the acute and the chronic changes occurring with exercise, as this knowledge facilitates exercise prescription as well as program design. Ultimately, the adaptation to training determines whether a resistance training program is effective and whether one is capable of a higher level of physiological function, performance, or both. A great deal of information on the adaptations to resistance training has been accumulated over the past several decades, and an understanding of these findings is important to the understanding of resistance training program design.

Physiological Adaptations

Before we start to discuss at length some of the basic elements of neuromuscular structure and function, let's examine what exactly is meant by *physiological adaptation*. First, if one has never trained the bench press exercise, the initial change in one repetition maximum (1RM) strength will be dramatic (e.g., 50% improvement in the first several weeks). However, after one has progressively trained for a long period of time (e.g., 24 months), the gains that are now made over several weeks are small (e.g., 3%) in comparison. This is because the potential for adaptation has been almost completed and now gains will start to slow down, even if training is optimal. In other words the "window of adaptation" is now much smaller as a result of prior training (Newton and Kraemer 1994). The physiological mechanisms that mediate strength gains (e.g., nervous system and muscle fiber adaptations) are now highly developed, and unless there is some increase in physiological potential (e.g., aging from 16 to 20 years) in which the genetic potential can change dramatically, improvements, though possible, will be slow. Thus, fitness gains or adaptations in the body do not take place at a constant rate throughout a training program.

The Motor Unit

The first step in adaptation to a resistance training program is to activate the muscles needed to produce force and lift a weight in an exercise session. In order for a muscle to be activated, neural innervation is necessary. The motor unit is composed of a neuron and all the muscle fibers its alpha neuron innervates; it is the functional unit of muscular activity under direct neural control. Each muscle fiber is innervated by at least one alpha motor neuron. The smaller the number of muscle fibers in a motor unit, the smaller the amount of force that can be produced by that motor unit when it is activated. The number of muscle fibers in a motor unit depends on the amount of fine control required for its function. For example, in muscles that stretch the lens of the eye, motor units may contain only 10 muscle fibers, whereas in the gastrocnemius, 1,000 muscle fibers may be found in one motor unit. On average for all of the muscles in the body about 100 muscle fibers are in a motor unit. Muscle function is controlled by the nervous system and starts with impulses being sent from the higher brain centers in the central nervous system, more specifically the motor cortex. Understanding motor unit recruitment is paramount to understanding the specificity of resistance exercise and training.

The central nervous system consists of more than 100 billion nerve cells. Neurons are involved in many more physiological functions (e.g., pain perception, brain functions, sweating, etc.) than just stimulating muscle to contract and therefore come in many shapes and sizes. Figure 3.1 is a schematic of a motor unit consisting of an alpha motor neuron and its associated muscle fibers. All neurons consist of three basic components: dendrites, soma, and axon. Basically, dendrites receive information, the soma processes the information, and axons send information out to other neurons or target cells. A motor neuron has relatively short dendrites and a long axon that carries impulses from the central nervous system to the neuromuscular junction.

Axons may be covered with a white substance high in lipid (fat) content called the myelin sheath. The myelin sheath is sometimes even thicker than the axon itself and is composed of multiple layers of this lipid substance. Nerve fibers possessing a myelin sheath are referred to as myelinated nerve fibers; those lacking a myelin sheath are called unmyelinated nerve fibers. The myelin sheath is created and maintained by

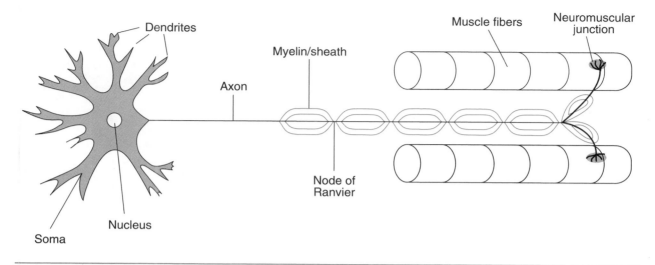

Figure 3.1 A motor neuron and the muscle fibers it innervates are called a motor unit.

Schwann cells. In a typical nerve there are about twice as many unmyelinated fibers as myelinated fibers. The smaller unmyelinated fibers typically are found between myelinated fibers. The myelin helps to insulate the nerve impulse conduction as it travels down the axon. This helps prevent impulses from being transferred to neighboring fibers. The myelin sheath does not run continuously along the length of the axon, but is segmented with small spaces about 2 to 3 micrometers (µm) in length where the membrane of the axon is exposed. These spaces occur about every 1 to 3 mm along the length of the axon and are termed nodes of Ranvier.

The movement of ions or charged molecules causes an impulse to move down the membrane of an axon or dendrite. The impulse in an axon causes the release of chemicals called neurotransmitters into the synapse (between neurons) or neuromuscular junction (the synapse between a neuron and a muscle fiber). The neurotransmitter binds to receptors on the dendrite or muscle fiber, which initiates a new electrical impulse. This new impulse then travels down the dendrite, or in the case of muscle fibers, initiates muscle action. In the case of the alpha motor unit, electrical stimuli for voluntary actions originate in the motor cortex and travel down the nervous system neuron to neuron until they reach the neuromuscular junction.

Neuromuscular Junction

The **neuromuscular junction** is the morphological structure that acts as the interface between the alpha motor neuron and the muscle fiber. Figure 3.2 is a schematic of the neuromuscular junction. All neuromuscular junctions have five common features: (1) a Schwann cell that forms a cap over the axon, (2) an axon terminal ending in a synaptic knob that contains the neurotransmitter acetylcholine (ACh) and other substances needed for metabolic support and function (e.g., ATP, mitochondria, lysosomes, glycogen molecules, etc.), (3) a junctional cleft or space, (4) a postjunctional membrane that contains ACh receptors, and (5) a junctional sarcoplasm and cytoskeleton that provides metabolic and structural support.

When an impulse reaches the end of the neuron side of the neuromuscular junction, it causes

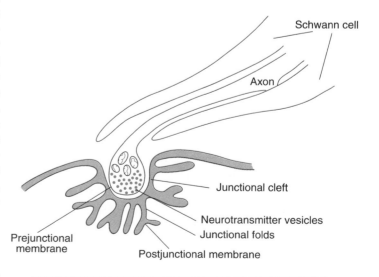

Figure 3.2 The neuromuscular junction in cross section.

the release of ACh. ACh is the primary stimulatory neurotransmitter for a motor neuron, and it is stored within the synaptic vesicles in the terminal ends of the axon. Approximately 50 to 70 ACh-containing vesicles are found per μm^2 of nerve terminal area. When the action potential reaches the axon terminal, calcium channels on the membrane of the synaptic knob open, causing the uptake of calcium ions (Ca^{++}). The increase in Ca^{++} concentration causes the release of ACh from the vesicles. The ACh diffuses from the prejunctional membrane across the synaptic cleft (about 50 nm wide) between the pre- and postjunctional membranes to the postsynaptic membrane.

On the postjunctional side of the neuromuscular junction the ACh binds to receptors located on the postjunctional membrane. The postjunctional membrane is a specialized part of the muscle cell's membrane and has junctional folds and ACh receptors. If enough ACh becomes bound to the postjunctional membrane receptors, the permeability of the membrane will increase and create a conducted ionic current with Ca^{++} as the ion predominately involved. This postsynaptic ionic current or electrical impulse is what initiates muscle action. The muscle fiber will continue to be activated (e.g., concentric, isometric, or eccentric muscle actions) as long as a sufficient amount of ACh is bound to the postsynaptic membrane receptors.

The ACh will eventually be destroyed by the enzyme acetyl-cholinesterase found at the base of the junctional folds of the junctional cleft. Destruction of ACh stops the stimulus needed for muscle fiber activation. The majority of by-products produced from the breakdown of ACh by acetyl-cholinesterase are taken up by the presynaptic membrane and used to produce new ACh.

Why is ACh needed at the neuromuscular junction? Why can't the ionic current of the neuron simply be conducted to the membrane surrounding the muscle fiber and thus stimulate muscle actions? Because the neuron is very small compared to a muscle fiber, the ionic current it conducts is insufficient to be directly transferred to the muscle fiber's membrane to stimulate the fiber. ACh is needed to cause an ionic current of sufficient strength (threshold) to be conducted by the muscle fiber's membrane and initiate muscle action. Figure 3.3 is a micrograph of a motor end plate showing several structural aspects of the neuromuscular junction (Deschenes et al. 1993).

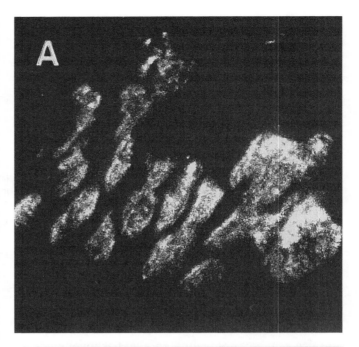

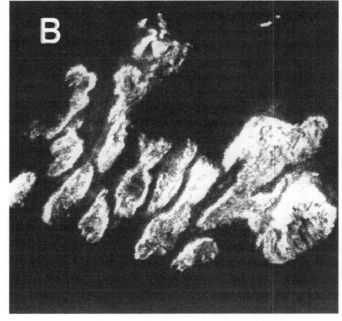

Figure 3.3 Neuromuscular junction stained for *(a)* presynaptic acetylcholine vesicles and *(b)* postsynaptic acetylcholine receptors. These images are magnified by 1,000.

Courtesy of Dr. Michael Deschenes' laboratory.

Conduction of Impulses

A nervous impulse is conducted in the form of electrical energy. When no impulse is being conducted, the inside of the neuron has a net negative charge, as compared to the outside of the neuron, which has a net positive charge. This arrangement of the plus and negative charges is termed the resting membrane potential. It is attributable to the distribution of molecules with electrical charges or ions and the impermeability of the resting cell membrane to these ions. Sodium (Na^+) and potassium (K^+) ions are the major molecules responsible for the membrane potential. Na^+ ions are predominantly located outside the neuron's cell membrane. K^+ ions are located mainly inside the neuron. There are, however, more Na^+ ions on the outside of the neuron than K^+ on the inside of the neuron giving the inside a less positive or net negative charge as compared to the outside of the neuron.

When an impulse is being conducted down a dendrite or an axon, the cell membrane of the neuron becomes permeable to both Na^+ and K^+ ions. Ions tend to move down a concentration gradient from areas where they are highly concentrated to areas where they are less concentrated. First, Na^+ ions move into the neuron giving the inside a plus charge compared to the outside of the neuron. This is termed depolarization, and such a reversal of electrical potential is called the action potential. The action potential lasts for only a brief period of time (milliseconds) because the membrane becomes permeable to K^+ ions. This results in K^+ ions leaving the interior of the membrane so that the interior of the membrane once again has a net negative charge relative to the exterior and is termed repolarization. The periods of permeability to both Na^+ and K^+ ions are very brief so that a relatively few ions actually move from the exterior to the interior and vice versa. An energy-dependent pumping system called the Na^+-K^+ pump is needed to maintain and restore the resting membrane potential after an impulse has been conducted. This pump actively removes Na^+ ions from the interior of the neuron and moves K^+ ions from the exterior to the interior of the neuron. This quickly restores the neuron to its original resting membrane potential in which there is a net negative charge on the inside. The process is repeated each time a neuron conducts a nervous impulse or action potential.

The type of nervous system conduction is related to whether the nerve is myelinated or unmyelinated. Myelinated nerves conduct their impulses using what is called saltatory conduction, and unmyelinated nerves use a conduction process called local conduction. The movement of the ions producing an action potential remains the same (as described earlier) for either type of conduction. In myelinated nerves the nodes of Ranvier allow the action potential to jump from node to node using saltatory conduction (*saltatory* means "to jump"). A significant amount of ions cannot move through the thick myelin sheath, but can easily move through the membrane at the nodes of Ranvier because of the low resistance to ionic current at the nodes of Ranvier. Saltatory conduction has two advantages. First, it allows the action potential to make jumps down the axon, thereby increasing the velocity of nerve transmission by five- to fiftyfold. Saltatory conduction results in the action potentials moving along at a velocity of 60 to100 m per second. Second, it conserves energy as only the nodes depolarize, which reduces the energy needed to reestablish the resting membrane potential.

Conversely, unmyelinated nerve fibers use a local circuit of ionic current flow to conduct the action potential along the entire length of the nerve fiber. A small section of the nerve fiber membrane depolarizes, and the continuation of local circuit ionic current flow causes nerve membrane depolarization to continue and the action potential travels down the entire length of the nerve fiber. The velocity of this type of nerve impulse conduction is much slower than that of myelinated nerve fibers, ranging from 0.5 to 10 m per second.

The neuron's diameter in part also determines the impulse conduction velocity. In general, the greater the diameter of a nerve fiber, the greater the conduction velocity. In myelinated nerve fibers, the impulse velocity increases approximately with the increase in the fiber diameter. In unmyelinated nerve fibers, the velocity of the impulse increases with the square root of the fiber diameter. Thus, as fiber diameter increases, conduction velocity of myelinated fibers increases substantially more than in unmyelinated fibers. The faster velocities of the larger myelinated fibers, such as the ones that innervate skeletal muscle, produce more rapid stimulation of muscle actions, but have higher thresholds for recruitment. Typically, type II skeletal muscle fibers (fast twitch) are innervated by larger-diameter axons than type I muscle fibers (slow twitch). Thus, motor units made up of type I fibers are typically recruited first due to the lower recruitment thresholds of their neurons. Motor units made up of type II fibers are recruited after the type I fibers because their larger axons have higher recruitment thresholds. This is termed the size principle of recruitment.

Motor Unit Activation and the Size Principle

A motor unit is composed of either all type I (slow-twitch) or all type II (fast-twitch) muscle fibers. However, the size and number of muscle fibers in each type of motor unit can vary, with some type I muscle fibers in type I motor units being larger than some type II motor units fibers. Yet force production demands are the key element in the outcome of a guided recruitment pattern. Typically, neurons innervating type I fibers are normally recruited first in a muscle action followed by the neurons innervating type II (type IIA followed by type IIB). Thus, the order of recruitment is normally type I first and then type II fibers if more force than the type I can generate is needed. There is however, some overlap between the last of the type I fibers recruited and the first of the type II fibers recruited and the last of the type IIA and first of the type IIB fibers recruited.

The muscle fibers in a motor unit are not all located adjacent to each other, but are spread out in the muscle in what are called microbundles of about 3 to 15 fibers. Thus, adjacent muscle fibers are not necessarily from the same motor unit. With disbursement of fibers in a motor unit, when a motor unit is activated, the "whole" muscle appears to be being activated. If fibers of a motor unit were all adjacent to each other when activated, only one portion or segment of the muscle would appear to be activated. Thus, disbursement of muscle fibers in a motor unit throughout the muscle allows the "whole" muscle to be activated rather than segments of the whole muscle.

Only the motor units that are recruited in an exercise produce force and will be subject to adaptational changes with exercise training. Thus, motor unit recruitment is of fundamental importance in the prescription of resistance exercise. Activated motor units stay facilitated for a time after use, which is very important for subsequent muscle contractions. That is, maximal or near-maximal contractions elicit a "postactivation potentiation" for subsequent muscle contractions occurring within several seconds to a few minutes after the high-intensity contraction (Hamada et al. 2000). This potentiation is more prominent in type II muscle fibers, and the mechanism involved is believed to be related to phosphorylation of myosin regulatory light chains during the maximal contraction, which renders actin and myosin more sensitive to calcium (Hamada et al. 2000). This neuromuscular potentiation has important ramifications for muscular performance and the recruitment of muscle fibers during exercise.

Another important concept is the all or none law. This means that when a threshold level for activation is reached for a specific motor unit, all of the muscle fibers in that motor unit are activated. If the threshold is not reached, then none of the muscle fibers in a motor unit are activated. Although this holds true for individual motor units, whole muscles, such as the biceps, are not governed by the all or none law. This is true because it is possible to activate only selected motor units within that muscle. This ability makes possible very fine control of the force produced. Motor units and their associated muscle fibers not activated generate no force and move passively through the range of motion made possible by the activated motor units. Without such a phenomenon of graded force production, there would be very little control of the amount of force that the whole muscle could generate and therefore poor control of body movements.

The fact that motor units follow the all or none law makes possible one method in which force variations produced by a muscle can be achieved. The more motor units within a muscle that are stimulated, the greater the amount of force that is developed. In other words, if one motor unit is activated, a very small amount of force is developed. If several motor units are activated, more force is developed. If all of the motor units in a muscle are activated, maximal force is produced by the muscle. This method of varying the force produced by a muscle is called multiple motor unit summation. The activation of motor units is based on the force production needs of the activity. For example, one might activate only a small number of motor units to perform 15 repetitions using 10 lb (4.5 kg) of an arm curl, as the resistance may only represent about 10% of maximal strength. Therefore, a small number of muscle fibers can provide the force to perform the exercise movement. Conversely, a 100-lb (45.4-kg) arm curl, which represents a 1RM, would require all of the available motor units to produce maximal force to perform the exercise movement.

Gradations of force can also be achieved by controlling the force produced by one motor unit. This is called wave summation. A motor unit responds to a single nerve impulse by producing a "twitch." A twitch (see figure 3.4) is a brief period of muscle activity producing force, which is followed by relaxation of the motor unit. When two impulses conducted by an axon reach the neuromuscular junction close together, the motor unit responds with two twitches. The second twitch, however, occurs before the complete relaxation from the first twitch. The second twitch summates with the force of the first twitch, producing more total force. This wave (twitch) summation can continue until the impulses occur at a high enough frequency that the twitches are completely summated. Complete summation is called tetanus and is the maximal force a motor unit can develop.

The order in which motor units are recruited in most cases is relatively constant for a particular movement (Desmedt and Godaux 1977). According to the size principle for recruitment of motor neurons, the smaller motor units—or what are called "low-threshold" (low electrical level needed for activation) motor units—are recruited first. Low-threshold motor units are composed of type I muscle fibers. Then, progressively higher threshold motor units are recruited based on the increasing demands of the activity. The higher-threshold motor units are composed predominantly of type II fibers. Heavier resistances (e.g., 3-5RM) require the recruitment of higher-threshold motor units than lighter resistances (e.g., 12-15RM). However, lifting heavier resistances will (according to the size principle) start with the recruitment of low-threshold motor units first (type I) and progressively move up the line until enough motor units are recruited to produce the needed force (see figure 3.5). Different motor units have different numbers of muscle fibers and different sizes of muscle fibers (i.e., cross-sectional area) leading to a variety of graded force production capabilities. Each muscle has different types and

numbers of motor units and not all individuals have the same array available to them (e.g., an advanced runner does not have large numbers of type II motor units for high force production).

Exceptions to the size principle may occur in very high velocity (ballistic) and high power outputs using highly trained movement patterns. In the animal world these are related to escape or catching movements (e.g., the flick of a cat's paw). In human sporting activities, a pitcher's fastball might be the type of sport skill that does not adhere to the size principle to enhance power production. In the case of a pitcher, then, rather than starting a training regime with the recruitment of low-threshold type I motor units, high-threshold type II motor units would be recruited first in order to allow faster movement velocity. Low-threshold motor units would not be recruited in the activity as they would slow down the movement. This process appears to be facilitated by inhibiting activation of the type I motor units, making it easier to go directly to the type II motor units. However, the applicability of not following the normal order of recruitment in humans remains speculative.

The determining factor of whether to recruit high- or low-threshold motor units is the total amount of force necessary to perform the muscular action. If a large amount of force is necessary either to move a heavy weight slowly or to move a light weight at a fast velocity, high-threshold motor units will be recruited. The higher-threshold motor units

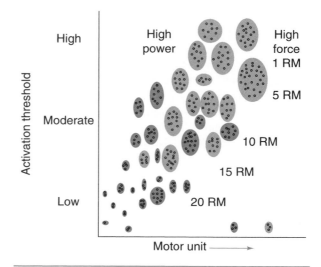

Figure 3.5 The size principle of motor unit activation.

Adapted, by permission, from J.E. Desmedt and E. Godaux, 1977, "Ballistic contractions in man: Characteristic recruitment pattern of single motor units of the tibialis muscle," *Journal of Physiology* 264: 673-694.

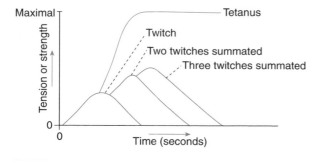

Figure 3.4 Gradations in force of one motor unit caused by wave summation.

have type II muscle fibers associated with them and typically contain a higher number of muscle fibers than lower-threshold motor units. Thus, their recruitment results in higher force or power production. Some type II muscle fibers can be found lower in the recruitment profile due to either a lower number of fibers or smaller type II muscle fibers associated with a certain motor unit.

The size principle order of recruitment ensures that low-threshold motor units are predominantly recruited to perform lower-intensity, long-duration (endurance) activities. Higher-threshold motor units are only used to produce higher levels of force, which result in greater strength or power. The size principle order of recruitment helps to delay fatigue during submaximal muscle actions because the high-threshold, highly fatigable type II motor units are not recruited unless high levels of force or power are needed. Likewise, the recruitment of the lower-threshold predominately type I fibers, which are less prone to fatigue unless high levels of force are needed, also helps to delay fatigue. Higher-threshold motor units would only be recruited when low force levels are needed if enough total work was performed to dramatically reduce glycogen stores in the lower-threshold motor units. However, this has not been typically observed with resistance exercise protocols. When the force production needs are low to moderate, motor units can be alternately recruited to meet the force demands (asynchronous recruitment). This means that a motor unit may be recruited during most of the first repetition with a light weight and then not or minimally recruited in the second repetition of a set. This ability to rest motor units when submaximal force is needed also helps to delay fatigue.

The higher-threshold motor units neurons recover more quickly (e.g., experience faster repolarization), allowing them to be activated more quickly in repeated actions than lower-threshold motor units. So, although the high-threshold type II motor units fatigue quickly, the ability of their neurons to recover quickly makes them ideal for repeated high-force, short-duration activities.

Recruitment order is important from a practical standpoint for several reasons. First, to recruit the type II fibers to achieve a training effect in these fibers, the exercise must be characterized by heavy loading, high power output demands, or both. Second, the order of recruitment is fixed for many movements including resistance exercise (Desmedt and Godaux 1977). If the body position

is changed, however, the order of recruitment can also change and different muscle fibers will be recruited (Grimby and Hannerz 1977; Matheson et al. 2001). The order of recruitment can also change for multifunctional muscles from one movement or exercise to another (Grimby and Hannerz 1977; Harr Romeny, Denier Van Der Gon, and Gielen 1982). The magnitude of recruitment of different portions of the quadriceps is different for the performance of a leg press versus a squat (Escamilla et al. 2001), and from one type of quadriceps exercise to another (Matheson et al. 2001). Likewise, the magnitude of recruitment of different abdominal muscles is different from one abdominal exercise to another (Willett et al. 2001). Variation in the recruitment order and magnitude of recruitment of different muscles may be one of the factors responsible for strength gains being specific to a particular exercise. The variation in recruitment order provides some evidence to support the belief held by many strength coaches that a particular muscle must be exercised using several different movement angles or exercises to develop completely.

Individuals do not all have the same compliment of motor units available to them. This along with differences in the total number of muscle fibers available allows for differences in force and power capabilities from individual to individual. With aging, some individuals may have only low-threshold motor units made up of predominantly type I muscle fibers in some muscles, which limits their power and force production capabilities. The type, number, and size of muscle fibers in the motor unit dictates the functional abilities of individual motor units and eventually the abilities of the total muscle.

Proprioception

Length and tension within muscles and tendons are continually monitored by specialized sensory receptors located within the muscles and tendons called **proprioceptors.** The length and tension of the muscles acting at a joint determine the joint's position. Thus, if the muscle length acting on a joint is known, the joint's position is also known, and changes in the joint's position can be monitored. The information proprioceptors gather is constantly relayed to conscious and subconscious portions of the brain and is important for motor learning (Hutton and Atwater 1992). Proprioceptors keep the central nervous system constantly informed of a movement or a series of movements.

Muscle Spindles

The two functions of **muscle spindles** are to monitor stretch or length of the muscle in which they are embedded, and to initiate a contraction to reduce the stretch in the muscle. The stretch reflex is attributed to the response of muscle spindles.

Spindles are located in modified muscle fibers and therefore are arranged parallel to normal muscle fibers. The modified muscle fibers containing spindles are called intrafusal fibers. These intrafusal fibers are composed of a stretch-sensitive central area (or sensory area) embedded in a muscle fiber capable of causing a contraction. If a muscle is stretched, as in tapping the patellar tendon to initiate the knee-jerk reflex or adding an external weight, the spindles are also stretched. The sensory nerve of the spindle carries an impulse to the spinal cord; here the sensory neuron synapses with alpha motor neurons. The alpha motor neurons relay a nerve impulse causing activation of the stretched muscle and its agonists. In addition, other neurons inhibit activation of antagonistic muscles to the stretched muscle. The stretched muscle shortens, and the stretch on the spindle is relieved. Performing strength training or plyometric exercises with prestretching takes advantage of this stretch reflex. This reflex is one explanation for greater force output after a prestretch.

Gamma motor neurons innervate the end portions of the intrafusal fibers, which are capable of shortening. Stimulation of these end portions by the central nervous system regulates the length and therefore the sensitivity of the spindles to changes in length of the extrafusal fibers. Adjustments of the spindles in this fashion enable the spindle to more accurately monitor the length of the muscles in which they are embedded.

Golgi Tendon Organs

Golgi tendon organs' main functions are to respond to tension within the tendon and, if it becomes excessive, to relieve the tension. These proprioceptors are located within the tendons of muscles and are consequently in a good location to monitor tension developed by a muscle.

The sensory neuron of a Golgi tendon organ travels to the spinal cord. In the spinal cord it synapses with the alpha motor neurons both of the muscle whose tension it is monitoring and of the antagonistic muscles. As an activated muscle develops tension, the tension within the muscle's tendon increases and is monitored by the tendon organs. If the tension becomes great enough that damage to the muscle or tendon is possible, inhibition of the activated muscle occurs and activation of the antagonist muscle(s) is initiated. The tension within the muscle is alleviated, and damage to the muscle or tendon avoided.

This protective function is not foolproof. It may be possible through resistance training to learn to disinhibit the effects of the Golgi tendon organs. The ability to disinhibit this protective function may be responsible in part for some neural adaptations and injuries that occur in maximal lifts by highly resistance trained athletes.

Nervous System Adaptations

Figure 3.6 presents a theoretical overview of the basic interactions and relationships among components of the neuromuscular system. A message is developed in the higher brain centers. This is transmitted to the motor cortex, where the stimulus for muscle activation is transmitted to a lower-level controller (spinal cord or brainstem). From there, the message is passed to the motor neurons of the muscle and results in a specific pattern of motor unit activation. Various feedback loops also exist that send information back to the brain. This process can help modify force production as well as provide communication with other physiological systems (e.g., endocrine). The high and low brain level commands can be modified by feedback from both the peripheral sensory and the high-level central command controller. Various adaptations in the communications among the various parts of the neuromuscular systems can be observed with resistance training. Differences in the neural activation of different resistance training programs can produce different types of adaptations such as increases in strength with little changes in muscle size (Ploutz et al. 1994).

When muscle attempts to produce the maximal force possible, typically all of the available motor units are activated. As discussed earlier, the activation of motor units is influenced by the size principle. This principle is based on the observed relationship between motor unit twitch force and recruitment threshold (Desmedt 1981). Force can be increased by recruiting more motor units; however, an increase in motor unit firing

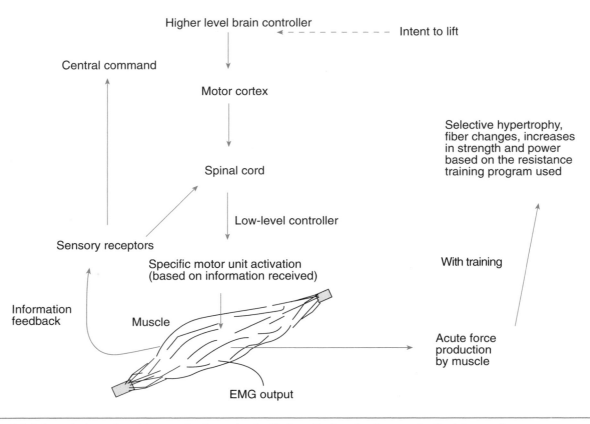

Higher level brain controller — — — — — — — — Intent to lift

Central command

Motor cortex

Selective hypertrophy, fiber changes, increases in strength and power based on the resistance training program used

Spinal cord

Low-level controller

Sensory receptors

With training

Specific motor unit activation (based on information received)

Information feedback

Muscle

Acute force production by muscle

EMG output

Figure 3.6 A theoretical overview of the neural pathways involved in the activation of and sensory feedback for muscle.

rate also increases force. These two factors result in a continuum of voluntary force in the muscle (Henneman, Somjen, and Carpenter 1985). Not only does maximal force production require the recruitment of all motor units including the high-threshold motor units, but also these motor units must be recruited at a high enough firing rate to produce maximal force (Sale 1992). Some have theorized that untrained individuals may not be able to voluntarily recruit the highest-threshold motor units or maximally activate their muscles (Carroll, Riek, and Carson 2001; Sale 1992). Thus, part of the training adaptation is developing the ability to recruit all motor units in a specific exercise movement.

Other neural adaptations also take place (Carroll, Riek, and Carson 2001). Activation of antagonists is reduced in some movements resulting in increased measurable force of the agonists. The activation of all motor units in all of the muscle(s) involved in a movement is coordinated or optimized to result in maximal force or power. Neuromuscular adaptations are made that allow the most effective control of the trained muscle(s)

in the context of coordination of the movement. This is true for both maximal and submaximal development of force.

Some advanced lifters or athletes may not follow the order of recruitment stipulated by the size principle. It may be possible to inhibit lower-threshold (i.e., slow) motor units and still activate the higher-threshold motor units in an attempt to enhance rate of force development and power production. This idea has been derived from observations during very rapid stereotyped movements and during voluntary eccentric muscle action in humans (Dudley and Harris 1992; Sale 1992). Dudley and colleagues (1990) demonstrated that the activation of knee extensors by the central nervous system during maximal efforts depends on the speed and type of muscle action. The central nervous system is also capable of limiting force by engaging inhibitory mechanisms, which may be protective in nature. Thus, training may result in changes in the order of fiber recruitment in both the agonists and antagonists or reduced inhibition, which may help in the performance of certain types of muscle actions.

Muscle Tissue Activation

Magnetic resonance imaging (MRI) allows for the visualization of whole muscle groups. Activated muscle can be observed via the color changes that exist in the images before and after exercise. Lighter areas represent areas in which muscle tissue has been activated with the exercise. This contrast shift has been shown to be directly related to force development from muscle actions evoked by both voluntary and surface electromyostimulation (Ploutz et al. 1994). A representative MRI image before and after multiple sets of 10RM leg press exercises is shown in figure 3.7.

MRI techniques have been used to examine changes in muscle activation due to training (Conley et al. 1997; Ploutz et al. 1994). Ploutz and colleagues (1994) used MRI technology and a specific program designed to increase strength with little or no change in muscle size over a 9-week training period. Training was performed 2 days a week. Each session consisted of high-intensity single knee extension exercise using the left quadriceps for three to six sets of 12 repetitions. Exercise-induced MRI contrast shifts were evoked by using five sets of 10 knee extensions for each resistance of 50%, 75%, and 100% of the maximum pretraining resistance that could be lifted for five sets of 10 repetitions. One repetition maximum (1RM) strength increased by 14% over the training period in the trained left thigh musculature and 7% in the right untrained thigh musculature. The left quadriceps femoris muscle cross-sectional area increased by 5%, and the right demonstrated no changes. This indicated that neural factors mediated much of the improvement in 1RM strength. Interestingly, the amount of muscle that needed to be activated in the posttraining test was less than that required to perform the same exercise protocol before training. This reduction in the amount of muscle needed to lift a given resistance in the posttraining state demonstrated that unless the resistance used is progressively increased over a training period, less muscle will be activated as muscular strength increases. It has also been shown that resistance training can result in changes in the muscles used to perform a submaximal task, such that some muscles that were active before training may not be significantly recruited to perform a submaximal task after training, yet activation can be increased to perform a maximal task (Conley et al. 1997).

These data also give insights as to why a classic modification of the progressive overload concept, specifically periodized training (i.e., variation in resistances and exercise volume used in training), may in fact be effective in providing recovery for certain muscle fibers. With increasing muscle strength over a training program, the use of heavy, moderate, and light resistances in training would allow for specific muscle fibers not to be taxed by the lifting required on light and moderate training days. Yet the increased stress per cross-sectional unit area of activated muscle could potentially elicit a physiological stimulus for strength gains and tissue growth (Ploutz et al. 1994). The heavy training days would maximally activate the available musculature, but by alternating the intensities over time, overtraining or a lack of recovery could be minimized (Fry, Allemeier, and Staron 1994; Fry, Kraemer, Stone et al. 1994). Such periodized training manipulations have been found to be important, especially as the training level becomes more demanding.

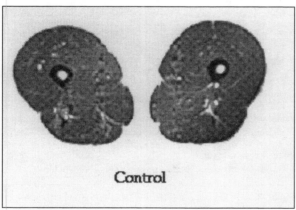
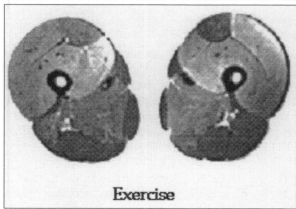

Figure 3.7 A cross-sectional magnetic resonance image (MRI) of thigh musculature before and after a heavy resistance workout. The white and lighter gray areas in the after-exercise scan represent muscle tissue that has been used to lift the weight. MRI allows examination of the extent to which specific parts of intact muscle have been activated with acute exercise.

Reprinted, by permission, from Dr. Gary Dudley, University of Georgia, and Dr. Lori Ploutz, Ohio University.

Changes in the Neuromuscular Junction

Morphological changes in the nervous system of humans with heavy resistance training remain unclear. Deschenes and colleagues (1993) provided insights into the adaptability of neuromuscular junctions (NMJ) with different intensities of exercise by examining the effects of high- versus low-intensity treadmill exercise training on the NMJ adaptations in the soleus muscle of rats. Both high- and low-intensity exercise running produced an increased area of the NMJ. Although NMJ hypertrophic responses were observed in both groups, the high-intensity group showed more dispersed, irregularly shaped synapses, and the low-intensity training showed more compact, symmetrical synapses. The high-intensity training group also exhibited a greater total length of NMJ branching when compared to the low-intensity and control groups. Thus, it might be hypothesized that heavy resistance exercise training would produce morphological changes in the NMJ. These changes may be of much greater magnitude than adaptations from endurance training due to the differences in required quanta of neurotransmitter involved with the recruitment of high-threshold motor units.

In a later study by Deschenes and colleagues (2000), rats either participated in a 7-week resistance training program or served as untrained controls. After the experimental period, the NMJs of soleus muscles, which in the rat is composed primarily of type I fibers, were visualized with immunofluorescent techniques (see figure 3.8), and muscle fibers were stained histochemically. The results indicated that resistance training significantly increased end plate perimeter length (15%) and area (16%), and significantly enhanced the dispersion of ACh receptors within the end plate region. Pre- and postsynaptic modifications to resistance exercise were highly related. No significant alterations in muscle fiber size or fiber type were detected. These data indicate that the stimulus of resistance training was sufficiently potent to remodel NMJ structure in type I muscle fibers, and that this effect cannot be attributed to muscle fiber hypertrophy or any changes in the muscle fiber–type myosin ATPase profile.

Time Course of Neural Changes: Initial Gains in Strength

The initial quick gains in strength due to training appear to be mediated by neural factors (Moritani

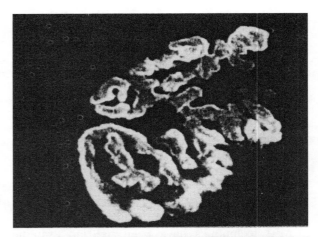
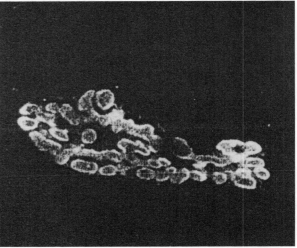

Figure 3.8 Type I (slow-twitch) and type II (fast-twitch) motor end plates of the neuromuscular junction.
Courtesy of Dr. Michael Deschenes' laboratory.

1992; Sale 1992). After a resistance training program there can be weak relationships between increases in strength and changes in muscle cross-sectional area (Ploutz et al. 1994), limb circumference (Moritani and DeVries 1979, 1980), and muscle fiber cross-sectional area (Costill et al. 1979; Ploutz et al. 1994; Staron et al. 1994), indicating that other factors are responsible for gains in strength. In one study, isometric training produced a 92% increase in maximal static strength, but only a 23% increase in muscle cross-sectional area (Ikai and Fukunaga 1970). On the basis of this kind of evidence scientists have concluded that neural factors have a profound influence on muscular force production (Carroll, Riek, and Carson 2001). Such neural factors are related to the following processes: increased neural drive (i.e., recruitment and rate of firing) to the muscle, increased synchronization of the motor units, increased activation of agonists, decreased activation of antagonists, coordination of all motor units and muscle(s) involved in a movement, and inhibition of the protective mechanisms of the muscle (i.e., Golgi tendon organs).

Neural factors and quality of protein changes (e.g., alterations in the type of myosin heavy chains and type of myosin ATPase enzymes) may explain some part of early (2 to 8 weeks) strength gains. Strength gains during this time are much greater than what can be explained by muscle hypertrophy. The specific type of program used may be one of the most important factors in initial strength gains due to neural factors because programs that are of very high intensity (>90% of 1RM), but low in total exercise volume (low number of sets) may not be an adequate stimulus for muscle tissue growth (Sale 1992). Therefore, strength gains may be more dependent on neural factors with these types of programs. If a program does promote muscle tissue growth, this may diminish the contribution of the initial neural adaptations to strength and power gains. However, typically muscle fiber hypertrophy has been shown to require more than 16 workouts to show significant increases (Staron et al. 1994). Thus, various types of training might be able to more quickly enhance the hypertrophy of muscle in the early phases (1 to 8 weeks) of training, thereby enhancing the hypertrophic contribution to strength and power gains. However, this has been observed in only a few studies (Cannon and Cafarelli 1987; Carolan and Cafarelli 1992; Thorstensson et al. 1976). The large majority of studies have demonstrated that in the early phases of a heavy resistance training program, increased voluntary activation of muscle is the largest contributor to strength increases (for reviews, see Moritani 1992; Sale 1992). After this period muscle hypertrophy becomes the predominant factor in strength increases, especially for younger men.

Neural Drive

Scientists have investigated neural drive to a muscle using integrated electromyogram (EMG) techniques (Häkkinen and Komi 1983; Kamen, Kroll, and Ziagon 1984; Moritani and DeVries 1980; Sale et al. 1983; Thorstensson et al. 1976). EMG techniques measure the electrical activity within the muscle and nerves and indicate the amount of neural drive (a measure of the number and amplitude of nervous impulses) to a muscle. In one of these studies, 8 weeks of dynamic constant external resistance weight training caused a shift to a lower level in the EMG-activity-to-muscular-force ratio (Moritani and DeVries 1980). Because the muscle produced more force with a lower amount of EMG activity, more force production occurred with less neural drive. Calculations predicted a 9% strength increase due to training-induced hypertrophy; in actuality, however, strength increased 30%. It is believed that this increase in strength beyond that expected from hypertrophy resulted from the combination of the shift in the EMG-to-force ratio and the 12% increase in maximal EMG activity. This and other research support the idea that an increase in maximal neural drive to a muscle increases strength. The studies reveal that less neural drive is required to produce any particular submaximal force after training; consequently there is either an improved activation of the muscle or a more efficient recruitment pattern of the muscle fibers. Some studies have demonstrated that improved activation of the muscle does not occur after training (McDonagh, Hayward, and Davies 1983). Therefore, a more efficient recruitment order is probably responsible for much of the increased force produced.

Sale and colleagues (1983) investigated the possibility that additional motor units can be recruited after strength training. As a mechanism to increase force production, this process assumes that an individual is not able to activate simultaneously all motor units in a muscle before training. Belanger and McComas (1981) found that this is true for some muscles but not for others and so could contribute to an increased force output in some, but not all, muscles.

Another neural factor that could cause increased force production is increased synchronization of motor unit firing. The greater the synchronization, the greater the number of motor units firing at any one time. It has recently been shown that synchronization of motor units results in an increase in EMG (65-130%) and an increase in force fluctuations (Yao, Fuglevand, and Enoka 2000), and synchronization is more prevalent during high-intensity contractions (Kamen and Roy 2000). Increased synchronization of motor units has been observed after strength training (Felici et al. 2001; Milner-Brown, Stein, and Yemin 1973). During submaximal force production, however, increased synchronization of motor units is actually less effective in producing force than asynchronous activation of motor units (Lind and Petrofsky 1978; Rack and Westbury 1969). Average force produced by synchronization with stimulations of 5 to 100% of maximum was not different from asynchronous firing (Yao, Fuglevand, and Enoka 2000). Thus, it is unclear whether greater synchronization of motor units produces greater force. Increased synchronization does, however, result in greater force fluctuations in simple isometric tasks (Carroll, Riek, and Carson 2001). This could decrease the steadiness of a muscle action, which could be detrimental to the performance in some activities.

Training has been shown to increase the period of time that all motor units can be tonically active from several to 30 seconds (Grimby, Hannerz, and Hedman 1981). An adaptation of this type may not cause an increase in maximal force, but it does aid in maintaining it for a longer period of time. It has also been observed that during maximal voluntary actions the high-threshold type II motor units normally do not reach stimulation rates required for complete tetanus to occur (DeLuca et al. 1982). If the stimulation rate to these high-threshold motor units were increased, the actual force production would also increase. Although neural adaptations clearly can increase strength, exactly how all of the neuronal mechanisms interact to bring about strength increases is not completely elucidated.

Inhibitory Mechanisms

Inhibition of muscle action by reflex protective mechanisms, such as the Golgi tendon organs, has been hypothesized to limit muscular force production (Caiozzo, Perrine, and Edgerton 1981; Wickiewicz et al. 1984). The effect of these inhibitory mechanisms can be partially removed by hypnosis. Ikai and Steinhaus (1961) found that force developed during forearm flexion by non-resistance-trained individuals increased 17% under hypnosis. In the same study, the force developed by highly resistance trained individuals under hypnosis was not significantly different from the force developed in the normal conscious state. The researchers concluded that resistance training may cause voluntary inhibition of these protective mechanisms. These protective mechanisms appear to be especially active when large amounts of force are developed, such as maximal

force development at slow speeds of movement (Caiozzo et al. 1981; Wickiewicz et al. 1984).

Information concerning protective mechanisms has several practical applications. Many resistance training exercises involve action by the same muscle groups of both limbs simultaneously, or bilateral actions. The force developed during bilateral actions is less than the sum of the force developed by each limb independently and has been shown to range from 3% to 25%, especially when fast contraction velocities are performed (Jakobi and Chilibeck 2001; Ohtsuki 1981; Secher, Rorsgaard, and Secher, 1978). The difference between the force developed during bilateral action and the sum of the force developed by each limb independently is called bilateral deficit. This bilateral deficit is associated with reduced motor unit stimulation of mostly fast-twitch motor units (Jakobi and Chilibeck 2001; Vandervoot, Sale, and Moroz, 1984). The reduced motor unit stimulation could be due to inhibition by the protective mechanisms and subsequently less force production. Training with bilateral actions reduces bilateral deficit (Secher 1975), thus bringing bilateral force production closer to the sum of unilateral force production or greater. Although bilateral exercise reduces the bilateral deficit, the performance of unilateral exercises may be important to maintain the deficit, for example, in sports in which force production of one limb independently is required in reciprocal movements. Unilateral exercises can be performed using dumbbells and some types of weight training equipment.

Knowledge of the neural protective mechanisms is also useful in understanding the expression of maximal strength. Neural protective mechanisms appear to have their greatest effect in slow-velocity/high-resistance movements (Caiozzo et al. 1981; Dudley et al. 1990; Wickiewicz et al. 1984). A resistance training program in which the antagonists are activated immediately before performance of the exercise is more effective in increasing strength at low velocities than a program in which precontraction of the antagonists is not performed (Caiozzo et al. 1983). The precontraction in some way partially inhibits the neural self-protective mechanisms, thus allowing a more forceful action. Precontraction of the antagonists can be used as a method both to enhance the training effect and to inhibit the neural protective mechanisms during a maximal lift. For example, immediately before a maximal bench press, forceful actions of the arm flexors and muscles that adduct the scapula (i.e., pull the scapula toward the spine) should make possible a heavier maximal bench press than no precontraction of the antagonists.

Neural Changes and Long-Term Training

The neural component may also play a major role in mediating strength gains in advanced lifters. In a study by Häkkinen, Pakarinen, and colleagues (1988c), minimal changes in muscle fiber size were observed in competitive Olympic weightlifters, but strength and power increased over two years of training. EMG data demonstrated that voluntary activation of muscle was enhanced over the training period. Thus, even in advanced resistance-trained athletes, the mechanisms of strength and power improvement may be related to neural factors. It must be kept in mind that the subjects in this investigation were competitive weightlifters who compete in body mass classification groups, and gains in muscle mass may not necessarily enhance their competitive advantage. Furthermore, the types of programs used by Olympic weightlifters are primarily related to strength and power development (Garhammer and Takano 1992; Kraemer and Koziris 1994). Other types of programs for bodybuilders or other athletes may have some similar characteristics related to power development, but must also be designed to meet muscle mass needs, specific sport performance needs, or both. Thus, training goals and specific protocols play a key role in the neural adaptation to resistance training.

Sale (1992) described this dynamic interplay of neural and muscular hypertrophy factors (see figure 3.9). A dramatic increase in the adaptation of neural factors is observed over the time course (e.g., 6 to 10 weeks) used for most resistance training studies in the literature. As the duration of training increases (>10 weeks), muscle hypertrophy eventually takes place and contributes more than neural adaptations to the strength and power gains observed. However, eventually muscle hypertrophy also reaches a maximum and plateaus. It is interesting to note that increases in muscle fiber cross-sectional area range from about 20% to 40% in most training studies. Few studies have training periods long enough to increase muscle fiber size beyond this level of change. Muscle fiber cross-sectional area changes do not necessarily reflect the magnitude of changes in the whole muscle cross-sectional area determined by image systems (MRI, CAT

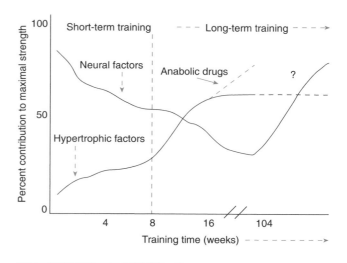

Figure 3.9 Dynamic interplay of neural and hypertrophic factors resulting in increased strength.

scans). This lack of relationship may be related to the possible need for several different exercises or training angles to stimulate the entire cross-sectional area of a whole muscle, whereas changes in a specific fiber may be brought about by only one exercise (Ploutz et al. 1994). Nevertheless, eventually strength and power gains derived from the "progressively and properly" loaded and activated musculature appear to be bounded by a genetic upper limit of neuromuscular adaptation (Häkkinen 1989).

Force-Velocity Curve

With strength training, ideally, the skeletal muscle **velocity and force-time curve** moves up and to the left (see figure 3.10). Yet this requires the optimal type of training configuration (e.g., periodization) in order to achieve changes in all phases of the force-velocity curve. Typically, periodized training strategies that address each of the components of the power equation (i.e., force and velocity) are used to maximize strength and develop power.

As the velocity of movement increases, the maximal force a muscle can produce concentrically (while shortening) decreases. This is empirically true. If an athlete is asked to perform a jump squat with the maximal amount of weight possible, the weight will move very slowly. But if the same athlete is asked to perform a jump squat with 30% of the maximal amount of weight, the bar moves at a faster velocity. Maximal velocity of shortening occurs when no resistance (weight)

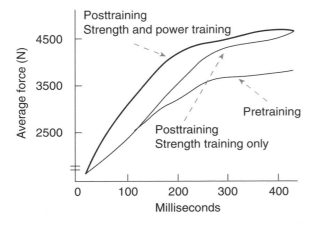

Figure 3.10 Response of the force-time curve for the squat movement to different types of resistance training programs.

is being moved or lifted. It is determined by the maximal rate at which cross-bridges can be formed and broken with the actin active sites. The force-velocity and force-time curves are important when examining various forms of weight training, such as power training, plyometric training, and isokinetic training.

Conversely, as the velocity of movement increases, the force that a muscle can develop eccentrically (lengthening) actually increases. This is thought to be due to the elastic component of muscle. However, the actual explanation for such a response remains unclear. It is interesting to note that eccentric force at even low velocities is higher than the highest concentric force or isometric force. Such high force development when using maximal eccentric muscle actions has been related to muscle damage in untrained individuals. However, it has been demonstrated that muscle exposed to repeated eccentric actions can adapt, and the damage per training session is reduced (Clarkson and Tremblay 1988; Gibala et al. 2000; Mair et al. 1995). Interestingly, eccentric force is not maximal at percentages of 1RM normally used for resistance training. Thus, the eccentric portion of the repetition may not be optimal in terms of strength gains.

The information concerning velocity at which training is performed points to four important conclusions (see the discussion of isokinetics in chapter 2). First, if the training program prescribes the use of only one velocity of movement, it should be an intermediate speed. Second, any training velocity increases strength within a range above and below the training velocity. Third, velocity-specific training may be needed for optimal performance

in some sports. Fourth, further research is needed to distinguish between the effects of neural factors and the effects of changes within the muscle fibers on the force-velocity curve.

Skeletal Muscle Fibers

Skeletal muscle fibers are unique as a cell in that they are multinucleated. Because of this basic fact, the protein that makes up the muscle fiber is under the control of different nuclei throughout the fiber. This has been called nuclear domains, meaning that different parts of the muscle fiber are controlled by different individual nuclei (Hall and Ralston 1989; Hikida et al. 1997; Pavlath et al. 1989) (see figure 3.11). Even more interesting is the fact that unless the number of nuclei is increased through mitotic division of activated satellite cells, muscle proteins may not be able to be added (Hawke and Garry 2001; Staron and Hikida 2001). Hypertrophy is not possible without an increase in the number of nuclei. The nuclei contain the DNA that genetically control the regulatory functions and adaptational abilities of each muscle cell.

Skeletal muscle is a heterogeneous mixture of several types of muscle fibers. Quantification of different biochemical and physical characteristics of the different muscle fibers has led to the development of several muscle fiber histochemical classification systems (Pette and Staron 1990). Although these classification systems appear similar, they are different. The characteristics of the type I and type II muscle fibers are shown in table 3.1.

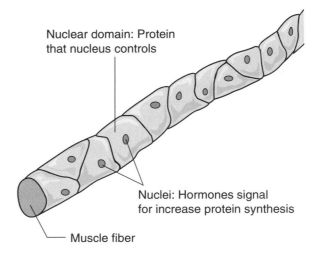

Figure 3.11 For muscular hypertrophy to occur, the number of nuclei in an individual muscle fiber must increase.

Table 3.1 Some of the Primary Muscle Fiber Type Classification Systems Seen in the Literature

Classification system	Theoretical basis
Red and white fibers	View of fiber color; the more myoglobin (oxygen carrier in a fiber), the darker or redder the color.
Fast twitch and slow twitch	Based on the speed and shape of the muscle twitch with stimulation. Fast-twitch fibers have higher rates of force development and a greater fatigue rate.
Slow oxidative, fast oxidative glycolytic, fast glycolytic	Based on metabolic staining and the characteristics of oxidative and glycolytic enzymes.
Type I and type II	Stability of the enzyme myosin ATPase under different pH conditions. The enzyme myosin ATPase has different forms, some of which result in quicker enzymatic reactions for ATP breakdown and thus higher cycling rates for that fiber's actin-myosin interactions.

Figure 3.12 presents how muscle fiber types are classified according to the most popular classification scheme using the histochemical myosin ATPase staining method. Myosin ATPase is the enzyme that is intimately involved in the cleaving of ATP to ADP, P_i, and energy. It is found on the heads of the myosin portion of the cross-bridges. This classification system is possible because different types of myosin ATPase are found in the different muscle fiber types. Different pH conditions result in different staining intensities of the different muscle fiber types. Myosin ATPase is an enzyme very specific to the cycling speed of myosin heads on the actin active sites; thus, it provides a functional classification representative of a muscle fiber's functional ability without the actual determination of "twitch speed."

The most common method of obtaining a muscle sample in humans is the muscle biopsy technique (see figure 3.13). A hollow stainless steel needle is used to obtain about 100 to 400 mg of muscle tissue (typically from a thigh, calf, or arm muscle). The sample is removed from the needle, processed, and then frozen. The muscle sample is then cut (sectioned) into consecutive (serial) sections and placed on cover slips for histochemical assay to determine the various muscle fiber types (Staron, Hagerman et al. 2001). Other variables (e.g., glycogen content of the fibers, receptor numbers, mitochondria, capillaries, other metabolic enzymes, etc.) can also be analyzed from a serial section of the biopsy sample.

Of great importance to the histochemical muscle fiber typing procedure is the fact that serial sections from the same muscle are placed into each of the preincubation baths, which consist of an alkaline (pH 10.4) and two acid (pH 4.6 and

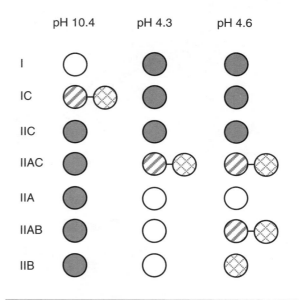

Figure 3.12 Myosin ATPase nomenclature for determination of type I and type II muscle fiber types. Hatching indicates intermediate staining between dark and light.

Courtesy of Dr. Robert S. Staron's laboratory.

4.3) baths before the rest of the histochemical assay. Ultimately, after the assay is completed, a muscle fiber is typed by comparing the fiber's color under each of the pH conditions (see figure 3.14).

In the classification system presented in figure 3.14, muscle fibers are classified as type I or type II. In addition, various muscle fiber subtypes (e.g., type IIA) can also be determined in both of the general type I and type II categories. The type I fiber is the most oxidative muscle fiber. Starting at the top and progressing toward the bottom in figure 3.12, each succeeding fiber type becomes

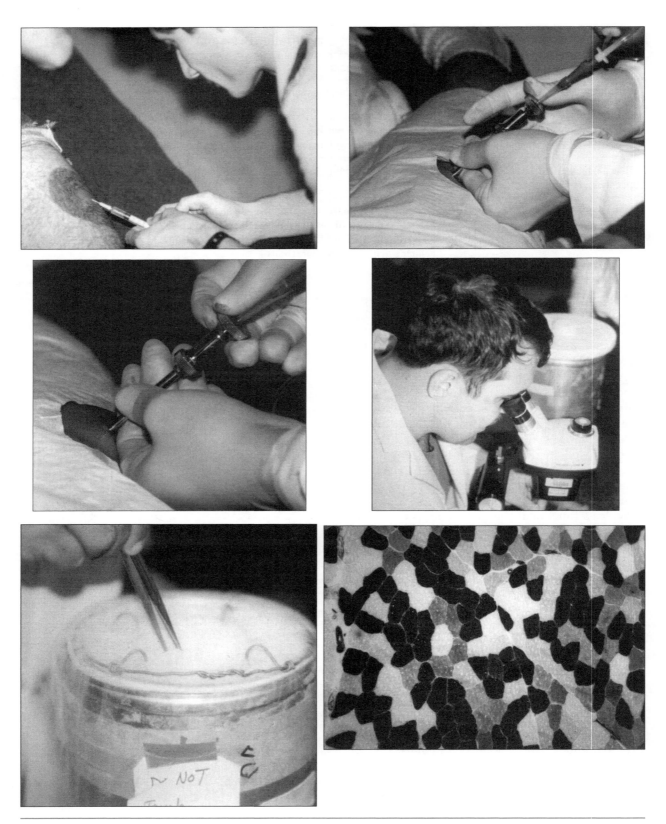

Figure 3.13 Obtaining and processing a muscle biopsy sample.
Courtesy of Dr. William Kraemer's laboratory.

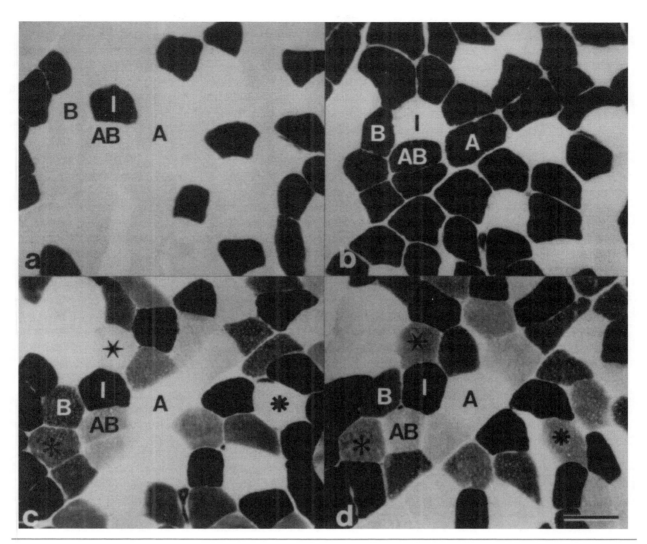

Figure 3.14 Myosin ATPase stained muscle fibers demonstrating types I, IIA, IIAB, and IIB fibers. *(a)* pH 4.3; *(b)* pH 10.4; *(c)* and *(d)* pH 4.6. ✳ and ✻ indicate fibers that stain slightly different in different serial sections of the same pH.

Courtesy of Dr. Robert S. Staron's laboratory.

less oxidative than the previous one. In figure 3.14 the various fiber subtypes can be seen in the muscle fibers after staining. Fiber subtypes are highly related to the type of myosin heavy chain (i.e., the most abundant protein in skeletal muscle) contained in the muscle's structure (Fry, Kraemer, Stone et al. 1994; Staron et al. 1991) and therefore related to the rate at which the cross-bridges can be cycled and so to "twitch speed."

Functional abilities have been associated with the classifications of fiber types because type II (white, fast twitch, fast oxidative glycolytic, fast glycolytic) and type I (red, slow twitch, slow oxidative) fibers have different metabolic and contractile properties. Table 3.2 shows that type

II fibers (fast twitch) are better adapted to perform anaerobic work, whereas type I fibers (slow twitch) are better adapted to perform aerobic work.

Type II fibers are suited to the performance of high-intensity, short-duration work bouts as evidenced by their biochemical and physical characteristics (see table 3.2). Such exercise bouts include a 40-m sprint, a 1RM lift, and sets with heavy resistance (2-4RM) of an exercise. These fiber types have a high activity of myofibrillar ATPase, the enzyme that breaks down ATP and releases the energy to cause fiber shortening. Type II fibers are able to shorten with a high contraction speed and have a fast relaxation time. These characteristics allow these fibers to develop

Table 3.2 Characteristics of Type I and Type II Muscle Fibers

Characteristic	Type I	Type II
Force per cross-sectional area	Low	High
Myofibrillar ATPase activity (ph 9.4)	Low	High
Intramuscular ATP stores	Low	High
Intramuscular PC stores	Low	High
Contraction speed	Slow	Fast
Relaxation time	Slow	Fast
Glycolytic enzyme activity	Low	High
Endurance	High	Low
Intramuscular glycogen stores	No difference	No difference
Intramuscular triglyceride stores	High	Low
Myoglobin content	High	Low
Aerobic enzyme activity	High	Low
Capillary density	High	Low
Mitochondrial density	High	Low

force in a short period of time or to have a high power output. Type II fibers rely predominantly on anaerobic sources to supply the energy necessary for muscle activation. This is evidenced by their high levels of ATP and PC intramuscular stores, as well as their high glycolytic enzyme activity. Type II fibers have a low aerobic capability as evidenced by their low intramuscular stores of triglyceride, low capillary density, low mitochondria density, and low aerobic enzyme activity. The fact that type II fibers rely predominantly on anaerobic sources of ATP and have low capabilities to supply ATP aerobically makes them highly susceptible to fatigue. Type II fibers are suited to perform activities in which a large power output is necessary and the activity is of short duration.

Type I fibers are more suited to the performance of endurance (aerobic) activities. Type I fibers have characteristics that include high levels of aerobic enzyme activity, capillary density, mitochondrial density, intramuscular triglyceride stores, and low fatigability. Type I fibers are ideal for the performance of low-intensity, long-duration (endurance) activities. Such activities include long-distance running and swimming, and long sets of an exercise (20 repetitions or more or super-slow contractions).

As discussed previously, several subtypes of type I and type II fibers have been demonstrated. Type IIA fibers possess good aerobic and anaerobic characteristics, whereas type IIB fibers possess good anaerobic characteristics but poor aerobic characteristics (Essen et al. 1975; Staron, Hagerman et al. 2001; Staron, Hikida, and Hagerman 1983). It now appears that the type IIB fibers may in fact be just a pool of unused fibers (with low oxidative ability) that upon recruitment start a shift or transformation ultimately to the type IIA fiber type (Adams et al. 1993; Staron et al. 1991, 1994). Dramatic reductions in the IIB fiber type occur with heavy resistance training, which supports such a theory. Type IIC fibers are very rare in humans and are more oxidative than type IIA and IIB fibers in several biochemical characteristics. Type IIAB fibers represent a hybrid or, in other words, a combination of both type IIA and B fiber types and may be a transition phase to an intermediate fiber type.

The type I muscle fiber has only one subtype, IC. There are very few type IC fibers (usually less than 5% of the total), and they are a less oxidative (aerobic) form of the type I fiber. With resistance training or anaerobic training, type IC fibers may increase in number due to the lack of an oxidative stress with the training modality.

Type II muscle fiber subtypes represent a continuum from the least oxidative type IIB to the more oxidative type IIC. The larger array of type II muscle fibre subtypes allows for a greater transformation among type II fiber subtypes with physical training (Ingjer 1969; Staron, Hikida, and Hagerman 1983; Staron et al. 1991, 1994). A number of older studies not using a full spectrum fiber type profile suggested that a fiber transformation may occur between the type I and type II fibers with exercise training (Haggmark, Jansson, and Eriksson 1982; Howald 1982). However, it now appears that the changes occur only within the subtypes of type I or type II fibers and that these early studies most likely were in error due to a lack of histochemical subtyping of all muscle fiber subtypes.

Sliding Filament Theory

How muscle contracted remained a mystery until an interesting theory was proposed in the middle of the 20th century. In 1954 a paper published in *Nature* by A.F. Huxley and R. Niedergerke and another by H.E. Huxley and E.J. Hansen provided the first fundamentally important insights that sarcomere shortening was associated with the sliding of myosin and actin filaments without these filaments themselves changing significantly in length. When the sarcomere shortens, myosin filaments remain stationary while myosin heads pull the actin filaments over the myosin filaments, resulting in the actin filaments sliding over the myosin filaments. A.F. Huxley (2000) overviewed a host of new findings on the dynamics of muscle contraction, but interestingly, the basic theory remains intact.

The contractile proteins are in fact held in a very tight relationship by the noncontractile proteins, which make up an extensive type of basket weave to keep the protein filaments of the sarcomere in place. The sarcomere is the basic muscle unit capable of developing force and shortening (see figure 3.15).

To understand the **sliding filament theory** of muscular activation, it is necessary to know the structural arrangement of skeletal muscle. Skeletal muscle is called striated muscle because the arrangement of protein molecules in the muscle give it a striped or striated appearance under a microscope (see figure 3.16). Muscle fibers are composed of sarcomeres stacked one on top of the other. At rest, there are several distinct light and dark areas creating striations within each sarcomere. These light and dark areas are due to the arrangement of the actin and myosin filaments, the major proteins involved in the contractile process. In the contracted (fully shortened) state, there are still striations, but they have a different pattern. This change in the striation pattern occurs due to the sliding of the actin over the myosin protein filaments.

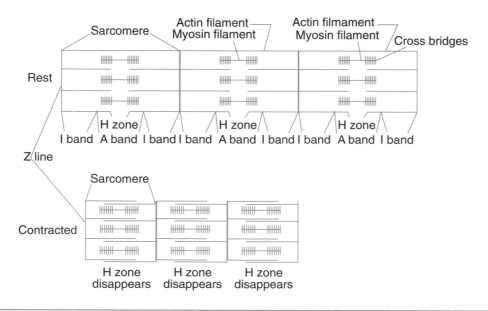

Figure 3.15 Sarcomere demonstrating the sliding filament theory. As the actin and myosin filament slide over each other, the entire sarcomere shortens, but the length of the individual actin and myosin filaments does not change.

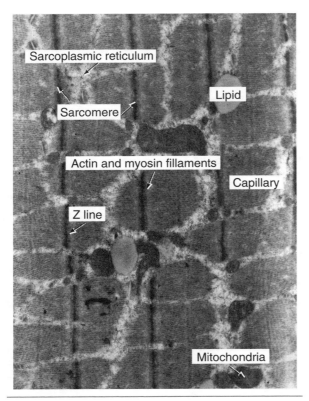

Figure 3.16 An electron micrograph demonstrating the striated appearance of human skeletal muscle and some structures present in it. Sarcomeres are fully shortened.

Courtesy of Dr. William Kraemer's laboratory.

A sarcomere runs from one Z line to the next Z line and is the smallest unit of a muscle fiber that can shorten. At rest there are two distinct light areas in each sarcomere: the H zone, which con-

tains no actin but does contain myosin; and the I bands located at the ends of the sarcomere, which contain only actin filaments. These two areas appear light in comparison to the A band, which contains actin and myosin filaments.

As the sarcomere shortens, the actin filaments slide over the myosin filaments. This causes the H zone to seem to disappear as actin filaments slide into it and give it a darker appearance. The I bands become shorter as the Z lines come closer to the ends of the myosin filaments. When the sarcomere relaxes and returns to its original length, the H zone and I bands return to their original size and appearance.

Phases of Muscle Action

Since the sliding filament theory was originally proposed, a great deal more has been discovered about how the protein filaments of muscle interact (Huxley 2000). At rest, the projections or cross-bridges of the myosin filaments touch the actin filaments, but cannot interact to cause shortening. The actin filament has active sites on which the myosin cross-bridges can interact with the actin to cause shortening. At rest, however, the active sites are covered by troponin and tropomyosin, two regulatory proteins that are associated with the actin filament (see figure 3.17).

When ACh causes an ionic current within the membrane surrounding the muscle fiber, it triggers the release of calcium ions (Ca^{++}) from the sarcoplasmic reticulum. The sarcoplasmic reticulum is a membranous structure that surrounds each muscle

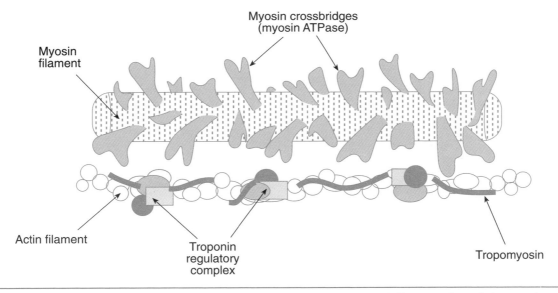

Figure 3.17 Schematic of a myosin and actin filament. The active sites are located on the actin filament underneath the troponin and tropomyosin molecules.

fiber. The released Ca++ binds to the troponin molecule, and this triggers a change in the troponin and tropomyosin that exposes the active sites on the actin. This is called the steric blocking model. With the active site now exposed, the myosin cross-bridges make contact with the active sites.

Contraction, or shortening of the sarcomere, can now take place. The attachment of the cross-bridge to the active site activates an enzyme (myosin ATPase) that breaks down an ATP (adenosine triphosphate) molecule located on the cross-bridge head and in so doing releases energy. ATP is an energy source for many cellular activities including muscle contraction. The released energy is used to cause the cross-bridge to swivel to a new angle or to collapse. The result of either of these two actions is to pull the actin over the myosin, causing the sarcomere to shorten. The tilt of the cross-bridge arm has been generally accepted as producing all of the force generation in muscle, but recent studies now implicate a much more complicated series of steps in the movement of the cross-bridge and possible roles for other factors such as nonmyosin proteins and temperature (for a detailed review, see Huxley 2000).

For further shortening to occur, the cross-bridge must break with the active site with which it is in contact and bind to another active site on the actin filament closer to the Z line. This is accomplished by reloading the cross-bridge with an ATP molecule. Once the cross-bridge is reloaded, it breaks the bond with the active site with which it is in contact and binds to a new active site closer to the Z line. The process of breaking contact with one active site and binding to another is termed recharging. ATPase breaks down the new ATP, causing the cross-bridge head to be cocked and ready for interaction with a new active site. Upon contact with a new active site, the myosin head again swivels forward or collapses. This causes the actin to slide further over the myosin, resulting in shortening of the sarcomere. This cyclical (or "ratcheting") process is repeated until either the sarcomere has shortened as much as possible or relaxation of the muscle takes place.

Relaxation of the muscle occurs when the impulse from the alpha motor neuron ends. This triggers the active pumping of Ca++ back into the sarcoplasmic reticulum. This pump mechanism requires energy from the breakdown of ATP to function. The troponin and tropomyosin assume their original position covering the active sites. The cross-bridges of the myosin filament now have no place at which to contact the actin and pull the actin over the myosin. With relaxation, muscle activity stops and the muscle may remain in the shortened position unless pulled to a lengthened position by gravity or an outside force, such as an antagonistic muscle, because muscle can only shorten and produce force.

Length-Tension (Force) Curve

The **length-tension (force) curve** (see figure 3.18) demonstrates that there is an optimal length at which muscle fibers generate maximal force. The total amount of force developed depends on the total number of myosin cross-bridges interacting with active sites on the actin. At the optimal length there is the potential for maximal cross-bridge interaction and thus maximal force. Below this optimal length, less tension is developed during activation because with excessive shortening there is an overlap of actin filaments such that the actin filaments interfere with each other's ability to contact the myosin cross-bridges. Less cross-bridge contact with the active sites on the actin results in a smaller potential to develop tension.

At lengths greater than optimal there is less and less overlap of the actin and myosin filaments. This results in less of a potential for cross-bridge contact with the active sites on the actin. Thus, if the sarcomere's length is greater than optimal, less force can be developed.

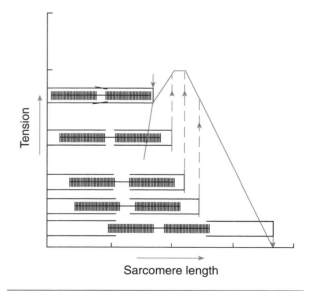

Figure 3.18 There is an optimal length at which a sarcomere develops maximal tension. At lengths less than or greater than optimal, less tension is developed.

Data from A.M Gordon, A.F. Huxley, and E. Julian, 1966, "The variation and isometric tension with sarcomere length in vertebrate muscle fibers," *Journal of Physiology* 7: 170-192.

The length-tension curve indicates that some prestretch of the muscle before initiation of a contraction will increase the amount of force generated. Many everyday and sporting activities do involve a prestretch. For example, every time the knee slightly bends before knee extension while walking, the quadriceps muscle is prestretched. Some power lifters attempt to use a prestretch by pulling their shoulders back (adducting the scapulas) and stretching the pectoral muscles before performing the bench press.

Bioenergetics

Bioenergetics concerns the sources of energy for muscle activity. Such terms as *aerobic* (energy production with oxygen) and *anaerobic* (energy production without the immediate need for oxygen) *training* have become popular among fitness enthusiasts, coaches, and athletes. There are two major sources to produce anaerobic energy (phosphocreatine system and anaerobic glycolysis) and one source to produce aerobic energy (oxidative phosphorylation). Knowledge of these energy sources and their interactions with each other is necessary to successfully plan a resistance training program that will optimally condition an individual for a particular sport or activity. Each sport activity will have a different energy demand and profile. Resistance training primarily enhances anaerobic and to a lesser extent aerobic metabolism.

ATP, the Energy Molecule

The source of energy for muscle activation is the adenosine triphosphate molecule or ATP. The main functional components of ATP are a sugar molecule called adenosine and three phosphate groups. When ATP is broken down to adenosine diphosphate (ADP, two phosphates) and a free phosphate molecule (P_i), energy is released. This energy is used for many different functions in the body including providing the energy for cross-bridge movement, thereby pulling the actin filaments across the myosin filaments to shorten the muscle. ATP is the immediate energy source for muscular actions (see figure 3.19). However, all three major energy sources supply ATP in different ways.

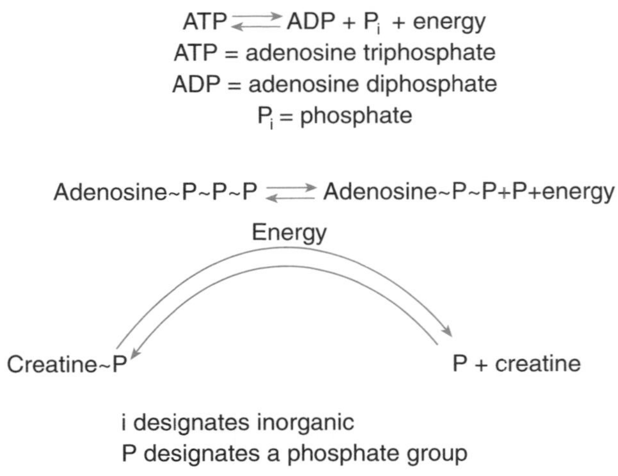

$$ATP \rightleftharpoons ADP + P_i + energy$$

ATP = adenosine triphosphate
ADP = adenosine diphosphate
P_i = phosphate

Adenosine~P~P~P $\rightleftharpoons$ Adenosine~P~P+P+energy
Energy
Creatine~P   P + creatine

i designates inorganic
P designates a phosphate group

Figure 3.19 When ATP breaks down to ADP, the derived energy can be used to perform muscular actions. When PC breaks down to P and C, the energy released is used to rebuild ATP.

Phosphocreatine Source

Stored within muscle and ready for immediate use to supply energy to the muscle are two compounds that chemically work together to allow fast energy availability—ATP and phosphocreatine (PC). PC is similar to ATP in that it also has a phosphate group and a high energy bond. In PC the phosphate group is bound to a creatine molecule. PC provides a convenient mechanism to help maintain ATP concentrations. When ATP is broken down to ADP and P_i, energy is released. This energy is used to produce muscular actions. However, when PC is broken down to creatine and P_i, the resulting energy is used to recombine ADP and P_i back into ATP (see figure 3.19). The rebuilt ATP can then be broken down again to ADP and P_i and the energy released used to perform more muscular actions. The energy released from the breakdown of PC cannot be used to cause muscle shortening because PC does not fit on the cross-bridges.

ATP and PC are stored within the muscle. There are, however, limited intramuscular stores of ATP and PC; this limits the amount of energy that the ATP-PC source can produce. In fact, in an all-out exercise bout, the energy available from the ATP-PC source will be exhausted in 30 seconds or less (Meyer and Terjung 1979). Depletion of intramuscular ATP and PC in some muscle fibers is the cause of the inability to perform two repetitions with a true one repetition maximum weight. One advantage of this energy source is that the energy is immediately available for use. A second advantage is that the ATP-PC source has a large power capacity, or is capable of giving the muscle a large amount of energy per second.

Because of the characteristics of the ATP-PC energy source, it is the primary source of energy for short-duration, high-power events. It supplies the major portion of energy to the muscles for such activities as a maximal lift, the shot put, the high jump, and the 40-yd dash. One of the reasons for continued heavy breathing after the completion of an intense short-duration exercise bout is that the muscular stores of ATP and PC must be replenished aerobically if the ATP-PC energy source is to be used again at a later time. The success of creatine supplementation for improving explosive and repeated burstlike activities underscores the importance of this energy source (Volek et al. 1999).

Anaerobic Glycolysis or Lactic Acid Energy Source

The extreme fatigue and nauseous feeling after several sets of a 10RM squat with only a minute rest between sets is due in part to the buildup of lactate. The breakdown of lactic acid in the muscle to lactate and its associated hydrogen ions causes concentrations of these compounds to increase in the muscle and blood. Lactate itself can contribute to fatigue by reducing the force the muscle is capable of producing (Hogan et al. 1995). Lactic acid breakdown causes the acid level of the body to build up and pH to decrease. With severe exercise, blood pH can go from a resting level of 7.4 to as low as 6.6 (Gordon et al. 1994; Sahlin and Ren 1989). This increase in hydrogen ions and decrease in pH are thought to be major contributors to fatigue (Gordon, Kraemer, and Pedro 1991).

Glycogen, a carbohydrate, is stored within the muscle. Glycogen is a long chain of glucose molecules. Glucose is a type of sugar. The energy necessary to make ATP is derived by splitting glucose molecules in half to yield two pyruvate molecules and release energy. The energy released from splitting each glucose molecule produces a net gain of two ATP. The pyruvate is then transformed into lactic acid. No oxygen is required for this process to take place, so this energy system is anaerobic.

The buildup of lactate in the muscle and blood has several side effects. One of these effects occurs when the lactate and hydrogen ion concentrations are high enough to affect nerve endings, causing pain. As the concentration of lactate increases, the interior of the muscle cells becomes more acidic. This can interfere with the chemical processes of the cell, including the processes of producing more ATP (Trivedi and Dansforth 1966) and altering membrane ion (sodium and potassium) permeability. This in turn results in hyperpolarization, which inhibits glycolysis through allosteric regulation of enzyme function, and the binding of Ca^{++} to troponin (Nakamaru and Schwartz 1972). The amount of energy that can be obtained from the lactic acid source is therefore limited due to the side effects of lactate, hydrogen ions, and decreased pH.

Despite the side effects of lactate accumulation, this energy source can produce a greater amount of energy than the ATP-PC source. Anaerobic glycolysis, however, cannot supply the muscle with as much energy per second as the phosphocreatine source and therefore is not as powerful.

The lactic acid energy source is a major supplier of ATP in all-out exercise bouts lasting from approximately 1 to 3 minutes (Kraemer et al. 1989). Such exercise bouts may include high-intensity sets at 10 to 12RM with very short rest periods (30 to 60 seconds) and the 400-m run. Heavy breathing continues after completion of these types of exercise bouts. This is in part due to the need to remove the accumulated lactate from the body.

Oxygen Energy Source

The oxygen energy source has received a lot of attention for many years. The major goal of jogging, swimming, and aerobic dancing is to improve cardiovascular fitness, which is analogous to improving oxidative phosphorylation. This energy source uses oxygen in the production of ATP and is therefore an aerobic energy source.

The oxidative phosphorylation system can metabolize carbohydrates (sugar) and fats. Significant amounts of protein are normally not metabolized. However, during long-term starvation and long exercise bouts significant amounts of protein (up to 10%) can be metabolized to produce energy (Dohm et al. 1982; Lemon and Mullin 1980; Tarnopolsky, MacDougall, and Atkinson 1988). Normally, at rest the body derives one-third of the needed ATP from metabolizing carbohydrates and two-thirds from fats. During physical exercise there is a gradual change to metabolizing more and more carbohydrates and less and less fats as the intensity of the exercise increases. During maximal physical exercise the muscle is metabolizing nearly 100% carbohydrates if sufficient carbohydrates are available (Maresh et al. 1989, 1992).

Aerobic metabolism of the carbohydrate glycogen begins in the same manner as it does in anaerobic glycolysis. Here, however, due to the presence of sufficient oxygen, the pyruvate is not converted into lactic acid, but enters into two long series of chemical reactions called Kreb's cycle and electron transport. These series of reactions eventually produce carbon dioxide, which is expired through the lungs, and water. The water is produced by combining hydrogen molecules with the oxygen that was originally taken into the body through the lungs. Thirty-eight molecules of ATP can be produced by aerobically metabolizing one glucose molecule. The aerobic metabolism of fats does not start with glycolysis. Fats go through a series of reactions called beta oxidation and then enter directly into Kreb's cycle. The end products of fat metabolism are similarly water, carbon dioxide, and ATP.

The maximal amount of energy that can be produced via aerobic metabolism is dependent on how much oxygen the body can obtain and use. Maximal aerobic power (VO$_2$peak) is the maximal amount of oxygen the body can obtain and use per unit of time. It is usually expressed either in absolute terms as liters of oxygen per minute (L O$_2 \cdot$min^{-1}), or in relative terms as milliliters of oxygen per kilogram (2.2 lb) of body weight per minute (ml O$_2 \cdot$kg$^{-1} \cdot$min^{-1}). VO$_2$peak in L O$_2 \cdot$min^{-1} does not take into account body mass. A larger individual might be expected to use more oxygen per minute solely due to his or her body size. Expressing VO$_2$peak in ml O$_2 \cdot$kg$^{-1} \cdot$min^{-1} places everyone on a scale relative to body mass. In this manner, comparisons can be made among individuals of different body mass.

Compared to the two anaerobic energy producing systems, the oxidative phosphorylation source is the least powerful. The aerobic energy source cannot produce enough ATP per second to allow the performance of maximal intensity exercise, such as a 1RM lift or a 40-m sprint. On the other hand, the aerobic energy source, due to the abundance of glycogen and fats and the lack of producing by-products that can inhibit performance, can supply virtually an unlimited amount of ATP over a long period of time. Therefore, it is the predominant energy source for long-duration, low-intensity activities. Such activities range from extremely long sets of an exercise at a low intensity (resistance) to distance running (e.g., the marathon or ultra-marathon). In addition, this energy source contributes a moderate to high percentage of the ATP during activities composed of high-intensity work interspaced with rest periods or high-intensity activities lasting longer than about 25 seconds, such as interval run training and wrestling. These activities result in very high blood lactate ranging from 15 to 22 mmol · L^{-1} (Serresse et al. 1988). Performance of these activities requires both the oxygen and lactate energy sources to contribute significant amounts of energy. During many activities one energy source provides the majority of needed energy, but all energy sources contribute some of the needed energy.

Repayment of the Anaerobic Energy Sources

After an intense exercise bout, the anaerobic energy sources must be replenished if they are to be used again at a later time. The anaerobic energy sources are replenished by the aerobic energy source. After cessation of an anaerobic activity, heavy breathing continues for a period of time, even though physical activity is no longer taking place. The oxygen taken into the body, above the resting value, is used to replenish the two anaerobic energy sources. This extra oxygen has been referred to as an "oxygen debt" or more recently the "excess postexercise oxygen consumption" or EPOC. Research suggests that aerobic fitness does aid in repayment of the anaerobic energy stores (Tomlin and Wenger 2001). Therefore, it may be prudent for weightlifters and anaerobic-type athletes to maintain at least average aerobic fitness to aid in recovery between anaerobic work bouts and so aid in maintaining the quality of training sessions and repeat performances, such as the repetitive sprints separated by short rest periods found in some sports.

Replenishing the ATP-PC Energy Source

Immediately after an intense exercise bout, there is a several-minute period of very heavy, rapid breathing. The oxygen taken into the body above normal resting oxygen consumption is used to aerobically produce ATP in excess of what is required at rest. Part of this excess ATP is immediately broken down to ADP and P_i; the energy released is used to combine P_i and creatine back into PC. Part of the excess ATP is simply stored as intramuscular ATP. This rebuilding of the ATP and PC stores is accomplished in several minutes (Hultman, Bergstrom, and Anderson 1967; Karlsson et al. 1975; Lemon and Mullin 1980). This part of EPOC has been referred to as the alactacid portion of the oxygen debt.

The half-life of the alactacid portion of the oxygen debt has been estimated to be approximately 20 seconds (DiPrampero and Margaria 1978; Meyer and Terjung 1979) and as long as 36 to 48 seconds (Laurent et al. 1992). Half-life means that within that time period 50% or half of the alactacid debt is repaid. So within 20 to 48 seconds, 50% of the depleted ATP and PC are replenished; in 40 to 96 seconds, 75% is replenished; and in 60 to 144 seconds, 87% is replenished. Thus, within approximately 3 to 4 minutes the majority of the depleted ATP and PC intramuscular stores are replenished.

If activity is performed during the alactacid portion of the oxygen debt, the rebuilding of the ATP and PC intramuscular stores will take longer. This is because part of the ATP generated via the aerobic source has to be used to provide energy to perform the activity. An understanding both of the alactacid portion of the oxygen debt and of the rebuilding of the ATP-PC energy source is important in the planning of a training program that involves short-duration, high-intensity work, such as heavy sets of an exercise. The ATP-PC energy source is the most powerful energy source and is therefore the major source of energy for maximal lifts and heavy sets. Several minutes of rest must be allowed between heavy sets and maximal lifts to replenish the ATP and PC intramuscular stores; otherwise, they will not be available for use in the next heavy set. If sufficient recovery time is not allowed between heavy sets or maximal lifts, the lift or set either will not be completed for the desired number of repetitions or it will not be completed with the desired speed or technique.

Replenishing the Lactic Acid Energy Source

The anaerobic energy source is also, in part, responsible for removing accumulated lactate from the body. However, in this case, the oxygen taken in above resting values is used in part to aerobically metabolize the lactate accumulated during activity. This produces energy needed by the tissues and is termed the lactacid portion of the oxygen debt.

The relationship between the lactacid portion of the oxygen debt and lactate removal has been questioned (Roth, Stanley, and Brooks 1988); however, many tissues of the body can aerobically metabolize lactate. Skeletal muscle active during an exercise bout (Hatta et al. 1989; McLoughlin, McCaffrey, and Moynihan 1991), skeletal muscle inactive during an exercise bout (Kowalchuk et al. 1988), cardiac muscle (Hatta et al. 1989; Spitzer 1974; Stanley 1991), kidneys (Hatta et al. 1989; Yudkin and Cohen 1974), the liver (Rowell et al. 1966; Wasserman, Connely, and Pagliassotti 1991), and the brain (Nemoto, Hoff, and Sereringhaus 1974) can all metabolize lactate. Up to 60% of the accumulated lactate is aerobically metabolized (Gasser and Brooks 1979). Portions of the remaining 40% are converted to glucose and protein, and a small portion is excreted in the urine and sweat (Ingjer 1969). The half-life of the lactacid portion of the oxygen debt is approximately 25 minutes (Hermansen et al. 1976). Thus, approximately 95% of the accumulated lactic acid is removed from the blood in 1 hour and 15 minutes.

If light activity (walking, slow jogging) is performed after a workout, the accumulated lactate is removed more quickly than if complete rest follows the workout (Hermansen et al. 1976; Hildebrandt, Schutze, and Stegemann 1992; McLoughlin, McCaffrey, and Moynihan 1991; Mero 1988). When light activity is performed after the activity, a portion of the accumulated lactate is aerobically metabolized to supply some of the needed ATP to perform the light activity. It also appears that accumulated lactate is removed from the blood more quickly if the light activity is performed by the muscles active during the exercise bout and not by the muscles that were inactive during the exercise bout (Hildebrandt, Schutze, and Stegemann 1992). The light activity must be below the individual's lactic acid threshold or the work intensity below which a significant increase in blood lactate occurs. For aerobically untrained individuals, lactic acid threshold is at approximately 50 to 60% of peak oxygen consumption. As aerobic condition increases, so does the lactic acid threshold.

Light activity between sets during a weight training workout has been shown to be beneficial (Corder et al. 2000). Six sets of squats (85% of 10RM) were performed with 4-minute rest periods between sets. During the rest period the lifters either sat quietly or pedaled a bike at 25% or 50% of peak oxygen consumption. Blood lactate was significantly lower when pedaling a bike at 25% peak oxygen consumption compared to the other two types of rest periods. Additionally, at the end of the workout during which a bike was ridden at 25% peak oxygen, more repetitions were performed in a set to volitional fatigue (65% of 10RM) at the end of the workout compared to the other types of rest periods. Thus, light work can aid in a weight training workout if the rest periods are of sufficient length. Because of this, it is recommended that, if practical, the rest period between sets in which lactate accumulation occurs (e.g., short rest period programs or circuit weight training) consist of light activity of the muscles used during the activity rather than complete rest.

Interaction of the Energy Sources

Although one energy source may be the predominant energy source for a particular activity (e.g., ATP-PC for a maximal lift, aerobic for running a marathon), all three sources supply a portion of the ATP needed by the body at all times. Thus, the ATP-PC energy source is operating even when the body is at rest, and the aerobic energy source is operating during a maximal lift. Even at rest some lactate is being released by muscles into the blood (Brooks et al. 1991). During a marathon, even though the majority of energy is supplied by the oxygen energy source, a small percentage of the needed energy is supplied by the ATP-PC and lactic acid energy sources.

Although all three energy sources supply some portion of the ATP necessary for any activity, as the duration and intensity of activity changes, the predominant energy source also changes. At one end of the spectrum are activities such as a maximal lift, the shot put, and a 40-yd (36.7-m) sprint. The ATP-PC energy source supplies the vast majority of energy for these activities. The lactic acid energy source supplies the majority of the necessary energy for activities such as sets of 20 to 25 repetitions, three sets of 10RM with 1-minute rest periods, and 200-m sprints. The aerobic energy source supplies the majority of the needed ATP for extremely long sets and 5-mile runs. However, all three energy sources are still producing some energy at all times.

There is no exact point at which one energy source provides the majority of ATP energy for an activity. Shifting in the percentage contribution from each particular energy source is based on the intensity and duration of the activity. For example, as a marathon runner climbs a hill and lactate accumulates in the body, the lactic acid source is contributing more energy to the performance of the activity. The contribution of all three energy sources to an activity is dynamic and changes as the intensity and duration of the activity changes.

Bioenergetic Adaptations

Increases in the activities of an energy source's enzymes can lead to more ATP production and use per unit of time. This could lead to increases in physical performance. Enzyme activity of the ATP-PC energy source (e.g., creatine phosphokinase and myokinase) has been shown to increase in humans after isokinetic training (Costill et al. 1979) and traditional resistance training (Komi et al. 1982; Thorstensson et al. 1976), and in rats after isometric training (Exner, Staudte, and Pette 1973). Costill and colleagues (1979) used two training regimes for the legs in their isokinetic study. The enzymes associated with the ATP-PC energy source showed significant increases of approximately 12% in the leg trained with 30-second bouts and insignificant changes in the leg trained with 6-second bouts. According to these findings, enzymatic changes associated with the ATP-PC energy source are linked to the duration of the exercise bouts; the changes do not take place with exercise bouts of 6 seconds or less. However, little change, no change, or a decrease in enzymes (creatine phosphokinase and myokinase) associated with the ATP-PC energy source have also been observed after resistance training (Tesch, Komi, and Häkkinen 1987; Tesch 1992). This emphasizes the point that the type of program will affect the enzymatic adaptations. In addition, most studies showing no change or a decrease in enzyme activity also reported significant muscle hypertrophy. This indicates that initially enzyme activity may increase in response to resistance training, but it may not change or decrease with subsequent training producing significant muscle hypertrophy due to protein dilution (e.g., a reduction in concentration per unit of muscle weight due to increased muscle cross-sectional area).

Costill and colleagues (1979) also demonstrated a significant increase in phosphofructokinase (PFK), an enzyme associated with the lactic acid energy source of 7% and 18%, respectively, in the

6-second- and 30-second-trained legs. Neither leg showed a significant increase in a second enzyme (lactate dehydrogenase) associated with the lactic acid energy source. The enzyme phosphorylase has also been shown to increase after 12 weeks of resistance training (Green et al. 1999). The enzymes PFK, lactate dehydrogenase, and hexokinase have also been shown to be unaffected by or to decrease after heavy resistance exercise training (Green et al. 1999; Houston et al. 1983; Komi et al. 1982; Tesch 1987; Tesch, Thorsson, and Colliander 1990; Thorstensson et al. 1976). Thus, the type of lifting protocol and the magnitude of muscle hypertrophy affect the adaptations of any of the enzymes associated with the lactic acid energy source, just as they affect the enzymes associated with the ATP-PC energy source.

Increases in the activity of enzymes associated with aerobic metabolism have been reported with isokinetic training in humans (Costill et al. 1979), isometric training in humans (Grimby et al. 1973), and isometric training in rats (Exner et al. 1973). Enzymatic changes associated with the aerobic energy source may also be dependent on the duration of individual exercise bouts (Costill et al. 1979). However, enzymes involved with aerobic metabolism obtained from pooled samples of weight-trained muscle fibers have not demonstrated increased activity (Tesch 1992), have been shown to decrease with resistance training (Chilibeck, Syrotuik, and Bell 1999), and have been lower in lifters compared to untrained individuals (Tesch, Thorsson, and Essen-Gustavsson 1989). Bodybuilders using high-volume programs, short rest periods between sets and exercises, and moderate-intensity training resistances have been shown to have higher citrate synthase activity in type II fibers than other types of lifters who train with heavier loads and take longer rest periods between sets (Tesch 1992). However, since bodybuilders typically perform aerobic exercise as well as resistance training, cross-sectional data should be viewed with caution. Again, the type of program may influence the magnitude of enzyme changes in the muscle.

An enzyme associated with all three energy sources, myosin ATPase, has shown only minor changes in pooled muscle fibers (Tesch 1992). The fact that various types of myosin ATPase exist and are altered with strength training may indicate that this enzyme is more important than the absolute concentration change.

Enzymatic changes associated with any of the three energy sources are dependent on the duration of individual sets rather than the total amount of work performed. For practical application, normal heavy resistance programs will have a minimal effect on enzyme activities over time. However, a training program that minimizes hypertrophy and targets specific energy systems will most likely result in increased enzyme activities.

Muscle Substrate Stores

One adaptation that can lead to increased physical performance is an increase in the fuel available to the three energy sources. In humans it has been demonstrated that after 5 months of strength training the resting intramuscular concentrations of phosphocreatine (PC) and ATP are elevated 28% and 18%, respectively (MacDougall et al. 1977), although this finding is not supported by other studies (Tesch 1992). Another study has shown that the resting PC to inorganic phosphate ratio increases after 5 weeks of resistance training (Walker et al. 1998). The concept that PC and ATP stores are not increased by performing resistance training is supported by normal concentrations of PC and ATP in athletes having a significant amount of muscular hypertrophy (Tesch 1992).

A 66% increase in intramuscular glycogen stores was shown after resistance training for 5 months (MacDougall et al. 1977). Bodybuilders have been shown to have approximately a 50% greater concentration of glycogen than untrained individuals (Tesch 1992). However, muscle glycogen content has also been shown to not change with resistance training (Tesch 1992). Several research studies have also shown that blood glucose levels do not change significantly during resistance training sessions (Keul et al. 1978; Kraemer et al. 1990). This indicates that the supply of glucose to muscle will not limit the performance of normal resistance training. Whether an increase in PC and ATP occurs with resistance training may depend on pretraining status, the muscle group examined, and the type of program performed. However, it is clear that skeletal muscle glycogen content can increase after resistance training and that blood glucose concentrations do not decrease during resistance training. This indicates that at least during one training session fuel availability for the lactic acid energy source is not a limiting factor to performance.

The aerobic energy source uses glycogen (carbohydrates), triglycerides (fats), and some protein to produce ATP. It has already been stated that intramuscular glycogen stores can be increased through strength training. The enhancement of triglyceride stores in muscles after resistance training remains equivocal, as decreased and no difference from normal triglyceride content in the muscles of trained lifters have been reported (Tesch 1992). Increased lipid content has been observed in the triceps, but not in the quadriceps after training (Tesch 1992). Thus, there may be differences in the response of different muscle groups in terms of triglyceride stores. Although dietary practices and the type of program may affect triglyceride concentrations, it can be speculated that because most resistance training programs are anaerobic in nature, intramuscular triglyceride concentrations are minimally affected by resistance training unless accompanied by significant weight or fat mass loss.

Myoglobin Content

Muscle myoglobin content may decrease after strength training (Tesch 1992). Thus, it has been postulated that long-term strength training may depress myoglobin content and therefore the ability of the muscle fibers to extract oxygen. Again, the initial state of training as well as the specific type of program and magnitude of hypertrophy may influence the effect of resistance training on myoglobin content.

Capillary Supply

An increased number of capillaries in a muscle helps support metabolism by increasing the potential blood supply to the muscle. With typical resistance training (three sets of 10 repetitions) over 12 weeks, McCall and colleagues (1996) observed significant increases in the numbers of capillaries per type I and type II fibers. However, because of fiber hypertrophy, no changes in capillaries per fiber area or per area of muscle was shown. Improved capillarization has been observed with resistance training of untrained subjects (Frontera et al. 1988; Hather et al. 1991; Staron et al. 1989; Tesch 1992). Hather and colleagues (1991) demonstrated that with different types of training (i.e., combinations of concentric and eccentric muscle actions), capillaries per unit area and per fiber increased significantly in response to heavy resistance training even with hypertrophy resulting in increased fiber areas. As with the selective hypertrophy of type II fibers shown by some studies, any increase in capillaries appears to be linked to the intensity and volume of resistance training. However, the time

course of changes in capillary density appears to be slow as studies have shown that 6 to 12 weeks may not stimulate capillary growth beyond normal untrained levels (Tesch 1992; Tesch, Hjort, and Balldin 1983).

Power lifters and weightlifters exhibited no change in the number of capillaries per muscle fiber. However, due to muscle hypertrophy these same athletes show a decrease in capillary density (i.e., the number of capillaries per cross-sectional area of tissue) when compared to nonathletic individuals (Tesch, Thorsson, and Kaiser 1984). Conversely, Kadi and colleagues (1999) reported a higher number of capillaries surrounding the type I muscle fibers in the trapezius muscles of elite power lifters. The capillary density was higher for the control subjects in the type IIA muscle fibers, indicating that hypertrophy affects capillary diffusion distances in some type II fibers. Schantz (1982) also proposed that the training performed by bodybuilders induces increased capillarization. Thus, it can be hypothesized that high-intensity, low-volume strength training actually decreases capillary density, whereas low-intensity, high-volume strength training has the opposite effect of increasing capillary density depending on the magnitude of hypertrophy. An increase in capillary density may facilitate the performance of low-intensity weight training by increasing the blood supply to the active muscle. The short rest periods used by many bodybuilders during their workouts result in large increases in blood lactate concentrations from resting concentrations of 1 to 2 to greater than 20 mmol · L^{-1} (Kraemer, Noble et al. 1987). A higher capillary density may increase the ability to remove lactate from the muscle to the blood, thereby allowing better tolerance to training under such high lactate conditions (Kraemer, Noble et al. 1987). This idea is supported by data demonstrating that bodybuilders could use a heavier resistance under the same lactate conditions as compared to power lifters (Kraemer, Noble et al. 1987). This indicates that greater clearance and buffering of lactate took place allowing for the superior performance of the bodybuilders in the lifting protocol. Since blood lactate concentrations observed with heavy resistance protocols used by power lifters and weightlifters are rarely above 4 mmol·L^{-1}, the physiological stimulus to increase capillarization may not be as great.

Thus, capillarization can be increased with resistance training, but any change may be dependent on the total training volume. However, the time required for this adaptation to take place may be greater than 12 weeks. An increase in the total number of capillaries can be masked by muscle hypertrophy resulting in no change in number of capillaries per fiber area or a decrease in capillary density. A high-volume program may cause capillarization to occur, whereas a low-volume program may not.

Mitochondrial Density

Few studies have examined the effect of resistance training on mitochondrial density. In a fashion similar to capillaries per muscle fiber, mitochondrial density has been shown to decrease with resistance training due to the dilution effects of muscle fiber hypertrophy (Luthi et al. 1986; MacDougall et al. 1979). The observation of decreased mitochondrial density is consistent with the minimal demands for oxidative metabolism placed on the musculature during most resistance training programs. Chilibeck and colleagues (1999) found that 12 weeks of resistance training resulted in significantly increased type I and II muscle fiber cross-sectional areas of 26% and 28%, respectively. Their analysis of mitochondria demonstrated that strength training results in reduced density of regionally distributed mitochondria (e.g., subsarcolemmal and intermyofibrillar mitochondrial density decreased similarly). The effect of resistance training on mitochondrial number and density does require further study. However, similar to enzyme activity and capillary density, mitochondrial density appears to decrease in response to resistance training due to a dilution effect caused by muscle fiber hypertrophy.

Muscle Enlargement

One of the most prominent adaptations to a resistance training program is the enlargement of muscles. Today, sport scientists, athletes, and coaches all agree that a properly designed and implemented strength training program leads to muscle growth. This growth in muscle size has been thought to be primarily due to muscle fiber **hypertrophy** or an increase in the size of the individual muscle fibers (Kraemer, Fleck, and Evans 1996; MacDougall 1992).

Muscle fiber **hyperplasia**, or an increase in the number of muscle fibers, is also one possible mechanism for increasing the size of muscle. The concept of hyperplasia after resistance training in humans has not been directly proven because of methodological difficulties (e.g., one cannot take out the whole muscle for examination), but it has been shown in response to various exercise protocols in birds and mammals (for reviews, see Antonio and Gonyea 1994; MacDougall 1992).

Hypertrophy

An increase in muscle size has been observed in both animal and human studies. In laboratory animals, muscle growth has occurred due to hypertrophy alone (Bass, Mackova, and Vitek 1973; Gollnick et al. 1981; Timson et al. 1985). Increased muscle size in strength-trained athletes has been attributed to hypertrophy of existing muscle fibers (Alway 1994; Alway et al. 1989; Haggmark, Jansson, and Svane 1978). This increase in the cross-sectional area of existing muscle fibers is attributed to the increased size and number of the actin and myosin filaments and the addition of sarcomeres within existing muscle fibers (Goldspink 1992; MacDougall et al. 1979), although it has been suggested that an increase in noncontractile proteins may also occur (Phillips et al. 1999). This is reflected by an increase in myofibrillar volume after resistance training (Luthi et al. 1986; MacDougall 1986). Interestingly, extreme muscle hypertrophy may actually reduce myofibrillar volume (MacDougall et al. 1982).

Not all muscle fibers undergo the same amount of enlargement. The amount of enlargement is dependent on the type of muscle fiber and the pattern of recruitment (Kraemer, Fleck, and Evans 1996). Muscle fiber hypertrophy has been demonstrated in both type I and II fibers after resistance training (McCall et al. 1996). However, most studies show a greater hypertrophy of the type II fibers than the type I fibers. Conventional weight training in humans (Gonyea and Sale 1982) and animals (Edgerton 1978) appears to hypertrophy, selectively, the type II muscle fibers to a greater degree than the type I muscle fibers. Studies do, however, indicate that it may be possible to selectively hypertrophy either the type II or the type I muscle fibers depending on the training regimen. Power lifters who train predominantly with high-intensity (i.e., heavy resistances) and low-volume (i.e., small number of sets and repetitions) have been shown to have type II fibers with a mean fiber area of 79 mm^2 in the vastus lateralis (Tesch, Thorsson, and Kaiser 1984). Conversely, bodybuilders who train predominantly with a lower intensity but a higher volume have been shown to have type II fibers with a mean fiber area of 62 mm$^2 \cdot 100$ in the same muscle (Tesch, Thorsson, and Kaiser 1984). In addition, bodybuilders have been shown to possess a lower total percentage of type II fiber area in the vastus lateralis than Olympic lifters and power lifters (50% vs. 69%, respectively) (Tesch and Larson 1982). Thus, the high-intensity, low-volume training of Olympic and power lifters and the low-intensity, high-volume training of bodybuilders may selectively hypertrophy the type II fibers and type I fibers, respectively.

The increase in muscle fiber size can be seen by examining a group of muscle fibers under a microscope after they have been stained using the myosin ATPase method at pH 4.6. In figure 3.20, a sample obtained from a woman's vastus lateralis (quadriceps muscle) is shown before (a) and after (b) an 8-week heavy resistance training program. The fibers are cut in cross-section, and the dark ones are the type I fibers, the intermediate dark fibers are type IIAB fibers or some hybrid between IIA and IIB fibers, and the white fibers are the type IIA muscle fibers. This woman obviously increased the size of all of her muscle fibers with heavy resistance training, especially the type II (fast-twitch) muscle fibers. One can easily observe the larger cross-sectional area increase (hypertrophy) pre- to posttraining. Muscle hypertrophy is one of the hallmarks of training adaptations to heavy resistance training protocols. However, muscle must be recruited in order to see protein accretion and such fiber size increases.

Adaptations in muscle fibers with heavy resistance training must be viewed from both a quality and quantity of the contractile proteins perspective (i.e., actin and myosin). With the initiation of a heavy resistance training program, changes in the types of muscle proteins (e.g., myosin heavy chains) start to take place within a couple of workouts (Staron et al. 1994). As training continues, the quantity of contractile proteins starts to increase as muscle fibers develop increased cross-sectional areas. In order to demonstrate a significant amount of muscle fiber hypertrophy, a longer period of training time (>8 workouts) is needed to increase the contractile protein content in all of the muscle fibers. Thus, short-term programs (4 to 8 weeks) may not result in very large changes in the size of muscles.

Muscle hypertrophy gives the lifter a potential advantage for producing greater force, but not velocity of contraction. With hypertrophy, the pennation angle of muscle fibers in pennate muscles increases to a certain extent. Increased angle of pennation is unfavorable for force production (see figure 9.3 on page 270). Kawakami, Abe, and

Fukunaga (1993) compared pennation angle of the triceps brachii in bodybuilders and untrained men and reported that the bodybuilders had significantly greater pennation angles (33 degrees vs. 15 degrees for long head, 19 degrees vs. 11 degrees for short head). Kearns, Abe, and Brechue (2000) reported that the pennation angles of the triceps (long head) (21.4 vs. 16.5 degrees), medial aspect of the gastrocnemius (23.6 vs. 21.3 degrees), and lateral aspect of the gastrocnemius (15.4 vs. 13.5 degrees) were greater in sumo wrestlers than in untrained men. Kawakami and colleagues (1995) reported an increase in pennation angle of the triceps brachii from 16.5 to 21.3 degrees after 16 weeks of resistance training. Aagaard and colleagues (2001) examined the effects of 14 weeks of resistance training and reported an increase in the pennation angle of the vastus lateralis from 8 to 10.7 degrees in addition to a 18.4% increase in type II muscle fiber area. In addition, a correlation between muscle angle of pennation and muscle volume ($r = 0.622$) has been observed (Aagaard et al. 2001) as well as significant correlations between muscle thickness and pennation angle in some (triceps long head and gastrocnemius medialis) but not other (vastus lateralis) muscles of elite power lifters (Brechue and Abe 2002). Therefore, muscle hypertrophy resulting from resistance training appears to alter pennation angle unfavorably for producing force in some muscles.

There appears to be a limit to how much the pennation angle of a muscle may increase. It has been suggested that with extreme hypertrophy (e.g., that attained by football players, bodybuilders, etc.) a plateau exists in pennation angle after which an increase in fascicle length may limit individual fiber pennation angle (Kearns, Abe, and Brechue 2000). That is, an increase in the number of sarcomeres in series has been proposed to limit changes in pennation angle (Kearns, Abe, and Brechue 2000). American football players (Abe, Brown, and Brechue 1999), sumo wrestlers (Kearns, Abe, and Brechue 2000), and sprinters (Kumagai et al. 2000) have longer fascicle lengths (both absolute and relative to limb length) of the triceps, vastus lateralis, and gastrocnemius muscles than untrained men. In addition, increased fascicle length has been implicated for increasing the force per cross-sectional area of muscle and velocity of contraction. Kumagai and colleagues (2000) reported that faster sprinters (e.g., 10.0-10.9 s 100-m times) had greater fascicle length and smaller angles of pennation in comparison to slower sprinters (11.0-11.7 s 100-m times).

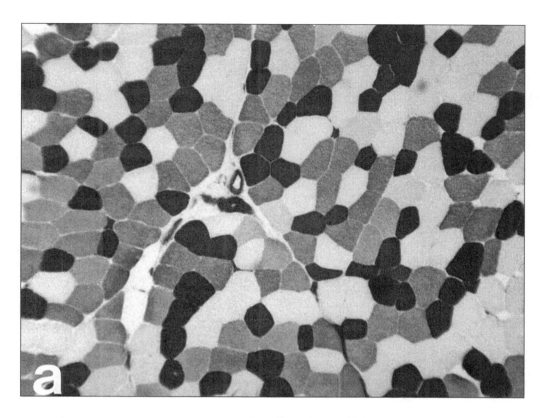

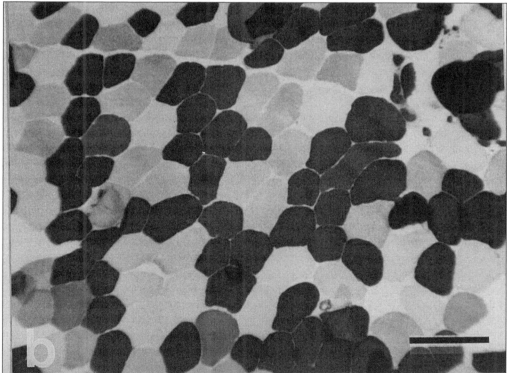

Figure 3.20 Muscle sample obtained *(a)* before and *(b)* immediately after an 8-week strength training program. Dark fibers are type I, intermediate dark fibers are type IIAB or a hybrid between IIA and IIB fibers, and light fibers are type IIA.

Data and micrograph courtesy of Dr. Robert S. Staron's laboratory.

Although genetic predisposition cannot be ruled out, it appears that either the addition of sarcomeres in series or an increase in sarcomere length may occur when a certain threshold of hypertrophy or a critical level of pennation angle has been reached (Kearns, Abe, and Brechue 2000).

Hyperplasia

Hyperplasia was first implicated as an adaptive strategy for muscle enlargement in laboratory animals (Gonyea 1980; Ho et al. 1980). Critics of these studies have claimed that methods of evaluation, damage to the muscle samples, as well as degenerating muscle fibers account for the observed hyperplasia. However, a few later studies attempting to correct for such problems still demonstrated increases in muscle fiber number (Alway et al. 1989; Gonyea et al. 1986).

Several studies comparing bodybuilders and power lifters concluded that the cross-sectional area of the bodybuilders' individual muscle fibers was not significantly larger than normal, yet these athletes possessed larger muscles than normal (MacDougall et al. 1982; Tesch and Larsson 1982). This indicates that these athletes have a greater total number of muscle fibers than normal, and hyperplasia may account for this increase. However, another study examining bodybuilders concluded that they possessed the same number of muscle fibers as the control group, but much larger muscles (MacDougall et al. 1984). This finding suggests that the large muscle size of bodybuilders is due to hypertrophy of existing muscle fibers rather than hyperplasia.

In a 12-week training study of men using both MRI and biopsy techniques to examine hypertrophy and the possible increase in cell number after a heavy resistance program, McCall and colleagues (1996) showed some evidence for hyperplasia in the biceps muscle despite hypertrophy accounting for the greatest portion of muscle enlargement. A study of hyperplasia in cats indicated that in order for hyperplasia to occur, the exercise intensity must be sufficient to recruit fast-twitch muscle fibers (type II fibers) (Gonyea 1980). It is possible that only high-intensity resistance training can cause hyperplasia and that type II muscle fibers may be targeted for this type of adaptation. More recently, power lifters have been shown to have higher numbers of myonuclei, satellite cells, and small-diameter fibers expressing markers for early myogenesis, thereby indicating hyperplasia (Kadi et al. 1999).

These effects appear to be enhanced by anabolic steroid use (Kadi et al. 2000), which potentially demonstrates an additional mechanism (e.g., more myonuclei means a greater number of androgen receptors available for interaction) for steroid-enhanced muscle growth.

Though limited data support hyperplasia in humans, there are indications that hyperplasia can occur as a result of resistance training. Because of these conflicting results, this topic continues to remain controversial, and further research on elite competitive lifters may help to resolve the controversy. Although hyperplasia in humans may not be the primary adaptational response of most muscle fibers, it might represent an adaptation to resistance training that is possible when certain muscle fibers reach a theoretical "upper limit" in cell size. It might be theorized that very intense long-term training may make some type II muscle fibers primary candidates for such an adaptational response. If hyperplasia does occur, it may only account for a small portion (e.g., 5-10%) of the increase in muscle size.

Protein Synthesis

Muscle hypertrophy is the result of an increase in protein synthesis, a decrease in protein degradation, or a combination of both. Protein synthesis increases after an acute bout of resistance exercise. When the amount of protein synthesized exceeds that which is degraded, then net protein accretion is positive and hypertrophy can occur. Hypertrophy in type II muscle fibers appears to involve an increase in the rate of protein synthesis, whereas hypertrophy in type I muscle fibers appears to involve a decrease in the rate of degradation (Goldspink 1992). When examining total-body protein synthesis during resistance exercise, Tarnopolsky and colleagues (1991) noted no changes. However, total-body measurements do not reflect changes at the muscle level. When measured in the biceps brachii and the vastus lateralis, protein synthesis is significantly elevated up to 48 hours postexercise (Chesley et al. 1992; MacDougall et al. 1992, 1995; Phillips et al. 1997). Phillips and colleagues (1997) reported that protein synthesis was elevated by 112%, 65%, and 34% respectively at 3, 24, and 48 hours post–resistance exercise. In addition, the protein breakdown rate was elevated by only 31%, 18%, and 1% at these same time points, indicating that muscle protein balance was elevated 23 to 48% over the 48-hour postexercise time period.

Training status of the individual plays a role in the post–resistance exercise change in protein synthesis. Phillips and colleagues (1999) examined the fractional rate of protein synthesis and breakdown in resistance-trained (at least 5 years of experience) and untrained men. Interestingly, they found that the rate of protein synthesis 4 hours postexercise was higher in untrained compared to trained individuals (118% vs. 48%, respectively). However, the rate of breakdown was also higher in the untrained men leading to a similar net protein balance of 37% and 34%, respectively, for the untrained and trained men. The researchers suggested that chronic resistance training reduces muscle damage, and consequently protein turnover.

Amino acid transport across the cell membrane and consequent uptake by skeletal muscle is important for enhancing protein synthesis. Biolo, Fleming, and Wolfe (1995) reported an increase in amino acid transport of 60 to 120% (depending on the amino acid) in the 3 hours after resistance exercise. Interestingly, arterial amino acid concentrations did not change, but rather a 90% increase in muscle blood flow accounted for much of the increase in amino acid transport. Growing evidence demonstrates the importance of blood flow in protein synthesis and muscle hypertrophy. Studies that have restricted blood flow and used light loading during resistance exercise (thereby increasing the concentrations of metabolites and the anaerobic nature of the exercise stimulus) have shown hypertrophy increases comparable to heavier loading, demonstrating the importance of blood flow and/or metabolite accumulation during resistance training to bring about adaptations (Rooney, Herbert, and Balwave 1994; Shinohara et al. 1998; Smith and Rutherford 1995). This may explain in part the efficacy of bodybuilding programs using moderate loading and high volume with short rest intervals for increasing muscle hypertrophy.

Muscle protein synthesis after resistance exercise depends heavily on amino acid availability, the timing of protein intake, and insulin concentrations in addition to other factors such as hormonal regulation (e.g., GH, testosterone, IGF-I, MGF), mechanical stress, and cellular hydration. The acute increases in protein synthesis appear to be influenced by changes at the nuclear level and by posttranscriptional modifications (e.g., an increase in protein synthesis independent of changes in RNA) by enhancing ribosome biogenesis, increasing the abundance of translation initiation factors, or both (Baar and Esser 1999; Jefferson and Kimball 2001). When insulin concentrations are elevated after resistance exercise (either by glucose intake or insulin infusion), the exercise-mediated acceleration of protein breakdown is reduced while synthesis rates are not significantly increased, thereby resulting in a net protein accretion of approximately 36% (Biolo et al. 1999; Roy et al. 1997). It is interesting to note that insulin increases have occurred after a resistance training session followed by postexercise supplementation with a carbohydrate-protein supplement (Williams et al. 2002). After resistance exercise, protein synthesis rate stimulated by amino acid intake is doubled when coinciding with increases in muscle blood flow (Biolo et al. 1997). A recent study has shown this effect to be greater when amino acids are taken before a workout to optimize amino acid delivery and transport during the workout because of greater blood flow (Tipton et al. 2001). These results indicate a potential ergogenic effect of glucose and amino acid intake before or directly after resistance exercise to maximize protein synthesis and recovery. In our laboratory we have found that amino acid supplementation attenuates muscle damage during the stressful early phases of overreaching (possibly by reducing protein degradation and enhancing recovery), which was crucial to maintaining muscle strength and power (unpublished observations of Dr. Kraemer's laboratory).

Based on these findings, Tipton and Wolfe (1998) proposed a model of protein metabolism during resistance exercise: (1) resistance exercise stimulates protein synthesis, (2) intracellular amino acid concentrations are reduced, (3) decreased amino acid concentrations stimulate protein breakdown and transport of amino acids into the muscle cell, (4) increased availability of amino acids further stimulates protein synthesis, and (5) tissue remodeling occurs. Therefore, it appears that optimal protein intake is crucial to optimizing recovery and performance as well as subsequent adaptation to resistance training.

Structural Changes in Muscle

Structural characteristics of muscle fibers after resistance training have been investigated. Despite the increase in myofilament number, the myofibrillar packing distance (i.e., the distance between myosin filaments) and the length of the sarcomere appear to remain constant after 6 weeks to 6 months of resistance training (Claassen et al. 1989; Luthi et al. 1986; MacDougall 1986). In addition, the ratio of actin to myosin filaments does not change after 6 weeks of resistance training (Claassen et al. 1989). The relative volume of the sarcoplasm, T-tubules, and other noncontractile tissue does not appear to change significantly as a result of resistance training (Alway et al. 1988, 1989; Luthi et al. 1986; MacDougall et al. 1984; Sale et al. 1987). Although increases in myofilament number take place, it appears that the spatial orientation of the sarcomere remains intact after resistance training. Thus, sarcomeres are added in parallel, contributing to the increase in muscle cross-sectional area and fat-free mass observed during resistance training. Additionally, fascicle length may increase with resistance training (see the section on hypertrophy) and has been significantly correlated with fat-free mass in elite male power lifters (Brechue and Abe 1986).

Other structural changes within skeletal muscle take place during resistance training. The sodium-potassium ATPase pump activity, which maintains sodium and potassium ion gradients and membrane potential, has been shown to increase by 16% after 11 weeks of resistance training (Green et al. 1999). Other structural characteristics do not appear to change during resistance training in young men and women. However, resistance training in the elderly appears to attenuate some of the age-related declines in muscle morphology. Resistance training has been shown to attenuate the age-related decreases in tropomyosin (Klitgaard et al. 1990), the maximal rate of sarcoplasmic reticulum calcium uptake (Hunter et al. 1999), sarcoplasmic reticulum calcium ATPase activity (Hunter et al. 1999; Klitgaard, Aussoni, and Damiani 1989), and calse-

questrin concentration (Klitgaard et al. 1989). These changes were not observed in younger populations (Green, Goreham et al. 1998; Green, Grange et al. 1998; Hunter et al. 1999; McKenna et al. 1996). These data indicate the importance of resistance training for limiting the age-related reductions in muscle structure and performance.

Muscle Fiber Type Transition

The quality of protein, which refers to the type of proteins found in the contractile machinery, has the ability to change its phenotypic profile with resistance training (Pette and Staron 2001). Much of the resistance training research focuses on the myosin molecule and examination of fiber types based on the use of the histochemical myosin adenosine triphosphatase (mATPase) staining activities at different pHs. Changes in muscle mATPase fiber types also give an indication of associated changes in the myosin heavy chain (MHC) content (Fry, Kraemer, Stone et al. 1994). We now know that a continuum of muscle fiber types exist and that transformation (e.g., type IIB to type IIA) within a particular muscle fiber subtype is a common adaptation to resistance training (Adams et al. 1993; Kraemer, Fleck, and Evans 1996; Staron et al. 1991, 1994). It appears that as soon as type IIB muscle fibers are stimulated, they start a process of transformation toward the type IIA profile by changing the quality of proteins and expressing different amounts of types and combinations of mATPase. Figure 3.21 shows the transformation process that occurs with heavy resistance training in the muscle fiber subtypes. Using this classification scheme for evaluating muscle fiber subtype changes, it is doubtful that under normal training conditions muscle fibers transform from type II

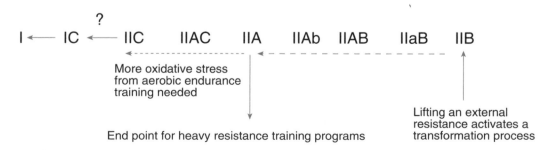

Figure 3.21 The process of muscle fiber type transformation. Changes in myosin ATPase and myosin heavy chain proteins underlie this process.

to type I (Kraemer, Patton et al. 1995). Thus, the old concept of trying to change muscle fiber types appears to be related to changes only within a fiber type (for reviews, see Kraemer, Fleck, and Evans 1996; Staron and Johnson 1993).

In a study by Staron and colleagues (1994), men and women performed a high-intensity resistance training protocol twice a week for 8 weeks. This protocol focused on the thigh musculature with heavy multiple sets of 6 to 8RM on one training day and 10 to 12RM on the other training day per week for several exercises (squat, leg press, and knee extension). Two-minute rest periods were used to allow for adequate rest between sets and exercises, but also to induce hormonal changes with the exercise protocol (Kraemer et al. 1990). Maximal dynamic strength increased over the 8-week training period without any significant changes in muscle fiber size or fat-free mass in the men or the women. This supports the concept of neural adaptations being the predominant mechanism in the early phase of training. It is interesting to note that a significant decrease in the type IIB percentage was observed in women after just 2 weeks of training (i.e., four workouts) and in the men after 4 weeks of training (i.e., eight workouts). Over the 8-week training program (16 workouts), the type IIB muscle fiber types decreased from 21% to about 7% of the total muscle fibers in both men and women. The alteration in the muscle fiber types was supported by myosin heavy chain (MHC) analyses. This study established the time course of specific muscular adaptations in the early phase of a resistance training program for men and women.

It is not known to what extent muscle fiber remodeling contributes to muscle strength; however, gradual increases in the number and size of myofibrils and perhaps the fast fiber type conversions of type IIB to IIA might contribute to force production. In addition, changes in hormonal factors (testosterone and cortisol interactions) are correlated with such changes in the muscle fibers (e.g., percentage shift in type IIA) and may help to mediate such adaptations. Many other changes that are taking place during muscle fiber remodeling in the early phase of training may influence when hypertrophy is initiated. Thus, the "quality" of the protein type generated in the remodeling of muscle may be an important aspect of muscular development, especially in the early phases of resistance training.

Longer studies of heavy resistance training have also examined changes in muscle fiber type and cross-sectional size with training. Staron and colleagues (1991) examined changes in skeletal muscle in women who trained for 20 weeks, detrained for 2 weeks, and then retrained for 6 weeks. Increases in muscle fiber cross section were seen with training. The percent of type IIB fibers decreased from 16% to 0.9%. This study also demonstrated that short detraining periods result in muscle fiber starting to return to pretraining values of muscle fiber cross-sectional areas, especially of type II fibers, and a conversion of type IIA back to type IIB fibers. Thus, the percent of muscle fiber types also return to pretraining values during detraining. In addition, it was demonstrated that retraining resulted in a quicker change in muscle size and conversion to type IIA fibers than when starting in an untrained condition. Thus, the concept used by athletes and coaches of "muscle memory" has some validity in the retraining of an individual after a period of detraining.

A series of studies using the same subject population examined the effect of resistance training on muscle strength, morphology, histochemical responses, and MHC responses (Adams et al. 1993; Dudley et al. 1991; Hather, Mason, and Dudley 1991). Three groups of men trained for 19 weeks. One group (CON/ECC) trained using both concentric and eccentric muscle actions, "normal" resistance training for four to five sets of 6 to 12 repetitions. A second group (CON) trained with only concentric actions for four to five sets of 6 to 12 repetitions, and a third group (CON/CON) used concentric-only actions but for 8 to 10 sets of 6 to 12 repetitions. Thus, the third group performed twice the training volume as the second group and the same amount of training volume if one normal repetition is viewed as two muscle actions. All groups showed significant gains in strength and an increase in the percent of type IIA fibers with an accompanying decrease in percent of type IIB fibers. Increases in type I fiber area occurred only in the CON/ECC group, and type II fiber area increased in both the CON/ECC and CON/CON groups. Capillaries per unit muscle fiber area increased only in the CON/CON and CON groups. The changes in type II fiber subtypes were paralleled by an increase in MHC IIA and a decrease in MHC IIB. The results indicate that hypertrophy, type II fiber type transformation, and capillaries per unit fiber area are all affected by muscle action type and training volume.

Satellite Cells and Myonuclei

Satellite cells and myonuclei may indicate cellular repair and formation of new muscle cells. In a very interesting study, Kadi and colleagues (1999) attempted to elucidate the cellular adaptations that occur in the trapezius muscle of drug-free elite power lifters with years of training. Ten elite power lifters and six control subjects had their cross-sectional area of muscle fibers and myosin heavy chain composition analyzed from muscle biopsy samples. In addition, a method was also developed for counting the number of myonuclei and satellite cell nuclei. As might be expected, the power lifters had dramatically larger fibers for all fiber types compared to controls. Novel to this investigation was the fact that the proportion of fibers expressing MHC IIA, cross-sectional area of each fiber type, number of myonuclei, satellite cells, and fibers expressing markers for early myogenesis were significantly higher in power lifters than in the control group. A significant correlation ($r = 0.80$) between the myonuclear number and the cross-sectional area was observed. Since myonuclei in mature muscle fibers are not able to divide, the authors suggested that the incorporation of satellite cell nuclei into muscle fibers resulted in the maintenance of a constant nuclear-to-cytoplasmic ratio or that the nuclear domain size was maintained. Interestingly, the presence of small-diameter fibers expressing markers for early myogenesis indicated the formation of new muscle fibers.

Kadi and Thornell (2000) also showed that 10 weeks of strength training can induce changes in the number of myonuclei and satellite cells in women's trapezius muscles. A 36% increase occurred in the cross-sectional area of muscle fibers. The hypertrophy of muscle fibers was accompanied by an approximately 70% increase in myonuclear number and a 46% increase in the number of satellite cells. Myonuclei number was positively correlated to satellite cell number, indicating that a muscle with an increased concentration of myonuclei will contain a correspondingly higher number of satellite cells. The authors suggested that the acquisition of additional myonuclei appears to be required to support the enlargement of multinucleated muscle cells after 10 weeks of strength training. Increased satellite cell content suggests that mitotic divisions of satellite cells produced daughter cells that became satellite cells.

Hikida and colleagues (2000) examined whether muscle fibers of elderly men can hypertrophy with strength training and, if so, whether they have the capacity to incorporate nuclei into the fibers. The sarcoplasmic area associated with each myonucleus was calculated in elderly men before and after 16 weeks of strength training, and compared to elderly control men. Muscle fiber type changes and myosin heavy-chain composition were also compared. All major fiber types (I, IIA, IIB) became significantly larger after training, and a transition of type IIB fibers to type IIA occurred with training. The area occupied by each fiber type correlated with myosin heavy chain percentage, and both of these changed similarly with strength training. The cytoplasm-to-myonucleus ratio increased, but not significantly ($p = .07$), with muscle fiber hypertrophy. The number of myonuclei per fiber and myonuclei per unit length of muscle fiber increased, but not significantly. Cross-sectional areas of the muscle fibers in untrained elderly men were much smaller than in untrained young men (when compared with earlier studies). Training increased the sizes of the elderly muscle fibers to that of the untrained young men. This hypertrophy of muscle fibers by 30% with training resulted in no change in the cytoplasm-to-myonucleus ratio. This suggests that the myonuclear population continues to adapt to growth stimuli in elderly muscles.

Roth and colleagues (2001) also examined satellite cell proportions and morphology in younger and older men and women with resistance training. Young men and women (20-30 years) and older men and women (65-75 years) completed 9 weeks of unilateral knee-extension exercise training 3 days per week with the contralateral leg serving as a control. All four groups demonstrated a significant increase in satellite cell proportion in response to resistance training (2.3% vs. 3.1% for all subjects combined) before and after training, respectively, with the older women demonstrating the greatest increase. Morphology data indicated a significant increase in the proportion of active satellite cells in after-training muscle samples compared with before-training samples and with control leg samples (31% vs. 6 and 7%). These results indicate that the proportion of satellite cells increases after resistance training in young and older men and women, with an exaggerated response in older women. Furthermore, the proportion of satellite cells that appear morphologically active increases as a result of resistance training.

The pattern of neural recruitment and the amount of muscle tissue recruited will determine whether cellular and whole muscle changes occur. When enough muscle is affected, body composition will be altered in the resistance-trained individual. The amount of muscle mass gained and fiber transformation consequent to a resistance training program will also be affected by an individual's genetic potential. In the future, long-term resistance training studies over several years with associated muscle biopsies will be needed to understand the cellular adaptations that take place after most of the muscle morphological changes have been made over the first 3 to 6 months.

Body Composition Changes

Body composition changes do occur in short-term resistance training programs (6 to 24 weeks). Table 3.3 depicts the changes in body composition due to various training programs. Normally the body is divided into two compartments when examining body composition. The terms *lean body mass* (LBM) and *fat-free mass* (FFM) are often used interchangeably. However, the two terms do have different definitions. LBM refers to essential fat plus all non-fat tissue, and FFM refers to only all non-fat tissue. Essential fat is the fat necessary to allow normal body functions. It is not possible to have 0% fat. Fat stores are needed to pad the heart, kidneys, and other vital organs; they also serve as structural components of membranes and as fuel stores for energy. With the commonly used means to determine body composition (hydrostatic weighing, skinfolds, dual energy absoptiometry), it is not possible to differentiate between essential fat and nonessential fat, so FFM is actually what is being determined. Fat weight is the weight of fat contained in the body. Total body weight equals FFM plus fat weight. For the purpose of comparison, fat weight is frequently expressed as a percentage of total body weight or percent body fat (% fat). For example, if a 100-kg (220-lb) athlete is 15% fat, his FFM, fat weight, and total body weight are related as follows:

$$\text{Fat weight} = 0.15 \times 100 \text{ kg}$$
$$= 15 \text{ kg}$$
$$\text{FFM} = \text{total body weight} - \text{fat weight}$$
$$= 100 \text{ kg} - 15 \text{ kg}$$
$$= 85 \text{ kg}$$

Normally the goals of a strength training program are to increase FFM and decrease fat weight and percent fat. Increases in FFM are normally viewed as mirroring increases in muscle tissue weight. Strength training induces decreases in % fat and increases in FFM (see table 3.3). Total body weight, for the most part, experiences small increases over short training periods. This occurs in both men and women using dynamic constant external resistance (DCER), variable resistance (VT), and isokinetic training (IK) with programs involving a variety of combinations of exercises, sets, and repetitions. Because of the variation in the numbers of sets, repetitions, and exercises and relatively small body compositional changes, it is impossible to reach concrete conclusions concerning which program is optimal for decreasing percent fat and increasing FFM. However, several studies report significantly greater changes in body composition with high-volume, multiple-set programs compared to low-volume, single-set programs (Kraemer et al. 2000; Marx et al. 2001) and suggest that periodized programs can result in greater changes in body composition than non-periodized programs (Fleck 1999).

Although some studies report larger increases in FFM, the largest increases in FFM consistently reported are a little greater than 3 kg (6.6 lb) in approximately 10 weeks of drug-free training. This translates into a FFM increase of 0.3 kg (0.66 lb) per week. When larger gains in FFM are shown, factors such as the trainees going through a natural growth period may be the cause. Although some coaches desire very large gains in body weight for their athletes during the off-season, this is impossible if that added body weight is going to be muscle mass.

Table 3.4 summarizes the results of studies investigating percent fat in bodybuilders and Olympic and power lifters. Average percent fat of these highly resistance trained males ranged from 4.1% to 15.6%, whereas female bodybuilders demonstrated an average of 9.0% to 20.4%. For the bodybuilders, these values significantly decreased as the competition day approached. All of these values are lower than the average percent fat of college-age males and females of 14% to 16% and 20% to 24%, respectively. Highly resistance trained athletes are therefore leaner than average individuals of the same age.

It should be noted, however, that the average off-season percent fat of most of the depicted groups of male athletes is above the essential fat levels of 6% (Sinning 1974). Female bodybuilders'

Table 3.3 Changes in Body Composition Due to Weight Training

Reference	Gender	Type of training	Length of training (weeks)	Days of training per week	Set and repetitions	Number of exercises	Total weight (kg)	LBM (kg)	% fat
					Changes based on type of training				
Withers 1970	F	DCER	10	3	40-55% 1RM/30 sec	10	+0.1	+1.3	-1.8
Withers 1970	M	DCER	20	3	40-55% 1RM/30 sec	10	+0.7	+1.7	-1.5
Fahey and Brown 1973	M	DCER	9	3	2 exercises 5 × 5, 2 exercises 3 × 5, 1 exercise 5 × 1-2	5	+0.5	+1.4	-1.0
Brown and Wilmore 1974	F	DCER	24	3	8 wk = 1 × 10, 8, 7, 6, 5, 4; 16 wk = 1 × 10, 6, 5, 4, 3	4	-0.4	+1.0	-2.1
Mayhew and Gross 1974	F	DCER	9	3	2 × 10	11	+0.4	+1.5	-1.3
Misner et al. 1974	M	DCER	8	3	1 × 3-8	10	+1.0	+3.1	-2.9
Peterson 1975	M	VR	6	3	1 × 10-12	20	—	-0.8	+0.6
Coleman 1977	M	IT	10	3	2 × 8-10RM	11	+1.7	+2.4	-9.1
Coleman 1977	M	VR	10	3	1 × 10-12RM	11	+1.8	+2.0	-9.3
Gettman and Ayres 1978	M	IK (60 deg/sec)	10	3	3 × 10-15	7	-1.9	+3.2	-2.5
Gettman and Ayres 1978	M	IK (120 deg/sec)	10	3	3 × 10-15	7	+0.3	+1.0	-0.9
Wilmore et al. 1978	F	DCER	10	2	2 × 7-16	8	-0.1	+1.1	-1.9
Wilmore et al. 1978	M	DCER	10	2	2 × 7-16	8	+0.3	+1.2	-1.3
Gettman et al. 1979	M	DCER	20	3	50% 1RM, 6 wk = 2 × 10-20, 14 wk = 2 × 15	10	+0.5	+1.8	-1.7
Gettman et al. 1979	M	IK	8	3	4 wk = 1 × 10 at 60 deg/sec, 4 wk = 1 × 15 at 90 deg/sec	9	+0.3	+1.0	-0.9

Study	Gender	Mode		Sets × reps				
Gettman, Cutler, and Strathman 1980	M	VR	20	3	2 × 12	9	-0.1	+1.6	-1.9
Gettman, Cutler, and Strathman 1980	M	IK (60 deg/sec)	20	3	2 × 12	10	-0.6	+2.1	-2.8
Hurley et al. 1984a	M	VR	16	3-4	1 × 8-12RM	14	+1.6	+1.9	-0.8
Hunter 1985	F	DCER	7	3	3 × 7-10	7	-0.9	+0.3	-1.5
Hunter 1985	F	DCER	7	4	2 × 7-10	7	+0.7	+0.7	-0.5
Hunter 1985	M	DCER	7	3	3 × 7-10	7	+0.6	+0.5	-0.2
Hunter 1985	M	DCER	7	4	2 × 7-10	7	0.0	+0.5	-0.9
Crist et al. 1988	M and F	DCER	6	5	—	—	+1.0	+2.0	-3.0
Bauer et al. 1990	M and F	SSC	10	3	4-7 × 20 sec	—	0	+1.0	-3.0
Staron et al. 1991	F	DCER	20	2	1 day/wk 3 × 6-8RM 1 day/wk 3 × 10-12RM	3	+2.0	+6.0	-4.0
Staron et al. 1989	F	DCER	18	2	3 × 6-8	4	0	+1.0	-1.0
Pierce et al. 1993	M	DCER	8	3	3 wk 3 × 10RM 3 wk 3 × 5RM 2 wk 3 × 10RM	10	+1.0	+1.0	-4.0
Butts and Price 1994	F	DCER	12	3	1 × 8-12RM	12	-0.1	+1.3	-2.2
Staron et al. 1994	M	DCER	8	2	M- 2 warm-up 6-8RM F- 2 warm-up 10-12RM	3	+0.7	+1.8	-2.1
Staron et al. 1994	F	DCER	8	2	M- 2 warm-up 6-8RM F- 2 warm-up 10-12RM	3	+1.3	+2.4	-2.9
Hennessy and Watson 1994	M	DCER	8	3	2-6 × 1-10	7	+2.9	+3.7	-1.4
Kraemer 1997	M	DCER	14	3 3	1 × 8-10 2-5 × 1-10	10 9	+1.4 +4.3	+2.7 +8.2	-1.5 -4.3

(continued)

Table 3.3 *(continued)*

Reference	Gender	Type of training	Length of training (weeks)	Days of training per week	Set and repetitions	Number of exercises	Total weight (kg)	LBM (kg)	% fat
Kramer et al. 1997	M	DCER	14	3	1 × 8-12 3 × 10 3 × 1-10	4 4 4	+0.2 +1.5 +0.3	+0.4 +1.1 +0	−0.1 +0.2 +0.2
Hoffman and Kalfeld 1998	F	DCER	13	4/wk 3 wk 1/wk 10 wk	3-4 × 8-12	4-6	+2.6	+3.1	−2.1
McLester et al. 2000	M and F	DCER	12	1	3 × 3-10	9	+0.4	+1.0	−0.6
McLester et al. 2000	M and F	DCER	12	3	1 × 3-10	9	+3.5	+4.6	−1.2
Mazzetti et al. 2000	M	DCER	12	2-4	2-4 × 3-12	7-8	+4.1	+1.4	+2.1
Kraemer, Keuning et al. 2001	F	DCER	12	3	2-3 × 10	10	−1.0	+3.6	−5.3
Kraemer, Mazzetti et al. 2001	F	DCER	36	2-3	1 × 8-12	14	—	+1.0	−2.5
Kraemer, Mazzetti et al. 2001	F	DCER	36	4	2-4 × 3-5 2-4 × 8-10 2-4 × 12-15	12	—	+3.3	−4.0
Lemmer et al. 2001	M	AR	24	3	upper body 1 × 15RM, lower body 2 × 15RM	8	+0.2	+2.0	−1.9
Lemmer et al. 2001	F	AR	24	3	upper body 1 × 15RM, lower body 2 × 15RM	8	+2.5	+1.9	+0.4
Marx et al. 2001	F	DCER	24	3	1 × 8-12RM	10	—	+1.0	−2.5
Marx et al. 2001	F	DCER	24	4	2-4 × 3-5 2-4 × 8-10 2-4 × 12-15	7-12	—	+3.3	−6.7

Changes based on type of training

AR = air resistance; DCER = dynamic constant external resistance; VR = variable resistance; SSC = stretch shortening cycle; IK = isokinetic.

Table 3.4 Percent Fat of Advanced Strength-Trained Athletes (Revised)

Reference	Caliber of athletes	% fat
	Men	
Fahey, Akka, and Rolph 1975	OL-national and international	12.2
Tanner 1964	OL-national and international	10.0
Sprynarova and Parizkova 1971	OL-national and international	9.8
Fry, Stone et al. 1995	OL-national and international	8.9
Katch et al. 1980	OL and PL-national and international	9.7
McBride et al. 1999	Ol-national PL-national	10.4 8.7
Fahey, Akka, and Rolph 1975	PL-national and international	15.6
Dickerman, Pertusi, and Smith 2000	PL-national and international	14.0 (record holder case study)
Fry et al. 1994a	OL-junior national	5.0
Katch et al. 1980	BB-national	9.3
Zrubak 1972	BB-national	6.6
Fahey, Akka, and Rolph 1975	BB-national and international	8.4
Pipes 1979	BB-national and international	8.3
Bamman et al. 1993	BB-regional (12 weeks pre) BB-regional (competition)	9.1 4.1
Manore, Thompson, and Russo 1993	BB-international	6.9
Kleiner, Bazzarre, and Ainsworth 1994	BB-national	5.0
Withers et al. 1997	BB-national (10 weeks pre) BB-national (competition)	9.1 5.0
Too et al. 1998	BB-regional (competition)	4.1
	Women	
Freedson et al. 1983	BB-national and international	13.2
Walberg-Rankin et al. 1993	BB-regional	12.7
Kleiner, Bazzarre, and Ainsworth 1994	BB-national	9.0
Alway 1994	BB-national and international	13.8
Alway 1994	BB-national	18.7
Van der Ploeg et al. 2001	BB-local (12 weeks pre) BB-local (competition)	18.3 12.7
Stoessel et al. 1991	OL-national and international	20.4

OL = Olympic lifters; PL = power lifters; BB = bodybuilders.

average percent fat of 13.2% is very close to the lower limit of female essential fat levels of 13 to 22% (Frish and McArthur 1974). Only a few studies report percent fat levels at or near essential fat levels, and generally these are for national- and international-caliber competitors. Women's essential fat levels may need to be higher than men to ensure normal functioning of the reproductive cycle (Frish and McArthur 1974). As they approach essential fat levels, many men and women become lethargic and moody. Additionally, when individuals approach or reach essential fat levels, a large portion of the weight they lose is FFM. This is true even in highly weight trained individuals such as bodybuilders, who continue to weight train while losing total body weight and fat weight (Too et al. 1998; Withers et al. 1997). Essential fat levels, therefore, are not to be viewed as ideal or target fat levels for athletes.

Endocrine System Responses and Adaptations

The endocrine system helps an organism adapt to its environment. The overall systematic interface of hormones with target cells, primarily muscle, is shown in figure 3.22. Hormonal influences are very important to both the acute response and the chronic adaptations associated with resistance training. A specific stimulus causes the release of a chemical messenger or hormone, targeted for specific tissue cells, into the blood. The hormone travels in the blood to the target cell (e.g., muscle), where it interacts and signals a metabolic change or adaptation. Hormones can also be released inside the cell itself for interaction with that cell. This is called an autocrine hormonal action. In addition, a hormone can be released from one cell and interact with another cell and never reach the circulatory system. This is called a paracrine hormonal action. Thus, hormones can interact with the cells of the body in a number of ways. Each of these mechanisms is involved with adaptations of the body to resistance training (Kraemer 1992b, 2000a).

Both the actions and the mechanisms of various hormones' actions are diverse (Kraemer 1988, 1992, 1994; Norris 1980). Hormones can affect almost every physiological function in the body. Cellular transport, enzyme synthesis, cell growth, protein synthesis, cell metabolism, and reproductive function are just a few physiological events that are mediated, in part, by hormonal actions. The close association of hormones to the nervous system makes the neural-endocrine system potentially one of the most important physiological systems related to resistance training adaptations. The type of resistance training workout used dictates the hormonal responses. Tissue adaptations are influenced by the changes in circulating hormonal concentrations after exercise. Thus, understanding this natural anabolic activity that takes place in the trainee's body is fundamental to successful recovery, adaptation, program design, training progression, and ultimately physical performance.

The endocrine system plays an important support function for adaptational mechanisms, ultimately leading to enhanced muscular force production (Kraemer 1988, 1992a, 1992b; Kraemer et al. 1991, 1992a, 1992b). It is well established that anabolic hormones (e.g., testosterone, insulin, growth hormones, and insulin-like growth factors) play various roles in enhancing tissue growth and development. In addition, gender differences (i.e., testosterone responses) in these hormonal concentrations and responses to exercise exist (Kraemer et al. 1993b). The key sequence of events is related to the effective stimulation of an endocrine, paracrine (local), and/or autocrine (within the target cell itself) endogenous response to the exercise protocol. These signals must then be received by the receptor mechanisms of the target tissues. The alteration of metabolism (typically protein) and the molecular mechanisms associated with cell transport phenomenon must then be translated to enhance synthesis, reduce degradation, or augment the cells' functional structure or secretory products leading to enhanced muscle mass, improved force production, or both.

Kraemer and colleagues (1990, 1991; Kraemer, Dziados et al. 1993; Kraemer, Fleck et al. 1993) determined that acute resistance exercise can increase circulating concentrations of hormones, but that hormones are differentially sensitive to different types of acute program variables. For example, the highest growth hormone, beta-endorphin, and cortisol concentrations were observed when 10RM multiple sets (3 sets) of exercises were performed separated by a short (1-minute) rest. Testosterone appears responsive to both a high-intensity, long-rest (3-minute) resistance (5RM) exercise protocol as well as to a 10RM, short-rest protocol. Thus, these series of studies showed that rest period length and the intensity of the resistance exercise can both affect the magnitude of the hormonal response to a workout. The following factors appear to determine whether anabolic hormone concentrations increase during a resistance exercise workout (Kraemer 1988, 1992a, 1992b):

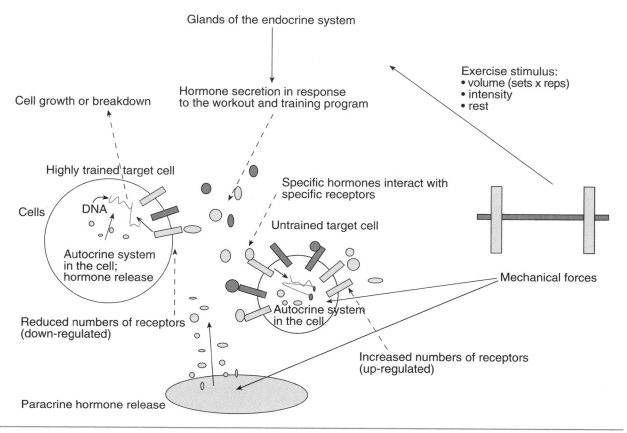

Figure 3.22 Endocrine interactions with cells. Resistance exercise stimulates the body's endocrine response by releasing hormones. These hormones interact with various cell receptors. Hormonal signals come from the endocrine, paracrine, and autocrine mechanisms and interact with the cell's DNA, resulting in the hormone's signal for either an increase or a reduction in protein synthesis.

- Amount of muscle mass recruited
- Intensity of the workout
- Amount of rest between sets and exercises
- Volume of total work
- Training level of the individual

Many different physiological mechanisms may contribute in varying degrees to the observed changes in peripheral blood concentrations of hormones, acute responses to resistance training, and chronic adaptations. These include the following:

- Fluid volume shifts. Body fluid tends to shift from the blood to the cells as a result of exercise. This shift can increase hormone concentrations in the blood without any change in secretion from endocrine glands. It has been hypothesized that regardless of the mechanism of increase, such concentration changes increase receptor interaction probabilities.

- Amount of synthesis and amount of hormones stored in glands. These factors can affect the release of, and therefore the concentration of, a hormone in the circulation.

- Tissue (especially liver) clearance rates of a hormone—that is, the time it takes a hormone to go through the circulation of the tissue. Hormones circulate through various tissues and organs, the liver being one of the major processing organs in the body. Time delays are seen as the hormone goes through the circulation in the liver and other tissues (e.g., lungs). The clearance time of a tissue keeps the hormone out of the circulation and away from contact with target receptors in other parts of the body or can degrade it making it nonfunctional.

- Hormonal degradation—that is, breakdown of the hormone itself.

- Venous pooling of blood. Blood flow back to the heart is slowed by pooling of blood in veins; the blood is delayed in the peripheral circulation due to intense muscle activity (muscle contractions greater than 45% of maximal). Thus, blood flow must recover during intervals when muscle activity is reduced. The pooling of the blood can increase the concentrations of hormones in the venous blood and also increase time of exposure to target tissues.

- Interactions with binding proteins in the blood. Hormones bind with specialized proteins in the blood that help with transport. Free hormones and bound hormones interact differently with tissue; ultimately, it is the free hormone that interacts with the membrane or other cellular receptors.

- Receptor interactions. All the previously mentioned mechanisms interact to produce a certain concentration of a hormone in the blood, which influences the potential for interaction with the receptors in target tissue. Receptor interaction is also affected by receptor affinity for a hormone and receptor density in the target cells. These factors all interact and result in the number of hormonal signals sent to the cell nucleus by the hormone-receptor complex or secondary messenger systems.

Another factor that can affect a hormone's concentration is when a sample is obtained. For example, increases in serum total testosterone are evident when blood is sampled during and immediately after protocols that use large-muscle group exercise (e.g., deadlift). When blood is sampled 4 hours or more after exercise and not immediately after it, other factors, such as diurnal variations (normal fluctuations in hormone levels throughout the day) or recovery phenomena can affect the magnitude or direction of the acute stress response (see figure 3.23).

Besides the anabolic function of hormones, many hormones help to meet the metabolic demands of acute strenuous exercise. Regulation of blood glucose concentrations, glycogen storage, and mineral metabolism are all mediated by hormonal actions. Table 3.5 provides a summary of the major hormones and their actions. Scientists are only just beginning to realize the complexity of the neuroendocrine system, as a myriad of interactions that occur among hormones and hormonal factors. Furthermore, endocrine function is highly integrated with nutritional status, nutritional intake, training status, and other external factors (e.g., stress, sleep, disease) that affect the remodeling and repair processes of the body. At this point the effects of resistance training on acute and chronic hormonal responses require

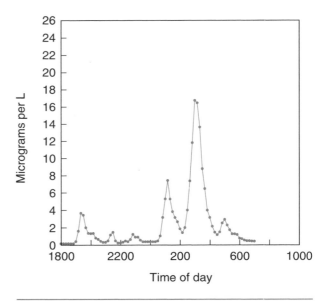

Figure 3.23 Circadian rhythm pattern of growth hormone.
Data courtesy of Dr. William Kraemer's laboratory.

a more detailed study. The challenge is to link physiological responses to chronic adaptations such as muscle hypertrophy and strength.

How paracrine (cell to cell release) and autocrine (within the cell release) changes are affected by heavy resistance training remains unknown due to methodological difficulties in determining the small changes in cells or in various intercellular spaces. Furthermore, research has been limited to those hormone forms that can be detected with an antibody assay (immunoreactive molecular forms), thus eliminating various forms that are not immunoreactive (e.g., some types of growth hormone). Finally, our understanding of how receptors on target tissues translate the endocrine message is just starting to develop. Each receptor can be differentially regulated in various fiber types in response to different exercise regimes (Bricourt et al. 1994; Deschenes et al. 1994). These responses at the target level of the cell (e.g., muscle, nerve, etc.) determine whether a hormonal message is realized. Thus, if the receptors are down-regulated, they will interact less with the hormone. If they are up-regulated, they will interact to a greater degree with the hormone. So the quantity of the hormone may not be as important as the number of receptors that effectively interact with the receptors in the target cells.

Endocrine Adaptations

Organs such as muscle and connective tissue are the ultimate target cells of most resistance training programs, but many adaptations occur within

Table 3.5 Selected Hormones of the Endocrine System and Their Actions

Endocrine gland	Hormone	Some actions
Testes	Testosterone	Stimulates development and maintenance of male sex characteristics, growth, and increased protein anabolism
Anterior pituitary	Growth hormone	Stimulates somatomedins release, protein synthesis, growth, and organic metabolism
	Adrenocorticotropin (ACTH)	Stimulates glucocorticoids release in adrenal cortex
	Thyroid-stimulating hormone (TSH)	Stimulates thyroid hormone synthesis and secretion
	Follicle-stimulating hormone (FSH)	Stimulates growth of follicles in ovary, seminiferous tubules in testes, ovum, and sperm production
	Luteinizing hormone (LH)	Stimulates ovulation and secretion of sex hormones in ovaries and testes
	Prolactin (LTH)	Stimulates milk production in mammary glands; maintains corpora lutea and stimulates secretion of progesterone
	Melanocyte-stimulating hormone	Stimulates melanocytes, which contain the dark pigment melanin
Posterior pituitary	Antidiuretic hormone (ADH)	Increase contraction of smooth muscle and reabsorption of water by kidneys
	Oxytocin	Stimulates uterine contractions and release of milk by mammary glands
Adrenal cortex	Glucocorticoids	Inhibit or retard amino acid incorporation into proteins (cortisol, cortisone, and so on); stimulate conversion of proteins into carbohydrates; maintain normal blood sugar level; conserve glucose; promotes metabolism of fat
	Mineralcorticoids	Increase or decrease sodium-potassium metabolism, increase (aldosterone, deoxycorticosterone, and so on) body fluid
Adrenal medulla	Epinephrine	Increases cardiac output; increases blood sugar, glycogen breakdown, and fat mobilization
	Norepinephrine (some)	Similar to epinephrine plus constriction of blood vessels
	Proenkephalins (e.g., peptide F, E,)	Analgesia, enhance immune function
Thyroid	Thyroxine	Stimulates oxidative metabolism in mitochondria and cell growth
	Calcitonin	Reduces blood calcium phosphate levels
Pancreas	Insulin	Stores glycogen, aids in the absorption of glucose
	Glucagon	Increases blood glucose levels
Ovaries	Estrogens	Develop female sex characteristics, exert system effects, such as growth and maturation of long bones
	Progesterone	Develops female sex characteristics; maintains pregnancy; develops mammary glands
Parathyroids	Parathormone	Increases blood calcium; decreases blood phosphate

the endocrine, paracrine, and autocrine systems as well. These changes are temporally related to changes in the target organs and the toleration of exercise stress. The potential for adaptation is great because of the many different sites and mechanisms that can be affected.

The hormonal mechanisms controlled by the endocrine system can be activated in response to an acute resistance exercise stress or be altered after a chronic period of resistance training. The mechanisms that mediate acute homeostatic changes typically respond to acute resistance exercise stress with a sharp increase or decrease in hormonal concentrations, in order to regulate a physiological function such as protein metabolism or immune cell activation. A more subtle increase or decrease usually occurs in chronic resting hormonal concentrations in response to resistance training. For example, the subtle increases in resting testosterone over the course of a resistance training program may help to mediate changes in protein synthesis, thus leading to increased muscle fiber size.

However, decreases in hormones can also be observed (e.g., testosterone decreases with ingestion of protein or a meal), which may indicate an increased uptake by the androgen receptor (Chandler et al. 1994; Kraemer, Volek et al. 1998). Thus, interpretation of circulating concentrations must be done with care, as it is the target tissue receptor that controls the use of a hormone from the circulation.

Anabolic Hormones

The primary anabolic hormones involved in muscle tissue growth and remodeling discussed in this section are testosterone, growth hormone, and insulin-like growth factors (IGF). Insulin also plays a key role, but it does not appear to be operational in normal ranges of protein metabolism (Wolfe 2000). Likewise, thyroid hormones are vital (i.e., without thyroid hormones chemical reactions cannot occur normally) to the biochemical reactions in many of the metabolic mechanisms regulated by other hormones (Greenspan 1994).

Because of its obvious anabolic properties, **testosterone** has been one of the primary hormones used as a physiological marker to evaluate the anabolic status of the body. In addition to its direct effects on muscle tissue, testosterone may indirectly affect the protein content of the muscle fiber by promoting growth hormone(s) release, which leads to IGF release from the liver as well as increased autocrine IGF-I and associated IGF family polypeptides (e.g.,

effects of testosterone on development of strength and muscle size are also related to its influence on the nervous system, which further facilitates neuroendocrine function and performance (Nagaya and Herrera 1995).

For example, testosterone can interact with receptors on neurons and increase the amount of neurotransmitters and influence structural protein changes leading to size changes of the neuromuscular junction. Each of these factors can enhance the force production capabilities of the muscle. These potential interactions with other hormones demonstrate the highly interdependent nature of the endocrine system in influencing the expression of strength.

How testosterone exactly interacts with the nucleus of the muscle cell remains a point of inquiry. After secretion, testosterone is thought to be transported to target tissues by a transport protein (e.g., sex hormone–binding globulin), after which it associates with a membrane-bound protein or cytosolic receptor, is activated, and subsequently migrates to the cell nucleus where interactions with nuclear receptors take place, resulting in protein synthesis. Kadi and colleagues (2000) reported some of the first insights into the expression of androgen receptors in highly trained power lifters (of which nine had used anabolic drugs). They found that androgen receptor–containing myonuclei vary among human skeletal muscles and that a higher androgen receptor content occurs in the trapezius than in the vastus lateralis. In addition, power lifters had a higher proportion of androgen receptors than untrained controls. Finally, those who used anabolic steroids had higher androgen receptor content than untrained controls and drug-free power lifters. Such cross-sectional data support the plasticity of androgen receptors in human muscle and its potential responsiveness to resistance training and anabolic drugs. Thus, the increases of the concentrations of testosterone may stimulate interactive use and help mediate adaptational changes.

Increases in peripheral blood concentrations of testosterone have been observed during and after many types of high-intensity endurance exercise protocols (Kraemer, Patton et al. 1995). Thus, variations in testosterone's cellular actions may be the result of differences in the cell membrane consequent to resistance exercise. In addition, the magnitude of muscle fiber recruitment (e.g., the size principle) and possible differences in receptor interactions under various exercise conditions due to the force differences on membranes may also play a vital role.

In addition, variation in the training stimulus may be important to see clear-cut differences in serum testosterone (Hickson, Hidaka et al. 1994).

In men several factors appear to influence the acute serum concentrations of total testosterone. The magnitude of increase during resistance exercise has been shown to be affected by the muscle mass involved and the exercise selection (Volek et al. 1997), the intensity and volume (Kraemer et al. 1990, 1991; Raastad, Bjoro, and Hallen 2000; Schwab et al. 1993), nutrition intake (i.e., protein and carbohydrate supplementation may attenuate the acute testosterone increases) (Kraemer, Volek et al. 1998), and training experience (Kraemer, Fleck et al. 1999). Large-muscle-mass exercises such as the Olympic lift (Kraemer et al. 1992), deadlift (Fahey et al. 1976), and jump squat (Volek et al. 1997) have been shown to produce significant elevations in testosterone. Collectively, this information indicates independently or in various combinations that the following exercise variables can increase serum testosterone concentrations:

- Large-muscle-group exercises (e.g., deadlift, power clean, squat)
- Heavy resistance (85-95% of 1RM)
- Moderate to high volume of exercise, achieved with multiple sets, multiple exercises, or both
- Short rest intervals (30 seconds to 1 minute)

The sequencing of exercises has not been studied. It has been suggested for strength training that large-muscle-mass exercises be performed before small-muscle-mass exercises (Kraemer and Ratamess 2000). Performance of large-muscle-mass exercises early in the workout may produce significant elevations in testosterone, which potentially may expose smaller muscles to a greater response than that resulting from performance of small-muscle-mass exercises only. However, further research examining this hypothesis is warranted.

The interaction of a resistance training program's intensity and volume affects the acute testosterone response. Raastad and colleagues (2000) examined two similar programs with the exception that one protocol used 70% of 3 to 6RM and the second used 100% of 3 to 6RM and reported significantly greater testosterone response after the high-intensity protocol. Schwab and colleagues (1993) compared a protocol of four sets of 6 repetitions (90-95% of 6RM) to four sets of 9 to 10 repetitions (60-65% of load used for a 6RM protocol) of the squat and reported similar increases

in testosterone after both protocols. However, testosterone did not significantly increase until after the fourth set. They concluded that a threshold of volume might be needed to elicit significant increases in testosterone. Bosco and colleagues (2000) made a similar observation when they reported significant increases in testosterone with high-volume resistance training, and no change during lower-volume resistance training (20 sets of 2 to 4 repetitions of half squats vs. 10 sets of 2 to 3 repetitions) in weightlifters. The authors also reported that testosterone concentrations decreased in a group of bodybuilders performing a high-volume protocol and increased in a group of weightlifters performing a lower-volume protocol (Bosco et al. 2000). Häkkinen and Pakarinen (1993) compared two squat training programs (20 sets of 1RM, and 10 sets of 10 repetitions with 70% of 1RM) and reported that significant increases in total and free testosterone occurred only in the higher-volume workout. An anaerobic glycolytic component for stimulating testosterone release may be evident, as Kraemer and colleagues (1990, 1991) reported that a bodybuilding program (moderate load, high volume) with short rest periods produced greater testosterone responses than high-load, low-volume training with long (i.e., 3-minute) rest periods. Therefore, it appears that programs high in volume with moderate to high intensity may be most effective for stimulating acute testosterone increases.

The age and training experience of individuals plays a critical role in the acute response of testosterone. Fahey and colleagues (1976) were unable to demonstrate significant increases among high school boys in serum concentrations of total testosterone. This was thought to be due to the nonresponsiveness of cells in the testes of young men. Older individuals, on the other hand, have been shown to produce significant elevations of testosterone during an acute bout of resistance exercise; however, the absolute concentrations are significantly lower than those of young adults (Kraemer, Häkkinen et al. 1998, 1999).

A certain level of training experience appears necessary to optimize the acute testosterone response. A report by Kraemer and colleagues (1992) suggests that increases in testosterone may occur if the resistance training experience of high school males (14-18 years) is 2 years or more. Kraemer, Staron, and colleagues (1998) were unable to demonstrate an acute increase during resistance exercise until previously untrained men completed at least 6 weeks of an 8-week program.

Therefore, training experience and age may affect the testosterone response.

Free Testosterone and Sex Hormone–Binding Globulin

Scant data are available concerning the acute exercise responses of free testosterone (testosterone not bound to a protein, such as sex hormone–binding globulin, for transport). Häkkinen and coworkers (Häkkinen, Pakarinen et al. 1987, 1988a) observed that free testosterone remained unaltered or decreased after resistance exercise training sessions. The so-called free hormone hypothesis says that only the free hormone interacts with target tissues. Still, the bound hormone significantly influences the rate of hormone delivery to a target tissue, such as muscle.

The role, regulation, and interaction of binding proteins and their interactions with cells also present interesting possibilities, especially with women, whose total amount of testosterone is very low in comparison with men. In fact, the binding protein itself may act as a hormone with biological activity. The biological role of various binding proteins appears to be an important factor in tissue interactions (Elkins 1990). These observations have demonstrated that changes in sex hormone–binding globulin and the ratio of this protein to testosterone are correlated to isometric leg strength and reflect the patterns of force production improvements in leg musculature (Häkkinen, Pakarinen et al. 1985).

Testosterone Responses in Women

For the most part, the majority of data on hormonal responses to resistance exercise and training have used college-age men. The testosterone hormonal response patterns during growth and development have traditionally been credited as responsible for the differences in muscular development and strength between men and women. To date, the majority of studies have shown that women typically do not demonstrate an exercise-induced increase in testosterone consequent to various forms of heavy resistance exercise (Bosco et al. 2000; Consitt et al. 2001; Häkkinen and Pakarinen 1995; Kraemer, Fleck et al. 1993; Stoessel et al. 1991). This may vary with individual women, as some women are capable of high adrenal androgen release. In one report, differences were observed in the resting baseline levels of testos-

terone between females who had performed 2 months of resistance training and inactive controls (Cumming et al. 1987). Still, other studies have been unable to demonstrate changes in resting serum concentrations of testosterone with training (Häkkinen et al. 1990; Häkkinen, Pakarinen, and Kallinen 1992). Yet in one of these studies a significant correlation was shown between resting total and free testosterone changes and maximal strength changes after training (Häkkinen et al. 1990). However, a recent study by Marx and colleagues (2001) reported significant elevations in resting serum testosterone with the response greater with higher-volume, periodized, multiple-set training compared to a single-set program during 6 months of training. It has also been shown that with greater statistical power using a large sample size, the small increase observed in women's resting testosterone increases significantly consequent to acute resistance exercise stress (Nindl, Kraemer, Gotshalk et al. 2001). Thus, the lack of prior detection of changes may well have been due to the small increases and the low number of participants in study samples. In addition, in studies with larger numbers of women, more women may be represented that have higher adrenal androgen content.

Long-Term Training Adaptations of Testosterone

We are still learning about the responses of testosterone to resistance training. It appears that training time, experience, and the overall stress related to training may be very important factors in altering the resting and exercise-induced concentrations of this hormone. In adult men, acute increases in testosterone are observed if the exercise stimulus is adequate (i.e., multiple sets, 5 to 10RM, and an adequate amount of muscle mass used). Häkkinen and colleagues (1988c) demonstrated that over the course of 2 years of training, increases in resting serum testosterone concentrations do occur, even in elite power athletes. This was concomitant to increases in follicle-stimulating hormone and luteinizing hormone, which are the higher brain regulators of testosterone production and release. Such changes may help augment the neural adaptations that occur for strength gain in highly trained power athletes.

In the study by Häkkinen, Pakarinen, and colleagues (1988c), the testosterone changes showed remarkable similarities to the patterns of strength changes; however, the ratio of sex hormone–

binding globulin to testosterone mirrored strength changes even more closely. It is interesting to hypothesize that in athletes with little adaptive potential for changes in muscle hypertrophy (i.e., highly trained strength athletes), changes in testosterone cybernetics may be a part of a more advanced adaptive strategy for increasing the force capabilities of muscle via neural factors. This may occur because of the potentiation of other hormonal mechanisms in tissue development or because of the enhancement of neural factors (Nagaya and Herrera 1995). Such differences in adaptational strategies appear essential to providing for further gains in performance over the course of a long-term training program. This may reflect the interplay of different neural and hypertrophic factors involved in mediating strength and power changes as training time is extended into years.

Androgen Precursors

The biosynthetic pathway of testosterone contains many steps. Some of the precursor molecules in these steps have been investigated during resistance training. The rationale is that a change in precursors may ultimately affect circulating testosterone concentrations and potentially the anabolic state of muscle tissue. Androstenedione and dehydroepiandrosterone (DHEA) are adrenal androgens that are testosterone precursors (Longcope 1996). These two compounds have received much attention in the literature because of their popularity as nutritional supplements and use in athletics (Pecci and Lombardo 2000). Studies have shown that recommended doses (100-300 mg/day) of these compounds do not increase circulating testosterone concentrations in healthy men (Ballantyne et al. 2000; King et al. 1999; Wallace, Lim, Cutler, and Bucci 1999), although the concentrations of DHEA, androstenedione, and luteinizing hormone were significantly elevated. Recently, Brown and colleagues (2002) showed that sublingual androstenediol increased serum free testosterone concentrations from 86.2 to 175.4 pmol/l and total testosterone from 25.6 to 47.9 nmol/l. However, the potential ergogenic effects of precursor hormones remain to be seen and require further examination particularly since many individuals consume higher than the recommended dose.

Adrenal androgens may play a greater role in women considering the low levels of testosterone present. At rest, women typically have higher concentrations of androstenedione than men (Weiss, Cureton, and Thompson 1983). However, androstenedione is significantly less potent than testosterone. Few studies have examined the acute response of testosterone precursors to resistance exercise. Using a program consisting of four exercises for three sets to failure with 80% of 1RM and 2-minute rest intervals, Weiss and colleagues (1983) reported increases in circulating androstenedione of 8 to 11% in both men and women in response to an acute bout of resistance exercise. However, little is known about the effect of acute increases in androstenedione on muscle strength increases and hypertrophy.

Chronic resistance training (e.g., 24 weeks of strength and power training) has been shown to decrease serum concentrations of the testosterone precursors 17-OH-progesterone, androstenedione, and DHEA (Alen et al. 1988). The impact of these findings is unclear, but may suggest a greater potential rate of androgen turnover in response to resistance training. Thus, the influence of these precursors during long-term resistance training is largely unknown and warrants further investigation.

Growth Hormone

Growth hormone (GH) is secreted by the pituitary gland, one of the most interesting endocrine glands. The main circulating isoform of GH (1-191 amino acids) is the 22 kD polypeptide hormone derived from the GH-N gene on chromosome 17 and is secreted by the anterior pituitary. In addition, other spliced fragments, including 22 kD missing residues 32-46 or missing residues 1-43 and 44-191 making 5- and 17 kD, respectively, have been identified. A host of other monomeric, dimeric, protein-bound, novel binding protein aggregates of GH, and chemically altered molecules have been identified and make up the superfamily of GH. The biological roles of these different isoforms and aggregates are now the focus of investigation, as the GH family of polypeptides and binding proteins have been implicated in the control of fat metabolism and growth-promoting actions. Nevertheless, the mediating events at the molecular level remain speculative. To date, studies have attempted to examine the concentrations in the blood, circulating changes with exercise, or recombinant GH administration, but scientific work is at the dawn of a new era in GH research (Hymer et al. 2000, 2001; McCall et al. 2000; Wallace et al. 2001). Thus, how the classic 22 kD GH interacts with receptors, physiological mechanisms, and integrated endocrine GH effects within the context of the superfamily of GH and binding proteins is not as well understood as previously thought.

The human GH superfamily of molecules is heterogeneous and includes the 22 kD monomer, the 20 kD mRNA splice variant, disulfide-linked homodimers and heterodimers of these monomers, glycosylated GH, high-molecular-weight oligomers, receptor-bound forms of GH, and hormone fragments resulting from proteolysis (Baumann 1991a). The distribution of 22 kD and non-22 kD isoforms varies in human blood and is thought to be due to differential metabolic clearance, circulating binding proteins, and the formation of GH fragments in peripheral tissues (Baumann 1991b). Because of the complex nature of the family of human GH molecules and its numerous physiological actions, it is possible that some of the effects of the hormone on lipid, carbohydrate, and protein metabolism; longitudinal bone growth; and skeletal muscle protein turnover may be controlled by different GH isoforms (Hymer et al. 2001; Rowlinson et al. 1996).

The effects of GH have essentially been investigated through the examination of the 22 kD immunoreactive polypeptide or recombinant form. The anabolic effects of GH on skeletal muscle are thought to have both direct and indirect influences. Although not yet completely understood, some of the effects of GH are thought to be mediated by stimulating the cell-released insulin-like growth factors (IGFs) (liver versus muscle types) via autocrine, paracrine, and/or endocrine mechanisms (Florini, Ewton, and Coolican 1996; Florini et al. 1996). Although the exact binding interactions with skeletal muscle remain unknown, some data have shown that GH does bind to skeletal muscle in pigs (Schnoebelen-Combes et al. 1996). However, exogenous GH administration in children and adults who are GH deficient has been shown to increase muscle mass and decrease body fat (Cuneo et al. 1991; Rooyackers and Nair 1997). These observations have led to the obvious conclusion that GH plays a significant anabolic role in skeletal muscle growth. Training adaptations are likely mediated by GH's effects on muscle protein synthesis (i.e., increases) and protein breakdown (i.e., decreases) (Fryburg and Barrett 1995). Also, GH is known to stimulate the release of available amino acids for protein synthesis in vivo, as well as the release of other growth factors (e.g., IGF-I) from muscle cells, thereby implicating GH in recovery

and tissue repair (Florini, Ewton, and Coolican 1996). The repair and remodeling after resistance exercise stress mediates the adaptive response of muscle. Moreover, studies have shown that increases occur in circulating GH concentrations during and/or after heavy resistance exercise in men (Kraemer et al. 1990), women (Kraemer, Fleck et al. 1993), and the elderly (Kraemer, Häkkinen et al. 1998), further indicating a potential stimulatory effect on GH secretion and enhanced potential for receptor interactions stress directed at improving muscular size, strength, and power consequent to heavy resistance exercise.

Hymer and colleagues (2001) examined the effects of acute heavy resistance exercise on biologically active circulating GH in young women via immunoassay versus bioassay techniques. The results from this study indicated that acute resistance exercise significantly increased the lower-molecular-weight GH isoforms (30-60 kD and < 30 kD) when measured by the immunofunctional assay (Strasburger et al. 1996), but not in the classic rat tibial line bioassay. However, acute circulatory increases have been observed in men for bioactive GH using the tibial line bioassay (McCall et al. 2000). Such data show that our understanding of the dynamics of pituitary function in response to exercise is starting to become more complex and requires further study. GH isoforms, aggregates, and binding proteins could be important hormonal factors for mediating adaptations in muscle consequent to resistance exercise and training. How such isoforms respond to different types of resistance training remains to be studied. One report shows that increases in tibial line GH occur with long-term resistance training in women, suggesting that higher-molecular-weight molecules are adaptive in nature (Rubin et al. 2000). To date, the exact mechanisms by which different GH molecules interact with their receptors to elicit their growth-promoting actions remains unclear.

An important, yet unanswered, question regarding the actions of GH is whether GH acts directly on skeletal muscle to stimulate its growth. The most convincing data to date is that tyrosine phosphorylation of JAK2 and STAT5 increased after intravenous GH administration in rats (Chow et al. 1996). Furthermore, it has remained difficult to demonstrate any specific binding of GH to skeletal muscle, and although we cannot rule out the possibility that GH does have a direct effect on skeletal muscle growth, this remains unclear (Florini, Ewton, and Coolican 1996). By measuring arterial and venous concentrations of GH during and after an acute bout of resistance exercise, Brahm and colleagues (1997) showed that GH uptake in skeletal muscle (quadriceps) increased significantly. These data, however, still do not eliminate any mediating indirect influences of the IGFs. The indirect effects of growth hormone on muscle growth and the numerous interactions between GH and the IGFs have been reviewed in detail (Florini, Ewton, and Coolican 1996), and it seems probable that many of the effects of GH are mediated in part by the actions of IGFs.

Various external factors, such as age, gender, sleep, nutrition, alcohol consumption, and exercise, all alter growth hormone release patterns (Giustina and Veldhuis 1998). The secretion of GH and thus the amount in the blood varies according to the time of day, with the highest levels observed at night during sleep (Giustina and Veldhuis 1998). Secreting pulses also have different amplitudes throughout the day, and exercise appears to increase their amplitude. It has been hypothesized that nocturnal increases are involved in various tissue repair mechanisms in the body. Thus, it is possible that GH secretion and release may directly influence adaptations of muscle and subsequent expression of strength.

Despite many unanswered questions, growth hormone is intimately involved with the growth process of skeletal muscle and many other tissues in the body. Not only is it important for normal development of a child, but it also appears to play a vital role in the body's adaptation to the stress of resistance training. The main physiological roles of growth hormones are as follows:

- Decreases glucose utilization
- Decreases glycogen synthesis
- Increases amino acid transport across cell membranes
- Increases protein synthesis
- Increases utilization of fatty acids
- Increases lipolysis (fat breakdown)
- Increases availability of glucose and amino acids
- Increases collagen synthesis
- Stimulates cartilage growth
- Increases retention of nitrogen, sodium, potassium, and phosphorus
- Increases renal plasma flow and glomerular filtration
- Promotes compensatory renal hypertrophy

Release and Binding of Growth Hormone

Growth hormone is released into the peripheral circulation, where it attaches to specific binding proteins that represent the extracellular domain of the GH receptor (Giustina and Veldhuis 1998). Growth hormone acts by binding to plasma membrane–bound receptors on the target cells. It is not known how extracellular domain binding of the receptor leads to a signal transduction in the cytosolic domain via such a short transmembrane sequence. Growth hormone binding may produce aggregates of receptors that traverse laterally in the fluid plasma membrane. Subsequently, the cell membrane–bound receptor also interacts and binds specifically with GH.

Human 22 kD GH has been shown to increase during resistance exercise and 30 minutes postexercise with the magnitude dependent on exercise selection (Kraemer et al. 1992), exercise intensity (Pyka, Wiswell, and Marcus 1992; Vanhelder et al. 1984), exercise volume (Häkkinen and Pakarinen 1993; Kraemer, Fleck et al. 1993), rest periods between sets (Kraemer et al. 1990, 1991; Kraemer, Patton et al. 1995), carbohydrate and protein supplementation (Chandler et al. 1994), and training experience in men (Kraemer et al. 1992). However, because not all resistance training programs will produce a significant elevation in serum 22 kD GH concentrations, a threshold volume and intensity may be needed (Vanhelder et al. 1984). High correlations have been reported between blood lactate and serum GH concentrations (Häkkinen and Pakarinen 1993), and it has been proposed that H$^+$ accumulation produced by lactic acidosis may be the primary factor influencing 22 kD GH release (Gordon et al. 1994). This finding is supported by an attenuated GH response after induced alkalosis during high-intensity cycling (Gordon et al. 1994). Hypoxia, breath holding, acid-base shifts, and protein catabolism all have been reported to influence GH release. Thus, the metabolic demands of resistance exercise play a significant role in GH concentrations.

Taylor and colleagues (2000) reported a greater acute increase in resistance-trained women than in nontrained women performing the same program. However, the trained women were capable of lifting greater loads, which may have affected the overall magnitude of exertion and so GH response. Studies have shown the acute GH response to be somewhat limited in older individuals (Craig et al. 1989; Kraemer, Häkkinen et al. 1999). However, it has been suggested that a major factor contributing to this limited GH response may be the magnitude of exertion. Pyka and colleagues (1992) also reported lower blood lactates in elderly subjects, thereby supporting the hypothesis that maximal effort is necessary for optimizing the exercise-induced secretion of GH. Resistance training over 12 weeks in the elderly has been shown to promote greater acute GH response to a resistance exercise protocol (Craig et al. 1989), suggesting that the greater response was due to an increased ability for exertion.

Moderate- to high-intensity programs high in total work using short rest periods appear to have the greatest effect on the acute 22 kD GH response compared to conventional strength or power training using high loads, low repetitions, and long rest intervals in men (Kraemer et al. 1990, 1991). Kraemer, Fleck, and colleagues (1993) reported similar results in women, although the resting concentrations of GH are significantly higher in women. Häkkinen and Pakarinen (1993) reported that 20 sets of 1RM in the squat only produced a slight increase in GH, whereas a substantial increase in GH was observed after 10 sets of 10 repetitions with 70% of 1RM. Multiple-set protocols have elicited greater GH response than single-set protocols in both sexes (Craig and Kang 1994; Gotshalk et al. 1997; Mulligan et al. 1996). These data indicate that programs moderate in intensity, but high in total work or volume using short rest intervals (e.g., bodybuilding programs or programs targeting local muscular endurance) may elicit the greatest acute increase in 22 kD GH concentrations probably due to high metabolic demands.

Recent studies have shown that the muscle action may affect the acute 22 kD GH response to resistance exercise. Kraemer, Dudley, and colleagues (2001) examined the GH response to performing concentric-only training or normal weight training consisting of concentric and eccentric muscle actions. The GH response was significant for the concentric-only training, but the acute response was greater for the normal weight training. This indicates that 22 kD GH is sensitive to the type of muscle actions used during resistance training, that higher brain centers (e.g., motor cortex) may play an active role in regulating 22 kD GH secretion during exercise stress, and that this regulatory mechanism appears to be sensitive to the specific type of muscle actions used during resistance training.

Training Adaptations of Growth Hormone

Longer sampling time periods (2 to 24 hours) will be needed to see if long-term resistance training will elicit changes in resting GH levels. In a recent study, Nindl, Hymer, and colleagues (2001) showed that changes in the pulsatile effects of GH did take place overnight. Resistance exercise (high volume, 50 sets total body) was performed at 3:00 PM and GH was measured 1 hour postexercise and throughout the night. GH was significantly elevated up to 30 minutes postexercise. However, pulsatility was different overnight compared to no exercise. It is the area under the time curve, which includes an array of pulsatile effects, that tells if changes in release have occurred. The maximum GH concentrations and pulse amplitudes were lower overnight after resistance exercise, although the total concentrations were similar to no exercise. This was evident throughout the early to middle segments of the night (i.e., 6:00 PM to 3:00 AM). However, from 3:00 AM to 6:00 AM, the mean GH concentrations were greater in the resistance exercise group.

The responses of GH to resistance training have not been studied extensively, but observations of normal single measures of resting concentrations of GH in elite Olympic lifters suggest little change (Häkkinen, Pakarinen et al. 1988c). Additionally, no changes in resting GH concentrations have been observed in several studies (Kraemer, Hakkinen et al. 1999; McCall et al. 1999; Marx et al. 2001). These data are consistent with GH's dynamic feedback mechanisms and its roles in the homeostatic control of several variables (e.g., glucose). This may also be due to the interactive effects of different GH molecules, aggregates, and variants with training. In addition, these data suggest that the acute response of GH to resistance exercise may be the most prominent mechanism for interacting acutely with tissue target receptors leading to adaptations. The exercise-induced increase has been significantly correlated with the magnitude of type I and type II muscle fiber hypertrophy ($r = 0.62$ to 0.74) after resistance training (McCall et al. 1999). These relationships could be indicative of a role for repeated acute resistance exercise–induced GH elevations on muscle adaptations. Changes in receptor sensitivity, different size GH molecules, differences in feedback mechanisms, IGF-I potentiation, and diurnal variations may also play significant roles in adaptations.

Insulin-Like Growth Factors

Many of the effects of GH are mediated through small polypeptides called insulin-like growth factors (IGFs), or somatomedins (Adams 1998). IGFs are secreted by the liver after GH stimulates liver cell DNA to synthesize them, a process that takes about 8 to 29 hours (Kraemer, Patton et al. 1995). Other factors, such as nutritional status and insulin levels, have also been shown to be important signal mechanisms for IGF release. The IGFs are structurally related to insulin and thus are members of the insulin/IGF peptide hormone family. The IGFs are small polypeptide hormones (70 and 67 amino acid residues for IGF-I and -II, respectively) that are secreted as they are produced and are not stored in large quantities in any organ or tissue. Similar to insulin, as well as other peptide hormones, the IGFs are synthesized as a larger precursor peptide that is posttranslationally processed into the final IGF-I or -II molecule. Because of their structural similarities, the IGFs can bind to insulin receptors and vice versa. Two IGF receptor types have been identified: type 1 and type 2. The binding affinities or the strength of binding among these molecules and their receptors are as follows: IGF-I binds type 1 > type 2 > IR (insulin receptor); IGF-II binds type 2 > type 1 > IR; and insulin binds IR > type 1 (Thissen, Ketelslegers, and Underwood 1994).

Nearly all IGFs in the circulation, and some IGFs in tissues (muscle), are bound to IGF-binding proteins (IGFBPs). These IGFBPs regulate IGF availability by prolonging their half-lives in circulation (~12-15 hours), controlling their transport out of circulation, and localizing IGFs to tissues (Collett-Solberg and Cohen 1996). Also, IGFBPs diminish the hypoglycemic potential of IGFs by limiting the concentrations of free IGF molecules in circulation (DeMeyts et al. 1994). Seven IGF-binding proteins (IGFBP 1-7) have currently been identified, but IGFBP-3 is the most common in the circulation with its primary role in the transport and bioactivity of the circulating IGFs (Zapf 1997). Together with IGF molecules, IGFBPs (-1, -2, -3, -4, -5, and -6) are produced and secreted by the liver as well as by most other cells including skeletal muscle (Florini, Ewton, and Coolican 1996; Frost and Lang 1999). Insulin-like growth factor binding protein-4 has a very high affinity for IGF-I, and has been shown to inhibit IGF-I's myogenic (i.e., differentiation) effects on skeletal muscle (Damon et al. 1998). Not surprisingly, resistance exercise appears to result in decreased human skeletal muscle IGFBP-4 mRNA, and increased muscle IGF-I mRNA (Bamman et al. 2001). Such results indicate that free IGF-I concentrations increase in skeletal muscle after mechanical loading, which is probably related to an increased need for processes related to tissue growth and repair. Together with the results from Borst and colleagues (2001), who demonstrated that long-term resistance training results in decreased circulating IGFBP-3 concentrations and increased circulating IGF-I concentrations, these studies suggest potential important roles for acute, local, and chronic systemic growth factor–mediated actions on skeletal muscle for strength and power adaptations.

In cell culture studies, IGFs have been shown to stimulate myoblast proliferation and differentiation, suppress proteolysis, increase glucose and amino acid uptake, and increase protein synthesis in various skeletal muscle cell lines (Florini, Ewton, and Coolican 1996). Several studies have also demonstrated the efficacy of the IGFs in increasing protein synthesis in human skeletal muscles (Fryburg 1994, 1996; Fryburg et al. 1995; Russell-Jones et al. 1994). These mitogenic (proliferation), myogenic (differentiation), and anabolic actions help to qualify the profound growth potentiating effects of the IGFs on skeletal muscle (Adams 1998; Florini, Ewton, and Coolican 1996).

The role of the IGFs in skeletal muscle growth as a mediator in the GH/IGF system has been well accepted for many years. This system is characterized largely by the fact that circulating GH is an important stimulus for IGF gene expression and release by the liver (Copeland, Underwood, and Van Wyk 1980). Although the liver is thought to be responsible for the majority of circulating IGFs, they are known to be produced by many other tissues and cells, including muscle (Goldspink 1999; Goldspink and Yang 2001). The extent to which circulating IGFs (endocrine) interact with skeletal muscle has been contested largely because most circulating IGFs (>75%) are bound as a ternary complex with IGF-binding protein-3 and an acid-labile subunit (~150 kD when bound), which apparently does not cross the capillary endothelium (Binoux and Hossenlopp 1988). As a result, it has been proposed that circulating IGFs exhibit only a minor effect on skeletal muscle adaptations to mechanical loading (Yarasheski 1994).

Support for the premise just discussed comes from recent resistance training studies that demonstrated no additive effects of exogenous GH treatment on serum total IGF-I concentrations on strength performance or on protein synthesis rates after exogenous GH administration with training in elderly subjects (Taaffe et al. 1994; Yarasheski et al. 1995). Possible shortcomings of these studies, however, may be related to the stimulatory effect that circulating GH is known to have on the secretion of IGFBPs from the liver, in particular IGFBP-3 (Florini, Ewton, and Coolican 1996). If the exogenous GH treatment resulted in increased IGFBP-3 concentrations (not measured), then the percentage of unbound, biologically active IGF-I may have remained essentially unchanged in these studies (Taaffe et al. 1994; Yarasheski et al. 1995).

Contrary to the argument against a role for circulating IGFs, Borst and colleagues (2001) recently reported a 20% reduction in circulating IGFBP-3 after 25 weeks of multiple-set resistance training. These data indicate that circulating IGFs may become more important for skeletal muscle adaptations with prolonged resistance training because circulating binding proteins decrease, thereby permitting an increased portion of unbound IGFs to cross the capillary endothelium and thus interact with muscle.

This trend for a decrease in IGF-binding protein elements has also been recently shown to begin within hours after a heavy resistance exercise bout. Nindl, Kraemer, and colleagues (2001) demonstrated that circulating concentrations of the acid-labile subunits begin to decrease 2 hours after a heavy resistance exercise bout, and are still lower than controls after 13 hours postexercise. Furthermore, Borst and colleagues (2001) reported a 20% increase in circulating IGF-I concentrations after training, and this is not the only study to demonstrate increasing circulating growth factors with long-term training (Kraemer, Aguilera et al. 1995). Long-term studies in women have shown elevations in resting IGF-I, particularly with high-volume training (Koziris et al. 1999; Marx et al. 2001). In addition, the increase in resting IGF-I was significantly greater with a high-volume, multiple-set program versus a single-set circuit-type program (Marx et al. 2001).

Thus, it appears that the volume and intensity of training are important for chronic IGF-I adaptations and that the IGF system undergoes adaptations with training that in turn improve the ability of the circulating IGFs to interact with skeletal muscle for cell growth and repair. Such adaptations in the endocrine actions of the IGFs on skeletal muscle could theoretically be mediated by, or simply complement, the autocrine/paracrine actions of the IGFs.

Support for autocrine/paracrine actions of the IGFs in muscle adaptational processes arise from the results of several studies that have shown significant hypertrophic effects of local IGF infusion directly into rat (Adams and McCue 1998) and human skeletal muscle (Fryburg 1994, 1996; Fryburg et al. 1995; Russell-Jones et al. 1994). Whether the local production and release of IGFs from skeletal muscle are influenced primarily by circulating GH or by other factors (e.g., mechanical loading) remains unclear. The role of GH in the stimulation of IGF secretion is supported by data showing that GH stimulates IGF-I gene expression in skeletal muscle of rats and pigs (Lewis et al. 2000; Loughna, Mason, and Bates 1992; Turner et al. 1988). However, this relationship is questionable because such a stimulatory influence of GH on muscle IGF has yet to be conclusively demonstrated in humans. GH-independent local IGF-I gene expression has also been demonstrated in skeletal muscle from several animal models including dwarf chickens, cattle, sheep, and pigs (Florini, Ewton, and Coolican 1996). Thus, the primary actions of the local IGFs on skeletal muscle do not appear to be influenced greatly by GH, and other factors (e.g., mechanical loading, stretch, etc.) may be more important for local IGF production and release (Adams 1998).

Recent reports describe the importance of a specific IGF-I isoform (also known as mechanogrowth factor) that is expressed by skeletal muscle in response to stretch, loading, or both (Bamman et al. 2001; Goldspink 1998; Goldspink and Yang 2001; Perrone, Fenwick-Smith, and Vandenburgh 1995). Stretch also has been shown to cause differentiated avian skeletal muscle cells in tissue culture to secrete IGFBPs in conjunction with IGFs, possibly for enhanced regulatory control of the actions of the IGF system on local muscle growth (Perrone, Fenwick-Smith, and Vandenburgh 1995). Bamman and colleagues (2001) recently showed that mechanical loading of human muscle (i.e., resistance exercise) results in increased muscle, but not serum IGF-I. (The results from this study also showed that the expression of skeletal muscle IGF-I mRNA in humans was greater after an eccentric as compared to a concentric bout of heavy squat exercise.) Thus, the eccentric component of resistance exercise appears to be a potent stimulus for the production and release of local growth factors in skeletal muscle.

Together, these data appear to emphasize the importance of mechanical loading–induced IGF isoforms for mediating muscle mass adaptations to resistance training; however, more studies examining these responses are needed. In particular, differences between slow eccentric training movements and explosive strength and power movements raise a question regarding the potential role of supramaximal eccentric exercise training (and the concomitant local IGF gene expression) to optimize explosive or maximal strength and power development. Perhaps such eccentric load–induced growth factors play a less significant role in explosive or maximal concentric strength and power development. This may help explain why many bodybuilding-type resistance training programs that emphasize higher volume (sets and repetitions) and slower, more controlled exercise movements (especially eccentric) are used more often for producing gains in muscle size, but not necessarily for strength and power performance.

Insulin

The ability of **insulin** to stimulate an increase in protein mass has been recognized since the 1940s when persons with type 1 diabetes (i.e., insulin-dependent) first began using insulin therapy to help regulate their blood glucose. Unfortunately, whether this increased protein mass in humans is due to increased protein synthesis, decreased protein degradation, or a combination of both remains unclear (Rooyackers and Nair 1997; Wolfe 2000). Results from most cell culture and animal model studies have demonstrated that insulin increases protein synthesis and decreases protein degradation (Rooyackers and Nair 1997). Results from other in vitro studies using human skeletal muscle cells have demonstrated that insulin increases protein synthesis, but protein degradation does not change (Rooyackers and Nair 1997). Even more confusing, results from in vivo studies in humans show mixed results, and appear to depend on the scientific methodology used to examine insulin's effects on protein metabolism. When tracer methodology is used to differentiate the balance between the arterial and venous concentrations of an essential amino acid such as phenylalanine (i.e., neither produced nor metabolized by skeletal muscle), the results from most studies have supported a decrease in protein degradation, but no change in protein synthesis (Biolo et al. 1999; Rooyackers and Nair 1997). It is believed that insulin-induced hypoaminoacidemia may help to explain the lack of an effect of insulin on protein synthesis rates, suggesting that insulin

would increase protein synthesis if intracellular amino acid concentrations were maintained or enhanced. Studies using amino acid infusion have in fact demonstrated a stimulatory effect of insulin on muscle protein synthesis (Biolo et al. 1999). Also, Wolfe (2000) argued that studies using tracer methodologies do not account for intracellular amino acids that originate from protein degradation, or amino acids that were originally released by protein degradation but were reincorporated into muscle protein before reaching the circulation. By accounting for such ongoing intracellular amino acid turnover processes (protein metabolism), more accurate measures of total protein synthesis and degradation appear to be possible (Biolo et al. 1995).

Although mechanistically unclear, physiological concentrations of insulin appear to increase protein synthesis as long as intracellular amino acid availability is maintained. The mechanisms by which insulin stimulates skeletal muscle protein synthesis include increases in the activation of enzymes, translation of mRNA, and gene transcription (Wolfe 2000). Changes in translational processes appear to occur first, however, with transcriptional processes activated later. Insulin can bind IGF receptors, and thus at higher concentrations such as after a large carbohydrate meal, this may also contribute to IGF type I receptor–mediated increases in protein synthesis.

The influence of insulin on protein degradation is implicated in its effects on two different protein degradation pathways: the ATP-dependent ubiquitin proteolytic system and lysosomal protein degradation (Wolfe 2000). It has been proposed that the ATP-dependent ubiquitin proteolytic system is suppressed by normal resting concentrations of insulin, but that this low-level suppression may not be altered by acute elevations in insulin concentrations (after meals) (Wolfe 2000). This type of ongoing regulation by insulin of the proteolytic breakdown system would thus help explain why, in the absence of insulin such as that observed with untreated insulin-dependent diabetes mellitus, muscle protein degradation is increased and muscle mass decreases over time.

Conversely, processes related to lysosomal protein degradation naturally increase after exercise (Kesperek et al. 1992). This may help to explain why a postexercise meal can reduce muscle protein degradation, since the meal would cause the pancreas to increase insulin secretion causing a transient physiologic hyperinsulinemia (Biolo et al. 1995). Thus, in normal daily life, resting insulin concentrations induce a low-level suppressive effect on protein degradation via reduced ATP-dependent ubiquitin proteolysis, but with acute exercise that typically results in lower circulating insulin, the inhibitory effects of insulin on lysosomal protein degradation are reduced and protein degradation increases transiently. At what levels insulin has the most dramatic effects on protein synthesis remains unclear, but it may only be during times of very low or very high levels of protein synthesis (Farrell et al. 2000; Szanberg et al. 1997).

Basal concentrations of insulin are not regulated by normal basal serum glucose concentrations (e.g. 80-100 mg/dl) and have been shown to be lower during regular strength training (Miller, Sherman, and Ivy 1984), overreaching (unpublished data from Dr. Kraemer's laboratory), and in bodybuilders with large muscle mass (Szczypaczewska, Nazar, and Kaciuba-Uscilko 1989). Thus, the role of insulin in resistance training adaptations in humans remains speculative as to the timing of its most important contribution to the protein accretion phenomenon.

Other Anabolic Factors

Although much research is still needed, it is becoming increasingly evident that other factors also potentiate skeletal muscle growth. Other hormones (e.g., angiotensin II, tibial peptide) and nerve factors (e.g., glial growth factor 2) have been implicated in skeletal muscle anabolic processes in animal and cell culture models. Angiotensin II is thought to be important for overload-induced cardiac and skeletal muscle hypertrophy. Gordon and colleagues (2001) recently demonstrated that angiotensin-converting-enzyme (ACE) inhibition in overloaded rat soleus muscle resulted in decreased hypertrophy (96%), whereas angiotensin II perfusion restored 71% of the hypertrophic response. The exact mechanism by which angiotensin II influences muscle hypertrophy has yet to be clearly elucidated, but concomitant changes in other factors (e.g., angiotensin II type 1 receptor density) appear to also be important. Ultimately, angiotensin II may very well be yet another important factor involved in the complex hormonal pathways associated with the intracellular signaling needed for tissue growth and repair after heavy resistance exercise.

Another less understood hormone, called tibial line peptide, was recently identified in human plasma and human postmortem pituitary tissue (Hymer et al. 2000). This peptide is proposed to be stored in a secretion granule associated with a specific subpopulation of GH cells, and it contains an amino acid residue sequence not found in human GH. Interestingly, this small peptide (~5 kD) demonstrated bioactivity in the tibial line bioassay, but not in the GH immunoassay. Thus, this peptide appears to be a biologically active hormone that is neither a GH isoform nor a fragment of the GH polypeptide family.

The importance of the nervous system to skeletal muscle function has been studied in detail, and it has generally been accepted that the type of motor unit innervating a skeletal muscle fiber (i.e., fast or slow) largely dictates the resultant fiber cell type (i.e., type I or type II) and its capacity for force production. Recently, evidence supporting myotrophic nerve factors that elicit growth and differentiation actions on muscle without direct physical contact has been mounting. The neuregulin family of neurotrophic proteins is characterized by glycosylated, transmembrane proteins including here gulin, neu differentiation factor, and glial growth factors (Florini et al. 1996b). Glial growth factor 2, unlike its fellow family members, is not a transmembrane protein, and thus it may function as a cell-released nerve factor. Florini and colleagues (1996) demonstrated that glial growth factor 2 is a potent myotrophic factor (i.e., stimulates growth and differentiation) in cultured myoblasts. Thus, at least in embryonic muscle cells, glial growth factor 2 may be important for the long-term regulation or maintenance of muscle protein accretion. Such long-term myotrophic effects are thought to be different from the well-accepted role that nerve impulses play in influencing muscle fiber type, therefore suggesting an autocrine/paracrine mechanism of action in glial growth factor 2.

Cortisol as a Primary Catabolic Hormone

Adreno-cortical steroid hormones, such as cortisol, were originally given the name glucocorticoids because of their effects on intermediary metabolism. This is because in the fasted state, cortisol helps to maintain blood glucose by stimulating gluconeogenesis and peripheral release of substrates, both of which are catabolic processes. In peripheral tissues, cortisol stimulates lipolysis in adipose cells and increases protein degradation and decreases protein synthesis in muscle cells, resulting in greater release of lipids and amino acids into circulation, respectively (Hickson and Marone 1993). Another important action of the glucocorticoids is local and systemic inflammatory mechanisms related to cytokine-mediated cortisol secretion via the hypothalamic-pituitary-adrenal axis (reviewed by Smith 2000). Perhaps the most notable function of the glucocorticoids, however, is their various roles in the body's response to stressful stimuli (i.e., injury, surgery, physical activity, etc.). Although evidence supporting other related concepts is mounting, Hans Selye's original general adaptation syndrome (i.e., stress-induced secretion of glucocorticoids enhances and mediates stress responses) remains a heavily researched topic (Pacak et al. 1998; Sapolsky, Romero, and Munck 2000; Selye 1936). Overall, the importance of the glucocorticoids to strength and power adaptations is related to their catabolic effects on skeletal muscle. With training, however, many hormones (e.g., testosterone) can override the elevations of cortisol observed as the androgen receptor becomes disinhibited (unpublished observations, Dr. Kraemer's and Dr. Deaver's laboratory groups) even at the level of the testis.

Although the specific mechanisms of catabolism are not completely understood, the numerous catabolic actions of the glucocorticoids are regulated by a complex integration of permissive, suppressive, stimulatory, and preparative actions that theoretically work together to help maintain (or reestablish) a homeostatic cellular environment and ultimately to help prevent any lasting deleterious effects of an acute stress on the body (Sapolsky, Romero, and Munck 2000). In this regard, resistance exercise can be thought of as an adaptive microtrauma that can lead to local acute inflammation, chronic inflammation, systemic inflammation, and ultimately to activation of the hypothalamic-pituitary-adrenal axis and the subsequent rapid increase in circulating cortisol concentrations for tissue repair and remodeling (Smith 2000).

Cortisol secretion responds quite rapidly to various stresses (e.g., exercise, hypoglycemia, surgery, etc.), typically within minutes. Although most inflammatory and blood-glucose regulatory actions of glucocorticoids may be directly associated with these rapid responses, changes in muscle protein turnover are mostly controlled by the classic steroid hormone–binding mechanism. Like testosterone, cortisol binds to a cytoplasmic receptor and activates a receptor complex so that it can enter the nucleus, bind specific hormone response elements on DNA, and act directly at the level of the gene. By doing this, cortisol alters transcription and the subsequent translation of specific proteins, but these processes take hours to days for completion.

Similar to other hormones, the biological activity of the glucocorticoids is regulated by the percentage of freely circulating hormone. About 10% of circulating cortisol is free, whereas approximately 15% is bound to albumin and 75% is bound to corticosteroid-binding globulin. The primary pathway for cortisol secretion begins with the stimulation of the hypothalamus by the central nervous system, which can occur as a result of hypoglycemia, the flight or fight response, or exercise. Cytokine-mediated cortisol release is implicated in high-volume and high-intensity exercise (especially eccentric muscle actions), and occurs as a result of adaptive microtrauma injury to the muscle tissue that causes the infiltration of white blood cells, such as neutrophils and monocytes, into the tissues (Smith 2000). The monocytes can then be activated in circulation, or in the tissues where they remain and become macrophages. Whether by circulating monocytes or tissue macrophages, these activated immune cells are capable of secreting hundreds of different cytokines that mediate local and systemic inflammatory processes. Interleukin-1 (IL-1) and IL-6 are proinflammatory cytokines secreted by activated monocytes (or macrophages) that are known to activate the hypothalamic-pituitary-adrenal axis (Kalra, Sahu, and Kalra 1990; Path et al. 1997). These cytokines interact with receptors on the hypothalamus and cause the sequential secretion of corticotropin-releasing hormone (CRH), adrenocorticotropic hormone (ACTH), and cortisol from the hypothalamus, anterior pituitary, and adrenal cortex, respectively (Smith 2000).

At each level of interaction (i.e., neutrophils to monocytes to cytokines to other cytokines to hypothalamus, etc.), all of these responses can be amplified dramatically, but the magnitude(s) will ultimately depend on the severity of the initial adaptive microtrauma (e.g., intensity of exercise). Severe inflammatory responses appear to occur only after severe injury, trauma, infection, very high-intensity resistance exercise, or very high-volume endurance training, and thus are implicated in the overtraining syndrome (Fry and Kraemer 1997; Smith 2000; Stone et al. 1991). However, daily exercise training is also associated with local and systemic cytokine responses at different levels, depending on the intensity of the exercise (Moldoveanu, Shephard, and Shek 2001).

Glucocorticoids are released from the adrenal cortex in response to exercise. Of these, cortisol accounts for approximately 95% of all glucocorticoid activity (Guyton 1991). Cortisol has catabolic functions that have greater effects in type II muscle fibers (Kraemer 1995). Studies have shown significant elevations in cortisol and ACTH during an acute bout of resistance exercise (Guezennec et al. 1986; Häkkinen, Pakarinen et al. 1988a, 1988b; Kraemer, Noble et al. 1987; Kraemer et al. 1992; Kraemer, Dziados et al. 1993; Kraemer, Fleck and Evans 1996; Kraemer, Fleck et al. 1999) with the response similar between men and women (Kraemer, Dziados et al. 1993), although one study reported an increase in cortisol in men but not women who performed the same protocol (Häkkinen and Pakarinen 1995). The acute cortisol response to resistance training appears to be independent of training status at least in adolescent weightlifters (Kraemer et al. 1992). Although it has been suggested that elevations in cortisol may attenuate the effects of testosterone (Cumming et al. 1987), no such relationships have been reported for resistance exercise–induced elevations.

Interestingly, programs that elicit the greatest cortisol response also elicit the greatest acute GH and lactate response. Significant correlations between blood lactate and serum cortisol ($r = 0.64$) have been reported (Kraemer, Patton et al. 1989). In addition, acute elevations in serum cortisol have been highly correlated ($r = 0.84$) to 24-hour postexercise markers of muscle damage (i.e., serum creatine kinase concentrations) (Kraemer et al. 1993). Metabolically demanding resistance training protocols (i.e., high volume, moderate to high intensity, with short rest periods) have shown the greatest acute cortisol response (Häkkinen and Pakarinen 1993; Kraemer et al. 1987, 1993), with little change shown with conventional strength and power training. Rest period length appears to be an important variable for eliciting a significant cortisol response (Kraemer et al. 1987, 1993). Kraemer, Clemson, and colleagues (1996) reported that performing eight sets of 10RM leg press exercise with 1-minute rest periods between sets elicited a significantly greater acute cortisol response than the same protocol using 3-minute rest periods. Therefore, although chronic high levels of cortisol have adverse effects, acute increases may be part of a larger remodeling process in muscle tissue.

Cortisol concentrations generally reflect the long-term training stress. Chronic resistance training does not appear to produce consistent patterns of cortisol secretion, as no change (Fry, Kraemer, Stone et al. 1994; Häkkinen, Pakarinen et al. 1987; Häkkinen, Pakarinen et al. 1988c; Häkkinen et al. 1990; Häkkinen, Pakarinen, and Kallinen 1992; Kraemer et al. 2002); decreases (Alen et al. 1988; Häkkinen, Pakarinen et al. 1985c; Kraemer, Staron et al. 1998; McCall et al. 1999; Marx et al. 2001); or increases (Häkkinen and Pakarinen 1991; Kraemer, Patton et al. 1995) have been reported during normal strength and power training and during overreaching in men and women. Nevertheless, Häkkinen, Pakarinen, and colleagues (1985c) reported greater reductions in resting serum cortisol after 24 weeks of strength training compared to power training. Marx and colleagues (2001) compared periodized multiple-set resistance training to single-set training over 6 months and reported that only the higher-volume group experienced a significant reduction in resting serum cortisol. Recently, Kraemer, Häkkinen, and colleagues (1999) reported that resting concentrations of serum cortisol decreased by the third week of a 10-week program in elderly individuals. An animal study has shown that cortisol concentrations may explain most of the variance ($\sim 60\%$) in muscle mass changes (Crowley and Matt 1996).

Thus, the acute cortisol response appears to reflect metabolic stress, whereas the chronic adaptation may be involved with tissue homeostasis involving protein metabolism (Florini 1987). A recent animal study has shown that resistance training allows the testosterone receptor to become less responsive to cortisol at the level of the testes (unpublished observations, Dr. Kraemer's and Dr. Deaver's laboratory groups).

Studies have used various ratios of cortisol and testosterone concentrations in the blood to estimate the anabolic status of the body during prolonged resistance training or with overtraining (Fry and Kraemer 1997; Häkkinen 1989; Häkkinen and Komi 1985c; Stone et al. 1991). The testosterone/cortisol ratio (T/C ratio) and/or free testosterone/cortisol ratios are the most used ratios, indicating the anabolic/catabolic status during resistance training. Thus, an increase in testosterone, a decrease in cortisol, or both would indicate increased tissue anabolism. However, this appears to be an oversimplification and is at best only a gross indirect measure of the anabolic/catabolic properties of skeletal muscle (Fry and Kraemer 1997). Several studies have shown changes in the T/C ratio during strength and power training, and this ratio has been positively related to performance (Alen et al. 1988; Häkkinen and Komi 1985c). Stressful training (overreaching) in elite weightlifters has been shown to decrease the T/C ratio (Häkkinen et al. 1987). Periodized, higher-volume programs have been shown to produce a significantly greater increase in the T/C ratio than low-volume, single-set programs (Marx et al. 2001). However, in an animal study in which the T/C ratio was manipulated to investigate muscle hypertrophy, Crowley and Matt (1996) reported that the T/C ratio was not a useful indicator of tissue anabolism. Thus, the popular use of the T/C ratio in monitoring overall anabolic and catabolic status of the human body has been shown to reflect some biological status with training. Although glucocorticoids represent the primary catabolic influence on muscle, how useful testosterone/cortisol ratios are for indicating anabolic/catabolic status remains unclear.

Connective Tissue

Physical activity increases the size and strength of ligaments, tendons, and bone (Fahey, Akka, and Rolph 1975; Stone 1992; Zernicke and Loitz 1992). As the skeletal muscles become stronger and can lift more weight, the ligaments, tendons, and bones must also adapt in order to support greater forces and weights. This concept is supported by significant correlations between muscle cross-sectional area and bone cross-sectional area in Olympic weightlifters with a mean of 5 years

of training (Kanehisa, Ikegawa, and Fukunaga 1998), which indicates that long-term participation in weightlifting results in increased bone and muscle cross-sectional areas.

Conroy and colleagues (1992) overviewed the basic characteristics of resistance training needed to alter healthy bone. Bone is very sensitive to mechanical forces such as compression, strain, and strain rate (Chow 2000). Such forces are common in resistance training (especially those observed for multiple-joint structural exercises) and are affected by the type of exercise, the intensity of the resistance, the number of sets, the rate of loading, the direction of forces, and the frequency of training. The majority of resistance training studies do show some positive effect on bone mineral density (Layne and Nelson 1999). However, bone has a tendency to adapt much more slowly (e.g., 6 to 12 months are needed to see a change in bone density) than muscle (Conroy et al. 1992).

Bone mineral density (BMD) increases as a result of resistance training, provided sufficient intensity and volume are performed (Kelley, Kelley, and Tran 2001) (see table 3.6). In a cross-sectional study, Conroy and colleagues (1993) demonstrated that elite junior weightlifters 14 to 17 years old who had been training for over a year had significantly higher bone density in the hip and femur regions than did age-matched control subjects. Even more amazing was that these young lifters had bone densities higher than adult men. In addition, bone density continued to increase over the next year of training (unpublished data).

Table 3.6 Bone Mineral Density Values for the Spine and Proximal Femur

Site	Bone mineral density (g · cm⁻²) Junior lifters	Controls	[% comparison to adult reference data] (% comparison to matched anatomical controls)
Spine	1.41 ± 0.20*#	1.06 ± 0.21	[113%] (133%)
Femoral neck	1.30 ± 0.15*#	1.05 ± 0.12	[131%] (124%)
Trochanter	1.05 ± 0.13*	0.89 ± 0.12	ND (118%)
Ward's triangle	1.26 ± 0.20*	0.99 ± 0.16	ND (127%)

Values are means ± 1 SD. * $P \geq 0.05$ from corresponding control data, # $P \geq 0.05$ from corresponding adult reference data. ND = no reference data available.

Adapted by permission from B.P. Conroy et al., 1993, "Bone mineral density in elite junior weightlifters," *Medicine and Science in Sports and Exercise* 25(10): 1105.

Dickerman, Pertusi, and Smith (2000) examined a current world record holder in the squat (1RM greater than 469 kg) and reported an average BMD of 1.86 g/cm² of the lumbar spine, which is the highest BMD reported to date. Tsuzuku, Ikegami, and Yabe (1998) reported significant differences in lumbar spine and whole-body BMD between young male power lifters and controls. In addition, a significant correlation was found between lumbar spine BMD and power lifting performance. In a later investigation, Tsuzuku and colleagues (2001) examined the differences between high- and low-intensity resistance training on BMD in young men and reported significantly greater BMD in the high-intensity group than in the low-intensity and control groups. There was no significant BMD difference between the low-intensity and control group except at the trochanter region. It appears that heavy resistance training is needed to see improvements in BMD. Because of the need for mechanical stress on bone for adaptation to occur, it has been recommended that three to six sets with 1 to 10RM loads of multiple-joint exercises be used with 1 to 4 minutes of rest between sets for optimal bone loading.

Resistance training is effective for increasing BMD in women of all ages. Nichols, Sanborn, and Love (2001) examined the effects of 15 months of resistance training on the BMD of adolescent girls (14-17) and reported that leg strength increased by 40%, which was associated with an increase in BMD of the femoral neck (1.035 to 1.073 g/cm²). Using a meta-analysis, Kelley and colleagues (2001) found that resistance training had a positive effect on the BMD at the lumbar spine of all women and at the femur and radius sites for postmenopausal women. Kerr and colleagues (2001) examined the effect of multiple-set strength training performed three times a week in older women and reported a significant effect at the intertrochanter hip site. This study demonstrated the effectiveness of a progressive strength program in increasing BMD at the clinically important hip site and generally in elderly women who are vulnerable to osteoporosis.

Physiological adaptations to ligaments and tendons after physical training do occur and may aid in injury prevention. Physical activity causes the increased metabolism, thickness, weight, and strength of ligaments (Staff 1982; Tipton et al. 1975). Damaged ligaments regain their strength at a faster rate if physical activity is performed after the damage has occurred (Staff 1982; Tipton et al.

1975). Both the attachment site of a ligament or tendon to a bone and the muscle-tendinous junction are frequent sites of injury. Research involving laboratory animals demonstrated that with endurance-type training the amount of force necessary to cause separation at these areas increases (Tipton et al. 1975). Human tendon fibroblasts subjected to mechanical stretch in vitro showed increased secretion patterns of growth factors (Skutek et al. 2001), indicating that stretch may have a positive effect on tendon and ligament tissue by cell proliferation, differentiation, and matrix formation. Thus, there is reason to believe that resistance training can affect ligaments and tendons.

Increasing the strength of the ligaments and tendons can help prevent possible damage to these structures caused by the muscle's abilities to lift heavier weights and develop more tension. These structures also appear to hypertrophy somewhat more slowly than muscle. Kubo and colleagues (2002, 2001) examined 8 and 12 weeks of resistance training of the plantar flexors and knee extensors, respectively, and reported that muscle size and strength increased significantly with no increase in tendon cross-sectional area. However, resistance training resulted in significant increases in tendon stiffness. They concluded that the training-induced changes in the internal structures of the tendon (e.g., the mechanical quality of collagen) accounted for the changes in stiffness and that increases in tendon cross-sectional area may take longer than 12 weeks. This may be a factor in anabolic steroid-induced musculotendinous injuries, as it has been hypothesized that large increases in muscle size and strength (and consequent training loads) may occur too rapidly to allow adequate connective tissue adaptation. Although it is now acknowledged that the dense fibrous tissues that make up tendons and ligaments respond to metabolic changes and are adaptable, no long-term research has been done examining the effects of heavy resistance exercise on these structures (Stone 1992; Zernicke and Loitz 1992).

The connective tissue sheaths that surround the entire muscle (epimysium), groups of muscle fibers (perimysium), and individual muscle fibers (endomysium) may also adapt to resistance training. These sheaths are of major importance in the tensile strength and elastic properties of muscle; they form the framework that supports an overload on the muscle. Compensatory hypertrophy induced in the muscle of laboratory animals also causes an increase in the collagen content of these connective tissue sheaths (Laurent et al. 1978; Turto, Lindy, and Halme 1974). Several researchers have reported that the biceps brachii of bodybuilders does not differ from age-matched control subjects in the relative amount of connective tissue (MacDougall et al. 1985; Sale et al. 1987), and that male and female bodybuilders possess similar relative amounts of connective tissue as control subjects (Alway, MacDougall et al. 1989). Thus, the connective tissue sheaths in muscle appear to increase so that the same ratio between connective and muscle tissue is maintained.

Resistance training has been found to increase the thickness of hyaline cartilage on the articular surfaces of bone (Holmdahl and Ingelmark 1948; Ingelmark and Elsholm 1948). One major function of hyaline cartilage is to act as a shock absorber between the bony surfaces of a joint. Increasing the thickness of this cartilage could facilitate the performance of this shock absorber function. Thus, connective tissue does appear to adapt to resistance training. However, the adaptation of connective tissue may take longer than the adaptation of skeletal muscle.

Cardiovascular Adaptations

Similar to skeletal muscle, cardiac muscle also undergoes adaptations to resistance training. Likewise, other aspects of the cardiovascular system, such as the blood lipid profile, also demonstrate adaptations. Adaptations and acute responses of the cardiovascular system to resistance training are especially important when weight training is performed by some special populations, such as seniors and individuals undergoing cardiac rehabilitation. As with all adaptations to resistance training, the response is dependent in part on training volume and intensity. Some of the cardiovascular system's adaptations brought about by resistance training, as well as other forms of physical conditioning, resemble the adaptations to hypertension (i.e., increased ventricular wall thickness and chamber size). When examined closely, however, differences exist between the adaptations to hypertension and those to resistance training. As an example, with hypertension, ventricular wall thickness increases beyond normal limits. With weight training, this rarely occurs and is not evident if ventricular wall thickness is examined relative to fat-free mass, whereas with

hypertension wall thickness increases are evident even when examined relative to fat-free mass. Differences in cardiac adaptations have resulted in the use of the terms *pathological hypertrophy* to refer to the changes that occur with hypertension and other pathological conditions and *physiological hypertrophy* to refer to the changes that occur with physical training.

Cardiovascular adaptations are caused by the training stimulus to which the cardiovascular system is exposed. Endurance training brings about different cardiovascular adaptations than resistance training. In general, these differences in adaptations are caused by the need to pump a large volume of blood at a relatively low blood pressure during endurance exercise, whereas during resistance training a relatively small volume of blood is pumped at a relatively high blood pressure. This difference between endurance and resistance training results in different adaptations.

Training Adaptations at Rest

Resistance training can affect virtually all the major aspects of cardiovascular function (see tables 3.7 and 3.8). Changes in cardiac morphology, systolic function, diastolic function, heart rate, blood pressure, and the lipid profile indicate both cardiovascular function and health, and cardiovascular risk.

Heart Rate

Resting heart rates of junior and senior competitive bodybuilders, power lifters, and Olympic lifters range from 60 to 78 beats per minute (Colan et al. 1985; Fleck and Dean 1987; George et al. 1995; Haykowsky et al. 2000; Smith and Raven 1986). The vast majority of cross-sectional data indicate that the resting heart rates of highly strength trained athletes are not significantly different from those of sedentary individuals (Fleck 1988, 2002). However, the resting heart rate of master-level power lifters has been reported to be 87 beats per minute, which was significantly higher than age-matched control subjects (Haykowsky et al. 2000) and lower than the average resting heart rates in highly resistance trained athletes (Saltin and Astrand 1967; Scala et al. 1987).

The majority of short-term (up to 20 weeks) longitudinal studies report significant decreases of approximately 4 to 13% and small nonsignificant decreases in resting heart rate (Fleck 2002). The mechanism causing a decrease in resting heart rate after weight training is not clearly elucidated.

Table 3.7 Chronic Resting Cardiovascular Adaptations From Resistance Exercise

Heart rate	No change or small decrease
Blood pressure	
Systolic	No change or small decrease
Diastolic	No change or small decrease
Rate pressure product	No change or small decrease
Stroke volume	
Absolute	Small increase or no change
Relative to BSA	No change
Relative to LBM	No change
Cardiac function	
Systolic	No change
Diastolic	No change
Lipid profile	
Total cholesterol	No change or small decrease
HDL-C	No change or small increase
LDL-C	No change or small decrease
Total cholesterol/HDL-C	No change or small decrease

However, decreased heart rate is typically associated with a combination of increased parasympathetic and decreased sympathetic cardiac tone. Some cardiovascular responses to isometric actions resemble typical weight training activity. During low-level isometric actions (30% of maximal voluntary contraction), both autonomic branches show increased activity (Gonzalez-Camarena et al. 2000). Thus, a decrease in resting heart rate as a result of weight training may not be due to the typical increase in parasympathetic cardiac tone and decrease in sympathetic cardiac tone, but rather to increased activity of both autonomic branches.

Blood Pressure

The majority of cross-sectional data clearly demonstrates highly strength trained athletes to have average resting systolic and diastolic blood pressures (Byrne and Wilmore 2000; Fleck 2002), although significantly above average (Snoecky et al. 1982) and less than average (Smith and Raven 1986) resting blood pressures have also been reported in weightlifters. Generally, short-term training studies have reported nonsignificant changes in resting systolic and diastolic pressures in normotensive individuals (Byrne and Wilmore 2000; Goldberg, Elliot, and Kuehl 1988, 1994; Lusiani et al. 1986). However, in normotensive individuals a significant decrease in resting systolic pressure (3.7%), but no significant change in resting diastolic pressure (Stone et al. 1983) and a significant decrease only in diastolic pressure (Hurley et al. 1988) have also been reported. In borderline hypertensive individuals significant decreases in both systolic and diastolic resting blood pressure have been reported after weight training (Hagberg et al. 1984; Harris and Holly 1987).

Decreased resting blood pressure, when it does occur after strength training, is probably related to decreased body fat and changes in the sympathoadenal drive (Goldberg 1989). The most likely explanations of hypertension, when it occurs in resistance-trained athletes, are essential hypertension, chronic overtraining, use of androgens, and/or large gains in muscle mass (Fleck 2002). Although body mass has been positively correlated to systolic blood pressure (Viitassalo, Komi, and Karovonen 1979), decreases in blood pressure have been shown with concomitant increases in fat-free mass (Goldberg et al. 1988; Stone et al. 1983), which indicates that gains in fat-free mass can occur without increases in resting blood pressure. The majority of both longitudinal and cross-sectional evidence indicates that weight training results in either no change or a small decrease in resting blood pressure in both normotensive and hypertensive individuals.

Rate Pressure Product or Double Product

Heart rate times systolic blood pressure is termed the *rate pressure product* or *double product*. It is an estimate of myocardial work and is proportional to myocardial oxygen consumption. A decrease in this variable is normally viewed as a positive adaptation to training. Short-term resistance training

Table 3.8 Cardiac Morphology Adaptations at Rest Due to Resistance Training

	Relative to		
	Absolute	**BSA**	**FFM**
Wall thickness			
Left ventricle	Increase or no change	No change	No change
Septal	Increase or no change	No change	No change
Right ventricle	No change	No change	No change
Chamber volume			
Left ventricle	No change or slight increase	No change or slight increase	No change or slight increase
Right ventricle	No change or slight increase (?)	No change or slight increase (?)	No change or slight increase (?)
Atrial	No change or slight increase (?)	No change or slight increase (?)	No change or slight increase (?)
Left ventricular mass	Increase or no change	No change	No change

BSA = body surface area (m²); FFM = fat-free mass (kg); ? = minimal data.

studies demonstrate significant decreases in resting rate pressure product after traditional weight training (Goldberg, Elliot, and Kuehl 1994) and after an Olympic-style weight training program (Stone et al. 1983). Although rate pressure product is not reported in many studies, any study showing a decrease in resting heart rate or systolic blood pressure would indicate a decrease in rate pressure product. Thus, weight training can decrease rate pressure product, which suggests that the left ventricle is performing less work and has a lower oxygen consumption at rest.

Stroke Volume

Stroke volume is the amount of blood pumped per heartbeat. An increase in resting stroke volume is viewed as a positive adaptation to training and is normally accompanied by a decrease in resting heart rate. No difference (Brown et al. 1983; Dickhuth et al. 1979) between highly strength trained males and normal individuals in absolute stroke volume, and greater values (Fleck, Bennett et al.1989; Pearson et al. 1986) in highly strength trained individuals have been reported. Increased absolute stroke volume, when present, appears to be due to a significantly greater end diastolic left ventricular internal dimension and a normal ejection fraction (Fleck 1988). A meta-analysis indicates that the caliber of athlete may influence absolute stroke volume, with national- and international-caliber athletes having a greater absolute stroke volume than lesser-caliber athletes (Fleck 1988). Although a few comparisons between highly resistance trained individuals and normal individuals show a significantly greater stroke volume relative to body surface area in the strength-trained individuals, the majority of comparisons show no significant difference between these two groups in stroke volume relative to body surface area (Fleck 2002). When a significant difference in stroke volume relative to body surface area is shown, the difference generally becomes nonsignificant when expressed relative to fat-free mass (Fleck 2002; Fleck, Bennett et al. 1989). Meta-analysis of stroke volume relative to body surface area demonstrates no difference by caliber of athlete (Fleck 1988). Thus, the greater absolute stroke volume in some national- and international-caliber highly strength trained athletes may be explained in part by body size. The preponderance of cross-sectional data indicates weight training to have no or little effect on absolute stroke volume or stroke volume relative to body surface area or fat-free mass. This conclusion is supported by a study reporting no change in absolute resting stroke volume after the performance of a short-term weight training program (Lusiani et al. 1986).

Lipid Profile

Both cross-sectional and longitudinal studies examining the effect of resistance training on the lipid profile are inconclusive. Literature reviews report resistance-trained male athletes to have normal, higher-than-normal, and lower-than-normal high-density lipoprotein cholesterol (HDL-C), low-density lipoprotein cholesterol (LDL-C), total cholesterol, and total cholesterol-to-HDL-C (Hurley 1989; Kraemer, Deschenes, and Fleck 1988; Stone et al. 1991). Reports on the lipid profile in strength-trained female athletes are also inconclusive, with positive changes (Elliot et al. 1987; Moffatt, Wallace, and Sady 1990) and no difference from normal reported (Morgan et al. 1986). The lipid profile of strength and power athletes has also been reported to show values indicative of increased cardiovascular risk (Berg, Ringwald, and Keul 1980). Short-term training studies using both male and female subjects are also inconclusive. Increases in HDL-C of approximately 10 to 15% and decreases in LDL-C of approximately 5 to 39% and decreases in total cholesterol of 3 to 16% in normolipidemic individuals have been demonstrated after short-term weight training programs (Hurley 1989). However, other longitudinal studies show no significant change in the lipid profile as a result of short-term resistance training programs (Hurley 1989; Kraemer, Deschenes, and Fleck 1988; LeMura et al. 2000; Staron et al. 2000).

All of the studies examining the effect of weight training on the lipid profile can be criticized. Limitations of the studies include inadequate control of age, diet, training program, and possible androgen use by the subjects; use of only one blood sample in determining the lipid profile; lack of a control group; not controlling for changes in body composition; and short duration. Wallace and colleagues (1991) demonstrated that an acute increase in HDL-C and a decrease in total cholesterol occurs 24 hours after a 90-minute resistance exercise session and that these levels do not return to baseline values by 48 hours after the exercise session. Many studies did not rule out this possible acute effect of the last training session. Because of these study limitations, conclusions must be viewed with some caution.

Weight training volume may have some effect on the lipid profile. Bodybuilders have been reported to have lipid profiles similar to runners. Power lifters, on the other hand, have lower HDL-C and higher LDL-C concentrations than runners when body fat, age, and androgen use (which has been shown to depress HDL-C concentrations) are accounted for (Hurley, Seals, Hagberg et al. 1984; Hurley et al. 1987). Over 12 weeks of training, middle-aged men showed the greatest positive changes in the lipid profile during the program's highest training volume phase (Blessing et al. 1987; Johnson et al. 1982).

How resistance training might positively affect the lipid profile has not been completely elucidated. Decreased percent body fat has been reported to positively influence the lipid profile (Twisk, Kemper, and van Mechelen 2000; Williams et al. 1994), and resistance training can decrease percent body fat. Resistance training may improve the oxidative capacity of skeletal muscle because of an increase in the activity of specific aerobic-oxidative enzymes (Wang et al. 1993). Such a change might occur due to fiber-type conversion from type IIB to type IIA (Staron et al. 1994) and an increase in capillaries per muscle fiber (McCall et al. 1996). Weight training could also negatively affect the lipid profile. Individuals with a higher percentage of type I muscle fibers tend to have a higher HDL-C concentration (Tikkanen, Naveri, and Harkonen 1996). Some resistance training programs have the greatest hypertrophic effect on type II fibers (Tesch 1987). The resulting decrease in the percentage area of type I fibers may unfavorably affect the lipid profile. Whether a change in the lipid profile occurs depends on the balance between factors that have a negative or positive effect.

Further research is needed before a conclusion can be reached concerning the effect of resistance training on the lipid profile. However, an aptitude for power or speed athletic events, including weightlifting, does not offer protection from cardiovascular risk in former athletes. On the other hand, an aptitude for endurance athletic events and continuing vigorous physical activity after retirement from competitive sport does offer protection against cardiovascular risk (Kujala et al. 2000). Therefore a prudent conclusion might be to encourage strength and power athletes to perform some aerobic training and follow dietary practices appropriate to bring about positive changes in the lipid profile. This may be especially important for long-term health after retirement from competition.

Cardiac Wall Thickness

Increased cardiac wall thicknesses are an adaptation to the intermittent elevated blood pressures during resistance training (Effron 1989). Both echocardiographic and magnetic resonance imaging (MRI) techniques (see figure 3.24) have been

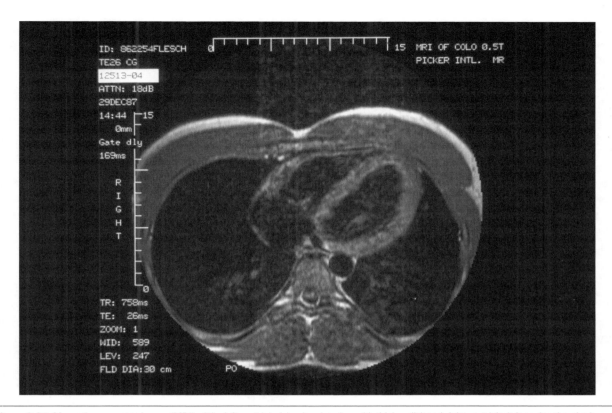

Figure 3.24 Magnetic resonance image (MRI) of the left ventricle (circular chamber with thick walls) and right ventricle (triangular chamber).
Courtesy of Dr. Fleck's laboratory.

used to investigate changes in cardiac morphology due to weight training. Several literature reviews have all concluded that highly strength trained individuals can have greater-than-average absolute diastolic posterior left ventricular wall thickness (PWTd) (Fleck 1988, 2002; Urhausen and Kindermann 1992) and diastolic intraventricular septum wall thickness (IVSd) (Fleck 1988, 2002; Perrault and Turcotte 1994; Urhausen and Kindermann 1992; Wolfe, Cunningham, and Boughner 1986). In general, absolute wall thickness in highly strength trained individuals rarely exceeds the upper limits of normal (Urhausen and Kindermann 1992; Wolfe, Cunningham, and Boughner 1986) and are normally significantly lower than in individuals with diseases such as aortic stenosis, obstructive cardiomyopathy, and extreme hypertension (Wolfe, Cunningham, and Boughner 1986). Increased ventricular wall thicknesses are also apparent in many other types of athletes. A ranking of 27 different sports places weightlifting as number eight in terms of left ventricular wall thickness (Spataro et al. 1994).

When cardiac wall thicknesses (PWTd and IVSd) of highly strength trained individuals are expressed relative to body surface area or to fat-free mass, rarely is there a difference from normal (Fleck 1988, 2002; Fleck, Bennett et al. 1989; Perrault and Turcotte 1994; Urhausen and Kindermann 1992). This is important because it indicates a physiological adaptation rather than an adaptation to a pathological disease state. The caliber of athletes may have some effect on ventricular wall thicknesses. A meta-analysis indicates IVSd thickness, but not PWTd to be affected by the caliber of the athlete, with national-, international-, and regional-caliber athletes having a greater IVSd thickness than recreational strength trainers (Fleck 1988).

Short-term longitudinal training studies also indicate that strength training can increase PWTd and IVSd; however, it is not a necessary outcome of all weight training programs (Effron 1989; Fleck 1988, 2002; Perrault and Turcotte 1994). The conclusion that not all resistance training programs result in an increase in ventricular wall thickness is supported by cross-sectional studies showing no significant difference from controls in ventricular wall thickness in female collegiate strength- and power-trained athletes (George et al. 1995) and junior and master national-caliber power lifters (Haykowsky et al. 2000).

Whether an increase in left ventricular wall thickness occurs probably depends on differences in the training performed. The highest blood pressures during a set to concentric failure occur during the last few repetitions of a set (Fleck and Dean 1987; MacDougall et al. 1985; Sale et al. 1994). Exercises involving large-muscle mass, such as leg presses, result in higher blood pressures than small-muscle-mass exercises (MacDougall et al. 1985). Therefore, whether sets are carried to concentric failure and the exercises performed may affect the occurrence of increases in ventricular wall thickness. Other factors that may affect whether changes in ventricular wall thickness occur include training intensity, training volume, the duration of training, and the rest periods between sets.

The effect of weight training on other cardiac chamber wall thicknesses has received considerably less attention than left ventricular wall thickness. However, a magnetic resonance imaging study reports no difference in systolic and diastolic right ventricular wall thickness between male junior elite Olympic weightlifters and age- and weight-matched controls (Fleck, Henke, and Wilson 1989). The same study did find the weightlifters to have significantly greater left ventricular wall thickness, which indicates that the right ventricle is not exposed to sufficiently elevated blood pressures to cause right ventricular wall hypertrophy.

Resistance training can result in increased left ventricular wall thickness, but it is not a necessary consequence of all resistance training programs. Increased left ventricular wall thickness, when apparent, is caused by the intermittent elevated blood pressures encountered during strength training. When expressed relative to body surface area or fat-free mass, generally no increase in left ventricular wall thickness is demonstrated. Additionally, increased left ventricular wall thickness rarely exceeds the upper limits of normalcy and is significantly below wall thickness increases resulting from pathological conditions.

Heart Chamber Size

An increase in ventricular chamber size or volume, which can occur from endurance training, is an indication of volume overload on the heart. The majority of cross-sectional data on highly strength trained athletes and longitudinal short-term training studies show resistance training to have little or no effect on absolute left ventricular internal dimensions, an indicator of chamber size (Fleck 1988, 2002; Fleck, Henke, and Wilson 1989; George et al. 1995; Perrault and Turcotte 1994; Urhausen and Kindermann 1992). This is true whether systolic or diastolic chamber dimensions are examined. Similar to left ventricular wall thickness, left ventricular internal dimensions in highly strength trained individuals normally do not exceed the upper limits of normal (Fleck 1988, 2002; Perrault and Turcotte 1994; Urhausen and Kindermann 1992; Wolfe, Cunningham, and Boughner 1986) and in most cases is not significantly different from normal when expressed relative to body surface area or fat-free mass (Fleck 1988, 2002; Urhausen and Kindermann 1992; Wolfe, Cunningham, and Boughner 1986).

Increases in cardiac chamber size do occur as a result of endurance training and participation in many other sports. A comparison of nationally ranked athletes in 27 different sports ranked weightlifters number 22 in terms of effect on left ventricular internal dimensions (Spataro et al. 1994). Although weight training may have a minimal effect on left ventricular internal dimensions, this variable should not decrease since that would indicate pathological pressure overload caused by hypertension or one of various forms of cardiomyopathy (Urhausen and Kindermann 1992). The slight increase or no change in left ventricular internal dimensions coupled with no change or an increase in left ventricular wall thickness is an important difference between weight training and pathological cardiac hypertrophy, in which a large increase in wall thickness is not accompanied by an increase in left ventricular internal dimensions (Urhausen and Kindermann 1992).

Meta-analysis indicates that the caliber of the athlete does not influence whether left ventricular internal dimension is significantly different from normal (Fleck 1988). Reports of nationally ranked junior and senior power lifters having normal left ventricular internal dimensions (Haykowsky et al. 2000) and of national-caliber strength-trained athletes having a left ventricular internal dimension not significantly different from normal (Dickhuth et al. 1979; Fleck, Bennett et al. 1989) also indicate that the caliber of the athlete has little effect on left ventricular chamber size. Since changes in ventricular volume are normally associated with a volume overload, it might be hypothesized that the type of weight training program performed would have an effect on left ventricular chamber size. A comparison of bodybuilders and weight lifters shows no significant difference between the two groups in left and right ventricular internal dimension, although the bodybuilders had slightly greater values. However, the bodybuilders, but not the weightlifters, had a greater absolute left and right ventricular internal dimension at rest (Deligiannis, Zahopoulou, and Mandroukas 1988) compared to normal. If expressed relative to body surface area or fat-free mass, left ventricular internal dimension of neither the bodybuilders nor the weightlifters was significantly different from normal. However, the right ventricular internal dimension of the bodybuilders was significantly different from normal when expressed relative to body surface area and fat-free mass. This same study also reported the left atrial internal dimension of both bodybuilders and weightlifters to be greater than normal in absolute terms and relative to body surface area and fat-free mass terms, with the bodybuilders having a significantly greater left atrial internal dimension than the weightlifters (Deligiannis, Zahopoulo, and Mandroukas 1988). This information indicates that the type of weight training program may affect cardiac chamber size, but the effect may be small.

Resistance training appears to result in a slight increase in cardiac chamber size. However, no difference from normal is generally apparent when examined relative to body surface area or fat-free mass. High-volume training programs may have the greatest potential to affect cardiac chamber sizes.

Left Ventricular Mass

An increase in ventricular mass can be brought about by an increase in either wall thickness or chamber size. The majority of data concerning left ventricular mass (LVM) has been obtained using echocardiographic techniques, and because of the assumptions used to calculate LVM, the information must be viewed with some caution. For example a change of 1 mm in left ventricular wall thickness can result in a significant increase of 15% in estimated LVM (Perrault and Turcotte 1994). The majority of cross-sectional studies on highly resistance trained athletes (Effron 1989; Fleck 1988, 2002; George et al. 1995; Haykowsky et al. 2000) and of longitudinal short-term training studies (Effron 1989; Fleck 1988, 2002; Wolfe, Cunningham, and Boughner 1986) demonstrated absolute LVM to be greater than normal in resistance-trained athletes or increased due to weight training. However, increased LVM is not a necessary outcome of all resistance training programs, and the difference is greatly reduced or nonexistent relative to body surface area or fat-free mass. Some data indicate that national- and international-caliber weight-trained athletes have a greater LVM than lesser-caliber athletes (Effron 1989; Fleck 1988).

The type of weight training program may influence how LVM is increased. Both bodybuilders and weightlifters have a significantly greater than normal absolute LVM; however, they are not significantly different from each other (Deligiannis, Zahopoulou, and Mandroukas 1988). Bodybuilders and weightlifters both also have significantly greater-than-normal left ventricular wall thicknesses. However, only bodybuilders have a significantly greater-than-normal left ventricular end-diastolic dimension (Deligiannis, Zahopoulou, and Mandroukas 1988). Thus, in bodybuilders the increased LVM is caused by both greater left ventricular wall thickness and chamber size, whereas in weightlifters the increase is caused for the most part only by greater-than-normal wall thickness. It could be hypothesized that a weight training program that increases both left ventricular wall thickness and left ventricular internal dimensions would result in the greatest increase in estimated left ventricular mass. Such a program may be a higher-volume weight training program.

Resistance training can increase absolute LVM; however, such an increase does not occur with all weight training programs. The increased LVM can be caused by an increase in either wall thickness or chamber size, or a combination of both, and may also be related to the type of program performed.

Cardiac Function

Abnormalities in systolic and diastolic function are associated with cardiac hypertrophy caused by pathological conditions, such as hypertension and valvular heart disease. This has raised concern that cardiac hypertrophy caused by resistance training may impair cardiac function. However, the majority of cross-sectional studies demonstrate that common measures of systolic function—percentage fractional shortening, ejection fraction, and velocity of circumferential shortening are unaffected by resistance training (Effron 1989; Ellias et al. 1991; Fleck 1988, 2002; George et al. 1995; Haykowsky et al. 2000; Urhausen and Kindermann 1992). However, it has also been reported that percentage fractional shortening is significantly greater in strength-trained athletes than in normal subjects (Colan et al. 1987), indicating enhanced systolic function. Short-term longitudinal training studies, on the other hand, show either no change (Lusiani et al. 1986) or a significant increase in percentage fractional shortening (Kanakis and Hickson 1980). The majority of studies indicate that weight training has no effect on systolic function, with minimal data indicating enhanced systolic function.

Diastolic function has received less attention than systolic function. However, cross-sectional data on highly weight trained individuals indicate no significant change from normal in diastolic function (Urhausen and Kindermann 1992). Power lifters competing at the national level, who have significantly greater absolute and relative-to-body-surface-area left ventricular mass, have been reported to have normal and even enhanced measures of diastolic function (peak rate of chamber enlargement and atrial peak filling rate) (Colan et al. 1985; Pearson et al. 1986). The use of anabolic steroids has been reported to be detrimental (Pearson et al. 1986) or to have no effect (Thompson et al. 1992) on measures of diastolic function. Differences in the results of these two reports may be due to the length of use and the type of anabolic steroid used.

A limited number of studies have examined the effect of resistance training on cardiac function. In general, resistance training appears to have no effect, or to slightly enhance, some measures of systolic and diastolic function.

Acute Cardiovascular Responses

The acute response to resistance training refers to physiological responses during one set of an exercise, several sets of an exercise(s), or one training session. Determining acute responses accurately can be difficult. Intra-arterial lines are necessary to accurately determine blood pressure because it is impossible with auscultatory sphygmomanometry to determine such things as blood pressure during the concentric and eccentric phases of repetitions. Finger plesmography has also been used to determine blood pressure continuously during resistance training. Cardiac impedance and echocardiographic techniques have been used to determine cardiac output, stroke volume, and left ventricular volumes, but these techniques also have limitations during physical activity. Thus, in some instances, conclusions drawn concerning the acute response to resistance training must be viewed with caution (see table 3.9).

Heart Rate and Blood Pressure

Heart rate and both systolic and diastolic blood pressures increase substantially during the performance of dynamic heavy resistance exercise (Fleck 1988; Hill and Butler 1991). This is true for machine, free weight, and isokinetic exercise (Fleck and Dean 1987; Iellamo et al. 1997; Kleiner et al. 1996; MacDougall et al. 1985; Sale et al. 1993, 1994; Scharf et al. 1994). Mean peak systolic and diastolic blood pressures as high as 320/250 mmHg and a peak heart rate of 170 beats per minute have been reported during

Table 3.9 Acute Response During Resistance Exercise Relative to Rest

	Portion of repetition	
	Concentric	Eccentric
Heart rate (no difference between concentric and eccentric)	Increase	Increase
Stroke volume (?) (eccentric value higher than concentric)	No difference or decrease	No difference or increase
Cardiac output (?) (eccentric value higher than concentric)	No difference or increase	Increase
Blood pressure (highest at exercise sticking point) 　Systolic increase 　Diastolic increase	Increase Increase	Increase Increase
Intrathoracic pressure (highest when a Valsalva maneuver is performed)	Increase	Increase

? = minimal data.

performance of a two-legged leg press set to failure at 95% of 1RM, in which a Valsalva maneuver was allowed (MacDougall et al. 1985). However, heart rate and blood pressure responses are also substantial even when an attempt is made to limit the performance of a Valsalva maneuver. For example, mean peak blood pressure values of 198/160 mmHg and a heart rate of 135 beats per minute during a single-legged knee-extension set performed to concentric failure at 80% of 1RM when a Valsalva maneuver is discouraged have been reported (Fleck and Dean 1987).

Both blood pressure (see figure 3.25) and heart rate increase as the set progresses, so the highest values occur during the last several repetitions of a set to volitional fatigue whether or not a Valsalva maneuver is allowed (Fleck and Dean 1987; MacDougall et al. 1985; Sale et al. 1994). When a Valsalva maneuver is allowed, the blood pressure and heart rate response is significantly higher during sets performed to volitional fatigue with submaximal resistances (50-95% of 1RM) than when a resistance of 100% of 1RM is used (MacDougall et al. 1985; Sale et al. 1994). When a Valsalva maneuver is discouraged, the blood pressure response is higher, but not significantly so, during sets at 90%, 80%, and 70% of 1RM compared to sets at 100% and 50% of 1RM to volitional fatigue (Fleck

and Dean 1987). The blood pressure and heart rate response during dynamic weight training appears to be similar to the response during isometric actions in that, as the duration of the activity increases, so does the heart rate and blood pressure response (Kahn, Kapitaniak, and Monod 1985; Ludbrook et al. 1978). Both the peak heart rate and blood pressure responses also appear to increase during submaximal sets to failure (50%, 70%, 80%, 85%, and 87.5% of 1RM) as the percentage of 1RM increases (Sale et al. 1994) and during three successive sets (see figure 3.25) to failure of the same exercise (Gotshall et al. 1999). Additionally, both the heart rate and blood pressure response increase with increased active muscle mass; however, the response is not linear (Falkel, Fleck, and Murray 1992; Fleck 1988; MacDougall et al. 1985).

During dynamic resistance exercise, higher systolic and diastolic blood pressures, but not heart rates, have been reported to occur during the concentric compared to the eccentric portion of repetitions (Falkel, Fleck, and Murray 1992; MacDougall et al. 1985; Miles et al. 1987). Therefore, the point in the range of motion during the eccentric or concentric portion of a repetition at which blood pressure is determined will affect the value. Using finger plesmography (see figure 3.26), Gotshall and colleagues (1999) showed that the highest systolic and diastolic blood pressures occur at the start of the concentric portion of the

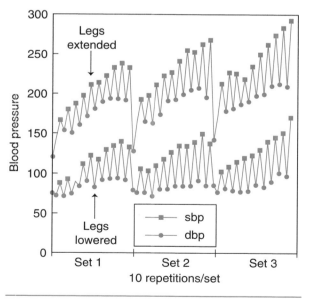

Figure 3.25 Blood pressure response increases during a two-legged leg press set to volitional fatigue as well as during three successive sets of 10 repetitions at a 10RM resistance.

sbp = systolic blood pressure; dbp = diastolic blood pressure.

Reprinted, by permission, from R.W. Gotshall et al., 1999, "Noninvasive characterization of the blood pressure response to the double-leg press exercise" *Journal of Exercise Physiology.* Available: www.css.edu/users/tboone2.

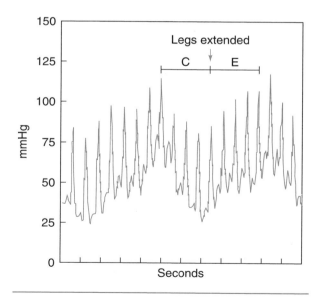

Figure 3.26 Blood pressure response during one complete repetition of a two-legged leg press exercise.

Reprinted, by permission, from R.W. Gotshall et al., 1999, "Noninvasive characterization of the blood pressure response to the double-leg press exercise" *Journal of Exercise Physiology.* Available: www.css.edu/users/tboone2.

leg press, with blood pressure decreasing as the concentric portion of the repetition progresses, until reaching its lowest point when the legs are extended. Blood pressure then increases as the legs bend during the eccentric portion of a repetition and again reaches its highest point when the legs are bent as far as possible. This indicates that the blood pressure response is highest at the sticking point of an exercise when the muscular contraction is nearest its maximal force.

Investigations with isokinetic exercise give some further insight into the acute blood pressure and heart rate response. Velocity of isokinetic contraction (30 to 200 degrees per second) has little effect on the blood pressure and heart rate response (Haennel et al. 1989; Kleiner et al. 1999), whereas isokinetic exercise performed with both a concentric and eccentric phase results in a higher peak blood pressure than concentric exercise only (Sale et al. 1993). Thus, many factors, including active muscle mass, whether sets are carried to volitional fatigue, the number of sets performed, the resistance used, where in the range of motion a measurement is obtained, and whether both concentric and eccentric muscular actions are performed, affect the blood pressure and heart rate response during dynamic resistance training.

Stroke Volume and Cardiac Output

Stroke volume and cardiac output responses determined by electrical impedance techniques during knee-extension exercise are shown to vary slightly depending on whether a Valsalva maneuver is performed. When attempts are made to limit the performance of a Valsalva maneuver, stroke volume and cardiac output during the concentric phase of the knee-extension exercise (12 repetitions with a 12RM resistance) are not elevated significantly above resting values (Miles et al. 1987). When a Valsalva maneuver is allowed during the knee-extension exercise (sets at 50%, 80%, and 100% of 1RM to fatigue), stroke volume is either significantly below resting values or not significantly different from resting values, and cardiac output is above resting values but not always significantly so (Falkel, Fleck, and Murray 1992). During the eccentric repetition phase when a Valsalva maneuver is not allowed, stroke volume and cardiac output are significantly increased above resting values. When a Valsalva maneuver is allowed, stroke volume during the eccentric phase is significantly above or not sig-

nificantly different from resting values, and cardiac output is always significantly greater than resting values. However, generally, with or without a Valsalva maneuver, stroke volume and cardiac output during the eccentric phase are generally higher compared to the concentric phase.

During squat exercise at 50%, 80%, and 100% of 1RM to fatigue, the stroke volume and cardiac output response are different between the eccentric and concentric repetition phases (Falkel, Fleck, and Murray 1992). During the eccentric phase, stroke volume is above resting values (sets at 50% and 100% of 1RM), but not always significantly so, or it is significantly below resting values (sets at 80% of 1 RM). Stroke volume during the concentric phase of all sets is significantly below resting values. Cardiac output during the eccentric phase during all sets is significantly above resting values, and during the concentric phase of all sets it is always above resting values, but not always significantly so.

Heart rate is not significantly different between the concentric and eccentric phases of a repetition (Falkel, Fleck, and Murray 1992; MacDougall et al. 1985; Miles et al. 1987). As discussed earlier, stroke volume is significantly greater during the eccentric compared to the concentric phase of repetition. Thus, the greater cardiac output during the eccentric compared to the concentric phase of a repetition is due solely to a greater stroke volume during the eccentric phase.

A general pattern for both large- (squat) and small- (knee extension) muscle-mass exercises for both stroke volume and cardiac output is that greater values occur during the eccentric compared to the concentric repetition phases. Stroke volume is generally below resting values during the concentric phase and generally above resting values during the eccentric phase. Cardiac output during the eccentric phase of both large- and small-muscle-mass exercises is generally above resting values. However, cardiac output during the concentric phase of large-muscle-group exercises may also be above resting values, but during small-muscle-group exercises can be either above or below the values.

Mechanisms of the Pressor Response

Several factors may influence the increase in blood pressure or pressor response during resistance training. Cardiac output can be increased above resting values during both the eccentric and concentric phases of resistance training exercise

(Falkel, Fleck, and Murray 1992), which may contribute to the increase in blood pressure during weight training.

Increased intrathoracic or intra-abdominal pressures may have an effect on the blood pressure response during resistance training (Fleck 1988). Intrathoracic pressure increases during resistance training exercise (Falkel, Fleck, and Murray 1992; MacDougall et al. 1985; Sale et al. 1994) especially if a Valsalva maneuver is performed. Increased intrathoracic pressure may eventually decrease venous return to the heart and so decrease cardiac output. During resistance exercise an indirect measure (mouth pressure) of a Valsalva maneuver and intrathoracic pressure indicates greater intrathoracic pressure in individuals showing a reduced cardiac output and stroke volume than in individuals showing indications of less intrathoracic pressure (Falkel, Fleck, and Murray 1992). The increase in intrathoracic pressure may limit venous return and so cardiac output, but at the same time it may cause a buildup of blood in the systemic circulation, causing an increase in blood pressure. Cardiac output and stroke volume can be above resting values during resistance training exercise. Therefore, to increase cardiac output and stroke volume during resistance training, it can be speculated that the increase in blood pressure and the powerful muscle pump during resistance exercise overcomes the decrease in venous return, which is due to an increase in intrathoracic pressure.

Increased intrathoracic pressure may have a protective function for the cerebral blood vessels similar to that thought to be active during a cough or strain (Hamilton, Woodbury, and Harper 1943). Any increase in intrathoracic pressure is transmitted to the cerebral spinal fluid because of the cerebral spinal fluid bearing on the intervertebral foramina. This reduces the transmural pressure of the cerebral blood vessels, protecting them from damage caused by the increase in blood pressure (MacDougall et al. 1985).

Increased intramuscular pressure during weight training exercise increases total peripheral resistance and occludes blood flow. Quite high intramuscular pressures (92 kPa) have been measured during static human muscular actions (Edwards, Hill, and McDonnell 1972). Although there is considerable intramuscular variability, static actions of 40 to 60% of maximum can occlude blood flow (Bonde-Peterson, Mork, and Nielsen 1975; Sadamoto, Bonde-Peterson, and Suzuki 1983). Increased intramuscular pressure

during muscular actions is the most probable reason for blood pressures being reportedly higher during the concentric compared to the eccentric portion of a repetition (Miles et al. 1987) and is probably responsible for blood pressure being the highest at the sticking point of a repetition (Gotshall et al. 1999).

Increased blood pressure during weight training may help maintain perfusion pressure and so help maintain blood flow despite an increased intramuscular pressure (MacDougall et al. 1985). This appears to be true at least for small human muscles (Wright, McCloskey, and Fitzpatrick 2000). After fatiguing a thumb muscle (adductor pollicis) by performing rhythmic isometric actions, blood pressure was increased by contracting the knee extensors. Eighteen percent of the isometric force lost due to fatigue of the small muscle was recovered for each 10% increase in blood pressure. The recovery of contractile force is probably related to an increase in perfusion pressure to the muscle. However, the applicability or magnitude of this mechanism to larger muscle groups is unclear.

Chronic Cardiovascular Adaptations During Exercise

Traditional cardiovascular training results in adaptations, such as reduced heart rate and blood pressure, that allow the performance of a given submaximal workload with less cardiovascular stress. A few studies have demonstrated a similar response for resistance (see table 3.10).

Heart Rate, Blood Pressure, and Rate Pressure Product

Several cross-sectional studies clearly demonstrate that resistance training can reduce cardiovascular stress during weight training and other exercise tasks. Male bodybuilders have lower maximal intra-arterial systolic and diastolic blood pressures and maximal heart rates during sets to voluntary concentric failure at 50%, 70%, 80%, 90%, and 100% of 1RM than sedentary subjects and novice (6 to 9 months of training) resistance-trained males (Fleck and Dean 1987). The bodybuilders were stronger than the other subjects, so they had a lower pressor response not only at the same relative workload, but also at greater absolute weight training workloads. Bodybuilders also had lower heart rates and rate pressure products, but not blood pressures, than medical

Table 3.10 Chronic Cardiovascular Adaptations During Exercise

	Absolute workload *	Relative workload *
Heart rate	Decrease	No change
Blood pressure Systolic Diastolic	 Decrease Decrease	 No change or decrease or increase No change or decrease or increase
Rate pressure product	Decrease	No change or decrease or increase
Stroke volume	Increase	?
Cardiac output	Increase	?
VO$_2$peak	Increase	?

* = minimal data and contradictory data; ? = unknown.

students during arm ergometry at the same absolute workload (Colliander and Tesch 1988). In addition, bodybuilders had a lower heart rate at the same relative workload (% 1RM) than power lifters during resistance training exercises (Falkel, Fleck, and Murray 1992). This indicates that high-volume programs may have the greatest effect on the pressor response during resistance training as well as other physical tasks. The lower pressor response shown by bodybuilders may be due in part to a smaller magnitude Valsalva maneuver during resistance exercise compared to power lifters (Falkel, Fleck, and Murray 1992).

Short-term training studies (12 to 16 weeks) also demonstrate cardiovascular adaptations during the performance of exercise tasks. Heart rate, blood pressure, and rate pressure product can all decrease as a result of weight training during bicycle ergometry, treadmill walking, and treadmill walking holding hand weights (Blessing et al. 1987; Goldberg, Elliot, and Kuehl 1988, 1994). Short-term training studies also demonstrate significant decreases in blood pressure and heart rate response during isometric actions (Goldberg, Elliot, and Kuehl 1994) and in both young adults (Sale et al. 1994) and 66-year-old adults (McCartney et al. 1993) during dynamic resistance training at the same absolute resistance. However, after 19 weeks of training the systolic and diastolic blood pressure response at the same relative resistance may be unchanged or even increased (Sale et al. 1994). It is important to note that the same relative resistance (percent of 1RM) after training is a greater absolute resistance. Maximal heart rate during all sets at the same relative resistance tended to be higher and tended to be lower at the

same absolute resistance, but not significantly so, after the 19 weeks of training. This longitudinal information demonstrates that weight training can reduce the pressor response during a variety of physical activities.

A decrease in heart rate, systolic blood pressure, or both during activity would result in a decreased rate pressure product. This indicates lower myocardial work and oxygen consumption. Both cross-sectional and longitudinal data indicate that weight training can reduce the rate pressure product during weight training as well as other physical tasks. This appears to be especially true at the same absolute workload before compared to after training. Thus, weight training can reduce cardiovascular stress during physical activity.

Stroke Volume and Cardiac Output

Weightlifters' cardiac output has been observed to increase to 30 L/minute, with stroke volume increasing up to 150 to 200 ml immediately after resistance training exercise, whereas untrained people show no significant change (Vorobyev 1988). Bodybuilders' peak stroke volume and cardiac output were significantly greater than those of power lifters during sets to voluntary concentric failure at various percentages (50%, 80%, and 100%) of 1RM of both the knee-extension and squat exercises (Falkel, Fleck, and Murray 1992). The bodybuilders' greater cardiac output and stroke volume were evident during both the concentric and eccentric phases of both exercises and may have been caused by the performance of a more limited Valsalva maneuver, resulting in a smaller elevation of intrathoracic pressure. During most of the squat and knee-extension exercise sets the bodybuilders demonstrated a higher maximal heart rate than the power lifters, indicating that cardiac output increased in the bodybuilders as the result of an increase in both stroke volume and heart rate. These results indicate that the type of resistance training program may affect the magnitude of any adaptation that results in the ability to maintain cardiac output during activity.

A short-term longitudinal training study indicates that training may have an effect on the magnitude of the Valsalva maneuver (Sale et al. 1994). After 19 weeks of weight training, esophageal pressures during a set at the same relative resistance (percent of 1RM) were unchanged. However, at the same absolute resistance, which is now a lower percent of 1RM after training, esophageal pressures during the first several repetitions of a set were reduced. This indicates a less forceful Valsalva maneuver during the first several repetitions of a set at the same absolute resistance after weight training. A reduction in the forcefulness of the Valsalva maneuver may allow stroke volume and cardiac output to increase compared to pretraining. Esophageal pressure during the last repetitions of the set was unaffected by training, and therefore did not alter stroke volume or cardiac output compared to pretraining values. These results indicate a differential effect on the forcefulness of a Valsalva maneuver during different repetitions of a set and therefore differing effects on intrathoracic pressure, venous return, and cardiac output during different repetitions of a set.

Both cross-sectional and longitudinal data indicate that stroke volume and cardiac output may increase during weight training in strength-trained individuals compared to untrained individuals. Any changes in stroke volume and cardiac output brought about by chronic weight training may be related to a reduction in the forcefulness of a Valsalva maneuver after training and the type of training performed.

Peak Oxygen Consumption

Peak oxygen consumption (VO_2peak) on a treadmill or bicycle ergometer is considered a marker of cardiovascular fitness. VO_2peak is minimally affected by heavy resistance training. Relative VO_2peak (ml/kg/min) of competitive Olympic weightlifters, power lifters, and bodybuilders ranges from 41 to 55 ml/kg/min (George et al. 1995; Kraemer, Deschenes, and Fleck 1988; Saltin

and Astrand 1967). These are average to moderately above average relative VO_2peak values. This wide range indicates that resistance training may increase relative VO_2peak, but that not all programs may bring about such an increase.

Insight into the type of programs that result in the greatest increase in VO_2peak can be gained by examining short-term training studies. Traditional heavy resistance training using heavy resistances for a few number of repetitions per set and long rest periods result in small increases or no change in VO_2peak (Fahey and Brown 1973; Gettman and Pollock 1981; Lee et al. 1990). An Olympic-style weightlifting program 7 weeks in length can result in moderate gains in absolute (l/min) VO_2peak (9%) and VO_2peak relative to body weight (8%) (Stone et al. 1983). In this study the first 5 weeks of training consisted of three to five sets of 10 repetitions for each exercise, rest periods between sets and exercises of 3.5 to 4.0 minutes, and two training sessions per day 3 days per week. Vertical jumps were performed 2 days per week for five sets of 10 repetitions. The majority of the increase in VO_2peak occurred during the first 5 weeks of the program. Training during the next 2 weeks was identical to the first 5 weeks, except that three sets of 5 repetitions of each exercise were performed. This 2-week training period resulted in no further gains in VO_2peak. The results indicate that higher-volume weight training may be necessary to bring about significant gains in VO_2peak. However, this conclusion must be viewed with caution because of the inclusion of vertical jump training in the total training program.

Circuit weight training generally consists of 12 to 15 repetitions per set using 40 to 60% of 1RM with short rest periods of 15 to 30 seconds between sets and exercises. This type of training resulted in gains in relative VO_2peak of approximately 4% in men and 8% in women during 8 to 20 weeks of training (Gettman and Pollock 1981).

For physical conditioning to elicit changes in VO_2peak, heart rate must be maintained at a minimum of 60% of maximum for a minimum of 20 minutes (American College of Sports Medicine 1998). Exercising heart rate and total metabolic cost during a circuit weight training session is significantly higher than during a more traditional heavy weight training session (Pichon et al. 1996). This may explain in part why circuit weight training elicits a significant increase in VO_2peak while little or no change is caused by a more traditional heavy weight training program. Additionally, the relatively long rest periods taken in a traditional heavy weight training program allow the heart rate to decrease below the recommended 60% of maximum level needed to bring about a significant increase in VO₂peak. Weight training programs intended to increase VO₂ should consist of higher training volumes and use short rest periods between sets and exercises.

The increase in VO₂peak caused by resistance training is substantially less than the 15 to 20% increases associated with traditional endurance-oriented running, cycling, or swimming programs. If a major goal of a training program is to significantly increase VO₂peak, some form of aerobic training needs to be included in the program. The volume of aerobic training necessary to maintain or significantly increase VO₂peak when performing weight training is minimal (Nakao, Inoue, and Murakami 1995). Moderately trained subjects minimally, but significantly, increased relative VO₂peak (3-4 ml/kg/min) over 1 to 2 years of weight training when performing only one aerobic training session per week of running 2 miles (3.2 km) per session. Individuals who performed only weight training during the same training period demonstrated a small but significant decrease in relative VO₂peak. No difference in maximal strength gains was demonstrated between the weight trainers that ran and those that did not.

Summary

Performance of resistance training exercise results in a pressor response that affects the cardiovascular system. Chronic performance of resistance training can result in positive adaptations to the cardiovascular system at rest and during physical activity. Factors such as the volume and intensity of training may influence to what extent any adaptation occurs. In the next chapter we will examine how to integrate the different components of a total conditioning program.

Key Terms

aerobic metabolism
all or none law
anaerobic energy producing systems
bioenergetics
connective tissue sheaths
cortisol
exercise specificity
Golgi tendon organs
growth hormone
hyperplasia
hypertrophy

insulin
insulin-like growth factors
length-tension (force) curve
motor unit
muscle biopsy technique
muscle spindles
myosin ATPase staining method
neuromuscular junction
proprioceptors
sarcomeres
size principle
skeletal muscle fibers
sliding filament theory
testosterone
type I (slow twitch)
type II (fast twitch)
velocity and force-time curve

Selected Readings

Fleck, S.J. 1988. Cardiovascular adaptations to resistance training. *Medicine and Science in Sports and Exercise* 20: S146-S151.

Fleck, S.J. 2002. Cardiovascular responses to strength training. In *Strength & power in sport*, edited by P.V. Komi. Oxford: Blackwell Science.

Gettman, L.R., and Pollock, M.I. 1981. Circuit weight training: A critical review of its physiological benefits. *Physician in Sportsmedicine* 9: 44-60.

Kraemer, W.J. 2000. Neuroendocrine responses to resistance exercise. In *Essentials of strength training and conditioning*, 2nd ed., edited by T. Baechle, 91-114. Champaign, IL: Human Kinetics.

Kraemer, W.J. 2000. Physiological adaptations to anaerobic and aerobic endurance training programs. In *Essentials of strength and conditioning*, 2nd ed., edited by T. Baechle, 137-168. Champaign, IL: Human Kinetics.

Kraemer, W.J., and Ratamess, N.A. 2000. Physiology of resistance training: Current issues. *Orthopaedic Physical Therapy Clinics of North America: Exercise Technologies* 9: 4.

Kraemer, W.J., Ratamess, N.A., and Rubin, M.R. 2000. Basic principles of resistance exercise. In *Nutrition and the strength athlete*, edited by C.R. Jackson. Boca Raton, FL: CRC Press.

Pette, D., and Staron, R.S. 2001. Transitions of muscle fiber phenotypic profiles. *Histochemistry and Cell Biology* 115: 359-372.

Rennie, M.J. 2001. How muscles know how to adapt. *Journal of Physiology* 535: 1.

Russel, B., Motlagh, D., and Ashley, W.W. 2000. Form follows function: How muscle shape is regulated by work. *Journal of Applied Physiology* 88: 1127-1132.

Staron, R.S., and Hikida, R.S. 2001. Muscular responses to exercise and training. In *Exercise and sport science*, edited by W. E. Garrett Jr. and D.T. Kirkendall. Philadelphia: Lippincott Williams & Wilkins.

Sueck, G.C., and Regnier, M. 2001. Plasticity in skeletal, cardiac, and smooth muscle. Invited review: Plasticity and energetic demands of contraction in skeletal and cardiac muscle. *Journal of Applied Physiology* 90: 1158-1164.

CHAPTER 4

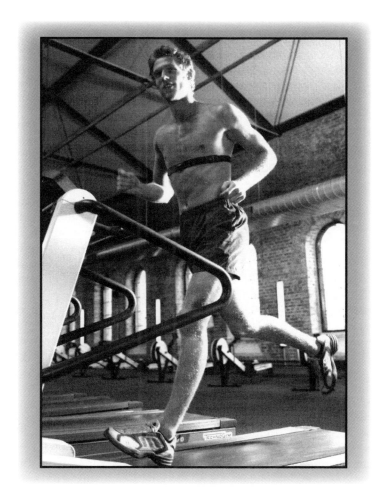

Integrating Other Fitness Components

When integrating the different fitness components into one total conditioning program, the most important concepts are prioritization and compatibility of training modalities. The timing and emphasis of each program component will affect the body's ability to adapt properly and achieve program goals. Proper exercise prescription is vital for the successful development of a total conditioning program.

Resistance training is only one form of conditioning and must be integrated into a total conditioning program, which can include a host of different conditioning programs customized to meet the training goals of the individual. Thus, a total conditioning program may have many components, including nutrition, resistance training, plyometrics, agility, cardiovascular endurance, speed development, flexibility, and skill training (see figure 4.1). Each type

Fitness
Components

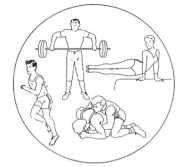

- Strength/Power
- Flexibility
- Cardiovascular endurance
- Local muscular endurance

Figure 4.1 The major components of physical fitness.

of resistance training program can interact differentially with a wide variety of other training components directed at improving physical function and performance.

In this chapter we will present an overview of the basic guidelines for exercise prescription in some of the primary conditioning modalities and review how resistance training interacts with these other exercise stimuli. The composition of a total conditioning program will change depending on the needs and goals of the individual. Training needs and goals will change over time and require both building and maintenance programs at different times in the program progression. Ultimately, each individual has a genetic ceiling for any trainable characteristic and an optimal exercise training program to reach their genetic ceiling.

Aerobic Training

The typical goal of aerobic conditioning is to improve peak oxygen consumption and associated cardiovascular functions to support endurance performance. A great deal of information exists regarding the effects and prescription of endurance exercise. This knowledge base spans from cardiac rehabilitation to elite distance running (American College of Sports Medicine 1998; Froelicher 1983). However, as Laursen and Jenkins (2002) note, we understand far less about the adaptations that take place in already highly trained endurance athletes. The ability to prescribe aerobic exercise is necessary to address the cardiovascular endurance needs of an individual undertaking a total conditioning program.

Aerobic endurance training programs can be either continuous or interval in nature. As we will discuss later in the chapter, in some cases high-intensity aerobic conditioning is not compatible with the maximal strength and power production needed in some sports. Interval programs are typically of higher intensity and also involve a higher degree of anaerobic metabolism due to the use of multiple exercise bouts and rest period lengths that may not allow complete recovery. Even short, high-intensity intervals are effective in promoting improvement in oxygen consumption (Knuttgen and Saltin 1972). For example, MacDougall and colleagues (1998) showed that 30-second maximum sprint efforts result in improvement in both anaerobic and aerobic enzymes related to energy production, maximum short-term power output, and peak oxygen consumption. The myth that one needs a long, slow, distance-running "aerobic base" before participating in other, more intense conditioning modalities most likely arises from the perceived need to use lower-intensity training during a "general conditioning phase," especially when starting with untrained individuals. However, the relationship between aerobic and anaerobic performances is limited and demonstrates that individuals who perform well in anaerobic tests do not necessarily perform well in aerobic tests (Koziris et al. 1996). This is most likely due to differences in body mass, the energy source best suited for a particular task, muscle fiber type, or training background. Nevertheless, whether using continuous or interval aerobic training methods, proper progression in the frequency, intensity, and duration is needed.

According to the American College of Sports Medicine (1998), "persons of any age may significantly increase their habitual levels of physical activity safely if there are no contraindications to exercise and a rational program is developed." Before starting a vigorous exercise program, a medical evaluation is useful. According to Wilmore and Costill (1994), a medical exam can have the following benefits:

■ Some people either should not be exercising or are considered at high risk and should be restricted to exercising only under close medical supervision. A comprehensive medical evaluation will help identify these high-risk individuals.

- The information obtained in a medical evaluation can be used to develop the exercise prescription.

- The values obtained for certain clinical measures such as blood pressure, body fat content, and blood lipid levels can be used to motivate the person to adhere to the exercise program.

- A comprehensive medical evaluation, particularly of healthy people, can provide a baseline against which any subsequent changes in health status can be compared.

- Children and adults should establish a habit of periodic medical evaluations because many illnesses and diseases, such as cancer and cardiovascular diseases, can be identified in their earliest stages when the chances of successful treatment are much higher.

As with any exercise program, the prescription of aerobic exercise should be individualized. Individuals who need more specific exercise prescriptions may benefit from a stress test to document their exact functional capacity and suggested training zone for heart rate monitoring. This is especially important for older adults or in individuals whose functional capacity is in doubt (e.g., those with cardiovascular pathologies). It can also provide very highly specific training data for elite athletes. The results of treadmill or cycle ergometry testing can be very helpful for individualizing exercise prescription for endurance training (see figure 4.2). The test modality should be specific to the exercise training or competition, even when "cross-training" is used. From this information the intensity of the exercise can be related to a heart rate value.

A **heart rate training zone** is typically prescribed to control the intensity of the aerobic exercise stimulus. An individual then performs steady state exercise within the training zone. Generally, the heart rate training zone is between 55 to 65% and 90% of maximal heart rate

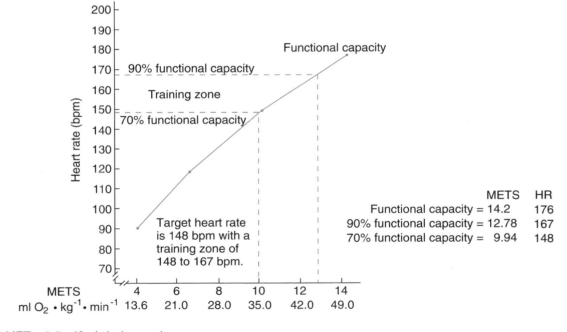

1 MET = 3.5 ml/kg/min (approx)

METS	HR
Functional capacity = 14.2	176
90% functional capacity = 12.78	167
70% functional capacity = 9.94	148

Stress test data

Heart rate	90	118	149	176
Work load (mph/% grade)	1.7/10	2.5/12	3.4/14	4.2/16
METS	4.0	6.6	10.0	14.2
Symptoms				Fatigue

Figure 4.2 Training zone of 70-90% of maximal capacity derived from an exercise stress test.

(American College of Sports Medicine 1998), with lower intensities typically used by untrained or aerobically unfit individuals. Energy demands are expressed in metabolic equivalents (METS) or as the amount of oxygen used.

One MET is equivalent to resting oxygen consumption, which is approximately $3.5 \, ml \cdot kg^{-1} \cdot min^{-1}$. For example, 10 METS represents an exercise intensity approximately 10 times the resting metabolic rate. An individual with a 10-MET functional capacity would have a peak oxygen consumption value of approximately $35 \, ml \cdot kg^{-1} \, min^{-1}$ (10 times $3.5 \, ml \cdot kg^{-1} \, min^{-1}$).

The functional capacity for a healthy individual is the end point of the test (e.g., voluntary exhaustion). Functional capacity could also be the point of the test at which no abnormal responses (e.g., abnormal EKG responses) are observed as is the case with cardiac patients. High MET values, which reflect high peak oxygen consumption values, are associated with the functional capacities of individuals who possess good cardiovascular endurance.

Despite the importance of individual exercise prescription, many individuals (most notably, coaches who are prescribing exercise for hundreds of athletes) do not have the resources available to obtain laboratory stress tests. For healthy individuals a training zone can be calculated using a percent of predicted maximal heart rate (see figure 4.3). Coaches and individuals must realize that for basic aerobic fitness, endurance training doesn't have to hurt to be effective. This is quite different from the competitive endurance athlete

who must use a much higher training intensity to prepare for competition. In addition, some athletes do not want to train at high-intensity, aerobic levels, as such training may inhibit the strength and power adaptations important for performance (Kraemer, Patton et al. 1995).

The duration and frequency of exercise also needs to increase progressively as the individual becomes more tolerant of exercise stress. For basic cardiovascular endurance fitness, the duration of exercise should last 20 to 60 minutes and be performed 3 to 5 days per week (American College of Sports Medicine 1998). Running, bicycling, cross-country skiing, stair climbing, ellipse training, aerobics (e.g., bench-step aerobics), and swimming are some of the most popular and effective cardiovascular conditioning modalities (Kraemer, Keuning et al. 2001). However, a degree of specificity is necessary if the conditioning modality is vital to sport skills (e.g., run training if conditioning for soccer). Table 4.1 gives a basic summary of endurance training ranges.

Improvement of aerobic capacity can be accomplished through interval training. However, because the intensity is higher, interval training is typically only used with individuals who already have completed a general aerobic conditioning phase in a periodized training program (Fardy 1977).

An endurance exercise training session has a warm-up, a training period, and a cool-down (see figure 4.4). The heart rate is checked and the pace of the exercise adjusted so that the individual is exercising within his or her training zone. The heart rate can be manipulated by the pace at which the individual exercises. Heart rate watches are often used to monitor heart rate. However, a 10-second pulse rate can be taken after a steady state exercise duration is achieved (usually 3 to 5 minutes). A pace test at the training heart rate over a specified distance can be conducted over a number of training sessions. Pace tests for running or cycling should be performed on flat terrain. Also, as fitness levels improve, it is important to check this pace against the heart rate response relationship. In figure 4.5 a 1-mile run is used, but shorter

---

$$220 - 20 = 200 \text{ bpm predicted max HR*}$$

$$70\% \text{ maximal HR} = 70\% \times 200 = 140 \text{ bpm}$$

$$90\% \text{ maximal HR} = 90\% \times 200 = 180 \text{ bpm}$$

70-90% maximal HR Training Zone = 140 to 180 bpm

Figure 4.3 Training zone based on predicted maximal heart rate.
*A conservative estimate of maximal heart rate can be calculated as 220 – age in years = max heart rate bpm.

Table 4.1 Basic Guidelines for Intensity, Frequency, and Duration of Aerobic Exercise			
Fitness level	Intensity (% of maximal heart rate)	Frequency per week	Duration of each session
Endurance athlete	70-90%	5-7 days	1-2 hours
Healthy individual	55-90%	3-5 days	20-60 minutes

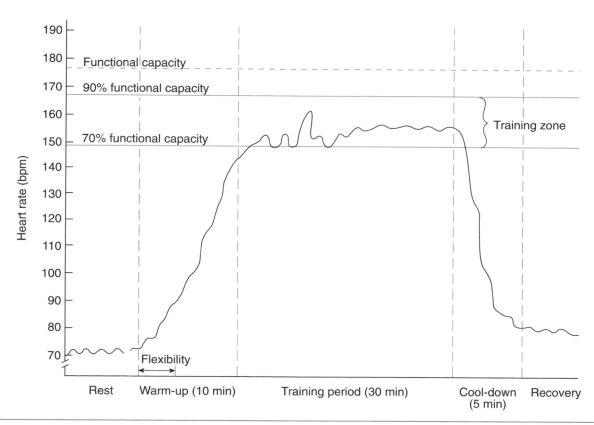

Figure 4.4 Heart rate response to warm-up, training period, and cool-down during an endurance training session.

Adapted from B.J. Sharkey, 1984, *Physiology of fitness* (Champaign, IL: Human Kinetics), 45.

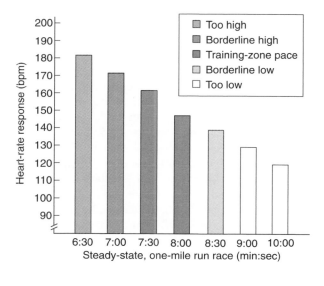

Figure 4.5 An individual's response to different paces of endurance steady state exercise. Target training zone is 148 to 167 bpm; training zone pace is 7:30 to 8:00 (min:sec) per mile.\

distances (e.g., one-half mile) can also be used to evaluate this relationship. A less-conditioned individual usually requires shorter pace distances to evaluate a training pace. It is important to ensure that steady state exercise is achieved at the selected distance (3 to 5 minutes of exercise duration after warm-up).

Interestingly, it has been estimated that peak oxygen consumption reaches the genetic ceiling of development within 6 to 12 months of aerobic training. Further increases in aerobic performance are therefore thought to be due to increasing the lactate threshold, improved running efficiency, improved race strategies, psychological toughening, improved acid buffering mechanisms, hemoglobin or hematological characteristics, respiratory system adaptations including improved respiratory muscle fitness, or improved force and power production capabilities (Laursen and Jenkins 2002; Markov et al. 2001). Slawinski and colleagues (2001) postulated that a reduction in stride rate variability may also influence endurance performance despite no change in the peak oxygen consumption of runners with training. Thus, endurance training, although marked by the classic marker of peak oxygen consumption, has many other factors contributing to success beyond this basic fitness variable.

Concurrent Strength and Endurance Training

Training adaptations are specific to the imposed training stimulus. So, how compatible are two different types of training that result in different adaptations when both types of training are performed concurrently? Our understanding of exercise training compatibility primarily relates to the concurrent use of aerobic endurance and strength training programs (Chromiak and Mulvaney 1990; Dudley and Fleck 1987). Studies examining such concurrent training provide the following conclusions.

- High-intensity endurance training may compromise strength, especially at high velocities of muscle actions.
- Power capabilities may be most affected by the performance of both strength and endurance training.
- High-intensity endurance training may negatively affect short-term anaerobic performance.
- The development of peak oxygen consumption is not compromised by a heavy resistance training program.
- Strength training does not negatively affect endurance capabilities.
- Strength and power training programs may benefit endurance performances by preventing injuries, increasing lactic acid threshold, and reducing the ground contact time during running.

The topic of exercise compatibility came to the attention of the sport science community when Hickson (1980) demonstrated that the development of dynamic strength may be compromised by concurrent performance of both resistance and endurance training. This study lasted only 8 weeks, so whether the reduction of strength development would continue over a longer training period was unknown. Because no periodization of either the resistance or the endurance training was used, and a relatively high training volume was performed, overtraining may have occurred

in the group that performed both types of training simultaneously. Conversely, in the group training for strength and endurance, improvement in aerobic capacity was not compromised compared to the group performing only endurance training.

Five years later Dudley and Djamil (1985) used a more conventional frequency of training and found only decrements in the magnitude of increase in angle-specific peak torque at fast velocities (160-278 degrees $\cdot$ sec^{-1}) of movement in a group simultaneously trained for strength and endurance as compared to a group trained only for strength. No decrements in angle-specific peak torque were observed at slow velocities (48-96 $\cdot$ sec^{-1}) of movement in the group that simultaneously trained for strength and endurance. This study was the first investigation to suggest that power may in fact be first affected by concurrent training over a short training period. Again, aerobic power of the combination training group was not compromised compared to a group trained for endurance only. These conclusions were supported by Hunter, Demmett, and Miller (1987), who examined simultaneous resistance training and endurance training over 12 weeks. Barbell squats were emphasized in this training program. An increase in strength of 39% was observed in the strength-only group, and the combined group increased by 24%. No impairment of peak oxygen consumption was observed, but strength at high velocities of movement was compromised in the endurance training group.

These early studies sparked an interest in the physiological compatibility of simultaneous strength and endurance training. Using various experimental protocols to explore adaptational responses to concurrent strength and endurance training, studies have shown that strength can be either compromised (Hennessy and Watson 1994; Nelson et al. 1990) or unaffected (Bell et al. 1991b; Hortobagyi, Katch, and LaChance 1991; Sale et al. 1990), whereas endurance capabilities are not affected. Other studies have reported that both strength and endurance capabilities can be attenuated especially over longer periods of concurrent training in trained athletes (Hennessy and Watson 1994; Nelson et al. 1990). Hennessy and Watson (1994) clearly demonstrated that strength, power, and speed performance may be most susceptible to "incompatibility" because of the high intensity and volume of training performed by highly trained athletes.

McCarthy and colleagues (1995) examined the effect of simultaneous strength and endurance training using a more realistic and typical 3-days-a-week routine. The strength training program consisted of four sets of 5 to 7 repetitions for eight exercises, and the endurance protocol consisted of 50 minutes of cycle exercise at 70% of the heart rate reserve. A strength-only group, endurance-only group, and combined group trained for 10 weeks. Subjects who performed the strength-only training or both types of training increased their 1RM squat, bench press, vertical jump, and maximal isometric knee-extension strength as well as their fat-free mass. The endurance group demonstrated no changes in these variables, but did increase peak oxygen consumption, as did the combined training group. The results of this study show that conventional training frequencies and programs are in fact compatible and further indicate that "overtraining" may be the ultimate cause of exercise incompatibility. Thus, whether concurrent strength and endurance training are compatible may depend on many factors such as training status, training intensity, and training volume.

Almost all of the studies used men as subjects, and only limited amounts of data are available on this issue in women. But in a study by Volpe and colleagues (1993) previously sedentary college-age women used conventional strength training (a periodized program) and endurance training (75% of predicted maximal heart rate) programs for 3 days per week over 9 weeks, and no incompatibility was observed for strength or endurance performances. One interpretation of these results is that training status does affect whether concurrent training is incompatible.

Concurrent Training and Cellular Changes

Few cellular data are available to provide insights into changes at the muscle fiber level with concur-

rent strength and endurance training (Nelson et al. 1990; Sale et al. 1990). The muscle fiber is faced with the dilemma of trying to adapt to the oxidative stimulus to improve its aerobic function and to the stimulus from the heavy resistance training program to improve its force production ability. So what happens to the muscle fiber population?

Kraemer, Patton, and colleagues (1995) examined changes in muscle fiber morphology over a 3-month training program in physically fit men. Training took place 4 days per week for 3 months. Both high-intensity strength and endurance training programs were varied throughout the week to provide a periodized training program to enhance recovery and prevent overtraining (i.e., a decrease in performance). Thus, the weight training program used two "heavy days" (i.e., 5RM) and two "moderate days" (10RM) per week, and the endurance training program used two "interval training days" and two "long duration run days" per week. Five participant groups were used to evaluate muscle fiber changes in the vastus lateralis muscle with training as follows: the strength (S) group performed a total-body strength training program; the combined (C) group performed the same total-body strength training program but also performed a high-intensity endurance training program; the upper-body combined (UBC) group performed only an upper-body strength training program and the high-intensity endurance training program; the endurance (E) group performed only the high-intensity endurance training; and a control group performed no training.

The data from the muscle fiber profile are depicted in figure 4.6 and shown in table 4.2. All training groups had a shift of muscle fiber types from type IIB to type IIA. The remaining type

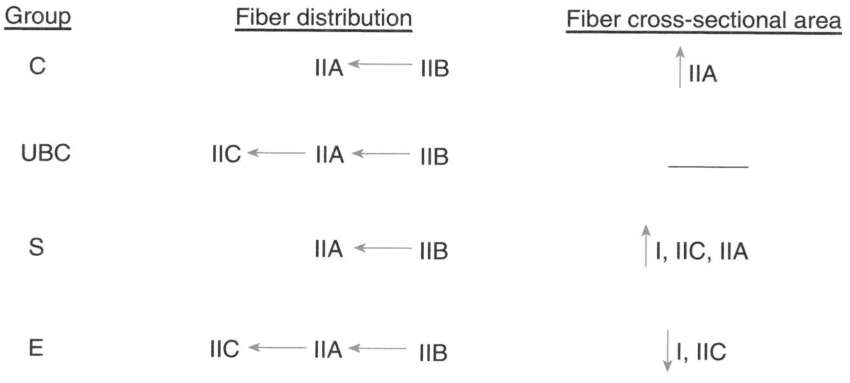

Group	Fiber distribution	Fiber cross-sectional area
C	IIA ← IIB	↑ IIA
UBC	IIC ← IIA ← IIB	———
S	IIA ← IIB	↑ I, IIC, IIA
E	IIC ← IIA ← IIB	↓ I, IIC

Figure 4.6 Fiber type changes with different types of training combinations

Adapted, by permission, from W.J. Kraemer et al., 1995b, "Compatibility of high intensity strength and endurance training on hormonal and skeletal muscle adaptations," *Journal of Applied Physiology* 78: 976-989.

Table 4.2 Muscle Fiber Characteristics Pre- and Posttraining

Group	C		S		E		UBC		Control	
	Pre	Post	Pre	Post	Pre	Post	Pre	Post	Pre	Post
% type										
I	55.6 (±11.1)	57.7 (±11.1)	55.21 (±11.7)	55.44 (±1.5)	54.1 (±5.9)	54.6 (±5.3)	50.6 (±8.0)	51.1 (±7.9)	52.0 (±11.5)	52.8 (±10.8)
IIC	1.9 (±2.2)	1.8 (±2.7)	2.4 (±1.6)	2.0 (±1.3)	0.9 (±0.6)	2.5* (±2.0)	1.3 (±1.0)	3.0* (±2.2)	1.6 (±0.9)	1.3 (±1.3)
IIA	28.4 (±15.4)	39.3* (±11.1)	23.3 (±11.5)	40.5* (±10.6)	25.75 (±4.8)	34.1 (±3.9)	25.5 (±4.2)	34.2* (±6.9)	25.6 (±1.6)	26.6 (±4.6)
IIB	14.11 (±7.2)	1.6* (±0.8)	19.1 (±7.9)	1.9* (±0.8)	19.2 (±3.6)	8.8* (±4.4)	22.6 (±4.9)	11.6* (±5.3)	20.8 (±7.6)	19.2 (±6.4)
Area (μm²)										
I	5008 (±874)	4756 (±692)	4883 (±1286)	5460* (±1214)	5437 (±970)	4853* (±966)	5680 (±535)	5376 (±702)	4946 (±1309)	5177 (±1344)
IIC	4157 (±983)	4658 (±771)	3981.2 (±1535)	5301* (±1956)	2741 (±482)	2402* (±351)	3050 (±930)	2918 (±1086)	3733 (±1285)	4062 (±1094)
IIA	5862 (±997)	7039* (±1151)	6084 (±1339)	7527* (±1981)	6782 (±1267)	6287 (±385)	6393 (±1109)	6357 (±1140)	6310 (±593)	6407 (±423)
IIB	5190 (±712)	4886 (±1171)	5795 (±1495)	6078 (±2604)	6325 (±1860)	4953 (±1405)	6052 (±1890)	5855 (±867)	5917 (±896)	6120 (±1089)

C = combined; S = strength; E = endurance; UC = upperbody combined.

* = p<0.05 from corresponding pretraining value.

Means (±SD).

Adapted, by permission, from W.J. Kraemer et al., 1995b, "Compatibility of high intensity strength and endurance training on hormonal and skeletal muscle adaptations," *Journal of Applied Physiology* 78(3): 976-989.

IIB fibers were not likely true type IIB fibers since the authors did not detect any type IIAB subtype. Ploutz and colleagues (1994) showed that if type IIAB fibers are not detected after high-intensity resistance training, the remaining type IIB fibers have a high concentration of aerobic enzymes and therefore may not be true IIB fibers. From this study the number of type IIB muscle fibers was lower after high-intensity strength training (group S) when compared to high-intensity endurance training including interval training (group E). This may be due to the greater recruitment of high-threshold motor units with heavy resistance training.

From an aerobic perspective it is interesting to note the small, but significant changes in the type IIC population of muscle fibers. The use of just upper-body strength training appears to negate the decreases in type I muscle fiber size in the legs with endurance training. This may be due to the legs' isometric muscle actions needed to support the upper body during resistance exercise. Muscle fiber cross-sectional areas show that changes occurred differentially across the continuum of exercise training modalities and were dictated by the type or combination of training stimuli to which the muscle was exposed. The muscle fiber adaptations observed in the C group were different from those in either the S or the E groups. This indicates that when two high-intensity training programs are used, with one focusing on high-intensity endurance training and the other on high-intensity strength training, the adaptive response at the level of the muscle fiber is not the same as when a single training mode is used.

In this study lower-body power was compromised in the C group, and the rate of strength development demonstrated a trend toward a compromised state in the C group as well. The response of the UBC group, however, clearly indicated that upper-body strength training is not affected by lower-body endurance training. This implies that training two different muscle groups, one for endurance and one for strength, can be done successfully. Consistent with several other studies, peak oxygen consumption was not diminished by the performance of both a high-intensity strength training program and an endurance training program (Dudley and Djamil 1985; McCarthy et al. 1995). Thus, the mechanisms of adaptation to resistance exercise depends on the global exercise stimuli presented to the activated musculature. In addition, concurrent training will begin to negatively affect strength increases in 2 to 3 months. Thus, at the cellular level a differential response to the simultaneous training occurred, and single training modes resulted in different muscle fiber changes than were observed with concurrent training.

In the 1970s, studies showing a reduction of mitochondrial density resulted in many runners avoiding resistance exercise programs. In a study by Chilibeck, Syrotuik, and Bell (2002) the effects of combined strength and endurance training for 12 weeks on mitochondria in muscle were examined in comparison to a nonexercising control group. The authors concluded that mitochondrial populations increase in number, but changes take place in different anatomical regions of the muscle. The intermyofibrillar region undergoes a linear increase with training, whereas the subsarcolemmal region undergoes a preferential increase late in the training program. The authors postulated that an increase in the late phase of a 12-week training program was the result of an increase in type I fibers in the exercise group. However, such increases in type I fiber numbers remain unclear at this point, as transformation of muscle fibers have been attributed either to a limited myosin ATPase profile leading to experimental errors in interpretation or to hyperplasia (see chapter 3). Nevertheless, the use of both types of training does not appear to reduce the oxidative potential at the cellular level, which was a fear of many endurance runners in the 1970s, when initial studies were published showing reductions in mitochondrial density using area measurement paradigms.

The physiological mechanisms that may mediate adaptational responses to concurrent training remain speculative, but appear related to alterations in neural recruitment patterns, attenuation of muscle hypertrophy, or both (Chromiak and Mulvaney 1990; Dudley and Djamil 1985; Dudley and Fleck 1987). Such physiological attenuation may, in fact, result in overtraining (i.e., decrease in performance) with longer periods of training (Hennessy and Watson 1994; Nelson et al. 1990). Conversely, concurrent exercise training, when properly designed, may just require a longer time for the summation of physiological adaptations. Trainees do not appear to be able to adapt optimally to both modes of training, as the programs needed to effectively alter high fitness levels may not be compatible. Thus, priority training may be important when several fitness components must be trained at the same time.

A multitude of factors (e.g., exercise prescriptions, pretraining fitness levels, exercise modalities, etc.) can affect the exercise stimulus and therefore the subsequent adaptational responses (Chromiak and Mulvaney 1990; Dudley and Fleck 1987; Sale et al. 1990). The majority of studies in the literature have used relatively untrained subjects to examine the physiological effects of simultaneous strength and endurance training (Chromiak and Mulvaney 1990; Dudley and Fleck 1987). Few data are available regarding the effects of simultaneous strength and endurance training on previously active or fit individuals who are able to tolerate higher intensity exercise training programs (Hennessy and Watson 1994). Thus, more study of this topic is needed, especially concerning the effect of concurrent training of trained individuals and females.

Exercise prescription must take into consideration the demands of the total program and ensure that the volume of exercise does not become counterproductive to optimal physiological adaptations and performance. Those involved in exercise prescription should keep the following points in mind:

- Training program sequences should be prioritized as they relate to training program goals. Individuals should not attempt to perform high-intensity and high-volume strength and endurance training concurrently.
- Periodized training programs with planned rest phases should be used to allow for adequate recovery from training sessions.
- A strength or power athlete should limit high-intensity aerobic training because the high oxidative stress accompanying high-volume or high-intensity endurance training appears to negatively affect power development.

Does Resistance Training Affect Endurance?

MacDougall and colleagues (1979) noted a decrease in mitochondrial volume density in the triceps muscle after a high-intensity strength training program. Because mitochondria are the site of aerobic energy production, any decrease in the volume density of mitochondria could theoretically decrease the oxidative capacity of the muscle. Thus, based on the results of this study, many distance runners did not perform resistance training fearing that it will compromise their endurance capabilities. A decrease in mitochondrial density after resistance training would appear to support this belief. What distance runners failed to recognize, however, was that resistance training offers other benefits, such as injury prevention and the elimination of the overuse phenomenon. Protein being removed from the type I and IIC muscle fibers with high-intensity endurance running (Kraemer, Patton et al. 1995) may result in injury and decreased performance over the long term.

One of the most consistent findings of concurrent training studies has been that even heavy resistance training does not impair endurance performance. In fact, several studies indicated that strength training may actually increase markers of endurance ability (Hickson et al. 1980, 1988; Marcinik et al. 1991). For example, after 12 weeks of weight training 3 days per week, peak cycling oxygen consumption was unchanged, but cycling lactate threshold and time to exhaustion were elevated 12% and 33%, respectively (Marcinik et al. 1991). Unfortunately, all of the previously cited studies used untrained or moderately trained individuals as subjects.

More recent studies, however, have shown that resistance training can improve endurance performance in trained athletes. Bastiaans and colleagues (2001) replaced part of the conditioning program typically dedicated to endurance training with explosive strength training in cyclists and reported that endurance performance was not compromised. However, the inclusion of explosive strength training negated a decrease in 30-second sprint ability shown with no explosive strength training. Sprint performance is important to cyclists during various parts of a race, such as the sprint at the end of the race. Paavolainen and colleagues (1999) equated the total training volume of two groups of elite distance runners.

However, in one group 32% of the total volume was dedicated to explosive strength training, and in the other only 3% was dedicated to explosive strength training; both groups trained for 9 weeks. Neither groups' peak oxygen consumption changed significantly. However, only the group that performed the additional explosive strength training significantly reduced 5K run time. These studies indicate that endurance performance is enhanced via neuromuscular mechanisms (e.g., enhanced stretch-shortening cycle activity and reduced contact time with the ground) independent of changes in aerobic capacity. Thus, resistance training programs that use moderate intensities (5-15RM) and emphasize injury prevention are appropriate for endurance athletes, do not negatively affect endurance performance, and may actually improve performance.

In sports that depend almost exclusively on one of the three energy sources, long-term intensive training of a second energy source may retard the development of the primary energy source. For example, distance runners depend heavily on the oxidative energy source, and extensive training of the adenosine triphosphate phosphocreatine energy source using resistance training may compromise the development of the oxygen energy source over long training periods (years). For the same reason, athletes who are highly dependent on strength/power may not want to heavily train the oxygen energy source. Whether this is due to overtraining resulting from the high volume and intensity necessary to train simultaneously for endurance and strength, or to some underlying physiological mechanism, is still unknown. It should be pointed out that many sports are not dependent on only one energy source (Fox and Mathews 1981). The needs analysis of individuals will dictate whether they would benefit from the training of multiple energy sources. In this case, the compatibility question may be a moot point; research should center on what mixture of strength and endurance training will cause the greatest possible gains in both parameters, when simultaneous training must be performed.

Anaerobic Sprint and Interval Training

Sprint performance is determined by the ability to accelerate, the magnitude of maximal velocity, and the ability to maintain velocity against the onset of fatigue. A complex interaction of the nervous system and muscle(s) to produce high-velocity movements and its interaction with resistance training to improve this ability has resulted in many different training paradigms (for review, see Ross, Leveritt, and Riek 2001). Fatigue of neural origin during and after sprint training may affect the optimization of the training session. McKenna and colleagues (1997) showed that 7 weeks of sprint interval training consisting of maximal 30-second bouts enhanced aerobic metabolism, improved anaerobic metabolism, and increased maximal sprint performances. All training-related changes suggested that fatigue was reduced during maximal effort sprinting. Conditioning with sprint intervals is quite different from using sprint intervals to improve speed in a given distance (e.g., 40 yd for an American football player). Thus, training programs must be separated between those related to speed development and those that use sprints to condition the cardiovascular and acid-base status of the body for toleration of such stress in competition.

Young, McDowell, and Scarlett (2001) clarified the fact that sprint speed is different from speed during agility runs of two or more directional changes. The training effect for unidirectional speed development does not transfer to multiple direction changes thought of as high-speed agility, which are typical of many sports. Thus, training programs need to be designed in order to target specific goals.

In addition to resistance training, other more sport-specific anaerobic training may be necessary. Some examples are sprinting and agility drills for football and sprint swimming for water polo. This type of training enhances both the motor skill and the conditioning component needed for performance in a particular sport. Thus, to improve sport performance, sport-specific movement needs to be performed in addition to resistance training even though anaerobic training adaptations are similar to those observed for resistance training (Burke, Thayer, and Belcamino 1994; Howald, 1982).

Interval Training

Conditioning is necessary to enhance speed or anaerobic endurance. Sprint activities of a few seconds require a higher power output than longer-duration sprints of 1 to 2 minutes (Wilmore and Costill 1994). Training needs to be related to both the distance and the duration of the activity performed in the particular sport. For a football lineman, 5- to 20-yd sprints (1 to 3 seconds) are appropriate, whereas a receiver may need to train using sprint distances ranging from 10 to 60 yd. An 800-m sprinter would need to train at distances and paces equivalent to the distance and pace needed in a race (Wilt 1968). This last program involves more interval-type training, which also emphasizes the aerobic component of the sport. It is important to differentiate between "quality" sprint training for maximal speed and "quantity" sprint conditioning for speed endurance and improvement of lactic acid buffering capacity.

Sprint Workouts

Sprint workouts should be performed 1 to 5 days per week depending on the sport (i.e., soccer vs. track and field sprinting) and the training cycle. A **sprint workout** should include the following:

- Warm-up
- Exercise at low loads for cardiovascular and muscular warm-up
- Technique drills
- Start drills
- A conditioning phase
- Cool-down

It is interesting to note from the data of Callister and colleagues (1988) that sprint training performed 3 days per week that consisted of three 100-yd (91.4-m) sprints followed by three 50-yd (45.7-m) sprints with a rest interval of 3 minutes and 90 seconds, respectively, between each sprint and 5 minutes between sets resulted in increases in sprint speed, but no increases in peak oxygen consumption over an 8-week training program. Conversely, when two sets of four sprint intervals of 20 seconds were separated by only 1 minute of rest, significant increases in the peak oxygen consumption were observed by the eighth week of a 10-week training program (Kraemer et al. 1989). Thus, the exercise-to-rest ratio is a vital factor in determining the effects of sprint intervals on increases in peak oxygen consumption or sprint speed. The concept of needing traditional aerobic training to increase peak oxygen consumption is incorrect, as this can be accomplished with sprint intervals when the exercise-to-rest ratio is low. The progression must be appropriate so the trainees can tolerate the exercise stress, which is a function of the exercise volume and intensity and the exercise-to-rest ratio used in the sprint interval program.

Shorter sprint training involves all-out exercise intensity. As the duration of the activity increases to longer sprint distances (e.g., 800 m), the pace becomes important and can be improved through interval training. Interval training can also be designed to address the aerobic metabolic needs necessary to perform longer sprints (e.g., 800 m). Figure 4.7 depicts a "power unit" workout, which is a symmetrical form of interval training. It consists of long units (distances longer than the race itself), short units (40 to 60 m) and kick units (approximate distances used for the kick in a race). Track and field coaches use the power unit workout to promote the development of race speed. The long units develop endurance at the race distance, and the short units develop leg speed. This program is typically performed during the preseason and in-season on grass (soft surfaces) and straightaways. An adequate endurance conditioning base is necessary before initiating such high-intensity workouts.

The importance of tolerating the high lactate concentrations associated with different sport activities (e.g., longer-duration sprinting and wrestling) necessitates training that increases lactate production and in turn enhances lactate removal (Brooks and Fahey 1984). Exercise intervals shorter than 20 seconds do not result in anaerobic energy source depletion when used with a recovery interval of a similar duration (Lamb 1978). This recovery interval allows trainees to repeat short sprints at near-maximal velocity. Therefore, recovery time between sprint distances must be carefully controlled (see table 4.3). For example, a sprint workout for basketball might include a 5-second exercise duration. From table 4.3 it is clear that each sprint has to be run at 100% intensity and that only a 5-second recovery period between sprints is allowed. Twenty to 30 intervals are required two to four times per week.

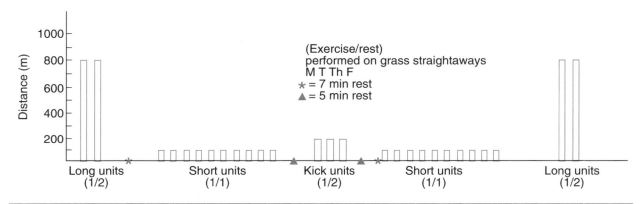

Figure 4.7 Anaerobic power unit workout.

Table 4.3 General Guidelines for Interval Training				
Exercise duration (min:s)	% intensity	Recover (min:s)	Number of intervals	Sessions per week
0:05	100	0:05	20-30	2-4
0:10	100	0:10	20-30	2-4
0:20	100	0:15	10-20	2-4
0:30	100	1:00-2:00	8-18	2-4
1:00	95-100	3:00-5:00	5-15	2-4
2:00	90-100	5:00-15:00	4-10	2-4
3:00	80-90	5:00-15:00	3-8	2-4

Adapted, by permission, from D.R. Lamb, 1978, *Physiology of exercise: Responses and adaptations* (Boston, MA: Allyn & Bacon), 167.

A training pace for sprint intervals can also be determined as a function of the individual's maximal 2-mile run time (see table 4.4). As with any exercise conditioning program, trainers must make good clinical decisions regarding the progress of a workout, and trainees must pay attention to their body's responses to the training stress.

Sprint training regimes using high-speed inclines have also been used to improve power and train the associated muscles used in sprinting. Studies have found that the average power and energy generated during hip flexion and extension in the swing phase were the greatest using incline sprint running. Thus, incline sprint training provides for enhanced muscular loading during both the swing and stance phases (Swanson and Caldwell 2000). In addition, the use of resistive devices for sprinting (e.g., weighted vest, sleds, towing devices) also appears beneficial for enhancing sprint performance.

Flexibility Training

Over the past 10 years a host of information has been accumulating on the role and use of **flexibility training** in conditioning programs. The emerging data on flexibility indicate that care is needed when addressing the flexibility needs in the warm-up. Different joint movements and time frames of use may each require different stretching techniques, and different types of or combinations of flexibility programs may be needed depending on the specific goal. The typical one-size-fits-all stretching program (e.g., static stretching) performed as a standard part of all warm-ups and cool-downs may not meet the specific needs of each situation.

Another question of continual interest is whether flexibility training can reduce injuries linked to physical activity. This has been an elusive concept to address because of experimental

Table 4.4 General Guidelines for Initial Paces for Distance and Interval Run Programs

Total two-mile run time (min)	Time for interval distance (min)		
	880 yds*	440 yds*	Mile*
10	2:30	1:15	6:50
11	2:45	1:22.5	7:30
12	3:00	1:30	8:00
13	3:15	1:37.5	8:40
14	3:30	1:45	9:20
15	3:45	1:52.5	10:00
16	4:00	2:00	10:40
17	4:15	2:07.5	11:20
18	4:30	2:15	12:00
19	4:45	2:22.5	12:50
20	5:00	2:30	13:20
21	5:15	2:37.5	14:00
22	5:30	2:45	14:40
	90-100% $\dot{V}O_2$max		70% $\dot{V}O_2$max

* = speeds are based on two-mile run time and percentage of maximal oxygen consumption.

Adapted, by permission, from Kraemer, W.J., et al., 1987, "The effects of various physical training programs on short duration high intensity load bearing performance and the army physical fitness tests," *USARIEM Technical Report*, 30/87 August.

difficulties. Pope and colleagues (2000) attempted to address this question during military training in a sample of 1,538 men. Two groups participated in a warm-up with only one group performing 20-second static stretches under supervision for each of six major muscle groups of the lower limbs. Ultimately, the inclusion of stretching did not affect the exercise-related injury incidence, and the authors found that fitness levels may be more important in the prevention of injury than flexibility. Smith and colleagues (1993) showed that both static and ballistic stretching can induce their own levels of soreness as exercise stresses but that ballistic stretching was associated with less soreness (DeVries 1980). Johansson and colleagues (1999) extended these findings by demonstrating that preexercise stretching did not provide any protective effect on delayed muscle soreness, tissue damage, or loss of force-production capabilities after a heavy eccentric protocol that typically induces significant muscle damage.

Thus, although stretching is an exercise stress important for range of motion capabilities, it may not be the primary factor in preventing injury. Stretching protocols can be viewed as a part of an acute warm-up strategy and also as a chronic type of training to improve the range of motion of a joint. Recent evidence indicates that these two views of stretching should not be combined, as stretching may affect some performance capabilities in certain warm-up protocols.

Chronic improvement in flexibility is an important component of physical fitness and needs to be addressed in the context of a resistance training program, especially when range of movement capabilities hamper normal function or sport performance. Stretching can be performed in both the warm-up and cool-down phases of a training session, but as will be explained in the next section, intense stretching in the context of all warm-ups may not be warranted because of its effects on the physical performance immediately after stretching.

For chronic training effects, stretching is normally performed each day and in some cases up to three times a day. Willy and colleagues (2001) also suggested that stretch training may have to be maintained, as its effects have been shown to be lost 4 weeks after the cessation of an effective 6-week training protocol. In addition, the resumption of training for the same length of time after cessation did not result in any gains beyond the end point of the first stretching program. This means that the participants essentially started

over in terms of flexibility. The length and retention of flexibility training adaptations remain relatively unstudied at this point, but care should be taken to consider flexibility maintenance programs once flexibility goals have been met because of the potential loss of range of motion that may occur if flexibility training is discontinued.

Essentially, there are four basic types of stretching techniques (Moore and Hutton 1980).

- Static stretching
- Dynamic range of motion (DROM) or ballistic stretching
- Slow movements
- Proprioceptive neuromuscular facilitation (PNF)

Deciding which technique to employ in a program depends on the amount of time available for stretching, the effectiveness of the flexibility technique, and the availability of a training partner.

Static Stretching

The most common type of stretching is the static stretching technique. This form of stretching requires the participant to voluntarily relax the muscle while elongating it, and then holding the muscle in a stretched position. This technique has become popular because it is easy to learn and effective (Moore and Hutton 1980). An example of the static technique would be the classic "toe touch," in which one bends over and tries to touch one's toes while keeping the knees straight. The movement is held at the point of minimal discomfort. Stretching must be performed progressively. Each time, the individual should try to reach farther to extend the range of movement and hold the stretch at the point of minimal discomfort. Subsequent stretching continues to improve the range of motion.

Static stretching is still one of the most effective and desirable techniques to use when comfort and limited training time are major factors in the implementation of a stretching program (Moore and Hutton 1980). Wiemann and Hahn (1997) showed that lower resting tension in the muscle is related to the individual's tolerance to a higher stretching strain, and this helps to bring about an improvement in the joint's range of movement with stretching exercises. In addition, Mohr and colleagues (1998) showed that during static stretching, the EMG activity during a given stretch position is low in some muscles being stretched, indicating a partial neural mediation with stretching. Brandy, Irion, and Briggler (1998) showed that static stretching is more than twice as effective as dynamic range of motion flexibility exercises for increasing hamstring flexibility (11- vs. 4-degree increase). In this study, dynamic range of motion training consisted of achieving a stretched position in 5 seconds, holding the stretch 5 seconds, and then returning to an unstretched position in 5 seconds, and static stretching consisted of one 30-second static stretch. Magnusson (1998) pointed out that the use of stretching to improve flexibility is a widespread practice, but the effectiveness of different programs may be related to the change in stretch tolerance rather than to the passive properties in muscle. In partial support of this theory, Magnusson, Aagaard, and Nielson (2000) showed that static stretching for 90 seconds did not alter the viscoelastic properties of muscle.

Many variations of this technique have been proposed, with stretch time ranging up to 60 seconds. However, Brandy, Irion, and Briggler (1997) showed that times beyond 30 seconds are not more effective when stretching is done each day. In another study, Roberts and Wilson (1999) showed that holding stretches for 15 seconds was more effective than holding them for 5 seconds for improving active range of motion, but not for passive range of motion. Thus, performing 15- to 30-second stretches three to five times appears to be optimal. McNair and colleagues (2001) showed that the greatest decreases in tension occurs in the first 20 seconds of a held static stretch of the ankle joint. They concluded that if relaxation of peak tension is the target goal, then held stretches are more effective than continuous passive-motion stretches. If the goal is to decrease stiffness, then continuous passive motion is a more effective method of stretching.

Ballistic and Dynamic Range of Motion Stretching

Ballistic stretching involves a "bouncing" or "bobbing" movement during the stretch; the final position in the movement is not held stationary. It can also involve the dynamic exercise range of motion specific to an event, such as a practice takeoff for long jump, bounds, and plyometrics. Ballistic stretching using no outside load gained popularity as a warm-up activity, but was less popular as a means to improve chronic joint range

of movement (Shellock and Prentice 1985). Tissue damage related to delayed-onset muscle soreness may be related to this type of stretching exercise (DeVries 1980). Ballistic stretching might be more appropriate as part of a dynamic warm-up after a general warm-up and a static type of stretch.

Continuous Passive Slow Movements

Continuous slow movements such as neck rotations, arm rotations, and trunk rotations are also a type of stretching activity. The value of using this type of stretching technique may be more important to warm-up activities than to achieving increases in flexibility. However, McNair and colleagues (2001) reported that, at the ankle joint, if the goal is to decrease stiffness, then continuous passive motion is more effective than static stretching. Continuous slow movement stretching might provide a better dynamic technique in warm-up activities than the more aggressive ballistic stretching. The pace of the warm-up activity may have to be titrated to a speed that provides metabolic and circulatory stimulation to promote acute movement ability. Chronic changes with this stretching are specific to the type of stretching used, and each has different applications in conditioning.

Proprioceptive Neuromuscular Facilitation (PNF) Techniques

Proprioceptive neuromuscular facilitation (PNF) stretching techniques have increased in popularity over the last 15 years as a method of improving flexibility (Cornelius 1985; Cornelius et al. 1992; Shellock and Prentice 1985). A number of different procedures have been proposed, including contract-relax and contract-relax/agonist contraction (Moore and Hutton 1980). The theoretical basis of these techniques is that the voluntary action of the agonist muscle provides neural activation resulting in reciprocal inhibition of the antagonist muscle, thus allowing greater range of motion. Etnyre and Lee (1988) made a comparative examination of static stretching and PNF techniques in men and women. After 12 weeks of training they found that all groups had improved in flexibility. Women had greater range of motion compared to men throughout the program, but their comparative increases were not greater than those of the men. PNF techniques were more effective for increasing the range of motion for both hip flexion and shoulder extension for both genders. Men showed better results with the contract-relax/agonist contraction method, whereas women showed no differences between PNF methods. There are several variations of PNF techniques, but the three major types are as follows (Shellock and Prentice 1985):

■ Slow-reversal-hold
■ Contract-relax/agonist
■ Hold-relax

Using the hamstring stretch as an example, the slow-reversal-hold technique is as follows: The trainee lies on his back, with his knee extended and his ankle flexed to 90 degrees. A partner pushes on the leg, passively flexing the hip joint until the trainee feels slight discomfort in the hamstring. The trainee then pushes for 10 seconds against the partner's resistance by activating the hamstring muscle. The hamstring muscles are then relaxed, and the antagonist quadriceps muscles are activated, while the partner applies force for 10 seconds to further stretch the hamstrings. The leg should move so there is increased hip joint flexion. All muscles are then relaxed for 10 seconds, after which time the stretch is repeated beginning at this new joint angle. This push-relax sequence is typically repeated at least three times.

The other two PNF techniques commonly used are similar to the slow-reversal-hold method. The contract-relax/agonist technique involves a dynamic concentric action before the relaxation/ stretch phase. In the earlier example the hamstrings are contracted so the leg moves toward the floor. The hold-relax technique uses an isometric contraction before the relaxation/stretch phase. Clark and colleagues (1999) showed that the hold-relax technique was more effective than the static stretch technique to improve the straight-leg raise range of motion, indicating that static stretch may not be the most effective for all types of flexibility requirements in a training program.

Osternig and colleagues (1990) examined acute changes in 10 high-intensity athletes, 10 endurance athletes, and 10 controls and demonstrated that the contract-relax/agonist procedure produced 89 to 110% greater hamstring EMG activity and 9 to 13% more knee joint range of motion than the contract-relax or stretch-relax PNF methods, respectively. Endurance athletes had 58 to 113% greater EMG activity in the hamstrings compared to the high-intensity and control groups, respectively. However, it is interesting to note that the endurance athletes attained significantly less range of motion than the other two groups in all cases. Short-term high-intensity activity may necessitate less hamstring resistance to knee extension than long-term endurance training (Osternig et al. 1990). The authors also concluded that decreases in muscle activity may not be related to increases in joint range of motion, and that factors other than muscle relaxation are important in achieving increased range of motion. The differential effects of different stretch techniques need to be considered for different athletic groups so that any stretch-induced injury can be avoided. Understanding of the various stretching techniques is vital to their proper use and application (for a review, see Etnyre and Lee 1987).

Moore and Hutton (1980) studied the different PNF techniques and noted that PNF has not proved to be superior to static stretching in all studies. Each technique is capable of improving flexibility. Individuals must be well motivated and have the time to perform PNF stretching. PNF methods (with the exception of the hold-relax technique) require a partner. Furthermore, individuals must learn the techniques, which can take some time. Moore and Hutton (1980) suggested that unless an individual is willing to tolerate the greater discomfort associated with PNF training, the use of static stretching is more appropriate. In addition, in some movements the position may be more important than using a static or PNF technique. Sullivan, Dejulia, and Worrell (1992) demonstrated this when they noted that the position of the pelvic tilt used in a hamstring flexibility program played a greater role in determining the improvement in the ranges of motion than the specific technique itself. This emphasizes the concept that most flexibility techniques are effective, but other factors may influence their appropriateness in a given program design.

Effects of Using Flexibility Protocols As a Part of Warm-Ups

The timing and compatibility of stretching techniques has been made more complex with the revisiting of a finding from the 1970s that stretching may inhibit strength performance. Several recent studies have demonstrated that each of the stretching techniques may inhibit force production. Therefore, we are just starting to learn about the specificity of the effect and how long it may persist. Nevertheless, careful consideration is needed for when to stretch and what types of activities are negatively affected by stretching. This may be especially important when choosing warm-up activities before performances that require force and power production.

PNF stretching can negatively affect vertical jump performance in women, but a general warm-up and one that also included typical static stretching did not have such an effect on jump performance (Church et al. 2001). Conversely, static stretching was found to negatively affect isokinetic knee extension torque production below 150 degrees per second (2.62 rad · s^{-1}), but not at higher velocities of movement for isolated joint force production (Nelson, Allen et al. 2001). In addition, the inhibition of maximal isometric torque production with static stretching is joint-angle specific to the stretch protocol used (Nelson, Guillory et al. 2001). Nelson and Kokkonen (2001) showed that ballistic stretching can also inhibit maximal strength. Young and Elliott (2001) found that static stretching produced significant decrements in drop jump performance, but a nonsignificant decrease in concentric explosive muscle performance. In contrast to other findings, the authors also observed that PNF stretching had no effect on concentric stretch-shortening cycle muscle performance. They speculated that for activities involving relatively short stretch-shortening cycle muscle function (e.g., the contact phase of sprinting or jumping with an approach), static stretching may have a detrimental effect on performance. If the other proposed benefits of a warm-up can be achieved by other methods, then the possible negative acute effect of stretching on force production can be eliminated.

Behm, Button, and Butt (2001) suggested that poststretch force decrements appear to be more related to inactivation of muscles affected by the stretch than to the changes in the elasticity often thought to be affected by stretching the musculo-connective tissue components. This will remain an important area of study for the next several years to further our understanding of how stretching can be used in warm-up activities and what mechanisms mediate the acute effects on performance.

Chronic increases in flexibility are obviously needed for some types of activities, such as high hurdling. However, how chronic changes in flexibility affect other types of performance is a difficult effect to experimentally examine, and it appears to be a separate issue concerning the use of flexibility training. Thus, for acute warm-up

protocols, the compatibility of the type of physical performance and the need for a stretching protocol as part of a warm-up needs to be carefully considered.

Does Resistance Training Affect Flexibility?

The concept of being muscle bound is often associated with resistance training. Some individuals and coaches believe that resistance training results in a decrease in flexibility. Little scientific or empirical evidence supports this contention, provided that stretching is performed as part of a total conditioning program (Todd 1985). As early as 1956, Massey and Chaudet demonstrated that heavy resistance training does not cause a decrease in flexibility. Thrash and Kelly (1987) examined the effects of weight training on the range of motion of the ankle, trunk, and shoulder joints before and after an 11-week resistance training program (three times per week, three sets of 8RM of exercises stressing all major muscle groups) and reported that significant increases were observed in ankle dorsiflexion and shoulder extension without any additional flexibility training. Thus, the authors concluded that a weight training program to develop muscular strength would not impair flexibility and might enhance certain ranges of motion.

The training program used, in addition to the initial level of flexibility, appears to be critical to the degree of flexibility an individual can achieve with resistance training. Beedle, Jesse, and Stone (1991) did show differences between various athletes who weight train, and these differences were related to the type of training program performed (e.g., Olympic weightlifting versus power lifting). Olympic weightlifters and control subjects had greater flexibility on five flexibility measures, indicating that power lifting may require muscle size increases that can partially limit range of motion (e.g., chest size increased so that one cannot touch the elbows in the front) (Kraemer and Koziris 1994). Such data support the contention that lifting alone may not promote flexibility in trained individuals.

Flexibility training may need to be performed in addition to some types of machine resistance training programs, especially in the elderly (Hurley 1995). Barbosa and colleagues (2002) recently showed that 10 weeks of resistance training improved flexibility only by 13% (as determined by the sit and reach test) in elderly women, and Fatouros and colleagues (2002) showed that 16 weeks of resistance training increased flexibility in some but not all joint movements in elderly men. These data demonstrate the initial responsiveness of individuals with low initial levels of flexibility and strength when beginning a resistance training program.

Conversely, it is interesting to note that ballet dancers improved their functional range of voluntary movement, which added to the aesthetics of their dance movements, by adding a resistance training program (Stadler, Noble, and Wilkerson 1990). Thus, whereas flexibility training may extend the functional range of motion, control of that range of motion is a function of strength and power development. Thus, resistance training and flexibility training appear to be complementary in certain situations.

Typically, heavy resistance training results in either an improvement or no change in flexibility (Massey and Chaudet 1956). Competitive weightlifters possess average or above-average flexibility in most joints (Beedle, Jesse, and Stone 1991; Leighton 1955, 1957). In a descriptive study of several groups of athletes, Olympic weightlifters were second only to gymnasts in a composite flexibility score (Jensen and Fisher 1979) and had better scores than power lifters or control subjects (Beedle, Jesse, and Stone 1991). Resistance training does not appear to necessarily result in a loss of flexibility, but flexibility training programs may be needed to enhance the range of motion. Furthermore, as muscle hypertrophy becomes extreme, one might have to add joint-specific range of motion flexibility training and monitor needed ranges of motion.

Still, in some cases, limited flexibility in range of motion may provide a competitive advantage for certain performances (e.g., power lifters in the bench press) (Kraemer and Koziris 1994). Competitive power lifters have limited flexibility, which may be due to the competitive task, especially in the upper body (i.e., bench press) (Beedle, Jesse, and Stone 1991; Chang, Buschbacker, and Edlich 1988), as lower-body flexibility has not been identified as a problem. To aid in maintaining or even increasing flexibility, the lifting technique should stress the full range of motion of both the agonist and antagonist muscle groups, and exercises should be done that strengthen both the agonists and antagonists of a joint to ensure strength balance. Recently, Kubo, Kanehisa, and Fukunaga

(2002) showed that resistance training increases the stiffness of the tendon structures as well as increases muscle strength and size, whereas static stretching results in changes in the viscosity of the tendon structures, but not in the elasticity. Thus, both types of training may be needed for increasing flexibility.

Summary

Muscular strength, flexibility, cardiovascular endurance, and local muscular endurance all play varying roles in health, fitness, and sport performance. Training for sport performance is considerably different from training for health and fitness. Also, better sport performance is not always associated with better health. This might be especially true as performances progress toward an elite level and risk of injury is high due to the high training volume and intensity.

Developing an overall conditioning program that addresses each fitness component is necessary. The needs analysis facilitates the determination of time and effort that needs to be spent on a specific fitness component. Although certain data suggest that some incompatibility exists between different fitness components, proper modification of the exercise program should address this issue. The shot-put champion may not spend a great deal of time performing cardiovascular endurance exercises, but that person may perform cardiovascular conditioning three days a week for 20 to 30 minutes to assist anaerobic recovery, maintain remedial aerobic fitness levels, or both. Even a small amount of aerobic training helps maintain or even increase peak oxygen consumption and has positive effects on the blood lipid profile of resistance training individuals over years of training (Nakaoi, Inoue, and Murakami 1995). Conversely, the champion cross country runner may not perform a high volume of resistance training, but may resistance train twice a week for 20 to 30 minutes with exercises for the ankles, quadriceps, hamstrings, shoulder, and back. These exercises help to prevent injury and improve postural muscle strength. The art and science of successful exercise prescription involve understanding all of the following:

■ The goals and objectives of training (needs analysis)
■ The fitness level of the individual (exercise testing)

- The variables involved with prescription and the stimulus/effect relationships of the exercise stimuli

- The training adaptations associated with different exercise stimuli

- The psychological ability to perform the exercise (interaction and training observations)

Proper exercise prescription can result in the successful design of exercise programs that address the specific component(s) of physical fitness needed by the individual for health, fitness, and performance. The program emphasis will shift according to the specific needs of the individual. It is important to understand, however, that no one form of training (e.g., resistance training) can produce all of the required training effects for every sport or individual. This chapter addressed how to develop a total conditioning program. How to individualize the resistance training program is discussed in the next chapter.

Key Terms

aerobic conditioning

ballistic stretching

cardiovascular endurance fitness

continuous slow movements

exercise training compatibility

flexibility training

functional capacity

heart rate training zone

interval training

MET

proprioceptive neuromuscular facilitation (PNF)

sprint performance

sprint workout

static stretching

stretching techniques

total conditioning program

Selected Readings

American College of Sports Medicine. 1998. Position stand: The recommended quantity and quality of exercise for developing and maintaining cardiorespiratory and muscular fitness, and flexibility in healthy adults. *Medicine and Science in Sports and Exercise* 30: 975-991.

Chromiak, J.A., and Mulvaney, D.R. 1990. A review: The effects of combined strength and endurance training on strength development. *Journal of Applied Sport Science Research* 4: 55-60.

Dudley, G.A., and Fleck, S.J. 1987. Strength and endurance training: Are they mutually exclusive? *Sports Medicine* 4: 79-85.

Hennessy, L.C., and Watson, A.W.S. 1994. The interference effects of training for strength and endurance simultaneously. *Journal of Strength and Conditioning Research* 8: 12-19.

Hutton, R.S. 1992. Neuromuscular basis of stretching exercises. In *Strength and power in sport*, edited by P.V. Komi, 29-38. Oxford: Blackwell Scientific Publications.

Koziris, L.P., Kraemer, W.J., Patton, J.F., Triplett, N.T., Fry, A.C., Gordon, S.E., and Knuttgen, H.G. 1996. Relationship of aerobic power to anaerobic performance indices. *Journal of Strength and Conditioning Research* 10: 35-39.

Laursen, P.B., and Jenkins, D.G. 2002. The scientific basis for high-intensity interval training: Optimizing training programs and maximizing performance in highly trained endurance athletes. *Sports Medicine* 32: 53-73.

Osternig, L.R., Robertson, R.N., Troxel, R.K., and Hansen, P. 1990. Differential responses to proprioceptive neuromuscular facilitation (PNF) stretch techniques. *Medicine and Science in Sports and Exercise* 22: 106-111.

Ross, A., Leveritt, M., and Riek, S. 2001. Neural influences on sprint running: Training adaptations and acute responses. *Sports Medicine* 31: 409-425.

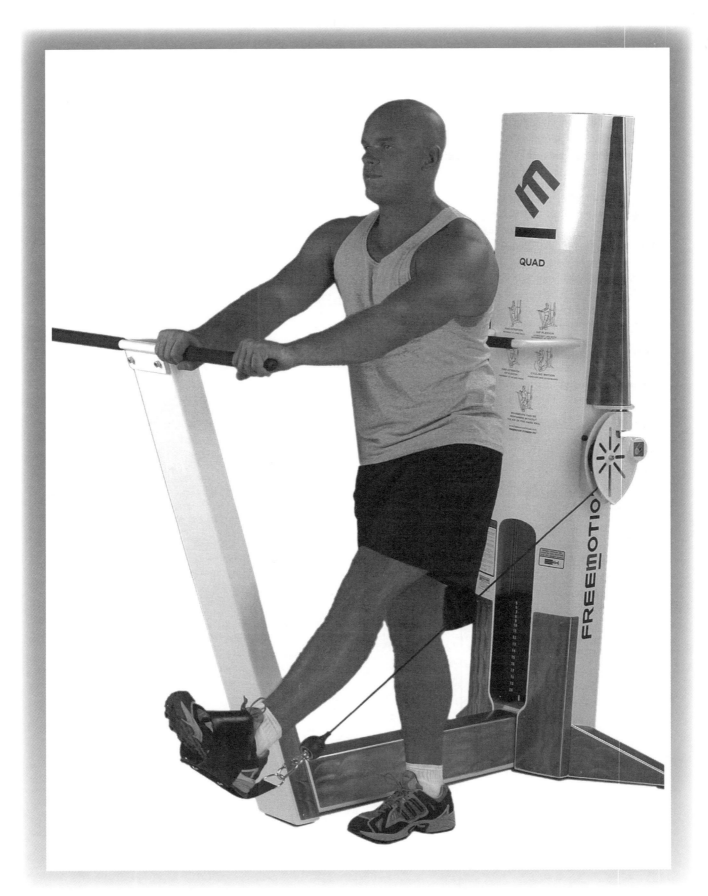

PART II

Exercise Prescription of Resistance Training

Many factors need to be considered when designing a resistance training program to successfully meet the needs and goals of a trainee. If the trainee is preparing for a sport or a particular activity, a general program specific to that sport or activity is developed. The general sport-specific program must then be individualized, however, to address the strengths and weaknesses of each individual. Chapter 5 examines factors that must be considered when individualizing a resistance training program. Chapter 6 discusses various types of resistance training systems and techniques that can be used to meet the needs of an athlete or a fitness enthusiast. In chapter 7 advanced training strategies, such as periodization and stretch-shortening cycle training or plyometric training, are examined. Such advanced training strategies are a necessary component for optimal fitness gains in experienced resistance trained athletes and fitness enthusiasts. Chapter 8 discusses detraining, or the reversal of training adaptations that take place when resistance training is reduced or stopped. Knowledge of detraining is useful in developing programs that will maintain training adaptations for as long as possible in a potential detraining situation, such as in-season programs for a particular sport. The information contained in part II will help you design optimal individualized resistance training programs.

CHAPTER 5

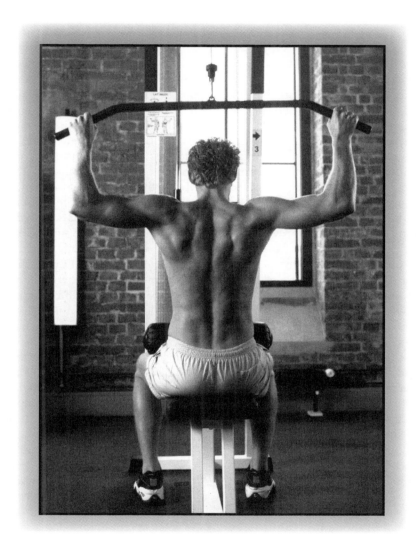

Developing the Individualized Resistance Training Workout

An individualized training program is needed to meet each person's specific goals of realizing optimal training adaptations and performance improvements. Historically, with resistance training comes the quest to the find the "best" training program. It is important to understand that what is best for one individual may not be best for another. Therefore, **program design** is a highly individualized process based on a sound understanding of the basic principles of resistance training. The process of program design should be based on the understanding of a specific paradigm that can be used to develop, prescribe, and modify a resistance training workout over time. In this chapter we will describe how to design a single resistance exercise protocol and what must be considered in this program design process.

Program Choices

Over the ages, strength has been the subject of myth, legend, and in modern times intense marketing strategies to promote sales of equipment and programs. Different systems of resistance training have been promoted with emotional and mythological fervor, often disregarding the underlying scientific facts or findings. In this era of "infomercial" claims, evaluating information about resistance training programs and determining their efficacy has become difficult. Desired gains of individuals are often unrealistic and lead to exercise nonadherence when improvements do not meet expectations. Substantial improvements are often evident in the early phases of training, but such changes cannot be expected to continue with long-term training. Thus, the challenge is designing resistance training programs that are both effective and realistic.

Debates rage in locker rooms, in muscle magazines, at conferences, and on Web sites concerning what constitutes the best resistance training program. This is not a simple question because the best program is really related to the exact training goals of the individual. Furthermore, training goals are related to the specific types of adaptations desired and the genetic potential of the individual to attain them. Finally, other factors such as age and gender will also affect the program effectiveness. Thus, the argument can be made that one best program of exercises, sets, reps, and load does *not* exist. The next question might be, Will the same training program still be effective at other points in time? Since training goals may change and trainees will become more fit, it is doubtful that the same program will result in the same magnitude of adaptations over time. Thus, the concept of progression is an important principle in resistance training. Program designers must use the major principles of resistance training (e.g., progressive overload, specificity, and variation) and pay special attention to making effective changes that meet the changing training goals and fitness level of each trainee.

With all of the variations in resistance training components, an almost infinite number of programs can be designed. If the program is based on sound scientific principles, it will have positive effects that will be related to the specific characteristics of the program design (i.e., the principle of specificity). For example, if a trainee uses light weights and performs a high number of repetitions, local muscular endurance will improve, but little improvement in muscular strength will occur (Anderson and Kearney 1982). This is an example of a specific training response. Such a response is predictable from our understanding of the physiological adaptations related to training with light loads. The program designer, however, must also consider the differences in the magnitude of the response to training among individuals. The initial exercise prescription should be made based on scientific understanding, the training goals, and the type of associated program element (e.g., light weight and a high number of repetitions in this example) needed to stimulate a change. However, the training response of each individual will vary, and modification of the exercise protocol may be needed if the desired effects are not observed after a period of training has been completed (e.g., the trainee may want to increase the number of repetitions per set). Each adaptation will take place on a different time line since neural adaptations happen rapidly and muscle protein accretion leading to muscle hypertrophy will take longer (see chapter 3). Thus, the expectations for change must be kept within the physiological context of each variable's adaptation time course.

Ultimately, some individuals may never be able to attain a high degree of improvement for a particular variable (e.g., large gains in muscle hypertrophy) because of their inherent genetic limitations. Nevertheless, the program design can be adjusted over time to optimize each person's physiological potential for a particular training goal. Although it may be possible to predict a certain type of adaptation from a specific program design variable such as intensity, individuals will vary in the magnitude of response over time. For example, one can predict that a program of three sets of 25 to 30 repetition maximum (RM) will result in improved muscular endurance, but one person may perform 18 repetitions while another person may perform 26 repetitions at 80% of 1RM after the same 12-week training program. If the prior level of training experience is the same for both individuals, physiological factors may account for the differences (e.g., muscle fiber type, neurological recruitment patterns) in performance increases. Earlier program variation (e.g., more sets and a higher number of repetitions) for the less responsive individual may be a more effective program progression. Here it is important to make a value judgment on the importance of the progression rate for a particular variable. Is there a sport or daily life performance impact for the individual who can perform only 18 repetitions in the test versus the individual who can perform 26 repetitions? Maybe 18 repetitions per set is in excess or not sufficient to have a performance impact for the sport or daily life activity in question.

Several questions remain: What is the person trying to excel at? How specific are the changes related to the testing outcome? Is the test specific for the task being trained for or is it just a general test? Here is where evaluation of the testing program (i.e., specific testing data) and the program design interface with each other, and where the desired training effects of the program must be evaluated individually. The absolute magnitude of a training response will vary individually with the same training program. Thus, general programs written for fitness, sports, or other activities should be viewed only as a starting point for an individual. One must then work to adjust the program design to match the training responses of the individual.

The key to successful program design is the identification of specific variables that need to be controlled in order to better predict the training outcomes. In fact, one study showed that using a personal trainer to control the progression of intensity resulted in greater strength gains than allowing the average trainee to make such decisions (Mazzetti et al. 2000). This underscores the most challenging aspect of resistance training prescription—that of manipulating the acute program variables. The development of individual training goals for specific training phases or cycles also becomes paramount in long-term program design. Thus, one is faced with making appropriate changes in the resistance training program over time to meet the program's changing goals. This necessitates making sound clinical or coaching decisions on program design and changes. These decisions are based on a valid initial program design, the ability to monitor and test for progress, and an understanding of the individual needs of the trainee. To do this requires a basic understanding of resistance training principles and the underlying theory of the program design process. One then must also understand the needs of the sport or activity and how to use testing data to monitor the training effects for each individual. Therefore, the dynamics of planning and changing the exercise prescription is vital for the ultimate success of any resistance training program (see figure 5.1).

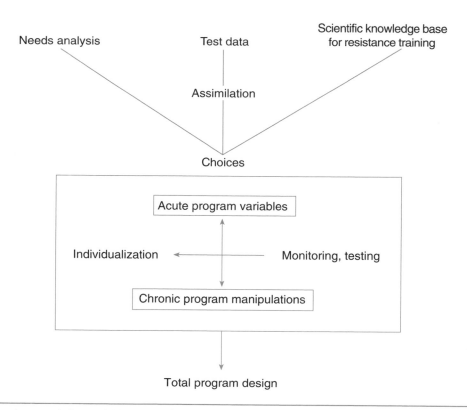

Figure 5.1 An exercise prescription model for resistance training.

Understanding the factors that go into creating the "exercise stimulus" is crucial to the success of the program design process. The creation of an effective exercise stimulus starts with the development of a single training session directed at specific trainable characteristics (e.g., force production, power, hypertrophy). Over time changes made in the acute program variables will create the progressions, variations, and overloads needed to achieve physiological adaptations and improved performances. Chronic training effects related to long-term progression using such concepts as periodization are developed by planning each workout correctly. Thus, the planning process always starts with the individual training session and the acute program variables chosen to address different goals. Quantifying the workout with testing can help in evaluating the progress made toward a specific training goal. However, training logs are the most fundamental evaluation tool for monitoring progress in a program.

In this chapter we will address the following components of program design: the needs analysis and then the acute program variables such as intensity, volume, rest intervals, exercise selection and order, repetition speed, and training frequency.

Needs Analysis

A needs analysis is a process that consists of answering a series of questions that assist in the design of a resistance training program (see figure 5.2) (Kraemer 1983b). Program designers should take the time to examine each of these questions in order to properly develop each of the acute program variables.

The major questions in a needs analysis are as follows:

- What muscle groups should be trained?
- What basic energy sources (e.g., anaerobic, aerobic) should be trained?
- What type of muscle action(s) (e.g., isometric, eccentric) should be trained?
- What are the primary sites of injury for the particular sport or activity, and what is the prior injury history of the individual?
- What are the specific needs for muscle strength, hypertrophy, endurance, power, speed, agility, flexibility, body composition, balance, and coordination?

Biomechanical Analysis to Determine Training Needs

The first question requires an examination of the muscles and the specific joint angles that need to be trained. For any activity, including a sport, this involves a basic analysis of the movements performed. An "eyeball" technique can be used to determine the movements and muscles used. A basic understanding of biomechanics will help

Needs Analysis

Exercise movements
- Specific muscles
- Joint angles
- Contraction mode
- Loading needs

Metabolism used estimated % contribution from:
- ATP-PC source
- Lactic acid source
- Oxygen source

Injury prevention
- Most common sites of possible injury
- Sites of previous injury

Acute Program Variables

Choice of exercise
- Structural
- Body part
- Muscle action type
- Muscle action velocity

Order of exercise
- Large-muscle group first
- Small-muscle group first (preexhaust)
- Arm to leg, arm to arm, or leg to leg

Number of sets

Rest periods
- Short: <1 minute
- Moderate: 1 to 3 minutes
- Long: >3 minutes

Load (intensity)

Figure 5.2 A detailed component model for the acute program variables. The needs analysis is an important preliminary step in making better decisions concerning the acute program variables.

to further define this analysis. Videotaping equipment or a variety of other image-capture devices can also shed light on the specific aspects of movement patterns involved in an activity. The movement pattern analysis includes a basic analysis of the muscles, joint angles, movement velocities, and forces involved. The decisions made at this stage will help define the choice of exercises, one of the acute program variables.

Because the principle of specificity is a major tenet in resistance training, understanding exactly what you are trying to mimic in the weight room is an important aspect of program design. Biomechanical analyses will allow you to choose specific exercises that use the muscles and types of muscular actions in a manner specific to the activity for which training is being performed. Specificity assumes that muscles used in the sport or activity must be trained in terms of the following:

- The joint around which movement occurs
- The joint range of motion
- The pattern of resistance throughout the range of motion
- The pattern of limb velocity throughout the range of motion
- The types of movements that occur (concentric, eccentric, isometric)

Resistance training for any sport or activity should include full range of motion exercises around all of the body's major joints. However, training designed for specific sports or activity movements should also be included in the workout to maximize the contribution of strength training to performance. The best way to select such exercises is to analyze the sport or physical activity biomechanically and to match it to exercises according to the previously mentioned variables. Although few such analyses of sports or activities have been performed, biomechanical principles can be used in a qualitative manner to select exercises intelligently. Increased recognition of the importance of movement-specific resistance training programs (e.g., functional training) over the past decade has led to the development of specific equipment (i.e., stability balls, wobble boards) and programs designed to improve core stability, rotational strength and power, balance, reaction time, speed, acceleration, and agility (Santana 2000).

Slow-motion videotaping or other types of video data allow a trainer to analyze a physical activity roughly in terms of the variables listed earlier. Dr. Everett Harman, a biomechanist for the U.S. Army's Research Institute of Environmental Medicine, developed the following steps to be used for this purpose:

1. View a video picture of an athletic performance or activity.

2. Select a movement that appears to involve high-intensity physical exertion critical to the performance (e.g., the impact of two football linemen, the drive portion of a sprint stride, the takeoff in a high-jump).

3. Identify the joints around which the most intense muscular actions occur. Running and jumping, for example, involve intense muscle actions at the knee, hip, and ankle. Intense exertion doesn't necessarily involve movement. Considerable isometric force may have to be applied to keep a body joint from flexing or extending under external stress.

4. Determine whether the movement is concentric, isometric, or eccentric. While force is being produced, the muscle shortens during a concentric muscle action, is held at a constant length by an external force during an isometric muscle action, and is lengthened by an external force during an eccentric muscle action.

5. For each joint identified, determine the range of angular motion. To do this, measure the angle between the two body segments adjacent to the joint with a protractor. See how the joint angle changes through the movement. Record the range of motion.

6. Try to determine where in the range of motion around each particular joint the most intense effort occurs. Sometimes facial grimaces or tense muscles seen on video pictures can help identify points of peak intensity. Record the joint angle of peak intensity.

7. Estimate the velocity of movement in the early, middle, and late phases in the range of motion. If using videotape, the time between frames in seconds is 1/frame rate. For example, if the rate is 30 frames per second, the interval time is 1/30 or 0.033 seconds. In a movement segment, the angular velocity equals degrees traveled divided by the total time. For example, if the limb moves 5 degrees in three frame intervals, the movement speed is $5/(3 \times 0.033) = 50$ degrees per second.

8. Select exercises to match the limb ranges of motion and angular velocities, making sure that the exercises are appropriately concentric, isometric, or eccentric. As an example, in a jump takeoff, the muscles of the supporting leg(s) usually perform an eccentric action. Some form of eccentric training could accomplish training of this part of the movement. In a jump, after the knee reaches its smallest angle and the jumper begins to extend the leg for takeoff, high-intensity concentric action occurs initially at slow movement speed. To train that part of the movement, perform concentric actions through the specific range of joint motion using heavy weights at slow speed. To train a faster part of the movement, use lighter weights at higher speeds for the specific range of motion. Stretch-shortening cycle training, with or without weight, could also be used to simulate the complete stretch-shortening cycle of a jump.

9. It is best to make the exercise the most difficult at the point in the range of motion at which intensity during the target activity is greatest. This can be accomplished by trial and error, or using the principle that during an exercise or any lifting movement involving little acceleration, the greatest resistance to movement around a joint occurs when the limb supporting a weight is horizontal and the weight is farthest from the joint's center of rotation (e.g., around the midpoint of an arm curl movement). The most difficult portion of an exercise is commonly termed the *sticking point.* Many commonly performed weight exercises can be modified to locate peak tension or sticking point at a desired joint angle. For example, a basic exercise such as the arm curl can be done standing or bending over or on a preacher bench to modify the angle at which peak tension occurs. To apply additional force to a muscle at a particular point in the range of angular motion, the individual can attempt to accelerate the weight as the limb travels through the target range of motion.

Ideally, the trainer then chooses exercises based on the analyses of specific muscles used, muscle action types, and joint angles. For general fitness and muscular development, the major muscle groups of the shoulders, chest, back, torso, and legs are usually always trained.

The principle of specificity is an overriding rule in the process of designing a resistance training program. Each exercise and resistance used in a program will have various amounts of transfer to the performance of an activity or sport. The amount of transfer will be related to the degree of specificity that can be achieved with the total program design and available equipment. When training for improved health and well-being, the specificity of the training will be related to choosing exercises that can affect a given physiological variable (e.g., bone mineral density). Other program variables (e.g., rest periods) will also interact to optimize the metabolic and hormonal systems for positive effects. Thus, one acute program variable will interact with other acute program variables to create an integrated workout. The acute program variables will be discussed in much greater detail later in this chapter.

The concept of **transfer specificity** refers to the fact that every training activity will have a certain amount of carryover to other activities in terms of specificity. Except for practicing the specific task or sport itself, few if any conditioning activities have 100% carryover. However, some activities have a much higher amount of carryover to another task than others because of greater specificity or similarities in neuromuscular recruitment patterns, energy sources, and biomechanical characteristics.

Sometimes several exercises and loading schemes are required to completely train a movement. In a vertical jump, for example, heavy squatting is important for developing maximal strength during both the eccentric and concentric phase of jumping, and high-velocity jump squats with light weight (30% of 1RM) are needed to enhance the rate of force development and acceleration through the concentric phase of jumping. Although practicing unloaded jumps will help develop the technical skill of the activity and contribute to improvements, loaded movements are also needed to enhance the physical development of the body's neuromuscular system for improving performance (Kraemer and Newton 2000).

Most sport skills cannot be loaded without changing the movement pattern or technique. The optimal training program maximizes the specificity of the training program to create the greatest carryover to the sport or activity targeted for improvement. Many factors contribute to performance development, including technique, coordination, force production, rate of force development, and the stretch-shortening cycle

(Newton and Kraemer 1994). Resistance training addresses some of these factors and so improves the physiological potential for performance.

Energy Sources to Be Trained

Performance of every sport or activity derives a percentage of needed energy from all three energy sources (Fox 1979). However, many activities derive the majority of needed energy from one energy source (e.g., energy for the 50 m sprint comes predominantly from intramuscular ATP and PC). Therefore, the energy sources to be trained have a major impact on the program design. Resistance training typically focuses on the improvement of energy utilization derived from the anaerobic energy sources (ATP-PC and lactic acid sources). Improvement of whole-body aerobic metabolism has not been a traditional goal of classic resistance training. Resistance training can contribute to improvement in aerobic training effects by its synergistic effects on reductions in cardiovascular strain, more efficient recruitment patterns, increased fat-free mass, and improved blood flow dynamics under work stress. This is especially true in some specific populations, such as seniors.

Muscle Actions to Be Trained

Decisions regarding the use of isometric, dynamic concentric, dynamic eccentric, or isokinetic exercise modalities are important in the preliminary stages of planning a resistance training program for sport, fitness, or rehabilitation. The basic biomechanical analysis described previously is used to decide what muscles to train and to identify the type of muscle action(s) involved in the activity. Most activities and resistance training programs use several types of muscle actions. For example, one factor that separates elite power lifters from less competitive power lifters is the rate at which the load is lowered in the squat and bench press (Madsen and McLaughlin 1984; McLaughlin, Dillman, and Lardner 1977). Elite power lifters lower the weight at a slower rate than less competitive lifters do, even though the former use greater resistances. In this case, some eccentric training may be advantageous for competitive power lifters. In wrestling, on the other hand, many holds involve isometric muscle actions of various muscle groups. Therefore, some isometric training may help in the conditioning of wrestlers. Kraemer, Fry, and colleagues (2001) noted that isometric grip strength and "bear hug" isometric strength are both dramatically reduced

over the course of a wrestling tournament. Thus, improvement in isometric endurance at high levels of force production may aid recovery and help performance.

Primary Sites of Injury

It is also important to determine the primary sites of injury in a sport or recreational activity, as well as to understand the injury profile of an individual. The prescription of resistance training exercises can be directed at enhancing the strength and function of tissue so that it better resists injury or reinjury, recovers faster when injured, and reduces the extent of damage related to an injury. The term prehabilitation has become popular. This term refers to preventing initial injury by training the joints and muscles that are most susceptible to injury in an activity. The prevention of reinjury is also an important goal of a resistance training program. Thus, understanding the sport's or activity's typical injury profile (e.g., knee joints in wrestling) and the individual's prior history of injury can help in properly designing a resistance training program. Resistance exercise stress causes muscle tissue damage, which stimulates hypertrophy and is mediated in part by many of the same inflammatory, immune, and endocrine processes that are involved in the repair of injured tissue. Resistance training may help to condition and prepare these systems for the more extensive repair activities needed for faster injury recovery as well as to help prevent injury as a result of stronger individual tissues (e.g. tendon, ligament, and muscle).

Various Muscle Components

Determining the magnitude of improvement needed for variables such as muscle strength, power, hypertrophy, endurance, speed, balance, coordination, flexibility, and body composition is an important step in the overall process of designing a resistance training program. It may seem reasonable to assume that a resistance training program should optimize all of these variables. To do so, various training phases may be included to train various fitness components at particular times during the total training program. On the other hand, improvements in all of these variables may not be needed in all cases. For example, many sports require a high strength-to-mass or a high power-to-mass ratio. In such cases resistance training programs are designed to maximize strength and power while minimizing increases in body mass. This is evident in sports that have weight classes such as weightlifting, power lifting, and wrestling and for sports that require maximal sprinting speed or jumping ability (e.g., high jump, long jump) in which increasing body mass may be detrimental to sprint speed as well as maximal jump height or distance. In addition, some sports benefit from increasing fat-free and body mass, such as American football, in which the force of impact is greater for a given body mass, assuming power is increased accordingly. Thus, the need for these components of muscular fitness must be evaluated in order to plan a proper resistance training program.

Program Design

After the needs analysis has been completed, a specific workout is designed, which leads to the development of workouts and a training program. These workout sequences should address the specific goals and needs of the individual. Acute program variables serve as the framework of one specific resistance training session. Approaches to the "chronic program manipulations" or periodization of the various acute program variables will be addressed in chapter 7. Understanding the effects of acute program variables is very important because individual training sessions make up all training programs.

Acute Program Variables

In 1983 Kraemer (1983b) developed an approach to evaluating each workout for a specific set of training variables. Using statistical analyses, he determined five specific acute program variable clusters, each of which contributed differently to making various workouts unique. The acute program variables are capable of providing a general description of any single workout protocol. By manipulating each acute program cluster in figure 5.3, a training session is designed. By manipulating the many acute program variable choices, an almost infinite number of workout protocols can be created. All training sessions result in specific physiological responses and eventually adaptations as a result of the choices made regarding each acute program variable.

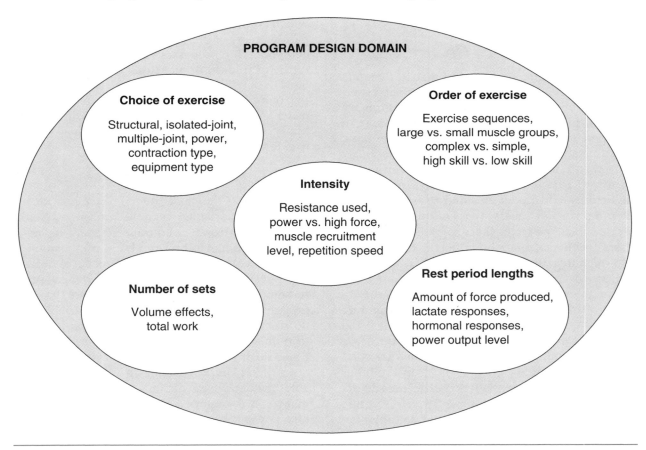

Figure 5.3 The clusters of acute program variables that can be manipulated in a resistance training program.

Choice of Exercise

As described in the needs analysis, the choice of exercise will be related to the biomechanical characteristics of the goals targeted for improvement. The number of possible joint angles and exercises are almost as limitless as the body's functional movements. A change in joint angle affects what muscle tissue is activated. Using magnetic resonance imaging (MRI) technology, Dr. Gary Dudley of the University of Georgia and Dr. Per Tesch of the Karolinska Institute in Sweden have shown that changes in the joint angles with the same exercise (e.g., toes pointing in, out, or straight forward during the knee-extension exercise) change the activation pattern of muscle (Tesch and Dudley 1994). Muscle tissue not activated will not benefit from resistance training. Exercises should be selected that stress the muscles and joint angles designated by the needs analysis.

Exercises can be arbitrarily designated as primary exercises and assistance exercises. Primary exercises train the prime movers in a particular movement and are typically major muscle group exercises (e.g., leg press, bench press, hang pull). Assistance exercises train predominantly one muscle group (e.g., triceps press, biceps curl) that aids in the movement produced by the prime movers. Exercises can also be classified as structural (i.e., multijoint) or body-part (i.e., isolated or single joint). Structural exercises include those whole-body lifts that require the coordinated action of several muscle groups. Power cleans, power snatches, deadlifts, and squats are good examples of structural whole-body exercises.

Exercises can also be classified as multijoint or multimuscle group exercises or exercises that require movement at more than one joint and the use of more than one muscle group. For example, the bench press involves movement of both the elbow and shoulder joints and is a multijoint or multimuscle group exercise. Some examples of other multijoint exercises are the lat pull-down, military press, and leg press. Exercises that attempt to isolate a particular muscle group are known as body-part, single-joint, or single-muscle-group exercises. Bicep curls, knee extensions, and knee curls are examples of isolated single-joint, single-muscle-group, or body-part exercises. Many assistance exercises can be classified as body-part, single-muscle-group, or single-joint exercises.

Structural or multijoint exercises require neural coordination among muscles and promote the coordinated use of multijoint and multimus-cle group movements. Chilibeck and colleagues (1998) recently showed that multijoint exercises require a longer initial learning or neural phase compared to single-joint exercises. It is especially important to include structural and multijoint exercises in a program when whole-body strength movements are required for a particular activity. Most sports and functional activities in everyday life (e.g., climbing stairs) depend on structural multijoint movements. In most sports whole-body strength and power movements are the basis for success, including all running and jumping activities, tackling in American football, a takedown in wrestling, and hitting a baseball. Many times, structural exercises involve the need for advanced lifting techniques (e.g., power cleans, power snatches), which require additional exercise technique coaching beyond simple movement patterns. Teachers and coaches should have experience with correctly teaching techniques or identify a professional with the ability to teach and supervise these lifts (e.g., a United States Weightlifting club coach) before including them in a training program. For individuals interested in basic fitness, structural exercises are also advantageous when training time is limited and it is necessary to train more than one muscle group with each exercise. The time economy achieved with structural and multijoint exercises is also an important consideration for an individual or team with a limited amount of time per training session.

Muscle Action

Concentric, eccentric, and isometric muscle actions influence the adaptations to resistance exercise. Greater force is produced during eccentric muscle actions with the advantage of requiring less energy per unit of muscle force (Bonde-Peterson, Knuttgen, and Henriksson 1972; Eloranta and Komi 1980; Komi, Kaneko, and Aura 1987). It has been known for some time that an eccentric component is needed to optimize muscle hypertrophy (Dudley et al. 1991; Hather, Mason, and Dudley 1991). This is why individuals (e.g., bodybuilders) have used such techniques as "heavy negatives," "forced negatives," and "slow negatives" in an attempt to maximize muscle hypertrophy. With pure eccentric resistance exercise, especially in untrained individuals, delayed-onset muscle soreness can be more prominent compared to concentric-only actions, isometric training, and normal weight training including a concentric and eccentric action (see the discussion of postexercise soreness in chapter 2). In addition, performing a high-intensity training session or performing new exercises at novel joint angles can result in greater muscle soreness when an eccentric action is involved. Dynamic strength improvements and hypertrophy are greatest when eccentric actions are included in a repetition (Dudley et al. 1991). So, normally, weight training is performed using both a concentric and an eccentric action.

Isometric muscle actions are less metabolically demanding and may be less conducive to hypertrophy increases than dynamic muscle actions (Ikai and Fukunaga 1970; Ryschon et al. 1997). Isometric strength increases are specific to the joint angles trained (i.e., *angular specificity*), but have shown carryover to other joint angles (see chapter 2). Thus, isometric actions can be used to bring about strength gains at a certain point in the range of motion of an exercise or movement (see the discussion of functional isometrics in chapter 6).

From a program design perspective an important aspect of muscle action type is strength specificity. Strength specificity means that the largest strength gains will be realized if training and testing are performed using the same muscle action type. For example, if training is performed in an isometric manner, large gains in strength will be realized if strength is tested in an isometric manner, but smaller gains will be shown if tested using another muscle action type. Thus, the types of muscle action used when performing an activity should be used in the training program for that activity.

Order of Exercise

For many years the order of exercise in resistance training programs consisted of performing large-muscle-group exercises before performing small-muscle-group exercises. It has been theorized that by exercising the larger muscle groups first, a superior training stimulus is presented to all of the muscles involved. This is thought to be mediated by stimulating a greater neural, metabolic, endocrine, and circulatory response, which potentially may augment the training with subsequent muscles or exercises later in the workout. This concept was also used in the sequencing of structural or multi- and single-joint exercises. In this system the more complex multijoint exercises (e.g., squats) were performed first followed by the less complex single-joint exercises (e.g., bicep curls). The sequencing rationale for this exercise order is that the exercises performed in

the beginning of the workout require the greatest amount of muscle mass and energy for optimal performance. Thus, this sequencing strategy focus on attaining a greater training effect for the large-muscle-group exercises.

If structural exercises are performed early in the workout, more resistance can be used since fatigue is limited. To examine this concept, the authors examined the workout logs of 50 American football players performing squats at the beginning of the workout and then at the end of the workout. The players used significantly heavier resistances (195 ± 35 versus 189 ± 31 kg) on heavy days (3-5RM) when they performed the squats first.

Sforzo and Touey (1996) investigated the use of the squat and bench press with different exercise orders. Session 1 began with multijoint exercises and ended with single-joint exercises for the same muscle groups (i.e., squat, leg extension, leg curl, bench press, shoulder press, and triceps push-down). Session 2 used the reverse order (i.e., leg curl, leg extension, squat, triceps push-down, shoulder press, and bench press). Each exercise was performed for four sets of 8RM with 2 minutes of rest between sets and 3 minutes of rest between exercises. On average, a 75% decline in bench press performance and a 22% decline in squat performance occurred when single-joint exercises were performed first. Factors such as inadequate recovery prior to the last exercise, inadequate rest periods between sets and exercises, a dramatically higher amount of exercise performed before the structural exercises, psychological fatigue, or increased physiological fatigue before the squat and bench press exercises may have contributed to the reduced performance.

Bodybuilders in the United States and weightlifters in the former Soviet Bloc countries have used different types of "preexhaustion" methods. This exercise order involves performing the small-muscle-group exercises before the larger-muscle-group exercises. For example, a single-joint exercise (e.g., dumbbell fly) is performed before a multijoint exercise (e.g., bench press). The theory is that the fatigued smaller muscles will contribute less to the movement, thereby placing greater stress on other muscle groups. For example, muscular exhaustion during the bench press exercise is often related to fatigue of the triceps muscles. Many bodybuilders include the bench press to maximize hypertrophy of the chest muscles. Therefore, the rationale for performing a single-joint exercise such as the dumbbell fly is to "preexhaust" the chest muscles so that exhaustion during the bench press may be related to chest muscle fatigue as opposed to fatigue of the triceps. The result is often a lowering in the amount of resistance used in the large-muscle-group exercise, which makes us question the use of preexhaustion for pure strength training. Another method of preexhaustion involves fatiguing synergistic or stabilizing muscles before performing the primary exercise movement. An example of this concept is performing lat pull-downs or military presses before performing the bench press exercise. Although typically used for hypertrophy training, the advantages and disadvantages of the preexhaustion system in optimizing strength and power gains remain anecdotal and need further direct study. However, some data do indicate that fatigue and its metabolites (e.g., lactic acid) may stimulate strength development (Shinohara et al. 1998; Smith and Rutherford 1995). Rooney, Herbert, and Balwave (1994) showed that continuous repetitions resulted in greater strength gains than when rest was taken between repetitions. Thus, accumulation of a metabolic factor(s) related to fatigue may be a physiological signal for adaptation. How this is related to preexhaustion techniques remains unclear for maximizing strength compared to a traditional sequencing method.

The priority system has also been used extensively in resistance training. When using the priority system, the training session goal(s) for the day focus on exercises performed first or early in the training session. Such order sequences allow the trainee to concentrate efforts, use heavier resistances for the exercises, and eliminate excessive fatigue during the performance of the priority exercises performed first in the training session.

A corollary to the priority system is the sequencing of power exercises (e.g., power cleans, plyometrics) so that they are performed early in a session. This allows the lifter to develop and train maximal power before becoming fatigued, which will hinder the development of maximal power. However, in some instances, power-type exercises may be performed later in the session for the purpose of improving anaerobic conditioning. For example, basketball players must not only have a high vertical jump, but they must also be able to jump during an overtime period when fatigued. In this instance, power exercises may be performed later in the session to train the ability to develop maximal power under conditions of fatigue (e.g., vertical jump ability in a fatigued state).

Another consideration in the exercise order is placing exercises that are being taught or practiced (especially complex movements) near the beginning of the exercise order. For example, if an athlete is learning how to perform power cleans, this exercise would be placed in the beginning of the workout so that learning the motor skills of the exercise will not be inhibited by fatigue.

The sequencing of exercises also involves the orders used in various types of circuit weight training protocols. The question of whether one follows a leg exercise with another leg exercise, or whether one should proceed to another muscle group has to be addressed. The concept of preexhaustion can come into play here. Alternate-muscle-group ordering, such as arm-to-leg ordering, allows for some recovery of one muscle group while another is performing an exercise. This is the most common order used in designing circuit weight training programs. Beginning lifters are less tolerant of arm-to-arm and leg-to-leg exercise orders or stacking exercises for a particular muscle group because of high blood lactate concentrations (10-14 mmol/L) especially when rest periods between exercises are short (10 to 60 seconds) (Kraemer et al. 1990, 1991). However, stacking exercises is a common practice among elite bodybuilders in an attempt to bring about muscle hypertrophy. Normally, an alternate order is used initially and then, if desired, a stacked order is gradually incorporated into the training session.

When functional strength is the emphasis, basic strength exercises such as the squat and bench press should be performed early in the workout. Training for enhanced speed and power entails performance of total-body explosive lifts such as the power clean and jump squat near the beginning of a workout. Improper sequencing of exercises can compromise the lifter's ability to perform the desired number of repetitions with the desired load. Therefore, exercise order needs to correspond with specific training goals. A few general methods for sequencing exercises for both multiple- and single-muscle-group training sessions are as follows:

- Large-muscle-group before small-muscle-group exercises
- Multijoint before single-joint exercises
- Alternating of push and pull exercises for total-body sessions
- Alternating of upper- and lower-body exercises for total-body sessions
- Exercises for weak points (priority) performed before exercises for strong points of an individual

■ Olympic lifts before basic strength and single-joint exercises

■ Power-type exercises before other exercise types

■ Most intense to least intense (particularly when performing several exercises consecutively for the same muscle group)

One final consideration for exercise order is the fitness level of the individual. As discussed earlier, training sessions should never be too stressful for an individual, especially a beginning trainee.

Number of Sets

All exercises in a training session need not be performed for the same number of sets. The number of sets is one of the factors affecting the volume of exercise (e.g., sets multiplied by reps multiplied by weight). Typically, three to six sets are used to achieve optimal gains in strength, and the physiological responses appear to be different with three versus one set of exercises in a total-body workout (Gotshalk al. 1997; Mulligan et al. 1996). It has been suggested that multiple-set systems work best for developing strength and local muscular endurance (Atha 1981; Kraemer 1997), and the gains will be made at a faster rate than those achieved through single-set systems (McDonagh and Davies 1984). In many training studies, one set per exercise performed for 8 to

12RM at a slow velocity has been compared to both periodized and nonperiodized multiple-set programs. In untrained subjects, several studies have reported similar strength increases between single- and multiple-set programs, and some have reported the superiority of multiple sets (see figure 5.4). The studies depicted in figure 5.4 all show the strength increases due to single set versus a variety of multiple set programs:

A—1 × 6 to 9RM vs. 3 × 6 to 9RM in moderately trained (MT) women (Schlumberger, Stec, and Schmidtbleicher 2001)

B—1 × 10 to 12RM vs. 3 × 10 to 12RM and a periodized program in untrained (UT) men (Stowers et al. 1983)

C—1 × 10 to 12RM vs. 3 × 6RM in UT men (Silvester et al. 1984)

D—1 × 8 to 12RM vs. a periodized program in UT women (Sanborn et al. 2000)

E—1 × 7 to 12RM vs. 2 and 4 × 7 to 12RM in MT men (Ostrowski et al. 1997)

F—1 × 10 to 12RM vs. 2 × 8 to 10RM in UT men (Coleman 1977)

G—1 × failure with 60 to 65% of 1RM vs. 3 × 6 (80 to 85% of 1RM) in UT men (Jacobson 1986)

H—1 × 8 to 20RM vs. 3 × 6 (75% of 1RM) in UT men (Messier & Dill 1985)

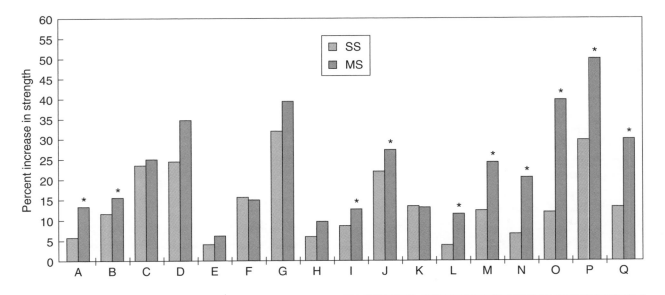

Figure 5.4 Comparison of muscle strength increases following single-set (SS) and multiple-set (MS) resistance training programs. Studies are arranged from short-term (6 weeks) to long-term (9 months).

* Indicates a difference between groups. Data presented are the mean percentage increases across all exercises used in testing for each study.

I—1 × 8 to 12RM vs. 3 × 8 to 12RM in resistance-trained (RT) men (Kraemer 1997)

J—1, 2, or 3 × 2, 6, or 10RM in UT men (Berger 1963d)

K—1 × 8 to 12RM vs. 3 × 8 to 12RM in MT men and women (Hass et al. 2000)

L—1 × 8 to 10RM vs. a periodized program in RT men (Kraemer 1997)

M—1 × 8 to 12RM vs. 3 × 10RM and a periodized program in RT men (J.B. Kramer et al. 1997)

N—1 × 8 to 10RM vs. a periodized program in RT men (Kraemer 1997)

O—1 × 8 to 12RM vs. a periodized program in UT women (Marx et al. 2001)

P—1 × 8 to 12RM vs. 3 × 8 to 12RM in UT men and women (Borst et al. 2001)

Q—1 × 8 to 12RM vs. a periodized program in RT women (Kraemer et al. 2000).

Studies examining resistance-trained individuals have shown multiple-set programs to be superior for strength, power, hypertrophy, and high-intensity endurance improvements (Kraemer 1997; Kraemer et al. 2000; J.B. Kramer et al. 1997; Marx et al. 2001; McGee et al. 1992). Figure 5.4 shows that most studies 14 weeks or longer (especially in trained individuals) demonstrate the superiority of varied, multiple-set programs for long-term improvement. These findings have prompted the recommendation from the American College of Sports Medicine (2002) for periodized multiple-set programs when long-term progression (not maintenance) is the goal. No study has shown single-set training to be superior to multiple-set training in either trained or untrained individuals. Therefore, it appears that both programs are effective for increasing strength in untrained subjects during short-term training periods (i.e., 6 to 12 weeks). However, some short-term and all long-term studies support the contention that training volume greater than one set is needed for further improvement and progression in physical development and performance. A recent extensive meta-analysis demonstrated that for both trained and untrained individuals, four sets per muscle group elicits maximal strength gains (Rhea et al. 2003). Interestingly, the meta-analysis showed untrained subjects show greater strength increases with increased volume (i.e., 1 vs. 4 sets). Still, the need for variation is also critical for continued improvement, and this includes the use of lower-volume training during some phases of the overall training program. The key factor is the use of periodization of training volume rather than the number of sets, which represents only one factor in a volume and intensity periodization model.

Considering the number of variables involved in resistance training, comparing single- and multiple-set protocols may be an oversimplification. For example, several of the aforementioned studies compared programs of different set numbers regardless of differences in intensity, exercise selection, and repetition speed. In addition, the use of untrained subjects during short-term training periods has also raised criticism of studies (Stone et al. 1998), as untrained subjects have been reported to respond favorably to most programs (Häkkinen 1985). Part of this has evolved because of the popularity of a specific single-set program (e.g., one set of 8 to 12 repetitions) that researchers desired to compare to other protocols. Single-set programs do produce strength gains, and untrained individuals show greater strength gains than trained individuals no matter what the training volume (Rhea et al. 2003). The greater strength gains shown by untrained individuals may mask any differences between programs of different training volumes, especially short-term studies of 6-12 weeks, in untrained subjects. However, single-set programs are effective during short time frames of 6-12 weeks (Keeler et al. 2001). Single-set programs can use training variation of exercise choice and other acute program variables. However, greater volume (within reasonable limits) may be needed beyond this initial training period to produce optimal improvements. In advanced lifters, further increases in volume may be counterproductive, but the correct manipulation of both volume and intensity seems to produce optimal performance gains and avoid overtraining (Häkkinen, Komi et al. 1987; Häkkinen, Pakarinen et al. 1988a).

Multiple sets of an exercise present a training stimulus to the muscle during each set. Once initial fitness has been achieved, a multiple presentation of the stimulus (three to four sets) with specific rest periods between sets, which allows the use of the desired resistance, is superior to a single presentation of the training stimulus. Some advocates of single-set programs believe that a muscle or muscle group can only perform maximal exercise for a single set; however, this has not been demonstrated. In fact, highly trained bodybuilders (Kraemer, Noble et al. 1987) and athletes trained to tolerate short rest period protocols (Kraemer 1997) can repeat multiple sets at a 10RM using the same resistance with as little as 1 minute of rest between sets.

The importance of the exercise volume (sets multiplied by repetitions multiplied by weight) is a vital concept of training progression. This is especially true in individuals who have already achieved a basic level of training or strength fitness. The interaction of the number of sets with the principle of variation in training, or more specifically "periodized training," may also help augment training adaptations. The time course of volume changes is important to the change in the exercise stimulus in periodized training. Use of a constant volume program may lead to staleness and lack of adherence to training. Ultimately, the variation of training volume (i.e., using both high- and low-volume protocols) to provide different exercise stimuli over a long-term training period will be important to provide rest and recovery periods. This is addressed in the discussion of chronic programming or periodization in chapter 7.

The number of sets performed per workout for multiple-set programs is highly variable and has not received much attention in the literature. In general, the total number of sets per workout will be affected by (1) the muscle groups trained and their consequent size (e.g. large- vs. small-muscle-mass exercises); (2) the intensity (fewer sets for high intensity and vice versa); (3) the training phase (i.e., whether the goal is strength, power, hypertrophy, or endurance); (4) the training frequency and workout structure (e.g., total-body vs. upper- or lower-body splits vs. muscle group split workouts); (5) the level of conditioning; (6) the number of exercises in which a muscle group is involved; and (7) the use of anabolic drugs (which enable lifters to tolerate higher-than-normal training volumes). Resistance training programs incorporating anywhere from 10 to 40 sets per workout are common. The number of sets is based on the individual lifter and depends on the needs analysis, administrative factors, and other aforementioned factors.

Rest Periods Between Sets, Exercises, and Repetitions

An understanding of the influence of rest periods on the stress of the workout and the amount of resistance that can be used has been a topic of study over the past 10 years. Rest periods between sets and exercises determine the magnitude of ATP-PC energy source resynthesis and the concentrations of lactate in the blood. The length of the rest period significantly increases the metabolic, hormonal, and cardiovascular responses to an acute bout of resistance exercise, as well as the performance of subsequent sets (Kraemer 1997; Kraemer, Dziados et al. 1993; Kraemer, Noble et al. 1987; Kraemer et al. 1990, 1991, 1997). Kraemer (1997) reported differences in performance with 3- versus 1-minute rest periods. All lifters were able to perform 10 repetitions with 10RM loads for three sets with 3-minute rest periods for the leg press and bench press. However, when rest periods were reduced to 1 minute, 10, 8, and 7 repetitions were performed, respectively. Figure 5.5 presents the blood lactate response to various exercise protocols that use rest periods of different lengths.

For advanced training emphasizing absolute strength or power, rest periods of 3 to 5 minutes are recommended for structural exercises (e.g., squats, power cleans, deadlifts) using maximal or near-maximal loads, whereas less rest may be needed for smaller-muscle-mass exercises or single-joint movements (American College of Sports Medicine 2002). For novice to intermediate lifting, 2 to 3 minutes of rest may suffice for structural lifts, as loading used during this stage of resistance training appears less stressful to the neu-

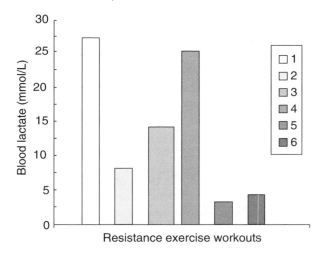

Immediate postexercise concentrations

Figure 5.5 Postexercise lactate responses to different resistance exercise protocols: (1) bodybuilding workout; (2) low-intensity circuit weight training; (3) high-intensity circuit weight training; (4) short-rest, high-intensity workout; (5) power lifting; and (6) Olympic weightlifting.

Data from Kraemer, Noble et al., 1987; Gettman and Pollock 1981; and Keul et al. 1978.

romuscular system (i.e., advanced lifters require resistances closer to their genetic potential where maximizing energy store recovery is crucial to the attainment of near-genetic-potential strength levels). Robinson and colleagues (1995) reported a 7% increase in squat performance after 5 weeks of training when 3-minute rest periods were used compared to only a 2% increase when 30-second rest periods were used. Pincivero and colleagues (1997) reported significantly greater strength gains (5-8%) when 160-second rest intervals were used compared to 40-second intervals.

Strength and power performance is highly dependent on anaerobic energy metabolism, primarily the phosphagen energy source. The majority of phosphagen repletion seems to occur within 3 minutes (Dawson et al. 1997; Fleck 1983; Volek and Kraemer 1996). In addition, removal of lactate and H^+ may require at least 4 minutes (Robinson et al. 1995). Performance of maximal lifts requires maximal energy substrate availability before the set with minimal or no fatigue, and this requires relatively long rest periods. Stressing the glycolytic and ATP-PC energy systems may enhance training for muscle hypertrophy (e.g., bodybuilding), and thus less rest between sets appears to be effective. Both types of protocols may be effective for optimizing strength and size.

Kraemer and colleagues (Kraemer, Fleck et al. 1993; Kraemer et al. 1990, 1991) used a combination of workouts to compare the impact of rest changes on blood lactate responses. The 5/3 workout consisted of using a 5RM resistance for all exercises with 3 minutes of rest between sets and exercises. The 5/1 workout consisted of using a 5RM for all exercises with 1 minute of rest between sets and exercises. The 10/3 and 10/1 workouts consisted of using 10RM with either a 3- or 1-minute rest between sets and exercises, respectively. Comparisons of the 5/1 to 5/3 and 10/1 to 10/3 workouts demonstrated the dramatic effect rest periods have on blood lactate concentrations. Short rest periods significantly elevated blood lactate concentrations compared to longer rest periods. Comparisons of the 5/1 to 10/1 and 5/3 to 10/3 workouts demonstrated the effects repetitions at an RM resistance and total work (repetitions multiplied by resistance multiplied by distance resistance moved) performed have on blood lactate concentrations. These comparisons indicated that higher volumes of work (10RM) result in higher blood lactate concentrations. The authors also noted that the effect of rest periods between sets and exercises, and on the total work performed, on blood lactate concentrations was similar for both genders.

These studies also indicated that a heavier resistance does not necessarily result in higher blood lactate concentrations. The amount of work performed and the duration of the force demands placed on the muscle(s) influence the blood lactate concentrations. The 10RM allows a higher number of repetitions and longer sets, and exercise still takes place at a relatively high percentage of the 1RM (75-85% of 1RM), which results in higher blood lactate concentrations. High force, which produces a greater time under tension per repetition, may also stimulate greater lactate responses compared to work-matched, higher-velocity, lighter-resistance, and higher-power protocols (Bush et al. 1999).

From a practical standpoint Tharion and colleagues (1991) demonstrated that short-rest programs can cause greater psychological anxiety and fatigue. This might be related to the greater discomfort, muscle fatigue, and high metabolic demands. The psychological ramifications of using short-rest workouts must also be carefully considered when designing a training session. The increased anxiety appears to be due to the dramatic metabolic demands characterized by short-rest workouts (i.e., 1 minute or less). Although the psychological demands are higher, the changes in mood states do not constitute abnormal psychological changes and may be a part of the arousal process before a demanding workout.

The frequent use of high-intensity workouts with short rest periods and heavy loading should be slowly introduced into a training program to enable a gradual improvement in toleration to increased muscle and blood acid levels (decreased pH), and improvements in acid-base buffer mechanisms (Gordon, Kraemer, and Pedro 1991). However, if such adaptations are vital to a sport (e.g., wrestling or 400- to 800-m track events), the progression from long to short rest period lengths may be needed for better performance. Usually such a program is performed within the context of a strength or power training program for a sport (e.g., two high-lactate workouts and two strength or power workouts in a week cycle) or as a preseason program for 8 to 12 weeks before the start of the wrestling or track season. Short rest period length is also characteristic of circuit weight training, but the resistances are typically lighter (i.e., 40-60% of 1RM) (Gettman and Pollock 1981). Such training does not result in as high a blood lactate concentration as short-rest-period, multiple-set 10RM sessions.

Lactic acid may not be the "bad by-product" we have thought it to be (Brooks and Fahey 1984). Although it may contribute to fatigue, it can be used as a source of energy. Furthermore, it does provide a relative comparison of the stress and accumulative use of the lactic acid energy source. The type of training session, including rest periods, will determine to a great extent the amount of lactic acid that is produced and removed from the body. Recent studies have also shown that lactic acid may be important for increases in muscle strength and hypertrophy (Shinohara et al. 1998; Smith and Rutherford 1995). Thus, the role of lactic acid during resistance training appears to be important depending on the training goals.

If a particular needs analysis identifies lactic acid as the primary energy source, the rest periods may be gradually shortened to allow the buildup of blood lactate, thus encouraging an increased tolerance and buffering of more acidic conditions. This type of training design (particularly for preseason training) may allow better tolerance for such anaerobic athletes as wrestlers, sprinters (400 to 800 m), and basketball players. Other anaerobic athletes, such as position baseball players, rely primarily on the ATP-PC energy source for energy production to perform their skills. Resistance training programs that elevate lactic acid concentrations may not be necessary to improve performance in these athletes. Careful manipulation of rest periods is essential to avoid placing inappropriate and needless stresses on the individual during training. Furthermore, because of the fatigue created by a high-volume, short-rest workout, such a workout should not occur immediately before a training session designed to develop skill in the sport or activity. Exceptions to this guideline may be in sports such as wrestling, in which all skills must be performed late in a match under conditions of high lactate concentrations.

Individuals training for improved local muscular endurance must (1) perform multiple repetitions (or long-duration sets), (2) train to and beyond the point of fatigue, or (3) minimize recovery between sets (i.e., train in a semifatigued state). For such individuals, high repetitions and shorter rest periods (30 to 90 seconds or less) for local muscular endurance training appear to be most effective (Anderson and Kearney 1982). The amount of rest taken between repetitions has only been partially addressed. Rooney and colleagues (1994) had subjects train using 6 to 10 consecutive high-intensity repetitions or 6 to 10 repetitions separated by 30-second rest periods; they reported significantly greater strength improvement with consecutive repetitions (56%) than with extended rest between repetitions (41%). These findings demonstrate that fatigue may contribute to the strength training stimulus. However, trainees desiring a high percentage of the peak velocity or power for each repetition in the workout may need to schedule rest periods after several repetitions of several sets.

Future research will need to address the aspect of rest between repetitions as the "quality" of each repetition begins to take on greater importance in producing gains in strength and power. A "rest-pause" training system may be one of the new directions for research into optimizing quality of the training session. New feedback systems on resistance exercise equipment that signal other performance factors beyond just the lifting of a weight allow us to evaluate the quality of each repetition based on the percent of peak velocity or maximal power. The concept of a quality repetition in a workout should come under more scrutiny and evaluation in the near future. Where the "fatigue" stimuli discussed earlier and the more "full recruitment" stimuli requiring a longer rest period will interface for optimal training effects remains to be determined. Most likely both styles of training may be needed to gain different aspects of strength, size, and power fitness. See figure 5.6 for a comparison of repetition quality under different repetition conditions.

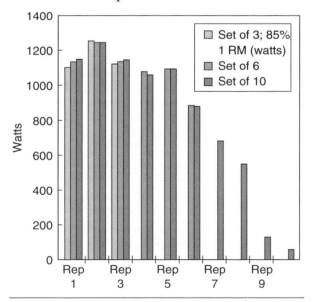

Figure 5.6 Power output from different numbers of repetitions in a set.

Courtesy of Dr. Kraemer's laboratory.

Resistance Used (Intensity)

The amount of resistance used for a specific exercise is probably one of the key factors in any resistance training program (McDonagh and Davies 1984). It is the major stimulus related to changes observed in measures of strength and local muscular endurance. When designing a resistance training program, a designer must choose a resistance for each exercise. The use of either repetition maximums (RMs) or the specific resistance that allows only a specific number of repetitions to be performed is probably the easiest method for determining a resistance. Typically, one uses a training RM target (a single RM target, 10RM) or RM target zone (a range such as 3-5RM). Then, as the strength level of the lifter changes over time, the resistance is adjusted so the lifter continues to use a true RM target or RM target zone resistance.

Research has supported the basis for an RM continuum (see figure 5.7) (Anderson and Kearney 1982; Atha 1981; Clarke 1973; McDonagh and Davies 1984; Weiss, Coney, and Clark 1999). This continuum simply relates RM resistances to the broad training effects derived from their use. An inverse relationship exists between the amount of weight lifted and the number of repetitions performed. Several studies have indicated that training with loads corresponding to 1 to 6RM was most conducive to increasing maximal dynamic strength (Berger 1962b; O'Shea 1966; Weiss, Coney, and Clark 1999). Although significant strength increases have been reported using loads corresponding to 8 to 12RM (Delorme and Watkins 1948; Kraemer 1997; Staron et al. 1994), this load range appears to be most effective for increasing

muscular hypertrophy (Kraemer, Fleck, and Evans 1996). Loads lighter than this (i.e., 12-15RM and lighter) have smaller effects on maximal strength in previously untrained individuals (Anderson and Kearney 1982; Weiss, Coney, and Clark 1999), but have proven to be very effective for increasing local muscular endurance (Stone and Coulter 1994). Contrary to early studies on resistance training, using a variety of training loads appears to be more conducive to increasing muscular fitness than performing all exercises with a constant resistance, such as a 6RM resistance. Therefore, periodized training in which load variation is included appears most effective for long-term improvements in muscular fitness (see chapter 7).

As lifters move away from the 6RM or less strength stimulus zone to lighter resistances and greater repetition numbers, their gains in strength diminish until they are negligible. The strength gains achieved above 25RM resistances are typically small to nonexistent in untrained individuals (Atha 1981; Anderson and Kearney 1982) and perhaps are related to enhanced motor performance or learning effects when they occur. A variety of individual responses due to genetic predisposition and pretraining status affect the training increases observed. But after initial gains have been made as a result of neural or learning effects, heavier resistances will be needed to optimize muscle strength and size gains. Power development will be discussed in detail in chapter 7, but power at different loads represents a maximal capability with a certain percent of 1RM, with maximal mechanical power typically achieved somewhere between 30 and 45% of 1RM (Kraemer and Newton 2000).

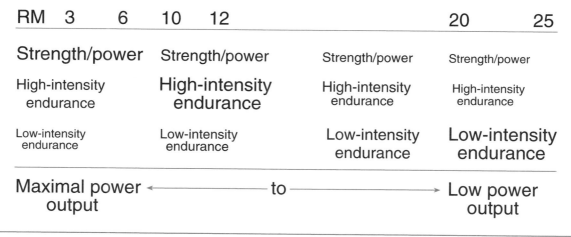

Figure 5.7 Theoretical repetition maximum continuum.

Using percentages of 1RM is another method of determining resistances for an exercise (e.g., 70% or 85%). If the trainee's 1RM for an exercise is 100 lb (45.4 kg), an 80% resistance would be 80 lb (36.3 kg). This method requires that the maximal strength in various lifts used in the training program be evaluated regularly. If 1RM testing is not undertaken regularly (e.g., each week), especially when beginning a program, the percentage of 1RM used in training will decrease, and therefore the training intensity will be reduced. From a practical perspective, use of percentages of 1RM as the resistance for many exercises may not be administratively effective because of the amount of testing time required. Use of an RM target or RM target zone allows the individual to change resistances to stay at the RM target or within the RM target zone, thus developing the characteristics associated with that portion of the RM continuum.

The use of percentages of 1RM resistances is warranted for lifts related to the competitive Olympic lifts of the clean and jerk, snatch, and variations. Since these lifts require coordinated movements and optimal power development from many muscles to result in correct lifting technique, the movements cannot be performed at a true RM or to complete momentary failure. Drastic reductions in velocity and power output experienced in the last repetition of a true RM set may not be conducive to correct technique in structural lifts related to the Olympic competitive lifts (e.g., power cleans, snatches, power snatches, hang cleans). Therefore, percentage of the 1RM is warranted to correctly calculate resistances for such lifts.

In two classic studies Hoeger and colleagues (1987, 1990) (see table 5.1) studied the relationship between the percentage of 1RM and the number of repetitions that both trained and untrained men and women could perform. This relationship varied with the amount of muscle mass needed to perform the exercise (i.e., leg presses require more muscle mass than knee extensions). When using machine resistances with 80% of the 1RM, previously thought to be primarily a strength-related prescription, the number of repetitions the subjects could perform was typically greater than 10, especially for large-muscle-group exercises such as the leg press. The larger-muscle-group exercises appear to need much higher percentages of the 1RM to stay within the strength RM zone, or any other zone, of the repetition continuum.

An example of how using the percentage of 1RM can result in less than an optimal resistance to increase strength is the following: An individual uses 80% of 1RM to perform a set of the leg press and performs 22 repetitions. This results in the question, Even though a high percentage of the 1RM was used, will performing 22 repetitions per set result in optimal strength increases? Based on the RM continuum, a 22RM is primarily related to development of local muscular endurance, not optimal development for strength and power.

Kraemer, Fleck, and colleagues (1999) showed that power lifters could lift 80% of their 1RM in the leg press for 22 repetitions or a 22RM, and untrained controls could perform only 12 repetitions at 80% of their 1RM or a 12RM. Such data, along with the data presented in the two studies by Hoeger and colleagues (1987, 1990), clearly indicate that the method used in determining the resistance to be used for specific exercises must be carefully considered for each muscle group and for each specific type of lift and the exercise mode used (e.g., free weight squat vs. leg press machine). In general, a certain percentage of the 1RM with free weight exercises will allow fewer repetitions than the same percentage of 1RM on a similar exercise performed on a machine. This is due, most likely, to the need for greater balance and control in three planes of movement with free weights. With machines, the control of movement is generally needed in only one spatial plane.

Charts or equations are often used to predict the 1RM from the number of repetitions performed with a submaximal load or to help determine an RM (e.g., from 1 to 10) from the 1RM resistance that can be lifted (Mayhew, Ball, and Bowen 1992; Morales and Sobonya 1996; Ware et al. 1995). Unfortunately, most of these charts and equations assume a linear relationship between these variables, and this is not the case. Thus, such charts and the resulting values should be used only as rough estimates of a particular resistance to use for an RM or to predict an individual's 1RM. A variety of prediction equations are available to predict 1RM, but these equations have the same inherent weaknesses as the prediction charts.

The amount of weight lifted per repetition or set is highly dependent on other variables such as exercise order, volume, frequency, muscle action, repetition speed, and rest period length (Kraemer and Ratamess 2000). Altering the training load can significantly affect the acute metabolic (Collins et al. 1989; Willoughby et al. 1991), hormonal (Kraemer 1992a; Kraemer et al. 1990, 1991), neural (Häkkinen, Alen, and Komi 1985; Sale 1992), and cardiovascular (Fleck 2002) responses to training. These factors further complicate the relationship between a certain percentage of 1RM and how many repetitions per set can be performed.

Table 5.1 The Number of Repetitions That Can Be Performed With a Set Percentage of RM

	40% $\bar{x} \pm SD$	60% $\bar{x} \pm SD$	80% $\bar{x} \pm SD$	1RM[b] $\bar{x} \pm SD$
Untrained males n = 38				
LP	80.1±7.9A[a]	33.9±14.2A	15.2±6.5A	137.9±27.2
LD	41.5±16.1B	19.7±6.1B	9.8±3.9B	59.9±11.6
BP	34.9±8.8B	19.7±4.9B	9.8±3.6B	63.9±15.4
KE	23.4±5.1C	15.4±4.4C	9.3±3.4BC	54.9±13.3
SU	21.1±7.5C	15.0±5.6C	8.3±4.1BCD	40.9±12.6
AC	24.3±7.0C	15.3±4.9C	7.6±3.5CD	33.2±5.9
LC	18.6±5.7C	11.2±2.9D	6.3±2.7D	33.0±8.5
Trained males n = 25				
LP	77.6±34.2A	45.5±23.5A	19.4±9.0A	167.2±43.2
LD	42.9±16.0B	23.5±5.5B	12.2±3.72B	77.8±15.7
BP	38.8±8.2B	22.6±4.4B	12.2±2.87B	95.5±24.8
KE	32.9±8.8BCD	18.3±5.6BC	11.6±4.47B	72.5±19.8
SU	27.1±8.76CD	18.9±6.8BC	12.2±6.42B	59.9±15.0
AC	35.3±11.6BC	21.3±6.2BC	11.4±4.15B	41.2±9.6
LC	24.3±7.9D	15.4±5.9C	7.2±3.08C	38.8±7.1
Untrained females n = 40				
LP	83.6±38.6A	38.0±19.2A	11.9±7.0A	85.3±16.6
LD	45.9±19.9B	23.7±10.0B	10.0±5.6AB	29.2±5.6
BP	—[c]	20.3±8.2B	10.3±4.2AB	27.7±23.7
KE	19.2±5.3C	13.4±3.9C	7.9±2.9BC	26.7±7.8
SU	20.2±11.6C	13.3±8.2C	7.1±5.2C	19.3±8.3
AC	24.8±11.0C	13.8±5.3C	5.9±3.6C	13.8±2.7
LC	16.4±4.4C	10.5±3.4C	5.9±2.6C	15.8±3.7
Trained females n = 26				
LP	146±66.9A	57.3±27.9A	22.4±10.7A	107.5±16.0
LD	81.3±41.8B	25.2±7.9CB	10.2±3.9C	34.8±6.0
BP	—[c]	27.9±7.9B	14.3±4.4B	35.6±4.9
KE	28.5±10.9C	16.5±5.3ED	9.4±4.3CD	40.3±10.2
SU	34.5±16.8C	20.3±8.1CD	12.0±6.5CB	23.8±6.4
AC	33.4±10.4C	16.3±5.0ED	6.9±3.1ED	17.3±3.8
LC	23.2±7.7C	12.4±5.1E	5.3±2.6E	21.7±5.0

LP = leg press (knees apart at a 100° angle for the starting position); LD = lateral pull-down (resistance pulled behind the head to the base of the neck); BP = bench press; KE = knee extension; SU = sit-up (horizontal board, feet held in place, knees at a 100° angle, and resistance held on chest); AC = arm curl (low pulley); LC = leg curl (to 90° of flexion).

[a] Letters indicate significantly different groupings: alpha level = 0.05; same letter = no difference.

[b] 1RM expressed in kg.

[c] Data unobtainable due to resistance limitations on the Universal Gym equipment.

Adapted, by permission, from W.W.K. Hoeger, et al., 1990, "Relationship between repetitions and selected percentages of one repetition maximum: A comparison between untrained and trained males and females," *Journal of Applied Sport Science Research* 4: 47-54.

The load required to increase maximal strength may be dependent on training status. Beginning lifters need a minimal load of 45 to 50% of 1RM to increase dynamic muscular strength (Baechle, Earle, and Wathen 2000). However, experienced lifters need greater loads. Häkkinen, Alen, and Komi (1985) reported that at least 80% of 1RM was needed to produce any further neural adaptations in experienced weight trainers. The need for increased intensity (percent of 1RM) or load as training progresses is shown by the results of a meta-analysis (Rhea et al. 2003). A mean training load of 60% of 1RM resulted in maximal strength in untrained individuals while a mean training load of 80% of 1RM produced maximal strength in trained individuals. Neural adaptations are crucial to resistance training, as they precede hypertrophy during intense training periods. Thus, a variety of loads and so percentage of 1RM appear necessary to optimally increase both neural function (i.e., increased motor unit recruitment, firing rate, and synchronization) and hypertrophy.

Repetition Speed

The speed used to perform dynamic muscle actions affects the adaptations to resistance training. Repetition speed is dependent on training load, fatigue, and goals and has been shown to significantly affect neural (Häkkinen, Alen, and Komi 1985; Häkkinen, Komi, and Alen 1985; Eloranta and Komi 1980), hypertrophy (Coyle et al. 1981; Housh et al. 1992), and metabolic (Ballor, Becque, and Katch 1987) adaptations to resistance training. Force production and repetition speed directly interact during exercise performance. Generally, concentric force production is highest at slower speeds and lowest at higher speeds. This relationship is graphically represented as a force-velocity curve. The implications of the force-velocity curve demonstrate that training at slow velocities with maximal tension is effective for strength training, and training at high velocities is effective for power and speed enhancement. This generally is the case; however, a variety of velocities may be most effective for both strength and power enhancement.

The speed with which repetitions are performed does change the repetitions' qualities (i.e., power output, maximal force). In a comparison of Smith machine bench press repetitions at 55% of 1RM with both the eccentric and concentric phases lasting 5 seconds (slow training velocity), 30% of 1RM with the concentric phase performed in a ballistic manner so that the bar was thrown into the air and then caught before performing the eccentric phase of each repetition (power training), and 6 repetitions with a 6RM resistance (traditional heavy weight training), differences in the qualities of repetitions were shown (Keogh, Wilson, and Weatherby 1999). Both the slow training velocity and power training resulted in significantly lower levels of force during both the eccentric and concentric phases of repetitions and lower levels of electromyographic (EMG) activity than the traditional heavy weight training. Time under tension during the slow training was significantly longer and during power training significantly shorter than during traditional heavy weight training. These results lead to speculation that such traditional weight training would lead to greater strength gains than the other two training methods and that slow velocity training might enhance local muscular endurance more than the other two training methods.

Similarly, self-paced pull-ups and push-ups result in more total work, more repetitions performed, and greater power output in less time than performing these exercises at a pace of 2 seconds each for the concentric and eccentric phases (2/2 cadence) and 2 seconds and 4 seconds, respectively, for the concentric and eccentric (2/4 cadence) phases (LaChance and Hortobagyi 1994). The number of repetitions, total work, and power output of the 2/2 cadence was midway between the self-paced and the 2/4 cadence. The self-paced cadence was at a faster repetition velocity than the other two cadences. The results indicate that improving set performance (i.e., number of repetitions or load) may best be accomplished with the use of moderate to fast speeds. Thus, repetition speed does affect repetition quality. Despite differences in repetition quality, comparison of slow-velocity training to traditional velocity training are inconclusive, with slow-velocity training shown to be both superior (Westcott et al. 2001) and inferior (Keeler et al. 2001) to traditional velocity training in terms of strength gains.

A distinction needs to be made between intentional and unintentional slow-speed repetitions. Significantly reducing RM loads is an inevitable result of intentionally performing repetitions slowly. Unintentionally slow lifting speeds are used during high-intensity repetitions (i.e., strength training) in which the loading, fatigue, or both are responsible for the longer repetition duration. For example, the concentric phase of a 1RM bench press and the last repetition of a 5RM set may last 3 to 5 seconds (Mookerjee and Ratamess 1999). This may be considered slow;

however, lifting the weight faster is not possible under these conditions. This type of unintentionally slow lifting speed may be crucial to maximal strength development.

Intentionally slow-speed repetitions must be performed with submaximal loads so the lifter has greater control of the repetition speed; such repetitions do result in longer time under tension. Thus, intentionally slow lifting may be most suitable for increasing local muscular endurance when the time under tension is greater than moderate and fast speeds.

In comparison, both fast and moderate lifting speeds can increase local muscular endurance depending on the number of repetitions performed and the rest between sets. Training with fast speeds is the most effective way to enhance muscular power and speed, and is also effective for strength enhancement (Morrissey et al. 1998), but such training is not as effective for increasing hypertrophy as slow or moderate speeds (Häkkinen, Komi, and Alen 1985). High-speed repetitions impose less metabolic demands in exercises such as the leg extension, squat, row, and arm curl compared to slow- and moderate-speed repetitions (Ballor et al. 1987). In addition, training for power is best accomplished through light loads (30% of 1RM) performed at maximal speeds (Wilson et al. 1993).

A popular technique used for both strength and power training is **compensatory acceleration** (Hatfield 1989; Wilson 1994). This requires the lifter to accelerate the load maximally throughout the exercise's range of motion (regardless of momentum) during the concentric repetition phase, striving to increase velocity to maximal levels. A major advantage of this technique is that it can be used with heavy loads and is quite effective, especially for multijoint exercises (Jones et al. 1999). Hunter and Culpepper (1995) and Jones and colleagues (1999) reported significant strength and power increases throughout the range of motion when lifters used compensatory acceleration, with the increases being significantly greater than those achieved when training at a slower speed (Jones et al. 1999).

Rest Periods Between Workouts (Training Frequency)

The number of training sessions performed during a specific time period (e.g., 1 week) may affect subsequent training adaptations (see the discussion of dynamic constant external resistance training in chapter 2). Frequency is best described as the number of times certain exercises or muscle groups are trained per week and is dependent on several factors such as volume and intensity, exercise selection, level of conditioning or training status, recovery ability, nutrition, and goals. Training with heavy loads increases the recovery time needed before subsequent sessions, especially for multijoint exercises (Baechle et al. 2000). The use of extremely heavy loads may require 72 hours of recovery, whereas moderate and light loads may require less recovery time (48 and 24 hours, respectively) (Zatsiorsky 1995). In addition, reduced frequency is adequate during maintenance training. Training 1 to 2 days per week may be adequate for mass, power, and strength retention (Baechle et al. 2000). However, this appears effective only for short-term periods, as long-term maintenance training (i.e., reduced frequency and volume) leads to detraining.

Heavy eccentric training requires greater recovery time between workouts. Loading during eccentric training (approximately 120-130% of 1RM) is substantially more than loading during normal weight training (see the discussion of eccentric training in chapter 2). Studies show that eccentric exercise is more likely to cause delayed-onset muscle soreness (DOMS) than concentric-only training (Ebbeling and Clarkson 1989; Fleck and Schutt 1985; Talag 1973). Eccentric training causes greater muscle fiber and connective tissue disruption, greater enzyme release, DOMS, and impaired neuromuscular function, which limits force production and range of motion (Saxton et al. 1995). Recovery times of at least 72 hours are required before initiating another session requiring several heavy sets or supramaximal eccentric lifts (Zatsiorsky 1995). A recent study of untrained subjects compared frequencies of 1 day per week to 2 to 3 days per week (Sorichter et al. 1997). Each session consisted of seven sets of ten 1- to 2-second eccentric-only contractions of the quadriceps muscles. Both training groups showed strength improvement after training. However, the results showed that eccentric training once a week was effective for maintenance, whereas eccentric training twice a week was more effective for strength increases. Thus, the inclusion of heavy eccentric repetitions may necessitate a change in frequency (or the muscle groups trained per session) to accommodate the greater muscle necrosis and needed recovery time between training sessions.

Numerous resistance training studies have used frequencies of 2 to 3 alternating days per week with untrained subjects (Dudley et al. 1991; Hickson, Hidaka, and Foster 1994). This has been shown to be a very effective initial frequency. If the resistance training is not excessive, only moderate amounts of delayed-onset muscular soreness should be experienced the day after the session. Some studies have shown that training 3 days a week is superior to training 2 days a week (Graves et al. 1989), whereas training 3 to 5 days a week was superior in other studies (Gillam 1981; Hunter 1985). A meta-analysis indicates that for untrained subjects a training frequency of 3 times per week of a muscle group produces maximal strength gains (Rhea et al. 2003). The progression from beginning to intermediate lifting does not necessitate a change in frequency, but may be more dependent on alterations in other acute variables such as exercise selection, volume, and intensity. However, intermediate lifters commonly train 3 to 4 days a week. Increasing training frequency allows for greater specialization (i.e., greater exercise selection per muscle group, greater volume in accordance with more specific goals, or both). Thus, an upper/lower body split or muscle group split routine is common. Similar improvements in performance have been observed between an upper/lower split routine and a total-body workout in untrained women (Calder et al. 1994). In addition, similar muscle groups or selected exercises are not recommended to be performed on consecutive days during split-routine workouts to allow adequate recovery and minimize the risk of overtraining.

Training frequency for advanced or elite athletes may vary considerably (depending on intensity, volume, and goals) and is typically greater than the training frequency of intermediate lifters. One aspect of frequency that must always be kept in mind is how many times per week a muscle group is trained. In many situations, the higher total frequencies of advanced lifters are achieved by performing sessions dedicated to specific muscle groups (i.e., body part programs). A meta-analysis showed the optimal frequency for trained individuals was 2 days per week per muscle group and not 3 days per week as shown for untrained individuals (Rhea et al. 2003). The lower frequency for the trained individuals was in part due to a higher training volume per session used by the trained compared to the untrained individuals. One study demonstrated that American football players training 4 to 5 days a week achieved better results than those self-selecting frequencies of 3 and 6 days

a week (Hoffman et al. 1990). However, each muscle group was only trained 2 to 3 days per week. Weightlifters and bodybuilders typically use high-frequency training (i.e., four to six sessions per week). Two training sessions per day have been used (Häkkinen, Pakarinen et al. 1988a; Zatsiorsky 1995) during preparatory training phases, which may result in 8 to 12 training sessions per week (see the discussion of two training sessions in one day in chapter 7). Frequencies as high as 18 sessions per week have been reported in Bulgarian weightlifters (Zatsiorsky 1995). The rationale for this high-frequency training is that frequent short sessions followed by periods of recovery, supplementation, and food intake allow for high-intensity training via maximal energy utilization and reduced fatigue during exercise performance (Baechle et al. 2000). Häkkinen and Kallinen (1994) reported greater increases in muscle size and strength when training volume was divided into two sessions per day as opposed to one in female athletes. In addition, exercises (i.e., total-body lifts) performed by Olympic lifters require technique mastery, which may increase total training volume and frequency. Elite power lifters typically train with frequencies of four to six sessions per week (Kraemer and Koziris 1994). It should be noted that training at these high frequencies would result in overtraining in most individuals. The individual must be able to tolerate the physical stress to avoid overtraining (Fry, Kraemer, van Borselen et al. 1994). However, the superior conditioning of these athletes, in combination with potential anabolic drug usage and possible genetic predisposition, enable them to successfully use very high-frequency programs. Advanced periodized training cycles use variations in training frequency to alter the exercise stimulus, enhance the exercise stimulus, and provide adequate recovery between sessions.

Training 3 days a week for all situations and sports is far from the optimal. The individual's needs and goals should determine the amount of exercise required to increase a particular physiological or performance variable. Progression in frequency is a key component to resistance training. Frequency of training will vary depending on the phase of the training cycle, the fitness level of the individual, the goals of the program, and the individual's training history. Careful choices need to be made regarding rest between training days. These choices are based on the planned progress toward specific training goals and the toleration of the individual to the program changes made. If an individual experiences excessive soreness the next morning, this may indicate that the exercise stress is too demanding. If this is the case, the workout loads, sets, rest periods between sets, and training frequency need to be evaluated and adjusted.

Summary of Acute Program Variables

A single resistance training workout can be described by these acute program variables:

- Exercise and muscle groups trained
- Order of exercise
- Number of sets and set structure (i.e., ascending/descending pyramid, constant repetition/resistance)
- Rest periods
- Load or resistance used
- Repetition speed

The configuration of these variables results in the exercise stimulus for a particular workout. Workouts must be altered to meet changing training goals and to provide training variation. Within this paradigm for the description of resistance exercise workouts, careful control of various components and their manipulation creates new and optimal training sessions (Kraemer 1983c). Because so many different combinations of these variables are possible, an almost unlimited number of workouts can be developed. Understanding the influence and importance of each of the acute program variables in achieving a specific training goal is vital to creating the optimal exercise stimulus.

Figure 5.8 overviews the program characteristics for some of the major resistance training goals and matches them with combinations of the acute program variables. Using the acute program variables to develop various workouts that enhance certain characteristics is vital to physical development. It is also possible to train different muscles or muscle groups in different ways resulting in workout programs for different muscle(s) with different training goals. For example, it is possible to train the chest musculature for maximal strength while training the leg musculature for power and the abdominal muscles for local muscular endurance. Proper manipulation of the acute program goals in developing a single workout and changing the workout over time (chronic program manipulations) are the bases of success-

ful program design. Thus, no one should use the same resistance training program over long-term periods. Claims of a program's "superiority" often seen in magazines, on the Internet, and elsewhere and companies that advocate the sole usage of their programs are typically based on marketing or self-promotion and should be viewed with caution.

The prescription of resistance training is both a science and an art. The key is to be able to translate the science of resistance training into the practical implementation in the weight room. Herein is the challenge of bridging the gap between science and practice. Ultimately, individualized programs provide for the most optimal changes and result in the best overall training response for the individual. A paradigm for exercise prescription has been developed and presented in this chapter and provides the framework for optimal design of resistance training programs. This paradigm may be viewed as a general-to-specific model of resistance training progression (American of College of Sports Medicine 2002). In this model, it is recommended that beginning programs be simple and basic until an adequate fitness and strength foundation is built. A simple program may be effective for improving all aspects of fitness, especially in untrained individuals. However, this is not the case with advanced training. With progression, more variation should be introduced. With advanced levels of training, great variation is needed as the principle of specificity is an important determinant of further fitness gains. That is, it is virtually impossible to improve in multiple variables of fitness (i.e., strength, size, power, endurance, speed, body composition) at this stage at one time. Thus, specific training cycles need to be included to address each of these variables individually and to ensure progression. While guidelines can be given, the art of designing effective resistance training programs comes from logical exercise prescription followed by evaluation, testing, and interaction with the trainee. Prescription of resistance training is a dynamic process that requires the strength and conditioning coach or personal trainer to respond to the changing levels of adaptations and functional capacities of the trainee with altered program designs to meet the changing training goals.

Training Potential

One of the major factors in training success and the gains made in any fitness variable are related

1RM Strength

- Choice of exercise and the specific movement patterns and types of muscle action needed are emphasized.
- Exercises to be emphasized are performed early in the training session.
- High-intensity (typically <10RM) resistances that are varied over time (periodized): for example, 1 to 5RM (heavy), 6 to 10RM (moderate), >10RM (light).
- Moderate to long rest periods (>2 minutes) depending on the weight being lifted.
- Moderate to high number of sets for the primary specific exercises (4-10) (e.g., the squat); low to moderate number of sets for assistance exercises (1-3).

Power

- Choice of exercise and the specific movement patterns for power development are typically related to multijoint structural movements (Olympic-type exercises such as power cleans, hang pulls, snatches, hang cleans). Eccentric actions are not emphasized in these types of lifts.
- Exercises to be emphasized are performed early in the training session.
- High-intensity (typically <10RM) resistances that are varied over time (periodized): 1 to 5RM (heavy), 6 to 10RM (moderate), >10RM (light). Rarely are more than 5 repetitions performed in a set, whether using a heavy, moderate, or light resistance. Power development lags behind strength. Therefore, in a specific set, the number of repetitions performed will be slightly lower than the number the RM resistance allows.
- Moderate to long rest periods between sets and exercises (>2 minutes).
- Moderate to high number of sets for power-oriented exercises (4-10); low to moderate number of sets for assistance exercises (1-3).

Hypertrophy

- Large variety of exercise choice or movement patterns. Includes a considerable amount of isolation exercises. Concentric and eccentric actions are important. Multiple exercise angles are used for each joint.
- Large variety of exercise order. Muscles to be emphasized are exercised early in the training session.
- Moderate to high intensity (6-12RM); higher numbers of repetitions are sometimes used, especially with supersetting (back-to-back sets for the same muscle group).
- Short rest periods between sets and exercises (<1.5 minutes).
- High total number of sets per muscle or muscle group (>3).

Local Muscular Endurance

- Choice of exercise and the specific movement patterns and types of muscle action needed for the sport action are emphasized.
- Muscles to be emphasized are exercised early in the training session.
- Low intensity (12-20RM).
- Moderate rest periods between sets and exercises (2 to 3 minutes) for long repetition sets (20 or greater) and short rest periods (30 to 60 seconds) between sets and exercises for lower repetition sets (12-19).
- Moderate number of sets (2-3).

Figure 5.8 Program characteristics for basic goals in resistance training.

Adapted from *Physical Therapy Practice*, vol 2, W.J. Kraemer and L.P Koziris, "Muscles strength training: Techniques and considerations," pp. 54-68, Copyright 1992, with permission from Elsevier.

to an individual's starting fitness level and genetic potential. Not everyone is capable of the 300-lb (136.3-kg) bench press or 20-in. (32-cm) arms or the "hard body" promoted in magazines and the media. However, everyone is capable of making gains and improving both physical development and performance. The magnitude of fitness gains differs based on each person's genetic potential and desire for a given attribute.

Progression Over Time

The initial gains made during resistance training are large compared to the gains made after several months or years of training. As training proceeds, the size of gains decrease as the trainee approaches his or her genetic potential (see the top of the curve in figure 5.9). Understanding this concept is important to understanding the adaptations and changes that occur over time. Furthermore, one can see that almost any resistance training program might work for an untrained individual in the early phases of training as the potential for gain is significant.

Window of Adaptation

The opportunity for improvement in a particular variable has been called the window of adaptation (Newton and Kraemer 1994). This means that the more potential you have for improvement (i.e., the more untrained you are), the greater your relative gains will be. In addition, it could also mean that the greater your genetic potential (e.g., the number of muscle fibers you have), the greater your absolute gains will be. The window

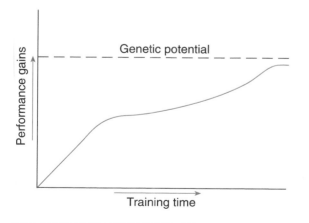

Figure 5.9 A theoretical training curve. Gains are made easily on the lower portion of the curve as individuals start to train and become slower as they approach their genetic potential.

of adaptation gets smaller and smaller as you train a specific variable and make improvements leading up to a theoretical "genetic ceiling." Therefore, if at the start of a training program, an individual already has a high level of adaptation or fitness, the starting window for adaptation will be small. Training expectations must therefore be kept in perspective in terms of both the relative gains that can be made in a specific fitness variable and the absolute gains that can be made starting with a specific genetic predisposition. Furthermore, all training adaptations are specific to the program performed, and not all training improvements are made in the same time frame (e.g., neural versus hypertrophy; see chapter 3) over a training program.

This concept is evident in highly trained athletes, who sometimes experience quite small gains in a performance variable over short training periods (e.g., 8 to 12 weeks). This is true for strength measures as well as for other performance measures such as sprint speed. Hoffman and colleagues (1990) demonstrated this phenomenon in a study in which college football players had a choice among different frequencies of training per week over a 10-week off-season conditioning program. The groups that chose 3 and 6 days a week made no gains in 1RM bench press (see table 5.2). The authors suggested that the 3-days-a-week program was not a sufficient stimulus to elicit significant strength improvements in already conditioned athletes who had participated in an intensive in-season heavy resistance training program. The lack of changes in 1RM bench press for players using a 6-days-a-week program was postulated to be the result of a short-term overtraining syndrome or overreaching. However, squat strength improved for all groups except the 3-days-a-week group, indicating that not all muscle groups (i.e., bench press vs. squat) will respond in the same manner to all training programs. Interestingly, none of the groups demonstrated an improvement in 40-yd (36.3-m) sprint times, which demonstrates how difficult it is for athletes who already have achieved a high degree of fitness in a particular variable to make improvements consequent to a short-term training. Nevertheless, while small changes (e.g., 0.1 second) in a 40-yd (36.6-m) dash may not be statistically significant, the practitioner should not overlook the practical importance of such an effect. Care must be taken to see that the changes for specific variables are at least responding in the desired direction (improvement). Thus, such

Table 5.2 Results of Performance and Anthropometric Testing in College Football Players Using a Selected Frequency of Training

Variable	Test	3 days	4 days	5 days	6 days
BW (kg)	Pre	80.3±5.1	94.2±12.7	99.2±14.4	112.3±12.4
	Post	79.6±6.4	93.1±12.0*	98.7±13.7	111.0±12.1
BP (kg)	Pre	107.2±11.6	127.7±13.9	131.1±20.1	143.9±12.0
	Post	109.1±28.7	132.2±14.5	135.3±9.0*	149.7±17.3
SQ (kg)	Pre	140.1±18.6	173.6±36.2	170.6±19.4	191.6±34.9
	Post	147.7±38.9	186.3±31.9*	183.4±22.1*	204.1±39.5*
40 (s)	Pre	4.83±0.14	5.01±0.22	4.97±0.23	5.23±0.20
	Post	4.82±0.19	4.97±0.18	4.93±0.24	5.18±0.20
VJ (cm)	Pre	70.2±7.7	65.9±8.4	64.5±8.6	59.9±6.7
	Post	71.7±7.6	66.0±8.8	66.0±7.9	62.5±7.1
2 MI (s)	Pre	933.1±49.7	945.0±61.3	960.8±99.3	982.2±65.0
	Post	811.1±77.1*	830.7±55.5*	834.2±84.8*	879.8±68.7*
SF (mm)	Pre	54.7±12.2	79.7±15.3	83.6±20.0	100.3±13.0
	Post	50.9±10.5*	72.9±12.7*	79.0±19.7*	92.4±15.2*
TH (cm)	Pre	56.0±2.5	59.5±4.6	59.8±4.6	63.9±3.4
	Post	56.7±1.6	61.4±3.5*	61.5±4.2*	65.0±3.2
CH (cm)	Pre	92.8±3.9	103.3±7.2	105.9±8.4	111.9±7.1
	Post	94.8±3.1*	105.5±6.9*	107.1±8.2*	112.3±6.1

$* = p < 0.05$

BW = body weight; BP = bench press; SQ = squat; 40 = 40-yd sprint; VJ = vertical jump; 2 MI = 2-mi run; SF = sum of skinfolds; TH = thigh circumference; CH = chest circumference.

Adapted, by permission, from J.R. Kraemer, et al., 1990, "The effects of self-selection for frequency of training in a winter conditioning program for football," *Journal of Applied Sport Science Research* 4: 76-82.

data and concepts indicate that the length of the training program, the fitness level of the athlete in a particular lift or performance task, genetic potential, and the frequency of training can all influence the training adaptations. The expectation of continual large strength or performance gains in all aspects of an athlete's sport-fitness profile is unrealistic.

Several recent studies have shown that differences in the rate of fitness improvement can be detected in both acute and chronic training. Even with short-term training, some programs are better than others in producing substantially greater changes in strength (Keeler et al. 2001; Schlumberger, Stec, and Schmidtbleicher 2001). Keeler and colleagues (2001) showed that over 10 weeks of training, a single-set program was superior to a superslow program in untrained women. Schlumberger and colleagues (2001) demonstrated that a three-set program was superior to a one-

set program over the first 6 weeks of training in trained women. These data indicate that the rate of improvement appears to be affected by the type and speed of the muscle action and the volume of training used in a program, even over the early phase of training.

Nevertheless, the accumulation or "banking" of training time is needed to see comprehensive and dramatic differences between different programs over longer training periods. Such long-term training adaptations are also more resistant to the effects of detraining. Two recent studies demonstrated this concept taking place over 6 to 9 months. In a 9-month study of collegiate women tennis players, a periodized training program was shown to be superior to a low-volume single-set training program in both the development of muscular strength and power as well as improvement in tennis serve ball velocity (Kraemer et al. 2000). In another study, a 6-month training program in untrained women showed similar findings in performance (e.g., 40-yd sprint speed), body composition, and strength and power measures, again demonstrating that a periodized multiple-set training program was categorically superior to a low-volume single-set circuit-type program (Marx et al. 2001). Thus, certain training principles (e.g., specificity, periodization, volume of exercise) appear to affect the rate and magnitude of fitness gains observed over a given training period. However, in both studies it took 2 to 3 months before superiority of the periodized program was shown in some fitness measures, demonstrating that long training periods may be needed before training programs show differences in fitness gains.

Setting Program Goals

In order to create an effective resistance training program design, specific program goals must be set. Factors such as age, physical maturity, training history, and psychological and physical toleration need to be considered in any goal development process and individual program design. In addition, designers must prioritize goals so that training programs do not compete for adaptation priority (e.g., endurance training reduces power development). Among the many common program goals in resistance training that are related to improvements in function are increased muscular strength, increased power, increased local muscular endurance, and improvements in physiological training effects (e.g., increase in lean tissue mass) (Kraemer and Koziris 1992). Other functional gains such as an increase in coordination, agility, balance, and speed are also common goals of conditioning programs, especially for athletes. In addition, it is becoming clear that such fitness attributes such as balance may also have important implications for injury prevention (e.g., limiting falls in older individuals). Other physiological changes related to increased fat-free mass through muscle hypertrophy or improvement of other physiological functions such as blood pressure, decreased body fat, and increased resting metabolic rate to help with long-term weight control are also goals of resistance training programs. Resistance training affects almost every physiological function and has the ability to enhance physical development and performance at all ages (Kraemer, Fleck, and Evans 1996).

For the most part, training goals should be testable variables (e.g., 1RM strength, vertical jump height) so trainers can judge objectively whether gains are made. Examination and evaluation of a workout log can be invaluable in evaluating the effects of various resistance training programs. Formal strength tests to determine functional changes in strength can be performed on a variety of equipment, including isokinetic dynamometers, free weights, and machines (Knuttgen and Kraemer 1987). Examining the results of specific tests can help both trainers and trainees modify the exercise program if improvements are not being made.

In some cases training for high-level sport performance does not coincide with improving an individual's health. Many elite athletes excessively train (e.g., lifting 7 days a week or running 100 miles in a week or training 4 to 6 hours a day) more than what is needed for optimizing health and general fitness. The goals in resistance training have to be put into the context of the desired outcome for the individual. For example, trying to gain maximal amounts of body mass (including fat and muscle) to be a lineman in American football may not be healthy; however, large athletes are sought after at the major college and professional levels (Kraemer and Gotshalk 2000). In this case, health and sport fitness may not be compatible. The competitive athlete must seriously consider whether training for a sport career will be detrimental to a healthy lifestyle after the career is completed. Still, not much is known about detraining the so-called "bulked up" athlete except to reduce body mass and eliminate some of the major risk factors for cardiovascular disease and diabetes (Kraemer 1983a; Mazzetti, Ratamess, and Kraemer 2000). Changing training goals after completion of a sport career is important to continued health and fitness.

Maintenance of Training Goals

A concept termed **capping** refers to training situations in which small gains will require very large amounts of time to achieve and in the long run are not necessary. This may be related to performance (e.g., bench press 1RM strength) or some form of physical development (e.g., calf girth). This is a difficult decision that comes only after an adequate period of training time and observation of the individual's potential for improvement. At some point, the trainer and trainee must make a value judgment as to how to best spend training time. When the decision is made not to devote further training time to developing a particular muscle characteristic (e.g., strength, size, power), the trainee enters into a maintenance training program. In maintenance programs we see the concept that all exercises need not be performed for the same number of sets, reps, and intensity despite the widespread use of such standardized programs. The training time saved by not spending as much training time on a certain characteristic can be used to address other training goals. Such program design decisions will allow various aspects of fitness to be developed and prioritized over a given training period.

Many examples of training "overkill" can be found in sports. For example, although the continued development of whole-body power is advantageous to an American football player, an exercise such as the bench press may not be a good measure of playing ability (Fry and Kraemer 1991). The physical attributes needed to bench press a great amount of weight are a large, muscular torso, including large chest and back musculature, and short arms. Large upper-body musculature is a positive attribute for American football players because of the sport's dependence on body mass. However, due to the advantages of taller players in today's game, especially as linemen, few elite football players have the short arms needed for great success in the bench press (Kraemer and Gotshalk 2000).

Should the bench press lift be used as a part of the exercise prescription for American football players? It should, but the expectations and magnitude of performance in that lift for each individual football player must be kept in perspective. Furthermore, the safe performance of this lift without injuring the shoulders is also a concern. Thus, each player's individual physical dimensions and size must be considered when developing short-term (e.g., bench press strength after a 10-week summer conditioning program) and especially long-term (e.g., bench press strength increase from the freshman to the senior year) goal development. Furthermore, the importance of a given lift to the performance of the sport should be evaluated. Spending extra time on the bench press to gain an extra 10 or 20 lb (4.5 or 9.1 kg) in the lift at the cost of not training, for example, hang cleans, which help develop the structural power vital for performance in football, would be an unwise use of training time (Barker et al. 1993; Fry and Kraemer 1991). For example, consider a player who has been training for over a year and has achieved a bench press 1RM of 355 lb (161.3 kg). The extra training time needed to achieve a 400-lb (181.1-kg) bench press may be better used

to train another lift (e.g., hang cleans), improve sprint speed or agility, or participate in more sport practice. Furthermore, the elite players may not have the physical dimensions (e.g., short arms) needed for a 400-lb (181.1-kg) bench press (Kraemer and Gotshalk 2000). Maintenance of the bench press may be called for in this case.

Making such training decisions are part of the many types of clinical or coaching decisions that must be made when monitoring the progression of resistance training. Are the training goals realistic in relationship to the sport or health improvement goal? Is the attainment of a particular training goal vital to the individual's success or health? These are difficult questions that need to be asked continually as training progresses.

Unrealistic Goals

Careful attention must be paid to the magnitude of the performance goal and how much training time will be needed to achieve it. Too often, goals are open ended and unrealistic. For many men the 23-in. (36.8-cm) upper arms, 36-in (57.5-cm) thighs, 20-in. (32.0-cm) neck, 400-lb (181.1-kg) bench press, or 50-in. (80.0-cm) chest are unrealistic goals because of genetic limitations. Women too can develop unrealistic goals. Many times this is in an opposite direction from men in that goals include drastic decreases in limb size and body shape to reflect the media culture's ideals for women. Again, based on genetics, such changes may not be possible in many women. Many women mistakenly believe that large gains in strength, muscle definition, and body fat loss can be achieved through the use of very light resistance training programs (e.g., 2- to 5-lb [0.9- to 2.3-kg] handheld weights) that attempt to "spot build" a particular body part or muscle. Although one may be able to "spot hypertrophy" a particular body part, it is not possible with resistances that are this light. Ultimately, for both men and women, it is a question of whether the resistance training program can stimulate the desired body changes. Those changes must be examined carefully and honestly.

Unrealistic expectations of equipment and programs also exist when they are not evaluated based on sound scientific principles. In today's "high-tech" and "big-hype" culture of infomercial marketing of products, programs, and equipment, the average person can develop unrealistic training expectations. In addition, movie actors, models, and elite athletes can also project a desired body image and performance levels, but for most people such upper levels of physical development, body type, and performance are unrealistic.

Proper goal development is accomplished by starting out small and making gradual progress. Goal setting is preceded by an evaluation of the individual's current fitness level. Most people make mistakes in goal development by wanting too much too soon, with too little effort expended. This is where frustration can begin from not seeing the expected gains, or injury and overtraining can occur from doing too much too soon. Making progress in a resistance training program requires a long-term commitment to a total conditioning program. In addition, proper nutrition and lifestyle behaviors can help support training goals and physical development. A careful evaluation of the training goals and the equipment needed to achieve them can avoid wasted time, money, and effort. Goals change, and resistance training programs must change along with them.

Prioritization of Training Goals

Although any strength training program will result in a host of concomitant adaptations in the body, prioritizing training goals will help a program designer create the optimal stimulus. For example, although performing four sets of 3RM in a particular exercise will enhance power by affecting the force component of the power equation, it does not address the velocity component of the equation. Thus, a program design that also has workouts (six sets of 3 reps at 30% of 1RM) or training cycles that address this goal will optimize power development. This becomes even more important as training progresses and the window of adaptation for performance decreases. Priorities for a specific goal can be set for a workout, a specific training phase or cycle, or a period of time (e.g., in-season). Many periodization models take this concept into consideration by manipulating the exercise stimuli used either over a training cycle (linear periodization) or in a workout (nonlinear periodization).

Although different resistance training programs can produce different effects in the body related to the production or support of force and the development of muscle, the careful examination of a conditioning program is crucial when other forms of exercise are included. Program designers must carefully consider the compatibility of training types as they relate to a specific goal. Placing too much emphasis on long-distance

running to maintain a low body mass in sports such as gymnastics or wrestling, for instance, can be detrimental to the power development vital for these sports. Conversely, the typical fitness enthusiast may not be as concerned with any negative effects on power development if the primary goal is body mass control and cardiovascular health. In this case, power capabilities take second place in the conditioning program. However, athletes who are serious about recreational basketball league play and performance, for example, may want to consider training for power to achieve cardiovascular fitness (such as in an interval training program) without compromising vertical jump power. Other types of conditioning elements must also be examined in the context of the resistance training program as well. These include plyometric training, sprint training, flexibility training, weight gain and weight loss programs, and sport practice and competitions.

Prioritization of training goals and the associated program designs must be considered in the more global context of the individual's entire exercise exposure. The key is to detect any competing exercise stimuli that will compromise recovery or physiological development of a specific high-priority training goal. The simultaneous development of training goals often requires careful partitioning of the program's design over time either within a week or within a training cycle.

Individualization

Each program must be designed to meet the individual's needs and training goals. The athlete, the teacher, the personal trainer, and the coach must all evaluate and understand the trainee's fitness level. Keep in mind, however, that a trainee's fitness level (e.g., 1RM strength test) should not be evaluated until it is known that the individual can tolerate the test demands and that the data generated are meaningful (Kraemer and Fry 1995). One of the most serious mistakes made in designing a workout is placing too much stress on the individual before he or she can tolerate it.

Progress in a resistance training program should follow the staircase principle (see figure 5.10). An individual begins a training session at a particular strength level. During the training session, strength decreases due to fatigue; at the conclusion of the session, strength is at its lowest point. After recovering from the first session, the individual should begin the next training session at a slightly higher strength level. This staircase

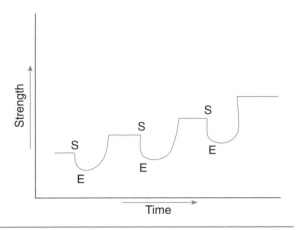

Figure 5.10 A resistance training program should allow for a staircase effect. *S* and *E* designate the start and end of a workout, respectively.

effect in fitness level should be observable as training sessions, weeks, months, and years progress. Designing training programs that allow for this staircase effect is the biggest challenge in the field of resistance training.

Computers have greatly enhanced our ability to monitor feedback and truly achieve individualized resistance training programs for large groups of people. When designing training programs for an athletic team or a large fitness facility, designers commonly distribute a generalized program for all to follow. Generalized programs will not produce the same results for each individual, and in sports even different positions require very different training programs (Kraemer and Gotshalk 2000). Thus, a general program written for a particular group of people or sport should be viewed as a starting point for each individual. Additions, deletions, changes, and progressions can then be applied to meet the unique goals of each individual. This applies to athletes as well as to individuals training for general fitness.

Case Study Exercise Prescriptions

The following case studies demonstrate manipulations of acute and chronic program variables. Each study offers one solution to the needs and goals of the case in question.

— Case Study One —

John just took a job at a senior high school as the head wrestling coach and physical education teacher. He was an avid weight trainer in college and felt this played a large role in his athletic career. John's undergraduate courses in exercise science stimulated an interest in strength training. On the basis of his interest and previous experience, he was appointed head of the high school's strength and conditioning program. John decided to develop a workout program for his wrestling team.

John started with a needs analysis for the sport and determined that the movements and joint angles involved with wrestling vary, but primarily involve the large muscles of the hips, legs, and back. Dynamic muscle actions are the most common, although a certain number of isometric actions take place during various wrestling moves. The energy is derived primarily from the lactic acid energy source and aerobic metabolism: Wrestling entails intense activity extended over 6 minutes with a limited amount of rest. His needs analysis for the wrestling team was as follows:

- **Muscle groups trained:** This sport requires overall physical training, but the large-muscle groups of the back, hips, and legs are especially important for the performance of most moves. Wrestling requires a great deal of dynamic strength and power, but also local muscular endurance.

- **Injury sites:** The main injury sites are the neck, shoulders, ankles, and knees.

- **Muscle actions:** Dynamic concentric and eccentric muscle actions are the primary movement types. Isometric muscle actions are used to a lesser extent.

- **Energy sources:** The lactic acid source is the major contributor of energy during a match with significant support from the aerobic source and the remainder derived from the ATP-PC source.

Off-Season Training

John designed the workout in table 5.3 for his wrestlers. The Monday-Wednesday-Friday program is designed to strengthen the various body parts of the wrestler using primarily body-part exercises and one structural exercise (squat). Exercises are ordered within a group to exercise the same body part at different joint angles. This exercise order combined with a short rest period (1.0 to 1.5 minutes) stresses the lactic acid energy source that results in an accumulation of lactic acid similar to what is observed during wrestling (12-20 mmol · L^{-1}). This workout is primarily used in the off-season and preseason before the wrestler is able to put much time in on the mat. Once the wrestler is in season, the use of such a high lactic acid workout program is less important

and may be performed only once a week, as the wrestling is providing the specific metabolic conditioning needs. Progression from 90-second rest periods to 1-minute rest periods is used at the start of the program to allow for the development of exercise toleration. The use of this type of program will reduce the symptoms of nausea, dizziness, and vomiting associated with the inability to tolerate the high levels of acidity that occur while wrestling. This type of workout helps the wrestler adapt to the high concentrations of lactic acid encountered during a wrestling match.

In order to address the structural strength needs of the wrestler, John also developed a Tuesday-Thursday training session. This is used at the onset of the program and is subject to chronic program manipulations (see table 5.4).

John designed this workout to develop explosive power in the legs, hips, and back. Structural exercises accomplish this goal. Adequate rest is given between sets and exercises to allow the use of heavy resistance to promote primarily strength and power gains.

Chronic Manipulations (Periodization)

Several possibilities for chronic manipulation exist in John's training program. As the season approaches, the number of repetitions can be decreased to 5 or 6, and even 2 or 3 repetitions for the structural exercises on the Monday-Wednesday-Friday and Tuesday-Thursday workouts. The rest periods between sets and exercises can be gradually decreased to 20 seconds for the body-part workouts (Monday-Wednesday-Friday). These two manipulations

Table 5.3 M-W-F Body-Part Workout (Stresses Lactic Acid and Energy Sources)

Bench press Upright row	10↓ 10↓ 10↓ 10↓ 10↓ 10↓ * * *
Lat pull-down Seated row	10↓ 10↓ 10↓ 10↓ 10↓ 10↓ * * *
Knee extensions Knee flexions	10↓ 10↓ 10↓ 10↓ 10↓ 10↓ * * *
Squats	10/ 5/ 5/ 5/ 5 → → → →
Sit-ups Knee-ups	50↓ 50↓ 20↓ 25↓ * *
Arm curls	10* 10* 10* → → →
Calf raises	10* 10* 10* → → →
Four-way neck isometrics	15 reps, 3-5 s each

/ = 2- to 5-min rest; * = 1-min rest; ↓ = alternating exercise order; → = do all sets of an exercise before moving to next exercise.

Note. All sets listed are at RM resistances.

Table 5.4 Tu-Th Structural Workout

Deadlifts	8/ 8/ 8/ 8/ 8/
Sit-ups	4 × 25
Split squats	10/ 10/ 10/ 10/
High pulls	8/ 8/ 8/ 8/

/ = 2- to 5-minute rests between sets and exercises.

Note. All sets listed are at RM resistances.

(continued)

Case Study One *(continued)*

help to peak strength levels while maintaining a high amount of stress on the lactic acid energy source. In addition, to create variation in training, one or two additional sets or one or two fewer sets at a higher intensity can be performed. This causes increases and/or decreases in the volume and intensity of the daily workouts helping to prevent the staleness portion of the general adaptation syndrome. Two- or three-week cycles in which the intensity (RM) is changed on the Tuesday-Thursday workouts (e.g., 10, 5, 3RM) and the rest between sets is altered on the Monday-Wednesday-Friday workouts (e.g., 60, 45, or 20 seconds) can also be used to add variation to the program. Wrestlers might also do the structural training program on Monday, Wednesday, and Friday and the high lactic acid program on Tuesday and Thursday once wrestling practice starts.

As the season approaches, John must focus training on the practice of actual wrestling skills. One way to decrease the time spent in the weight room is to decrease the number of sets and repetitions along with the rest periods. This may be a key consideration for the in-season program. Another way to accomplish this is to increase the number of structural workouts at the expense of the body-part workouts, with the goal being to eventually stop performance of the body-part workouts altogether and perform only three structural workouts per week. Since structural exercises stress several muscle groups at once, all major muscle groups are stressed in a shorter period of time than they would be in body-part workouts. Structural workouts become vital during the in-season program as do injury prevention exercises for the neck, knees, shoulders, and ankles. Therefore, these exercises should compose the majority of in-season exercises.

Individual Considerations

John realized that all of his wrestlers did not have the same level of experience with resistance training and physical conditioning. He therefore made individual modifications in the beginning resistances and rest periods until each of his wrestlers could tolerate the basic body-part and structural sessions. He also developed an individual workout card system and later a computer program to individualize the workouts of each wrestler so that each could make progress. He also ran teaching sessions in the weight room to instruct his athletes on the basic techniques of the lifts. One of his wrestlers had a chronic shoulder problem from the previous season. In this case, John added some rehabilitation exercises for the shoulder after consultation with the school's athletic trainer and later a few more exercises for the shoulder area to improve the athlete's overall shoulder strength. Some of the heavier wrestlers had very low aerobic fitness. For these John developed some basic aerobic fitness programs for use during the off-season program. All of his wrestlers were on aerobic fitness programs to facilitate better recovery between rounds and between matches (especially during tournaments). In addition, in the preseason he used an interval sprint program to enhance anaerobic as well as aerobic capacities. Finally, John stressed off-season weight control after appropriate body composition analysis and consultation with the team physician. This helped his wrestlers find their optimal weight.

— Case Study Two —

Maelu was primarily interested in a personal fitness program. She was actively involved in an aerobic running program and was ready to include a resistance training program to balance her conditioning activities, improve her upper-body strength, and prevent lower-limb injury during aerobic exercise. Her basic needs analysis indicated a need for additional upper-body strength along with quadriceps, hamstring, and calf exercises to aid in her injury prevention program. Based on the needs analysis, she developed the workout in table 5.5.

This program is designed to achieve moderate strength gains in the upper-body musculature. Two minutes of rest are allowed between both sets and exercises. Initially, light resistances are used to aid in developing proper exercise technique. The resistances are then increased until RM resistances are used for the desired number of repetitions. Because of the allowance of long rest periods, the training session can be performed in multiple-set fashion

(Maelu completes all sets of an exercise before performing the next exercise) or in a circuit format. Initially Maelu performs only one exercise per body part and one or two sets of each exercise until her tolerance to the workouts improves.

Chronic Changes

Maelu is not a competitive athlete and therefore is not attempting to prepare for a particular competition or season. She is interested in general fitness, and the purpose of her resistance training is to increase upper-body strength and improve lower-body strength to prevent injury. The major goals of chronic manipulations (classic strength and power periodization) are to prepare the individual for a particular season or competition and to ensure optimal or maximal continued gains in fitness and strength. Because these are not the goals of Maelu's program, a great deal of chronic manipulation is unnecessary. However, recent data (Kraemer et al. 2000; Marx et al. 2001) showing enhanced strength and power development as a result of undulating periodization indicate that she should try using heavy days with 3 to 5RM and 6 to 8RM resistances 1 or 2 days per week at points in her training program.

Maelu may, however, consider two other chronic manipulations of her program. One is to periodically substitute different exercises that stress the same muscle group for exercises already in her program. Examples of this are substituting squats or leg presses for knee extensions and knee flexions, bench presses for military presses, and bent-over rowing for lat pull-downs. This will help to keep the program from becoming tedious. Finally, Maelu should continually try to shorten her rest periods. This will decrease the amount of time necessary to complete a workout and improve Maelu's local muscular endurance.

Table 5.5 Training for Case Study 2

Chest exercise	
Bench press	12, 10, 10
Back exercise	
Lat pull-down	10, 10, 10
Abdomen exercises	
Bent-leg sit-ups	15, 15
Knee-ups	15, 15
Arm/shoulder exercises	
Military press	12, 10, 10
Arm curls	12, 10, 10
Leg exercises	
Knee extensions	15, 15, 15
Knee flexions	15, 15, 15
Toe raises	15, 15

— Case Study Three —

Joan is a women's collegiate volleyball coach. After a rather poor season last year, she decided to initiate an off-season resistance training program to help improve the team's performance. Joan has ideas as to what the goals of a resistance training program for women's volleyball should be. To make these goals more specific, however, she conducted a literature search concerning women's volleyball and discovered that several training factors have been found to be related to performance, including vertical jumping ability (Fleck et al. 1985; Gladden and Colacino 1978; Spence et al. 1980), upper-body and arm strength (Morrow et al. 1979), and low percentage of body fat (Fleck et al. 1985; Morrow et al. 1979). The goals of Joan's program are to increase vertical jumping ability and upper-body strength and to decrease the percentage of body fat. The exercises chosen to fulfill the needs are outlined in table 5.6.

Because of the arrangement of the weight room and limited time, Joan decided to run the program as a timed circuit allowing 30 seconds to perform the exercise and 1 minute of rest between exercises. She placed the athletes in groups of three, which provided spotters for each exercise and assistance in changing the resistance needed for each exercise. The athletes would begin training using a 10RM; when they could complete all three circuits of an individual exercise with the 10RM, she would increase the resistance. Resistance training was performed on Monday, Wednesday, and Friday. Joan also had team meetings in which she discussed proper diet and caloric balance. The aim of these meetings was to educate her players in the role these factors play in weight control and athletic performance.

Chronic Manipulations

Joan decided to start the resistance training program 9 weeks before the onset of the volleyball season. She decided to incorporate the concept of periodization: For the first 4 weeks the team performed the original workout; weeks 5, 6, and 7 called for exercises at 8RM; and for the last two weeks the team performed the exercises at 5RM. The rest periods diminished from 50 seconds to 40 seconds and finally to 30 seconds during the last 2 weeks of the program. In addition, for the last 5 weeks of the program the team performed plyometric jumping exercises on Tuesday, Thursday, and Saturday. Joan also found that an alternative workout using only structural exercises or integration and substitution of various structural exercises into her 3-days-a-week program could benefit the development of total body power and single leg strength. Such exercises are hang cleans, hang pulls, spilt squats, side squats, power snatches, lunges, and push presses.

Table 5.6 Training for Case Study 3		
	Sets	Repetitions
Hang cleans	3	5
Incline press	3	10
Squats	3	10
Lat pull-downs	3	10
Sit-ups	3	20
Toe raises	3	10
Wrist curls	3	10
Back extensions	3	10
Leg extensions	3	10
Leg curls	3	10

Summary

The combination of various program variables make up the exercise stimuli configuration that is presented to the body. The purpose of program design is to produce the most effective combination of training variables to create the desired stimuli so that adaptation will occur specifically in the manner desired. In many ways the prescription of resistance exercise has for a long time been more of an art than a science, leading to many myths, fads, and systems that are related more to philosophy than to fact. However, the growing number of scientific studies on resistance training continues to expand our understanding and can play a vital role in the exercise prescription process by providing guidelines for proper prescription. No matter how much science is available, the responsibility for making sound decisions concerning each program will rest with the coach, the personal trainer, or the individual. In each case a greater understanding of the knowledge base will help with training guidelines and offer initial answers to questions of program design. Program decisions should be based on a sound rationale and have some basis in scientific fact. This chapter addressed the developmental process of program design. We will cover chronic programming of resistance training, most notably periodization of training, in chapter 7. The next chapter offers descriptions of many systems of resistance training that have evolved over time. The framework presented in this chapter will help you understand each of these systems.

Key Terms

acute program variables
body-part exercises
capping
choice of exercise
compensatory acceleration
isolated single-joint exercises
needs analysis
prehabilitation
program design
progression
repetition speed
RM target
RM target zone
single-muscle-group exercises
specificity
structural or multijoint exercises
transfer specificity
window of adaptation

Selected Readings

American College of Sports Medicine. 2002. Position stand. Progression models in resistance training for healthy adults. *Medicine and Science in Sports and Exercise* 34: 364-380.

Calder, A.W., Chilibeck, P.D., Webber, C.E., and Sale, D.G. 1994. Comparison of whole and split weight training routines in young women. *Canadian Journal of Applied Physiology* 19: 185-199.

Hoffman, J.R., Kraemer, W.J., Fry, A.C., Deschenes, M., and Kemp, M. 1990. The effects of self-selection for frequency of training in a winter conditioning program for football. *Journal of Applied Sport Science Research* 4: 76-82.

Jones, K., Hunter, G., Fleisig, G., Escamilla, R., and Lemak, L. 1999. The effects of compensatory acceleration on upper-body strength and power in collegiate football players. *Journal of Strength and Conditioning Research* 13: 99-105.

Keogh, J.W.L., Wilson, G.J., and Weatherby, R.P. 1999. A cross-sectional comparison of different resistance training techniques in the bench press. *Journal of Strength and Conditioning Research* 13: 247-258.

Kraemer, W.J. 1997. A series of studies: The physiological basis for strength training in American football: Fact over philosophy. *Journal of Strength and Conditioning Research* 11: 131-142.

Kraemer, W.J., Duncan, N.D., and Harman, F.S. 1998. Physiologic basis for strength training in the prevention of and rehabilitation from injury. In *Rehabilitation in sports medicine*, edited by P.K. Canavan, 49-59. Stamford, CT: Appleton and Lange.

Kraemer, W.J., and Fry, A.C. 1995. Strength testing: Development and evaluation of methodology. In *Physiological assessment of human fitness*, edited by P. Maud and C. Foster. Champaign, IL: Human Kinetics.

Kraemer, W.J., and Gómez, A.L. 2001. Establishing a solid fitness base. In *High-performance sports conditioning*, edited by B. Foran, 3-16. Champaign, IL: Human Kinetics.

Kraemer, W.J., and Gotshalk, L.A. 2000. Physiology of American football. In *Exercise and sport science*, edited by W.E. Garrett and D.T. Kirkendall, 798-813. Philadelphia: Lippincott, Williams & Wilkins.

Kraemer, W.J., Mazzetti, S.A., Ratamess, N.A., and Fleck, S.J. 2000. Specificity of training modes. In *Isokinetics in human performance*, edited by L.E. Brown, 25-41. Champaign, IL: Human Kinetics.

Kraemer, W.J., and Nindl, B.A. 1998. Factors involved with overtraining for strength and power. In *Overtraining in athletic conditioning*, 69-86. Champaign, IL: Human Kinetics.

Kraemer, W.J., and Newton, R.U. 2000. Training for muscular power. In *Clinics in sports medicine*, edited by J. Young, 341-368. Philadelphia: W.B. Saunders.

Kraemer, W.J., and Ratamess, N.A. 2000. Physiology of resistance training: Current issues. In *Orthopaedic physical therapy clinics of North America*, edited by C. Hughes, 467-513. Philadelphia: W.B. Saunders

Kraemer, W.J., Ratamess, N.A., and Rubin, M.R. 2000. Basic principles of resistance training. In *Nutrition and the strength athlete*, 1-29. Boca Raton, FL: CRC Press.

Mazzetti, S.A., Kraemer, W.J., Volek, J.S., Duncan, N.D., Ratamess, N.A., Gómez, A.L., Newton, R.U., Häkkinen, K., and Fleck, S.J. 2000. The influence of direct supervision of resistance training on strength performance. *Medicine and Science in Sports and Exercise* 32: 1043-1050.

Mazzetti, S.A., Ratamess, N.A., and Kraemer, W.J. 2000. Pumping down: After years of bulking up, when they graduate, strength-trained athletes must be shown how to safely detrain. *Training and Conditioning* 10: 10-13.

Pearson, D., Faigenbaum, A., Conley, M., and Kraemer, W.J. 2000. The National Strength and Conditioning Association's basic guidelines for the resistance training of athletes. *Strength and Conditioning Journal* 22 (4): 14-30.

Sforzo, G.A., and Touey, P.R. 1996. Manipulating exercise order affects muscular performance during a resistance exercise training session. *Journal of Strength and Conditioning Research* 10: 20-24.

CHAPTER 6

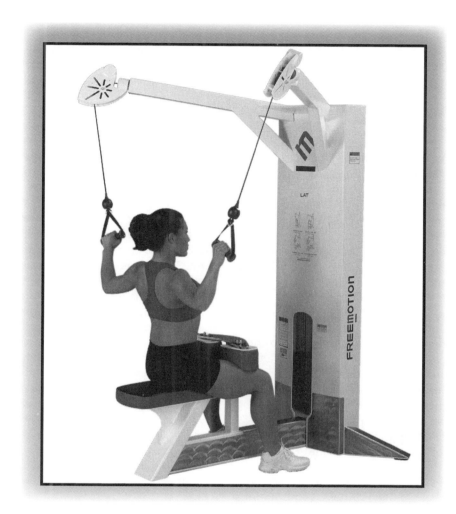

Resistance Training Systems and Techniques

Most resistance training systems and techniques were originally designed by strength coaches, power lifters, Olympic weightlifters, bodybuilders, or personal trainers to meet the needs and goals of a specific group, with the majority originally designed for young, healthy adults. The needs and goals of a group include not only training outcomes, such as increased strength or changes in body composition, but also administrative concerns, such as total training time available or equipment availability.

The fact that a system or technique has been used by enough people to have name recognition indicates that it has had success in bringing about desired training adaptations for a particular group. However, virtually any weight training system or technique, when performed consistently, will bring about training adaptations over short training periods, especially in untrained individuals. Generally, specific systems and techniques are popular not because they have been shown scientifically to be superior to other systems or techniques in terms of bringing about changes in strength, power, or body composition. Rather, they are popular because an individual, group, or company has marketed them. A system or technique may also be popular with a specific group because of administrative considerations, such as requiring less time to perform than another system or technique.

A great deal of speculation exists about why various systems and techniques are effective or how certain systems physiologically cause particular training adaptations. Generally, more research is needed, especially in resistance-trained individuals, concerning the effectiveness of all training systems and techniques. In particular, long-term studies (i.e., 6 to 9 months or longer) are needed to demonstrate whether a particular system or technique brings about continued gains in fitness or results in a training plateau after several months of training. Knowledge of the various systems and techniques is of value when attempting to design a training program to meet the training goals and needs as well as the administrative concerns for a particular individual or group. Different systems and techniques are also of value when a person encounters a training plateau, because a change in training is one way to move beyond a training plateau.

The variety of training systems and techniques demonstrates the vast array of acute training variable combinations that have been used and demonstrates the almost limitless combinations of acute training variables possible. Many practitioners adapt one training system or technique and then apply only that system to all individuals for long periods. Performance of nonvaried training over months of training can lead to a training plateau in strength, power, and body composition (Kraemer et al. 2000; Marx et al. 2001; Willoughby 1993). Additionally, indefinite use of one system or technique can result in a strength plateau after different training durations (Willoughby 1993). Thus, indefinite use of a single system or technique can lead to less-than-optimal fitness gains, and strength gains may plateau after different training durations for different muscle groups. The use of different training systems and techniques is one way to bring training variation into a program and therefore help to avoid training plateaus.

One common mistake novice practitioners make is to assume that a system or technique used by a champion bodybuilder, power lifter, Olympic weightlifter, or other type of athlete is best for a novice lifter or recreational athlete. Programs used by elite athletes are often too intense or have training volumes that are too high for the novice lifter or recreational athlete. It may have taken years of training for elite athletes to achieve the fitness levels necessary to tolerate the programs they are currently using. Elite strength and power athletes also have a genetic potential for superior strength, muscle hypertrophy, or both that allows them to tolerate the intense or high-volume programs they are currently using and still achieve gains in strength, power, and hypertrophy.

A training record is invaluable for determining which training system or variation of a system or technique works best for an individual, group, or team. Without a detailed record of workouts, a person will not remember enough details to repeat the progression of a program that was successful in bringing about fitness gains. Furthermore, the sets, repetitions, exercises, and resistances used in a program need to be documented for use in planning the next training session. Training records answer many questions concerning an individual's response to a particular program, including which system or technique works best and how long the trainee can continue with that particular system before reaching a plateau. Training logs are also motivational for many people because progress is documented and easily seen over the course of weeks or months of training.

Single-Set System

The **single-set system**, the performance of each exercise for one set, is one of the oldest resistance training systems. A single-set system described in 1925 (Liederman 1925) consisted of using heavy resistances and a few repetitions per set with a 5-minute rest between exercises. Single-set systems are still popular, and a single-set system of 8 to 12 repetitions per set to volitional fatigue has been recommended as a time-efficient way to develop and maintain muscular fitness in the recreational weight trainer or fitness enthusiast (American College of Sports Medicine 1998). Single-set systems do result in significant increases in strength and significant changes in body composition

(American College of Sports Medicine 1998). Some studies comparing nonvaried multiple-set systems to a nonvaried single-set system report no significant difference in fitness gains in up to 25 weeks of training (American College of Sports Medicine 2002; Leighton et al. 1967; Starkey et al. 1996). However, studies also report significantly greater gains in fitness with nonvaried multiple-set systems compared to nonvaried single-set systems (American College of Sports Medicine 2002; Burst et al. 2001; Kramer et al. 1997). Comparisons of various multiple-set periodized systems to nonvaried single-set systems in all cases show the periodized systems to result in greater increases and in most cases significantly greater increases in strength, increases in motor performance, and body composition changes (Fleck 1999; Kraemer et al. 1997, 2000; Marx et al. 2001).

Thus, a single-set system, although resulting in significant fitness gains, is not the best overall system. Single-set systems are a reasonable choice for individuals with very little time to dedicate to resistance training, and for athletes during an in-season program or any other training phase when they have less time to dedicate to resistance training.

Express Circuit

Personal trainers sometimes develop express circuits for clients with minimal time available for resistance, as well as any other type of fitness training. Express circuits are typically a variation of a single-set system. Normally, one set of 6 to 12 repetitions of each exercise is performed with 30 seconds to 1 minute of rest between exercises. Express circuits can use both multijoint and single-joint exercises and typically involve one exercise for each major muscle group. An express circuit has all the advantages and limitations of a single-set system.

Multiple-Set System

A multiple-set system can involve performing multiple sets with the same resistance; with varying resistances (i.e. heavy-to-light, light-to-heavy); with varying numbers or the same number of repetitions per set; and with all, some, or no sets carried to volitional fatigue. Virtually any training system that consists of more than one set of an exercise can be classified as a multiple-set system. One of the original multiple-set systems consisted of two to three warm-up sets of increas-ing resistance followed by several sets at the same resistance. This training system became popular in the 1940s (Darden 1973) and appears to be the forerunner of the vast array of multiple-set systems of today.

Although multiple-set systems have been shown to produce fitness gains in such areas as strength and body composition, performance of a multiple-set system with no change in training variables for long periods of time can result in a plateau in strength (Willoughby 1993). Additionally, comparisons (see chapter 7) of periodized multiple-set systems and nonvaried multiple-set systems have generally shown the periodized systems to result in greater fitness gains (Fleck 1999).

Bulk System

The bulk system refers specifically to a multiple-set system of three sets of 5 to 6 repetitions, normally with a 5 to 6RM resistance per exercise. A comparative study of 10 resistance training systems and techniques did include the bulk system (Leighton et al. 1967). The major weaknesses of the study were the fact that all of the systems and techniques, except for an isometric system, trained dynamically, but strength was tested isometrically, and the fact that untrained individuals served as subjects. Nevertheless, some insight can be gained from this investigation. This study trained college students twice a week for 8 weeks. Each group was composed of 20 to 29 individuals. The exercises performed with each system were the two-armed arm curl, two-armed arm press, lat pull-down, half squat, sit-up, side bend, leg press, knee curl, toe raise, and bench press. Isometric or static maximal strength was determined pre- and posttraining. The bulk system was one of the most effective systems in causing increases in the isometric strength of the back and legs over the short 8-week training period (see table 6.1). Therefore, this system may be valuable for increasing general leg and back strength during short-term training periods, such as immediate preseason training for a sport.

Circuit System

A circuit system consists of a series of resistance training exercises performed in succession with minimal rest (15 to 30 seconds) between exercises. Approximately 10 to 15 repetitions of each exercise are performed per circuit with a resistance of 40 to 60% of 1RM. Generally, several

Table 6.1 Comparison of Isometric Strength Gains Due to Nine Resistance Training Systems

	Bulk	Cheat system	Delorme	Descending half-triangle	Double progressive	Isometric[a]	Oxford	Supersetting	Triset
Elbow flexion	8*	23*	9*	11*	7	0	7*	12*	25*
Elbow extension	9	66**	16	9**	25*	35*	28**	9	30**
Back and leg	24**	27*	0	24*	13	−5	11	21*	17*

Strength values given are percent change pre- to posttraining; ** = significant increase pre- to posttraining at 0.01 level of significance; * = significant increase pre- to posttraining at 0.05 level of significance; [a] = isometric training consisted of one maximal action 6 seconds in duration; Oxford is a heavy-to-light system; Delorme is a light-to-heavy system.

Adapted, by permission, from J.R. Leighton, et al., 1967, "A study of the effectiveness of ten different methods of progressive resistance exercise on the development of strength, flexibility, girth and body weight," *Journal of the Association for Physical and Mental Rehabilitation* 21: 79.

circuits of the exercises are performed. When one set of each exercise is performed, the training protocol would more likely be termed an express circuit. The exercises can be chosen to train any muscle group. This system is very time efficient with large numbers of people because each piece of equipment is virtually in constant use. It is also very time efficient for an individual with a limited amount of training time.

The use of 40 to 60% of 1RM for performing 10 to 15 repetitions for some exercises will result in the set not being performed close to volitional fatigue and therefore may limit gains in maximal strength. In untrained males, untrained females, trained males, and trained females, the number of repetitions in a set carried to volitional fatigue of the leg press ranges from 78 to 146 repetitions with 40% of 1RM and from 34 to 57 repetitions with 60% of 1RM (Hoeger et al. 1990). Substantially more than 10 to 15 repetitions per set of the lat pull-down can also be performed at these percentages of 1RM. Thus, if one goal of a circuit system is to increase maximal strength, it may be advisable to increase the percentage of 1RM used in many exercises, or to design the circuit using 10 to 15RM resistances for the exercises.

One proposed benefit of a circuit system is improved cardiovascular fitness. This benefit is in part related to the use of short rest periods between exercises, which result in the heart rate remaining elevated during the entire circuit. Short-duration (8 to 20 weeks) circuit systems increase peak oxygen consumption approximately 4% and 8% in men and women, respectively (Gettman and Pollock 1981). This is substantially less, however, than the 15 to 20% increase in peak oxygen

consumption caused by traditional running, cycling, or swimming cardiovascular conditioning programs over the same time period. If subjects are already physically active or aerobically fit, even less improvement in peak oxygen consumption can be expected from a circuit system.

If one goal of a weight training system is to increase cardiovascular endurance, then a variation of a circuit is the system of choice. However, if a major goal of the total conditioning program is to maximally improve cardiovascular fitness, then a traditional endurance-training component, such as running, cycling, or swimming, needs to be included in the total training program.

Peripheral Heart Action System

This system is a variation of the circuit system. A training session using the peripheral heart action system is divided into several sequences (Gaja 1965). A sequence is a group of four to six different exercises, each for a different body part. The number of repetitions per set of each exercise in a sequence varies with the goals of the program, but normally 8 to 12 repetitions per set are performed. One training session consists of performing all the exercises in the first sequence three times in a circuit fashion. The remaining sequences are then performed one after the other in the same fashion as the first sequence. An example of the exercises in a peripheral heart action training session is given in table 6.2.

Because the heart rate is kept relatively high with a peripheral heart action system, it is very fatiguing. The short rest periods and maintenance of a relatively high heart rate make this program

Table 6.2 Example of a Four-Sequence Peripheral Heart Action Training Session

Body part	Sequence			
	1	2	3	4
Chest	Bench press	Incline press	Decline bench	Chest fly
Back	Lat pull-down	Seated row	Bent-over row	T-bar row
Shoulders	Military press	Upright row	Lateral raise	Front shoulder raise
Legs	Squat	Knee extension	Back squat	Split squat
Abdomen	Sit-up	Crunch	Roman chair sit-up	V-up

very similar to normal circuit training. Therefore, the peripheral heart action system is a good resistance training system for increasing cardiovascular fitness as well as local muscular endurance.

Triset System

The triset system is similar to the peripheral heart action system in that it incorporates groups or sequences of exercises. As the name implies, it consists of groups of three exercises. The exercises performed in a triset are for the same major body segment, such as the arms or the legs, but can train different muscle groups. Little or no rest between exercises is allowed, and normally three sets of each exercise are performed. The exercises constituting a triset are, for example, arm curls, triceps extensions, and military presses. Trisets have been shown to be a very effective system for increasing static strength (see table 6.1). The short rest periods and the use of three exercises in series for a particular body part or segment make this a good system when a training goal is to increase local muscular endurance.

Double Progressive System

In the double progressive system both the number of repetitions per set and the resistance used are varied. During the first several sets the resistance is held constant while the number of repetitions per set is increased until a specified number of sets has been performed. The resistance is then increased and the number of repetitions per set decreased until the number of repetitions performed has returned to the number performed in the first set. This process is then repeated for each exercise performed. An example of this system is given in table 6.3. Of the systems compared in table 6.1 the double progressive system appears

Table 6.3 Example of the Double Progressive System

Set	Repetitions	Resistance (lb)
1	4	120
2	6	120
3	8	120
4	10	120
5	12	120
6	10	140
7	8	160
8	6	175
9	4	185

to be one of the least effective for increasing isometric strength. The double progressive system is very time consuming. Additionally, the first sets performed appear to be warm-up sets, because they are not performed to volitional fatigue because more repetitions in successive sets with the resistance used can be performed. Although minimal, research indicates that the use of the double progressive system is unwarranted.

Multipoundage System

Safe performance of a multipoundage system with free weights requires one or two spotters to assist during a training session. If machines are used, spotters may not be needed. The trainee performs 4 or 5 repetitions at a 4 or 5RM resistance. Then the resistance is decreased, and the trainee performs another set of 4 or 5 repetitions.

This procedure is continued for several sets (Poole 1964). The number of sets possible depends on the original resistance used and the goals of the program. Some bodybuilders believe that this system results in increased vascularity and that the large volume of training that can be performed in a short period of time contributes to the development of muscular hypertrophy. The performance of several sets of an exercise in rapid succession probably results in high intramuscular concentrations of lactic acid, making this a good system for increasing local muscular endurance.

Breakdown Training

Breakdown training is similar to the multipoundage system in that the resistance is decreased to allow the performance of additional repetitions. After the trainee performs a set to voluntary muscular fatigue, the resistance is immediately reduced so that an additional 2 to 4 repetitions can be performed. Westcott (1994) reported increases in strength as a result of breakdown training. In this study, beginning weight trainers performed one set of 10 to 12 repetitions at a 10 to 12RM resistance for 1 month. During the next month of training half of the subjects continued with this program while the other half performed breakdown training. After reaching volitional fatigue, the resistance of the subjects performing breakdown training was reduced by 10 lb (4.5 kg) and they performed an additional 2 to 4 repetitions. The average increase in resistance used for training was 7 lb (3.2 kg) more with breakdown training at the end of the 2 months of training. The study did not statistically analyze if this difference between groups was significant. Because one group performed the same training program for the entire 2 months of training while the other group performed one type of training for 1 month and another type (breakdown training) for the second month, these results could be interpreted to mean that training variation and not breakdown training per se resulted in the additional strength gain. However, the project does indicate that breakdown training can increase strength in untrained individuals.

Superpump System

Proponents of the superpump system believe that advanced bodybuilders need to perform 15 to 18 sets for each body part per training session to achieve the desired muscular development

and definition (Page 1966). To achieve this high number of sets, anywhere from one to three exercises per muscle group are performed per training session. This system uses 15-second rest periods between sets of 5 to 6 repetitions (Page 1966). All repetitions are performed with strict adherence to correct exercise technique, and each muscle group is trained two to three times per week. The superpump system may be effective for advanced lifters who desire greater muscular hypertrophy of the arms, chest, and shoulders. This system may be too fatiguing to use when training the large muscles of the legs and back (Darden 1973).

Triangle System

Many power lifters and individuals interested in increasing 1RM lifting ability use triangle or pyramid systems. A complete triangle or pyramid system begins with a set of 10 to 12 repetitions with a light resistance. The resistance is then increased over several sets so that fewer and fewer repetitions are performed, until only a 1RM is performed. Then the same sets and resistances are repeated in reverse order, with the last set consisting of 10 to 12 repetitions (see figure 6.1). Generally, the resistance used and the number of repetitions performed are close to RMs. Any combination of repetition numbers per set can be termed a pyramid system as long as the number of repetitions per set increases initially and then decreases.

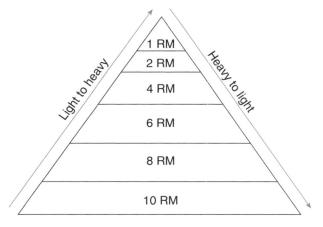

Figure 6.1 Performing sets that progress from light to heavy resistances is a light-to-heavy system (ascending half-pyramid). Performing sets that progress from heavy to light resistances is a heavy-to-light system (descending half-pyramid). A full pyramid, or triangle, consists of both the ascending and descending portions of the pyramid.

Light-to-Heavy System

As the name implies, the light-to-heavy system involves progressing from light to heavy resistances. One variation of this system became popular in the 1930s and 1940s among Olympic lifters (Hatfield and Krotee 1978). It consists of performing a set of 3 to 5 repetitions with a relatively light resistance. Five pounds (2.3 kg) are then added to the resistance, and another set of 3 to 5 repetitions is performed. This is continued until only 1 repetition can be performed. The Delorme regime, one of the earliest systems scientifically examined, consists of three sets of 10 repetitions with the resistance progressing from 50%, to 66%, and then to 100% of 10RM in successive sets; this can be termed a light-to-heavy system. This system causes significant increases in strength over short-term training periods (Delorme, Ferris, and Gallagher 1952; Delorme and Watkins 1948). The Delorme system was evaluated in the study depicted in table 6.1 and demonstrated a significant increase in isometric elbow flexion, but no significant increases in isometric elbow extension or back and leg strength.

Another type of light-to-heavy system is the ascending half-triangle or ascending half-pyramid (see figure 6.1). In this system only the first half of a triangle system (progressing from higher numbers of repetitions per set with a light resistance to smaller numbers of repetitions per set with heavier resistances) is performed. A variation of an ascending half-triangle system was one of the more effective systems for increasing isometric back and leg strength in the study depicted in table 6.1.

Heavy-to-Light System

In a heavy-to-light system, after a few warm-up sets, the heaviest set is performed, and then the resistance is reduced for each succeeding set. The Oxford system, a relatively old training system, is a heavy-to-light system consisting of three sets of 10 repetitions progressing from 100%, to 66%, and then to 50% of 10RM in each succeeding set. Significant gains in strength have been demonstrated with the Oxford system (McMorris and Elkins 1954; Zinovieff 1951). The Oxford system was evaluated in the study depicted in table 6.1 and demonstrated significant increases in isometric elbow flexion and elbow extension, but a nonsignificant change in back and leg strength. Comparisons of the heavy-to-light Oxford system and the light-to-heavy Delorme system are equivocal in terms of strength gain. One study found the heavy-to-light system to be superior to the light-to-heavy system in strength gains, but indicated that further research is necessary (McMorris and Elkins 1954). The study depicted in table 6.1 found little difference between the two systems for increasing isometric elbow-flexion strength, but found that the heavy-to-light Oxford system was superior to the light-to-heavy Delorme system for increasing isometric elbow extension and back and leg strength.

Some heavy-to-light systems can also be termed a descending half-triangle or descending half-pyramid (see figure 6.1). In this type of heavy-to-light system the first set performed is the heaviest set with the fewest repetitions; the resistance is then decreased and the number of repetitions increased.

Exercise Order Systems

Exercise order systems dictate the order in which exercises are performed. There are two major types of exercise order. The first is the **alternating muscle group order**, in which the trainee alternates exercises for different muscle groups. The second requires performing exercises for the same muscle group in succession and is commonly termed the **stacking exercise order**. All exercise order systems are some derivation of these two concepts.

Compound-Set System

The compound-set system is used by some bodybuilders to develop muscular hypertrophy (Hatfield 1981). This system involves alternating muscle groups as is done in many fitness and circuit weight training programs. For example, when using this system, the trainee performs one exercise for one muscle group and then, after little or no rest, another exercise for a muscle group in a different part of the body. This alternating of exercises for different muscle groups continues until the trainee has completed the desired number of sets. As in any system using alternating muscle groups, the first muscle group partially recovers while the second is being exercised, and vice versa. As an example, arm curls and knee extensions may be alternated in the compound-set system. The use of little or no rest period between exercises allows the performance of a large number of sets in a relatively short period of time, making this system a good choice for lifters with a minimal amount of training time.

Flushing

This system was developed by bodybuilders to produce hypertrophy, definition, and vascularity. The number of exercises, sets, repetitions per set, and rest periods is not clearly defined. Flushing involves performing two or more exercises for the same muscle group or for two muscle groups in close proximity to each other. The hypothesis behind flushing is to keep blood in the muscle group or groups for a long period of time. It is believed that this will help develop muscle hypertrophy. Many bodybuilders do train a muscle group with several exercises in succession during the same training session, so practical experience indicates that this practice may result in hypertrophy. It is unknown how blood flow mediates changes in hypertrophy, and such mechanisms are speculative. One hypothesis is that higher blood flow allows more of the body's natural anabolic factors found in the blood, such as growth hormone or testosterone, to bind to receptors in muscle and connective tissue. Another hypothesis is that increased blood flow increases the temporary hypertrophy caused by fluid leaving the blood plasma and entering the muscle. The temporary hypertrophy caused by weight training is also called the "pump." Increased cell volume as a result of increased water content has been shown to be one of the regulating factors of protein synthesis (Waldeger et al. 1997). Over time this could result in increased muscle hypertrophy. However, such speculation lacks sound supporting scientific evidence.

Priority System

The priority system can be applied to virtually all resistance training systems. It involves performing the exercises that apply to the training program's major goal(s) first in a training session, so that the trainee can perform these exercises with maximal intensity. For example, if single-joint exercises involving the muscles in the squat or bench press are performed before these exercises, total force (repetitions times weight lifted) is less and fatigue rate is greater in the bench press and squat (Sforzo and Touey 1996). The same is true for the single-joint exercises if the order is reversed. If exercises relating to the program's major goal(s) are performed late in the training session, fatigue may prevent the trainee from using maximal resistances for the desired number of repetitions, which may limit adaptation to the training.

For example, a bodybuilder's weakest muscle group in terms of definition and hypertrophy may be the quadriceps group. Using the priority concept, exercises for the quadriceps group would be performed at the beginning of the training session. A basketball coach may decide that a power forward's greatest weakness is lack of upper-body strength, which causes the player to be pushed around under the boards. Thus, major upper-body exercises would be placed at the beginning of the training session for this player. Likewise, an American football player may want to promote strength and power development of the hips and low back, and therefore would perform exercises meant to develop this characteristic, such as hang cleans and squats, at the beginning of the training session.

Supersetting Systems

Supersetting has evolved into two distinct systems. One system uses several sets of two exercises for the agonist and antagonistic muscle groups of one body part. Examples of this type of supersetting are arm curls alternated with triceps extensions or knee extensions alternated with knee curls. Significant increases in strength from this type of supersetting have been reported (see table 6.1). Of the nine systems compared in table 6.1, this type of supersetting is one of the most effective for increasing back and leg isometric strength.

The second type of supersetting is similar to the triset system. This type involves performing one set of two to three exercises in rapid succession for the same muscle group or body part (e.g., lat pull-downs, seated rows, and bent-over rows). This type of supersetting has resulted in significant strength gains, changes in body composition, and increases in vertical jump performance when performed as part of a periodized weight training program (Kraemer 1997).

Both types of supersetting typically involve sets of 8 to 10 or more repetitions with little or no rest between sets and exercises. Supersetting has been popular among bodybuilders, suggesting that these systems result in muscular hypertrophy. Because of the short rest periods between sets and the exercises used, blood lactic acid probably increases substantially, indicating that these systems increase local muscular endurance.

Split Routine System

Many bodybuilders use a split routine system and perform several exercises for the same body part in a training session to encourage hypertrophy. Because this is a time-consuming process, not all body parts are exercised in a single training session. This has led to training various body parts on alternate days, or a split routine. Many variations of the split routine are possible. An example of a split routine would be training the arms, legs, and abdomen on Monday, Wednesday, and Friday and the chest, shoulders, and back on Tuesday, Thursday, and Saturday. The example system allows the performance of several exercises for a body part in a training session of reasonable length, but means that training is performed 6 days per week.

Variations of the split routine system can be developed so that training sessions take place 4 or 5 days per week. Even though training sessions are quite frequent, sufficient recovery of muscle groups between training sessions is possible because body parts are not trained on successive days. A split routine system allows the training intensity for a particular body part or group of exercises to be higher than would be possible if the four to six sessions were combined into two or three long sessions of equivalent training volume. It is also possible to develop split routines in which the total training volume per body part is higher than that in a typical total body training session because in a split routine each training session is dedicated to a smaller number of body parts or muscle groups.

In highly strength trained athletes (e.g., college football players) short-term (10-week) strength gains in the bench press and squat exercises in part depend on the use of assistance exercises (Hoffman et al. 1990). Split routines can allow performance of more assistance exercises and so may also be useful for enhancing strength development.

A comparison of a total body training routine and a split system routine in young women who were previously not weight trained demonstrated no significant differences between groups in 1RM ability, fat-free mass, or percent body fat changes (Calder et al. 1994). The total-body group performed four upper-body (five sets, 6-10RM) and three lower-body (five sets, 10-12RM) exercises per session twice a week for 20 weeks. The split-routine group used the same exercises and set repetition scheme, but performed both the upper- and the lower-body exercises 2 days per week for a total of four training sessions on 4 different days per week. The results indicate that total-body and split-routine systems using the same total training volume produce similar results in healthy young women during the first 20 weeks of training.

Blitz or Isolated Split System

The blitz or isolated split system is a variation of the split routine system. Rather than training several body parts during each training session, only one body part is trained per session. The duration of the training session is not reduced. Thus, more sets and exercises per body part can be performed. An example blitz system is to perform all arm, chest, leg, trunk, back, and shoulder exercises on Monday through Saturday, respectively. Some bodybuilders have performed this type of program in preparation for a contest. A short-duration blitz program may also be appropriate if an athlete's performance is limited by the strength of a particular muscle group or groups. A long jumper might perform a variation of a blitz program for the legs before the start of the season, which might involve training only the legs 2 days per week.

Isolated Exercise System

This system devotes an entire training session to a single exercise (Horvath 1959). For example, on Monday only the bench press is performed; Tuesday, the squat; Thursday, the lat pull-down; and Friday, the deadlift. Other exercises can be added to achieve as many training days or sessions per week as desired. A resistance is selected that allows 8 to 10 repetitions to be performed. The trainee then performs set after set of that day's exercise for as many sets and repetitions as possible in 1 to 1.5 hours. A 1-minute period is allowed between sets.

The isolated exercise system is very fatiguing for the muscle group(s) involved, and a great deal of stress is placed on the joints involved in each exercise performed. This system is not recommended for more than 6 consecutive weeks (Horvath 1959). Similar to the blitz system, variations of this system may be appropriate for a short duration if an athlete's performance is limited by one particular muscle group. Some bodybuilders have used this program in an attempt to stimulate hypertrophy of a particular muscle or muscle group. However, the effectiveness of the system remains uninvestigated. Long-term use of this system may result in an overuse or overtraining syndrome of the muscle group(s) or joints involved. Therefore, a strong rationale for using this system is needed, and careful monitoring of trainees using this system is crucial.

Training Techniques Applicable to Other Systems

Many training techniques can be used when performing virtually all training systems. For example, trainees can perform partial repetitions when using any training system (e.g., a single-set system or a multiple-set system). The following training techniques are applicable to most types of training systems.

Cheating Technique

The cheating technique is popular among bodybuilders. As the name implies, it involves cheating or breaking strict exercise form (Weider 1954). As an example, rather than maintaining an erect upper body when performing standing barbell arm curls, the lifter uses a slight torso swing to start the barbell moving from the arms-straight position. The torso swing is not grossly exaggerated, but is sufficient to allow the trainee to lift 10 to 20 lb (4.5 to 9.1 kg) more resistance than is possible with strict exercise form. The barbell curl has a bell-shaped strength curve, with the arms-fully-extended position being a very weak position. The strongest position is when the elbow joint is at approximately a 90-degree angle. When barbell curls are performed with strict form, the maximum resistance that can be lifted depends on the resistance that can be moved from the weak, fully extended position. With a constant resistance, therefore, the muscles involved in flexing the elbow are not maximally active during the stronger positions of the exercise's range of motion. The goal of cheating is to allow the use of a heavier resistance, which will force the muscle(s) to develop a force closer to maximal through a greater portion of the exercise's range of motion and thus enhance strength and size gains. Cheating can also be performed at the end of a set once volitional fatigue has occurred.

Lifters should be cautious when using the cheating technique. The heavier resistance and the cheating movement can increase the chance of injury. As an example, the torso-swinging movement when performing arm curls can place additional stress on the low back.

Comparisons of strength gains due to the cheating technique versus those due to various other training systems and techniques indicate that this technique is quite effective (see table 6.1). The cheating technique was one of the most effective techniques in increasing elbow flexion, elbow extension, and back and leg isometric strength. This technique can be used in conjunction with many other training systems; for example, a lifter could cheat during the last set of a multiple-set system.

Exhaustion-Set Technique

An exhaustion set is a set performed until no further complete repetitions with good exercise technique can be completed. Synonymous with exhaustion sets are the terms *carrying sets to volitional fatigue, sets to failure,* and *sets to concentric failure.* Exhaustion sets can be incorporated into virtually any training system. Advocates of exhaustion sets believe that with this technique more motor units are recruited and therefore receive a training stimulus than when sets are not performed to exhaustion. This in turn will lead to greater strength and hypertrophy gains than when sets are not carried to exhaustion. Many training studies and programs describe the training using a term indicating that sets are performed until volitional fatigue. The use of a repetition maximum (RM) or an RM training zone (i.e., 4-6RM) in a training program indicates that sets were carried to exhaustion.

Fitness gains can be achieved when all sets in a training program are carried to momentary exhaustion. However, significant strength, motor performance, and body compositional changes have also been shown when some, but not all, sets in a training program were carried to exhaustion (Marx et al. 2001; Stone et al. 2000). Significantly greater gains in strength have also been reported when no sets in multiple-set programs are carried to failure compared to a single-set program in which all sets were carried to momentary muscular failure (Kramer et al. 1997). In fact, these studies reported greater fitness gains with periodized programs in which not all sets were carried to exhaustion compared to single-set and multiple-set programs in which all sets were carried to exhaustion. It is important to note that in these studies, even though some sets were not carried to complete exhaustion, the number of repetitions performed and resistances used resulted in sets being performed close to volitional fatigue. Sets to exhaustion or at least close to exhaustion do appear to be necessary to bring about fitness gains.

In some exercises, such as power cleans or power snatches, even though a set may not be carried to complete exhaustion, fatigue of some motor units has occurred. Even if another repetition can be performed with good exercise technique, maximal velocity with which the bar is moving may be decreased, indicating fatigue of some motor units. A slowing of maximal velocity in these exercises may be indicated by a greater knee angle when the bar is caught. Thus, from the perspective of maximal achievable bar velocity, the set has been carried to a point of momentary exhaustion of some motor units.

Burn Technique

The burn technique is an extension of the exhaustion-set technique. This technique can be incorporated into any other training system. After a set has been performed to momentary concentric failure or to exhaustion, the lifter performs half or partial repetitions. Normally 5 to 6 partial repetitions are performed, which cause an aching or burning sensation, giving this system its name (Richford 1966). The burning sensation is likely due in part to an increased intramuscular concentration of lactic acid. Similar to the forced repetition technique (discussed next), advocates of the burn technique believe that by performing partial repetitions in a fatigued state, more motor units will be fatigued resulting in greater gains in strength and hypertrophy. Some believe this technique is especially effective in training the calves and arms.

Forced Repetition or Assisted Repetition Technique

One form of the forced repetition or assisted repetition technique is an extension of the exhaustion-set technique. After a trainee has completed a set to exhaustion, training partner(s) assist the trainee by lifting the resistance just enough to allow completion of 2 to 4 more repetitions. Assistance is only provided during the concentric or lifting phase of repetitions, as it is still possible to perform the eccentric or lowering phase without assistance. To some weight trainers, forced repetitions has also come to mean a type of heavy negative training. With this forced repetition technique 2 to 3 repetitions are performed with a resistance that is greater than or close to the one repetition maximum (1RM) for the exercise. Similar to the first forced repetition technique described, assistance is provided by spotters during the concentric but not the eccentric phase of repetitions.

Advocates of forced repetitions believe that because the muscle is forced to continue to produce force after concentric failure or with a resistance greater than can be lifted during the concentric phase of a repetition, more motor units within the muscle will be fatigued and further gains in strength, hypertrophy, and local muscular endurance will be achieved. Lifters who can lift greater weights in the bench press and squat do lower the resistance more slowly than lifters who lift a lighter resistance (Madsen and McLaughlin 1984; McLaughlin, Dillman, and Lardner 1977). Because the eccentric phase of a repetition is performed without assistance during forced repetitions, it can be hypothesized that this technique may be of value in developing the neural adaptations necessary to lower a heavy resistance with good exercise technique. Therefore, this technique may be of value when attempting to increase the maximal weight possible for one repetition (1RM) in exercises, such as a bench press, in which performing the eccentric portion of a repetition at a slow velocity is advantageous because at a slow velocity the resistance develops little momentum.

Westcott (1995) reported gains in the strength of recreational lifters using assisted repetitions after sets had been carried to exhaustion over 6 weeks of training. This report did not statistically evaluate the gains made with assisted repetitions compared to another training system. A study comparing a single-set circuit system (8-12RM) with forced repetitions to a three-set circuit system without forced repetitions showed that the three-set circuit system resulted in significantly greater gains in bench press and leg press 1RM and the number of repetitions at 80% and 85% of 1RM in the bench press and leg press, respectively (Kraemer 1997). Although confounded by the difference in the number of sets performed, the results do demonstrate that a three-set circuit system results in significantly greater gains in strength than a single-set circuit system with forced repetitions.

Forced or assisted repetitions must be used with caution because muscular soreness may easily develop, especially in lifters not accustomed to this technique. Additionally, because the forced repetitions are performed under conditions of fatigue (after a set has been carried to exhaustion or with a weight too heavy to complete the concentric phase of all repetitions in the set), the lifter will encounter acute discomfort and must attempt to complete the forced repetitions despite discomfort. The spotters need to be extremely attentive and capable of lifting all of the resistance being used if the lifter loses proper exercise technique or is completely fatigued and cannot develop enough muscular force to complete a repetition.

Partial Repetition Technique

A partial repetition is a repetition performed within a restricted range of motion of an exercise. Normally, partial repetitions are performed for both the concentric and eccentric phases of a repetition for 1 to 5 repetitions per set with more than 100% of 1RM for a complete repetition. The amount of weight that it is possible to use for a partial repetition depends on the strength curve of the exercise (i.e., ascending, descending, or bell shaped) and the range of motion in which the partial repetition is performed. Advocates of the partial repetition technique believe that by using very heavy weights within a restricted range of motion, trainees will increase their maximal strength.

Partial repetitions have been used successfully to increase isometric strength within the partial repetition range of motion and the full range of motion of an exercise in subjects who had limited range of motion (Graves et al. 1989, 1992). In healthy weight-trained males, one bench press training session including both full range of motion and partial range of motion repetitions resulted in a significant increase in the partial repetition 1RM (4.8%) and 5RM (4.1%) weights, but no significant change in the full range of motion 1RM and 5RM weights (Mookerjee and Ratamess 1999). The partial repetition range of motion used for the bench press was from an elbow angle of 90 degrees to completion of a repetition. The increase in the partial repetition maximum weights was probably due to neural adaptations, such as more muscle fiber recruitment within the partial repetition range of motion. Functional isometric training has been shown to increase full range of motion 1RM strength only when the training is performed at the sticking point of an exercise (see the discussion of the functional isometric technique). This is related to the joint angle specificity of isometric training.

The lack of improvement in full range of motion RM weights with only one training session in healthy individuals may be related to neural joint angle specificity of the partial repetition technique. In healthy individuals, partial repetitions do appear to increase maximum strength very quickly within the range of motion of the partial repetition. However, in healthy individuals, the effect of long-term training using the partial repetition technique on maximum strength within the range of motion of the partial repetition and on full range of motion maximum strength remains to be investigated. Thus, if a trainee wants to quickly increase maximum strength within a certain range of motion of an exercise, partial repetitions may be appropriate. As with any training technique in which heavy resistances are used, attentive spotters and proper safety procedures are necessary when performing partial repetitions.

Superslow Systems

Superslow systems involve performing repetitions at a slow velocity. The total length of a repetition may range from 10 to 60 seconds. Proponents of superslow systems believe that the increased amount of time that a muscle is under tension enhances strength development and hypertrophy. Superslow systems typically use isolated joint or machine exercises in which the movement velocity throughout the range of motion can be controlled. Typically only one or two sets of 1 to 6 repetitions of an exercise are performed in a training session.

Eight weeks of one set of slow positive or concentric emphasis training in beginning lifters has shown slightly greater increases (27 vs. 22 lb, or 12.2 vs. 10 kg) than a typical single-set system in the average weight lifted (Westcott 1994). The results of the comparison were not statistically analyzed. The slow concentric emphasis training consisted of performing 4 to 6 repetitions taking 10 seconds for the concentric phase and 4 seconds for the eccentric phase of each repetition. The typical single-set system consisted of 8 to 12 repetitions taking 2 seconds for the concentric and 4 seconds for the eccentric phase of each repetition.

Six weeks of training with either slow negative (eccentric) or slow positive (concentric) emphasis training showed similar increases (22 vs. 26 lb, or 10 vs. 12 kg) in the average weight lifted (Westcott 1995). The results were not statistically analyzed and are confounded by the use of different exercises for the two training systems, but do indicate that both systems can increase strength. Training with both systems consisted of performing 4 to 6 repetitions of one set. During slow eccentric training, the eccentric phase of a repetition lasted 10 seconds while the concentric phase lasted 4 seconds. The length of the eccentric and concentric phases of a repetition was reversed for the slow concentric training.

An acute comparison of the bench press using a superslow variation and a traditional heavy weight training system indicated no advantage of the superslow system (Keogh, Wilson, and Weatherby 1999). The superslow variation consisted of using 55% of 1RM and performing both the concentric and eccentric phases of a repetition in 5 seconds. This resulted in fatigue in approximately 6 repetitions. The traditional heavy weight training system consisted of 6 repetitions at a 6RM resistance. Time under tension was significantly longer with the superslow system due to the slow velocity with which repetitions were performed. Blood lactate 3 minutes after a set was not significantly different between the two training systems. However, electromyographic (EMG) activity of the pectoralis major and triceps brachii during both the eccentric and concentric phases of repetitions was significantly less with the superslow system compared to the traditional heavy weight training system. This was true during the first, middle, and last repetition of the set. This indicates less muscle fiber recruitment with the superslow system.

Small Increment Technique

Resistance is traditionally increased when a certain number of repetitions per set can be performed. With free weights and plate-loaded machines, normally the smallest resistance increase is 2.5 lb (1.1 kg). With weight stack resistance training machines, the smallest resistance increase can be quite large (10 lb [4.5 kg] or more), especially if weights that attach in some manner to the weight stack are not available. The small increment technique uses smaller than normal increases in resistance. A short-duration (8-week) training study demonstrated that the small increment technique resulted in 1RM gains in the bench press and triceps press that were equivalent to those resulting from a more traditional increase in resistance technique (Hostler, Crill et al. 2001). With the small increment technique the resistance was increased 0.5 lb (0.22 kg) when 7 or 8 repetitions could be performed per set and 1 lb (0.44 kg) when 9 or more repetitions could be performed per set. During training, the resistance was increased with the small increment

technique approximately four times as often for the bench press and twice as often for the triceps press. The use of a small increment technique may improve the level of satisfaction of novice lifters and increase the likelihood of continuing a program by providing positive feedback of increasing resistance at a rapid rate. This system may also be helpful to experienced lifters currently experiencing a training plateau (Hostler, Crill et al. 2001).

Specialized Systems and Techniques

Specialized systems and techniques are designed to produce a particular training goal in advanced lifters. Typically, the goals of advanced lifters involve either increasing 1RM or producing muscle hypertrophy. These systems and techniques are normally recommended only for advanced lifters who have already mastered exercise technique and have made substantial physiological adaptations to weight training.

Functional Isometrics

Functional isometrics attempt to take advantage of the joint-angle specificity of strength gains caused by isometric training (see the discussion of isometrics in chapter 2). Functional isometrics entail performing a dynamic concentric action for a portion of the concentric phase of a repetition, until the resistance hits the pins of a power rack (see figure 6.2). The trainee then continues to attempt to lift the resistance with a maximal effort, performing an isometric action for 5 to 7 seconds. Note that in figure 6.2 pins in the power rack are also set at the lowest portion of the range of motion for the safety of the lifter.

The objective of this system is to use joint-angle specificity to cause increases in strength at the joint angle at which the isometric action is performed. The joint angle chosen to perform the isometric action is normally the sticking point (the weakest point in the concentric range of motion) for the exercise. The maximal amount of resistance that can be lifted concentrically in any exercise is determined by the amount of resistance that can be moved through the sticking point. It is thought that increasing strength at the sticking point will increase 1RM. The need to perform the isometric action at the sticking point of an exercise is supported by research.

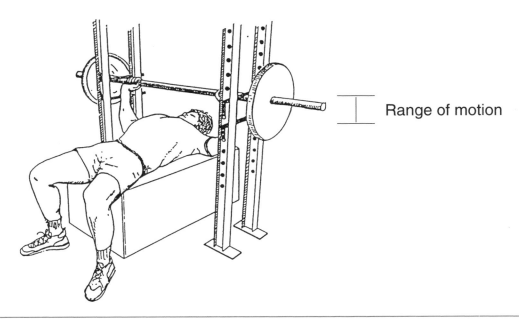

Range of motion

Figure 6.2 Functional isometrics used at the sticking point in the bench press. The top pin is placed at the exact point in the range of motion desired to be trained. The bottom pin is placed at the lowest point in the range of motion.

Short-term training studies comparing a training program using functional isometrics and a normal dynamic resistance training program indicate that significantly greater increases in 1RM bench press (19% vs. 11%, Jackson et al. 1985) and squat (26% vs. 10%, O'Shea and O'Shea 1989) occur when the functional isometrics are performed at or near the exercise's sticking point. However, in both the bench press and the squat, when the functional isometrics are performed at an elbow or knee angle of 170 degrees, which is not near the sticking point for either of these exercises, no significant difference in 1RM increases were noted compared to a normal dynamic resistance training program (Giorgi et al. 1998).

Many power lifters use this system without a power rack during the last repetition of a heavy set (e.g., 1-6RM). They attempt to perform as great a range of motion in the concentric phase of the last repetition as possible, and when they cannot lift the weight further, they continue to produce force isometrically at the exact angle at which the sticking point occurs. This type of training requires very attentive spotters. Lifters must know the sticking point in their range of motion to optimize training. This system is appropriate when the major goal of the program is to increase the 1RM capability of a particular exercise.

Negative System

During most resistance exercises the negative, or eccentric, portion of the repetition is lowering the resistance. During this phase the muscles involved are actively lengthening so that the lifter can lower the resistance in a controlled manner. Conversely, in most exercises the lifting of the resistance is termed the positive, or concentric, portion of the repetition.

It is possible to lower more weight in the negative portion of a repetition than is lifted in the positive portion. Thus, it is possible to use more than the 1RM for a complete repetition when performing negative training. Negative training involves lowering or performing the eccentric portion of repetitions with more than the 1RM for a complete repetition. Negative training can be done by having spotters help the lifter raise the weight, which the lifter then lowers unassisted. It can also be performed on some resistance training machines by lifting the weight with both arms or legs and then lowering the resistance with only one arm or leg. On some machines it is possible to lift the weight with both the arms and legs and then lower the weight using just the arms or just the legs. Negative training is also possible on some electronic weight machines. Proper exercise technique and safe spotting techniques must be used for all exercises performed in a heavy negative fashion.

Ranges of 105 to 140% of the concentric 1RM have been proposed for use during negative training. In a study by Nichols and colleagues (1995), seniors (mean age 68 years) safely used a range of 115 to 140% of the concentric 1RM during the eccentric phase of repetitions of six different machine-type exercises. Carpinelli and Gutin (1991) reported that during negative-only knee extensions, 11.7 repetitions can be performed with 120% of a normal (concentric/eccentric repetition) 1RM. The resistance used for negative training may depend on whether a machine or free weights are used. Heavier negative resistances may be possible with machines since they reduce the need for balancing the resistance.

In the study of seniors mentioned earlier, subjects safely used a negative system variation when training for 12 weeks with six different machine-type exercises (Nichols et al. 1995). Subjects used the predicted 1RM to perform the concentric and eccentric portions of repetitions, respectively, as follows: leg press, 50% and 57.5%; chest press, 50% and 70%; lat pull-down, 50% and 70%; seated row, 50% and 70%; fly, 60% and 70%; and shoulder press, 45% and 56.25%. All exercises were performed for three sets of 10 repetitions, except for the leg press, which was performed for four sets of 10 repetitions. Compared to a training group that performed all exercises for three sets of 12 repetitions except for the leg press, which was performed for four sets of 12 repetitions, the only significant difference in predicted 1RM was in the shoulder press. Both training groups significantly improved in strength compared to a control group in the shoulder press, lat pull-down, and fly exercises, whereas only the group performing the negative system variation made significant strength gains in the seated row. The results indicate that this negative system variation can be used safely in seniors, but that little advantage in strength gains is likely after 12 weeks of training.

Advocates of negative training believe that the use of more resistance during the negative portion of the exercise results in greater increases in strength. Neural adaptations may be part of the benefit of heavy negative training. In a comparison of maximal-eccentric-only versus maximal-concentric-only training, Hortobagyi and colleagues (1996) reported that electromyographic (EMG) activity during maximal eccentric actions is enhanced 86% after maximal eccentric training but only 11% after maximal concentric training. During maximal concentric actions, EMG activity is increased 8% and 12% after eccentric and concentric training, respectively. An increase in EMG activity during maximal eccentric actions may be advantageous, as discussed under forced or assisted repetitions, for increasing 1RM strength. Doan and colleagues (2001) also showed that performing a heavy eccentric repetition (105% of concentric 1RM) immediately before performing a concentric action results in a significantly heavier concentric 1RM. This indicates that the eccentric action may enhance the neural facilitation of the concentric movement. Thus, some evidence suggests that heavy eccentric training may result in neural adaptations that may enhance strength.

Competitive Olympic weightlifters training over 12 weeks have shown increased lifting ability when performing negative training (Häkkinen and Komi 1981). Lifters performing 25% of the eccentric actions in their training with 100 to 130% of the 1RM concentric action significantly increased 10% in the snatch and 13% in the clean and jerk. Lifters performing their normal training over this same time frame improved 7% in the snatch and 6% in the clean and jerk. The improvement in the clean and jerk shown by lifters performing negative training was significantly greater than that in the group performing normal training. Both groups also improved significantly in various measures of isometric strength, concentric and eccentric force during a leg press–type movement, and knee extension, but there was no significant difference between groups. The performance of these competitive athletes is measured by 1RM in the snatch and clean and jerk. Thus, negative training did offer them some competitive advantage.

Superoverload System

The superoverload system is a type of negative weight training. Partial repetitions are performed using 125% of the 1RM resistance. For example, if an individual's 1RM in the bench press is 200 lb (90.7 kg), 250 lb (113.4 kg) is used (200 lb [90.7 kg] × 1.25 = 250 lb [113.4 kg]) for the partial repetitions. Spotters help the lifter get the weight in the straight-arm position of the bench press. The lifter lowers the weight as far as possible before lifting the weight back to the straight-arm position without assistance from the spotters. The lifter performs 7 to 10 such partial repetitions per set. After the partial repetitions, the lifter lowers the resistance slowly to the chest-touch position, and the spotters help lift the weight back to the straight-arm position. Normally, three such sets per exercise are performed in a training session.

The superoverload system has been shown to be as effective as conventional weight training in developing 1RM strength (Powers, Browning, and Groves 1978). After 8 weeks of training, 3 days per week with at least 1 day of rest between training sessions, the superoverload system resulted in 1RM bench and leg press increases equal to those resulting from conventional weight training. Because resistances greater than 1RM are used in this training type, spotters are mandatory when using free weights. It is also possible to use some machines with this system. As with the negative system, the resistance may be lifted with both arms or legs and the partial repetitions performed with only one arm or leg.

Rest-Pause Technique

The rest-pause technique involves using near-maximal resistances (close to 1RM) for multiple repetitions. Between repetitions the lifter puts the weight down and rests for short periods of time. As an example, the lifter performs 1 repetition of an exercise with 250 lb (113.4 kg), which is near the 1RM for the exercise. The lifter then puts the weight down, rests 10 to 15 seconds, and then performs another repetition(s) with 250 lb (113.4 kg). This is repeated four or five times. If the lifter cannot perform a complete repetition, spotters assist just enough to allow completion of the 4 or 5 repetitions. Only one set of an exercise is performed, but two to three exercises per muscle group may be performed in the same training session. Proponents of this technique believe that using a resistance close to 1RM for multiple repetitions results in the greatest possible strength gains.

A variation of the rest-pause technique has been shown to result in significant strength gains over 6 weeks of training with three training sessions per week, but the strength gains were not as large as with a more conventional program (Rooney, Herbert, and Balwave 1994). The rest-pause technique consisted of performing one set of 6 to 10 repetitions at a 6RM weight with 30-second rests between repetitions. Strength gains of the rest-pause technique were compared to one set of 6 repetitions using a resistance of 6RM. Both groups trained using a seated arm curl (elbow flexors). Both groups experienced significantly greater increases in 1RM than a control group. However, the 1RM increase shown by the normal or no-rest-between-repetitions group (56%) was significantly greater than the increase shown by the rest-between-repetitions group (41%). Increases in maximal isometric strength of both groups were significantly greater than that of the control group; however, the difference between the rest and no-rest training groups was not significantly different. The results indicate that this variation of a rest-pause technique was not as effective in increasing dynamic strength as a no-rest-between-repetitions system and resulted in equivalent isometric strength gains.

Complex or Contrast Loading System

Complex training is the performance of one set of a strength exercise, such as the squat, and then, after a very short rest period, performance of a power-type exercise, such as the vertical jump (Fleck and Kontor 1986). The goal of this type of training is to enhance short-term power output (i.e., the ability to jump higher or throw a ball farther). Recently, the term *contrast loading* has replaced the term *complex training*. The goal of contrast loading is the same as that of complex training. However, contrast loading typically consists of alternating sets of a strength-type exercise, such as the bench press or squat with a resistance greater than 85% of 1RM, with sets of a power-type exercise, such as the bench throw or vertical jump using a resistance of 30 to 45% of 1RM. Proponents of this type of training believe that a neural adaptation, such as an increased ability to recruit muscle fibers or inhibition of neural protective mechanisms (Golgi tendon organs) is caused by the heavy resistance–type exercise and expressed in the power-type exercise, resulting in a greater power output. However, the exact mechanism by which power is increased during the power-type exercise is undefined.

Variations of contrast loading have been shown to enhance power output in well-trained athletes (Baker 2001a) and in a case study of

Table 6.4 Acute Program Variables of Various Training Systems

Training system	Repetitions/set	Resistance	Acute program variables				
			Choice of exercise	Order of exercise	Rest between sets or exercises	Sets per exercise	
Blitz	Normally 8-10	Normally 8-10RM	One muscle group/day	NS	NS	Multiple	
Breakdown	10-12	10-12RM	NS	NS	Several seconds	Normally 1	
Bulk	5-6	5-6RM	NS	NS	NS	3	
Burn	After a set to failure, 5-6 more partial reps are performed	RM to failure	NS	NS	NS	NS	
Cheat system	NS	>1RM or after set to volitional fatigue	NS	NS	NS	NS	
Circuit	10-15	40-60% of 1RM	NS	NS	15-30 s	1-3	
Compound set	NS	NS	NS	Alternating 2 muscle groups in different body parts	A few seconds	NS	
Complex or contrast loading	3-6	>85% of 1RM and 30-45% of 1RM	1 strength and 1 power	Strength followed by power exercise	1-3 min	1 to several	
Double progressive	NS	Constant resistance with increasing reps, then increasing resistance with decreasing reps	NS	NS	NS	NS	
Exhaustion set	NS	RM for desired number of reps	NS	NS	NS	NS	
Express circuit	6-12	Normally 6-1RM	One for each major muscle group	NS	30-60 s	1	
Flushing	NS	NS	2 or more for the same muscle group consecutively	NS	NS	NS	

(continued)

Table 6.4 (continued)

Training system	Repetitions/set	Resistance	Choice of exercise	Order of exercise	Rest between sets or exercises	Sets per exercise
			Acute program variables			
Forced repetition	After a set to failure, 2-4 assisted reps are done	NS	Exercise movement can be assisted	NS	NS	NS
Functional isometrics	NS	NS	After some concentric movement, a 5- to 7-s isometric action is performed	NS	NS	NS
Heavy-to-light	NS	Progresses from heavy to light	NS	NS	NS	NS
Isolated exercise	8-10	8-10RM	1 exercise/day	NS	1 min	As many as possible in 1-1.5 hr
Light-to-heavy	NS	Progresses from light to heavy	NS	NS	NS	NS
Multiple set	NS	NS	NS	NS	NS	2 or more
Multipoundage	4-5	4-5RM initially, then reduced to allow 4-5 more reps per set	NS	NS	NS	Several
Negative	NS	>1RM	NS	NS	NS	NS
Partial repetitions	1-5	>100% 1RM	Must be able to perform a partial range of motion	NS	NS	NS
Peripheral heart action	Normally 8-12	NS	Sequence of 4-6 exercises each for different body part	NS	None or little	NS
Priority	NS	NS	NS	Perform most important exercises first in session	NS	NS
Rest-pause	1-5	Near 1RM	NS	NS	10-15 s	NS

Single-set	4-10	4-10RM	NS	NS	30-60 s	1
Small increment	NS	Increased 0.22-0.44 kg (0.5-1 lb) when set can be completed	NS	NS	NS	NS
Split routine	NS	NS	Different muscle groups each session	NS	NS	NS
Superoverload	7-10 partial	>1RM	NS	NS	NS	3
Superpump	5-6	5-6RM	1-3 per muscle group	NS	15 seconds	15-18 per body part
Superset 1	Normally 8-12	Normally 8-12RM	Agonist and antagonist	Agonist and antagonist	None	Several
Superset 2	Normally 8-12	Normally 8-12RM zone	Several for same muscle group	NS	None to little	1 to several
Superslow	1-5	NS	NS	NS	NS	1-2
Triangle	NS	Light to heavy, back to light	NS	NS	NS	Several
Triset	NS	NS	3 for a body part	NS	None to little	3

NS = not specified.

an elite springboard diver (Baker 2001b). In the first of these studies, on one occasion a subject performed two sets of six vertical jumps with an 88-lb (40-kg) barbell on the shoulders, and one set of vertical jumps of 3 repetitions with a 132-lb (60-kg) barbell on the shoulders between the sets of six vertical jumps. On a second occasion the subject performed only the two sets of six vertical jumps. Rest between sets of vertical jumps was 2 to 3 minutes. Power output in the second set of six jumps with 88 lb (40 kg), after performing the set with the heavy or contrast load, increased 5.4% compared to the second set of vertical jumps when no contrast load set was performed. This demonstrated that in some way the heavy contrast load increased power output. However, the long-term effects of contrast load training on power output in competitive-type settings (i.e., not immediately after the heavy contrast load) needs to be investigated.

Summary

The potential for creating different and new resistance training systems and techniques appears almost infinite. All of the systems and techniques discussed in this chapter were designed to address specific training goals. They evolved from a variety of sources, including bodybuilding, power lifting, Olympic weightlifting, and personal trainers. When groups realize their desired adaptations using certain systems and techniques, they continue to use them. Some equipment companies promote resistance training systems and techniques that suit their equipment characteristics or that fit into marketing strategies. Commercial magazines promote and publish new and different training systems and techniques based on the need to increase the magazine's circulation. Each system or technique should be able to be described in terms of its acute program variables (see table 6.4). However, for most systems and techniques the acute program variables were never completely defined. This may explain why training responses to a given system or technique vary considerably.

Popular or fad training systems and techniques should be described and evaluated in terms of their acute program variables and their ability to address the needs of a specific population or sport. Additional sport science research is needed to evaluate the efficacy of virtually all training

systems and techniques. The choice depends on the goals of the program, time constraints, equipment availability, and how the goals of the resistance training program relate to the goals of the total fitness program. A major goal of any training system or technique is to bring about desired physiological adaptations, which are the subject of the next chapter.

Key Terms

alternating muscle group order
multiple-set system
negative training
single-set system
stacking exercise order
triangle or pyramid system

Selected Readings

Baker, D. 2001. A series of studies on the training of high-intensity muscle power and rugby league football players. *Journal of Strength and Conditioning Research* 15: 198-209.

Calder, A.W., Chilibeck, P.D., Webber, C.E., and Sale, D.G. 1994. Comparison of whole and split weight training routines in young women. *Canadian Journal of Applied Physiology* 19: 185-199.

Fleck, S.J., and Kontor, K. 1986. Complex training. *National Strength and Conditioning Association Journal* 8: 66-69.

Gettman, L.R., and Pollock, M.L. 1981. Circuit weight training: A critical review of its physiological benefits. *Physician and Sportsmedicine* 9: 44-60.

Giorgi, A., Wilson, G.J., Weatherby, R.P., and Murphy, A. 1998. Functional isometric weight training: Its effects on the development of muscular function and the endocrine system over an 8-week training period. *Journal of Strength and Conditioning Research* 12: 18-25.

Jackson, A., Jackson, T., Hnatek, J., and West, J. 1985. Strength development: Using functional isometric in isotonic strength training program. *Research Quarterly for Exercise and Sport* 56: 324-337.

Keogh, J.W.L., Wilson, G.J., and Weatherby, R.P. 1999. A cross-sectional comparison of different resistance training techniques in the bench press. *Journal of Strength and Conditioning Research* 13: 247-258.

Leighton, J., Holmes, D., Benson, J., Wooten, B., and Schmerer, R. 1967. A study of the effectiveness of ten different methods of progressive resistance exercise on the development of strength, flexibility, girth and body weight. *Journal of the Association of Physical and Mental Rehabilitation* 21: 78-81.

Mookerjee, S., and Ratamess, N. 1999. Comparison of strength differences and joint action durations between full and partial range-of-motion bench press exercise. *Journal of Strength and Conditioning Research* 13: 76-81.

Nichols, J.F., Hitzelberger, L.M., Sherman, J.G., and Patterson, P. 1995. Effects of resistance training on muscular strength and functional abilities of community-dwelling older adults. *Journal of Aging and Physical Activity* 3: 238-250.

O'Shea, K.L., and O'Shea, J.P. 1989. Functional isometric weight training: Its effects on dynamic and static strength. *Journal of Applied Sport Science Research* 3: 30-33.

Rooney, K.J., Herbert, R.D., and Balwave, R.J. 1994. Fatigue contribute to the strength training stimulus. *Medicine and Science in Sports and Exercise* 26: 1160-1164.

Stone, M.H., Potteiger, J.A., Pierce, K.C., Proulx, C.M., O'Bryant, H.S., Johnson, R.L., and Stone, M.E. 2000. Comparison of the effects of three different weight-training programs on the one repetition maximum squat. *Journal of Strength and Conditioning Research* 14: 332-337.

CHAPTER 7

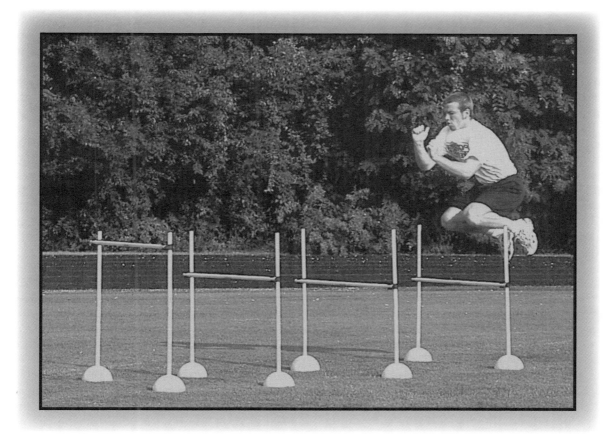

Advanced Training Strategies

The search for advanced training strategies probably began shortly after the development of the first resistance training programs. After performing a resistance training program for a short period of time and making substantial gains in strength and hypertrophy, someone probably wondered, What can I do to improve my current weight training program? The search for advanced training strategies that began at that point continues today. The popularity of advanced training strategies is demonstrated by a survey of National Football League strength and conditioning coaches indicating that 69% use some type of periodized training and 94% use plyometric exer-

cises in their total training programs (Ebben and Blackard 2001).

Advanced training strategies are necessary in part because as an individual becomes more physically fit, gains in fitness slow and training plateaus occur. Advanced training strategies are also necessary to optimally develop some fitness variables, such as power and muscular rate of force development, in highly fit individuals. Although new training strategies are developed frequently by coaches, personal trainers, and strength conditioning specialists, most are not studied scientifically. The advanced training strategies discussed in this chapter are periodization of strength training, power training, and plyometric or stretch-shortening cycle training. All of these training strategies have received a significant amount of attention from the sport science community. Therefore, there is sufficient research from which to draw conclusions and develop training guidelines.

Periodization of Resistance Training

Periodization of training refers to planned changes in the acute training program variables of exercise order, exercise choice, number of sets, number of repetitions per set, rest periods between sets and exercises, exercise intensity, and number of training sessions per day in an attempt to bring about continued and optimal fitness gains. Sport scientists, coaches, and athletes of the former Eastern Bloc countries of the Soviet Union and East Germany are credited with developing and researching the concepts of periodization. However, anecdotal evidence also indicates that athletes were performing periodized programs in the United States, Europe, and other Western countries as early as the 1950s.

The main goals of periodized training are optimizing training adaptations during short periods of time (e.g. weeks, months) as well as long periods of time (e.g. years, an entire athletic career). Some periodized plans also have as a goal to peak physical performance at a particular point in time, such as a major competition. Another goal of periodized training is to avoid training plateaus. Comparative studies of nonvaried programs and periodized programs in which serial testing was performed demonstrate that nonvaried programs can result in training plateaus (see table 7.1), whereas periodized programs result in more consistent fitness gains.

Manipulation of resistance training's acute training program variables results in a virtually limitless number of possibilities and so a limitless number of both short- and long-term training strategies. To date, the sport science community has investigated two major types of periodized resistance training: classic or traditional strength/power periodization and undulating periodization.

Classic Strength/Power Periodization

Classic strength/power periodization is what most individuals think of when they hear the term *periodized resistance training*. Classic strength/ power periodization follows a general trend of decreasing training volume and increasing training intensity as training progresses (see figure 7.1). For weight training this means that a relatively high total number of repetitions is performed at a low intensity when training is initiated, and as training progresses, the total number of repetitions performed decreases and training intensity increases.

When this type of training was first developed, only one or two major sport competitions took place per year, such as national or world championships. Thus, the training plan followed a yearly or six-month cycle in an attempt to peak physical performance at major competitions. This resulted in training volume reaching its lowest point and training intensity its highest point once or twice a year corresponding with major competitions. However, to allow for some physical and psychological recovery before the major competition, the highest training intensity occurred a short time before the major competition. Skill training for a particular sport or activity followed a very similar trend in terms of training intensity, except that it normally reached its highest intensity slightly closer to a major competition.

Each major training phase for athletes preparing for these yearly or twice-yearly competitions, then, lasted approximately 3 to 4 months. Anecdotal evidence and research indicate substantial strength and performance gains are possible with shorter training phases. Thus, the training plan time frame has since evolved to the point that training phases now last anywhere from 2 to 6 weeks. Thus, the time needed for one complete training cycle (i.e., performance of all training phases) is approximately 8 to 24 weeks. Studies examining classic strength/power periodization use these shorter training phases.

Terminology describing various time periods developed along with periodized training concepts. A macrocycle typically refers to one year of training, and a mesocycle refers to 3 to 4 months of a macrocycle. A microcycle typically refers to 1 to 4 weeks within a mesocycle. Several different terminologies describing specific training phases also developed (see figure 7.1). For example, a mesocycle using classic European terminology is the preparation phase. The training pattern and terminology most frequently used in sport science studies examining classic strength/power periodization is the American strength/power terminology. Typically, regardless of the terminology used, training phases have specific training goals normally in large part described by their names. For example, in the American strength/power terminology the peaking

Table 7.1 Percent Changes Between Various Training Periods Demonstrating Training Plateaus With Nonperiodized Training

	Bench press 1RM		
	Pre to 12 weeks	Pre to 24 weeks	12 to 24 weeks
Undulating perdiodization	23[ac]	47[ac]	19[b]
1 set × 8-12 reps	12[a]	12[a]	0
	Leg press 1RM		
Undulating perdiodization	21[ac]	32[ac]	9[c]
1 set × 8-12 reps	8[a]	11[a]	3
	Bench press reps at 80% 1RM		
Undulating perdiodization	14[ac]	24[ac]	9[b]
1 set × 8-12 reps	2	10[a]	8
	Leg press reps at 80% 1RM		
Undulating perdiodization	35[ac]	65[ac]	22[b]
1 set × 8-12 reps	16[a]	19[a]	2
	Wingate peak power		
Undulating perdiodization	14[ac]	27[ac]	12[b]
1 set × 8-12 reps	1	4	4
	Sit-ups in 1 min		
Undulating perdiodization	26[ac]	42[ac]	13[b]
1 set × 8-12 reps	8[a]	13[a]	2
	Vertical jump power		
Undulating perdiodization	24[ac]	40[ac]	13[b]
1 set × 8-12 reps	9[a]	10[a]	1
	40-yd sprint		
Undulating perdiodization	−3[ac]	−6[ac]	−3[b]
1 set × 8-12 reps	+1	−1	−1

a = significant difference from pretest; b = significant difference from 12 weeks; c = significant difference from one-set group.

Data from J.O. Marx et al. "Low-volume circuit versus high-volume periodized resistance training in women." *Medicine and Science in Sports and Exercise* 33: 635-643, 2001.

(continued)

Table 7.1 (continued)

	Bench press 1RM				
	Pre to 4 weeks	Pre to 16 weeks	4 to 8 weeks	8 to 12 weeks	12 to 16 weeks
Classic strength/power periodization	7[a]	24[ab]	4	8	5
5 × 10RM	5[a]	8[a]	0	1	2
6 × 8 RM	7[a]	10[a]	−2	2	3
	Squat 1 RM				
Classic strength/power periodization	9[ac]	33[ab]	3	9	12
5 × 10RM	4[a]	15[a]	3	3	5
6 × 8 RM	10[ac]	22[ac]	2	7	3

a = significant increase from control group; b = significant difference from other two groups; c = significant difference from 5 × 10RM group.

Data from D.S. Willoughby. "The effect of meso-cycle-length weight training programs involving periodization and partially equated volumes on upper and lower body strength." *Journal of Strength and Conditioning Research* 7: 2-8, 1993.

	Bench press 1RM			
	Pre to 16 weeks	Pre to 36 weeks	16 to 24 weeks	24 to 36 weeks
Undulating periodization	22[a]	25[a]	0[a]	4[ac]
1 set × 8-12 reps	10[a]	10[a]	0[a]	0[a]
	Leg press 1RM			
Undulating periodization	11[a]	18[a]	5[ab]	3[ac]
1 set × 8-12 reps	6[a]	7[a]	0[a]	0[a]
	Shoulder press 1RM			
Undulating periodization	19[a]	28[a]	7[ab]	2[ac]
1 set × 8-12 reps	14[a]	14[a]	3[a]	−3[a]
	Vertical jump			
Undulating periodization	26[a]	48[a]	6[a]	17[ac]
1 set × 8-12 reps	5	5	0	0
	Wingate power			
Undulating periodization	8	14[a]	4	3
1 set × 8-12 reps	0	0	0	0
	Serve velocity			
Undulating periodization	21[a]	23[a]	2[ab]	0[a]
1 set × 8-12 reps	4	4	3	−3

a = significant difference from pretest; b = significant difference from 16 weeks; c = significant difference from 24 weeks.

Data from W.J. Kraemer et al. "Influence of resistance training volume and periodization on physiological and performance adaptations in collegiate women tennis players." *American Journal of Sports Medicine* 28: 626-633, 2000.

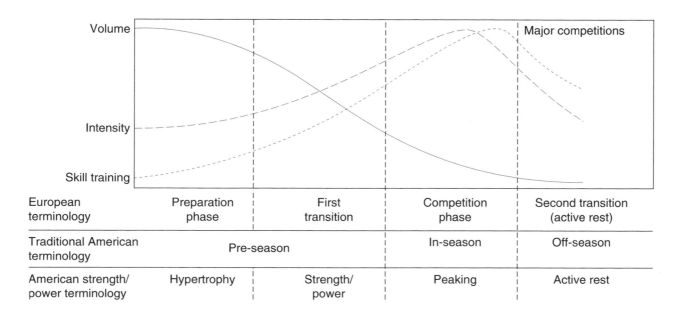

European terminology	Preparation phase	First transition	Competition phase	Second transition (active rest)
Traditional American terminology	Pre-season		In-season	Off-season
American strength/ power terminology	Hypertrophy	Strength/ power	Peaking	Active rest

Figure 7.1 Strength/power training model pattern of volume intensity.

phase's major goal is to maximize or peak the expression of strength or power.

Active recovery phases are incorporated into the classic strength/power periodization model. However, active recovery does not mean complete cessation of physical activity or training, nor is this phase typically very long. This would result in substantial deconditioning, and the trainee would then have to spend training regaining his former physical condition, rather than improving it. Active recovery phases normally consist of a reduction in training volume and intensity rather than cessation of training. Long active recovery phases may be incorporated into some programs and are dependent on the individual sport and athlete's requirements and may relate to the level of training and experience of the athlete. For example, a few weeks of active recovery by an experienced and successful athlete immediately after a major competition or competitive season may not be detrimental.

Because the American strength/power periodization terminology and model are used most frequently in studies examining classic strength training periodization, a more detailed description of each training phase is warranted (see table 7.2). Note that training volume decreases and intensity increases from the hypertrophy to peaking training phases. Additionally, note that a range of sets and repetitions per set exists for each exercise. So, although training volume and intensity do follow a general trend of decreasing

and increasing as training progresses, variations in volume and intensity can and do occur on a daily or weekly basis in most training plans. The variation in number of sets and repetitions also allows for variation in volume and intensity in specific exercises. For example, a particular individual may have different intensities and volumes for specific muscle groups or exercises based on her individual needs and goals. Although the general pattern of the American strength/power periodized plan is used by sport science studies, a wide variation in training phase length, number of sets, and number of repetitions per set has been used in training studies (see table 7.3).

Undulating Periodization

Undulating periodization is a more recent type of periodization than the classic strength/power model. A major goal of the strength/power model is to peak strength and power immediately at the end of the peaking phase. However, for sports or activities with long seasons in which competitive success depends on performance throughout the entire season, development and maintenance of physical fitness during the entire season is important. Peaking strength and power for major competitions normally occurring at the end of the season is also important. However, without success during the season, qualification for major tournaments and competitions does not occur.

Table 7.2 Classic Strength/Power Periodization Model

	Training phase				
	Hypertrophy	**Strength**	**Power**	**Peaking**	**Active rest**
Sets	3-5	3-5	3-5	1-3	Light physical activity
Reps/set	8-12	2-6	2-3	1-3	
Intensity	Low	Moderate	High	Very high	
Volume	Very high	High	Moderate	Low	

Adapted, by permission, from M.H. Stone, H. O'Bryant, and J. Garhammer, 1981, "A hypothetical model for strength training," *Journal of Sports Medicine* 21: 344.

Therefore, the primary goals of a training model for sports or activities with long seasons, such as volleyball, basketball, baseball, and soccer, should be to develop physical fitness to ensure success during the season and yet continue to develop fitness throughout the season.

Undulating models are gaining popularity in sports and activities with long seasons for several reasons. A typical strength/power training program sometimes results in strength and power peaking immediately before the season, yet the major competitions occur at the end of the season. On the other hand, performing high-volume training during the initial portion of the season to attain peak strength and power at the end of the season might result in residual fatigue and thus poor performance at the start of the season. This could result in the athlete not qualifying for a major competition or tournament at the end of the season.

Undulating periodization varies training volume and intensity so that fitness gains occur over long training periods, such as long seasons, and treats peaking of physical fitness at a certain point in time as a minor training goal. With **undulating periodization,** training intensity and volume are varied by using different RM or near-RM training zones. Typically, three training zones are used, such as 4 to 6RM, 8 to 10RM, and 12 to 15RM zones. A very heavy resistance training zone such as 1 to 3RM could also be included in an undulating model, although inclusion of such a training zone has not been studied scientifically. The training zones are varied on a training session, weekly, or biweekly manner. The training zones are not necessarily sequentially performed, however, so training intensity or volume follows a pattern of consistently increasing or decreasing over time. In undulating training models typically multijoint exercises use all training zones, whereas some sessions composed of predominantly single-joint exercises use only the 8 to 10RM training zone.

For example, an undulating model using three training zones and two different types of training sessions could be as follows: A Monday and Thursday session predominantly composed of multijoint exercises including power-type exercises, such as power cleans, would use all three training zones, while a session performed on Tuesday and Friday using some multijoint exercises, but predominantly single-joint exercises, would always use the 8 to 10RM zone. Another undulating pattern of intensity and volume would be always performing the same exercises in three sessions during a week, with multijoint exercises using all three training zones and single-joint exercises using only the 8 to 10RM training zone. Obviously, many other undulating patterns are possible.

Many different patterns of training volume and intensity can be developed using periodization concepts including combining various aspects of the classic strength/power and undulating models. For example, a classic strength/power model during the off-season and early preseason of a sport can ensure that strength and power peak immediately before the season. An undulating model during late preseason and in season can then help not only to maintain, but also to increase fitness during the season so that strength and power contribute maximally to success throughout the entire season. Unfortunately, mixing these two training models has not been studied by sport scientists.

Comparative Studies

When examining any comparison of weight training programs, we must consider both the length of the study and the training status of the subjects (see chapter 3). During the first 4 to 6 weeks of any realistic weight training program, substantial gains in strength will occur because of neural adaptations. Other physiological adaptations, such

Table 7.3 Strength/Power Periodized Training Studies

Reference	Mean age (yr) and sex	Training length (wk)	Frequency per week	Sets × reps	Intensity	Exercises trained	Test(s)	Percent increase
Stone et al. 1981	High school M	6	4	Multiple sets 3 × 6	Progressed at own rate	Squats and 5 others	Squat Vertical jump	?* ?*
				Classic periodization 3 wk 5 × 10 1 wk 5 × 5 1 wk 3 × 3 1 wk 3 × 2	Progressed at own rate	Squats and 5 others	Squat Vertical jump	?*a ?*a
Stowers et al. 1983	College M	7	3	1 × 10	10RM	Combination of 8	Bench press Squat Vertical jump	7* 14* 0
				3 × 10	10RM	Combination of 8	Bench press Squat Vertical jump	9* 20* 1
				Classic periodization 2 wk 5 × 10 3 wk 3 × 5 2 wk 2 × 3	RMs	Combination of 8	Bench press Squat Vertical jump	9* 27*b 10*
O'Bryant et. al 1988	19 M	11	3	3 × 6	81-97% of pretrain 1RM	Squat and 8 others	Squat Cycle power	32* 6*
				Classic periodization 4 wk 5 × 10 4 wk 3 × 5, 1 × 10 3 wk 3 × 2, 1 × 10	70-117% of pretrain 1RM	Squat and 8 others	Squat Cycle power	38*a 17*a
McGee et al. 1992	19-20 M	7	3	1 × 8-12	8-12RM	Combination of 7	Cycling to exhaustion Squat reps to exhaustion	12 46
				3 × 10	Close to 10RM	Combination of 7	Cycling to exhaustion Squat reps to exhaustion	15* 71*
				Classic periodization 2 wk 3 × 10 3 wk 3 × 5 2 wk 3 × 3	Close to RMs	Combination of 7	Cycling to exhaustion Squat reps to exhaustion	29* 74*

(continued)

Table 7.3 *(continued)*

Reference	Mean age (yr) and sex	Training length (wk)	Frequency per week	Sets × reps	Intensity	Exercises trained	Test(s)	Percent increase
Willoughby 1992	20 M	12	2	3 × 10	Pretrain 10RM	Bench press and squat	Bench press Squat	8* 13*
				3 × 6-8	6-8RM	Bench press and squat	Bench press Squat	17*c 26*c
				Classic periodization 4 wk 5 × 8-10 4 wk 4 × 5-7 4 wk 3 × 3-5	RMs	Bench press and squat	Bench press Squat	28*d 48*d
Willoughby 1993	20 M	16	3	5 × 10	79% 1RM	Bench press and squat	Bench press Squat	8* 14*
				6 × 8	83% 1RM	Bench press and squat	Bench press Squat	10* 22*e
				Classic periodization 4 wk 5 × 10 4 wk 4 × 8 4 wk 3 × 6 4 wk 3 × 4	79% 1RM 83% 1RM 88% 1RM 92% 1RM	Bench press and squat	Bench press Squat	23*f 34*f
Baker, Wilson, and Carlyon 1994a	19-21 M	12	3	5 × 6 core exercises 5 × 8 all others	RMs	Combination of 17	Bench press Squat Vertical jump	12* 26* 9*
				Classic periodization 4 wk 5 × 10 core, 3 × 10 all others 4 wk 5 × 5 core, 3 × 8 all others 3 wk 3 × 3, 1 × 10 core, 3 × 6 all others 1 wk 3 × 3 core, 3 × 6 all others	RMs	Combination of 17	Bench press Squat Vertical jump	12* 27* 4*

				2 wk undulating periodization 2 wk 5 × 10 core, 3 × 10 all others 2 wk 5 × 6 core, 3 × 8 all others 2 wk 5 × 8 core, 3 × 10 all others 2 wk 5 × 4 core, 3 × 6 all others 2 wk 5 × 6 core, 3 × 8 all others 2 wk 4 × 3 core, 3 × 6 all others	RMs	Combination of 17	Bench press Squat Vertical jump	16* 28* 10*
Herrick and Stone 1996	20-24 F	15	2	3 × 6	6RM	6	Bench press Squat	25* 46*
				Classic periodization 8 wk 3 × 10 1 wk off 2 wk 3 × 4 1 wk off 2 wk 3 × 2	RMs	6	Bench press Squat	31* 54*
Kraemer 1997	20 M	14	3	1 × 10, forced reps	8-10RM	9	Bench press Hang clean Vertical jump Wingate power	3 4* 3* 0
				Classic periodization 3 wk 2-3 × 8-10 2 wk 3-4 × 6 2 wk 5 × 1-4 Repeat all weeks	50% of 1RM 70-85% of 1RM 85-95% of 1RM	12	Bench press Hang clean Vertical jump Wingate power	11*g 19*g 17*g 14*g
Schiotz et al. 1998	24 M	10	4	4 × 6 core exercises 3 × 8 all others	Initially 80% of 1RM then progress at subject's pace	2 core and 5 assistance	Bench press Squat	5 11*

(continued)

Table 7.3 (continued)

Reference	Mean age (yr) and sex	Training length (wk)	Frequency per week	Sets × reps	Intensity	Exercises trained	Test(s)	Percent increase
				Classic periodization 2 wk 5 × 10 core, 3 × 10 assistance 1 wk 3 × 10, 1 × 8, 1 × 6 core, 3 × 10 assistance 1 wk 2 × 8, 3 × 5 core, 3 × 8 assistance 1 wk 1 × 8, 1 × 6, 3 × 5 core, 3 × 8 assistance 1 wk 1 × 8, 4 × 5 core, 3 × 8 assistance 1 wk 1 × 8, 2 × 5, 1 × 3, 1 × 1 core, 3 × 6 assistance 1 wk 2 × 5, 1 × 3, 1 × 2, 1 × 1 core, 3 × 6 assistance 2 wk 2 × 3, 4 × 1 core, 3 × 4 assistance	Initially 50% pretrain 1RM then progress at subject's pace	2 core and 5 assistance	Bench press Squat	8* 10*
Stone et al. 2000	College M	12	3	5 × 6	6 RM, mean 67% of pretrain 1RM	6	Squat	10
				Classic periodization wk 1-4 major 5 × 10, 3 × 10 assistance wk 5-8 5 × 5 major, 3 × 8 assistance wk 9-11 3 × 3, 1 × 10 major, 3 × 6 assistance wk 12 3 × 3 major, 3 × 6 assistance	RMs, mean 61% of pretrain 1RM	6	Squat	15*

Study	Age/Sex	Duration (wk)	Days/wk	Program	Intensity	Exercises	Exercise tested	% change
				Classic periodization wk 1-2 5 × 10 major, 3 × 10 assistance wk 3-4 3 × 5, 1 × 10 major, 3 × 10 assistance wk 5 3 × 3, 1 × 5 major, 3 × 10 assistance wk 6-8 3 × 5, 1 × 5 major, 3 × 5 assistance wk 9 5 × 5, 1 × 5 major, 3 × 5 assistance wk 10 3 × 5, 1 × 5 major, 3 × 5 assistance wk 11 3 × 3, 1 × 5 major, 3 × 5 assistance wk 12 3 × 3 major, 3 × 5 assistance	Heavy/light days, hevay days use RM, mean 72% of pretrain 1RM	6	Squat	15*
Rhea et al. 2002	21 M	12	3	Classic periodization wk 1-4 3 × 8 RM wk 5-8 3 × 6 RM wk 9-12 3 × 4 RM	RMs	5 exercises	Leg press Bench press	14* 26*
Rhea et al. 2002				Undulating periodization daily day 1 3 × 8 RM day 2 3 × 6 RM day 3 3 × 4 RM	RMs	5 exercises	Leg press Bench press	29*f 56*f

* = significant change pre- to posttraining

a = significant difference from 3 × 6 group

b = significant difference from 1 × 10 and 3 × 10 groups

c = significant difference from 3 × 10 group

d = significant difference from 3 × 10 and 3 × 6-8 groups

e = significant difference from 5 × 10 group

f = significant difference from 5 × 10 and 6 × 8 groups

g = significant difference from 1 × 8-10 group

f = significant difference from classic periodization

as changes in the quality of the muscle proteins, can also be dramatic during the first several weeks of a training program. These very quickly occurring physical adaptations can result in substantial strength increases. For example, Prevost, Nelson, and Maraj (1999) noted a 22% increase in strength in untrained males after only 2 days of isokinetic training at 4.71 rads per second. Thus, in short-term studies, any significant difference between training programs in strength and power or short-term high-intensity anaerobic endurance (i.e. Wingate cycling test) is difficult to achieve because all realistic weight training programs will result in significant gains in strength initially. These initial strength gains may mask any real difference between the training programs. This is especially true when untrained individuals are trained. Conversely, if superiority of one training program over another is demonstrated in a short-term study, it may merely mean that the superior program brings about quicker neural adaptations or fiber-type transformations, and any differences between programs may be nonexistent with longer-term training. This may be especially true if no gains in muscle fiber cross-sectional area or fat-free mass are demonstrated.

Another issue to consider in a discussion of comparative studies is the fact that most use untrained or moderately trained individuals as subjects. This limits the applicability of the studies to highly trained individuals or athletes. Strength and power increases occur at a much slower rate in highly trained individuals compared to moderately trained individuals (Häkkinen et al. 1989). Thus, assuming that the magnitude of change and rate of change in variables such as strength from studies using untrained subjects are directly applicable to highly trained individuals is tenuous. It is also important to note that not all muscle groups will respond at the same rate or with the same magnitude after a specific resistance training program, including periodized programs (see tables 7.1, 7.3, and 7.4). For example, over 16 weeks of strength/power periodized training, the increase in strength shown in the bench press was substantially less than that shown in the squat after 4, 8, 12, and 16 weeks of training (Willoughby 1993). Thus, trainers should be cautious about assuming that a particular training program will result in the same rate and magnitude of adaptations in different muscle groups or different exercises. Nevertheless, a sufficient number of studies comparing periodization models to nonvaried training models have been performed so

that we can form conclusions concerning the effectiveness of periodized models. This is not to imply, however, that further study of periodized models is not needed.

Strength/Power Periodization Training Studies

Comparative studies of strength/power periodization to single-set and multiple-set nonvaried programs demonstrate that periodization can result in significantly greater strength gains (see table 7.3). Most comparisons used healthy young males as subjects. However, one study did show greater percentage gains in strength in women with periodized training, but no significant difference between the periodized and multiple-set training program was shown (Herrick and Stone 1996). Although most studies used untrained individuals, several studies using moderately trained or trained individuals indicated that strength/power periodization does result in significantly greater strength gains than nonperiodized programs. For example, defining trained as the ability to bench press 120% and squat 150% or greater of total body weight, Willoughby (1992, 1993) showed that periodized training resulted in greater strength gains than nonvaried multiple-set programs. It has also been shown that high school (Stone, O'Bryant, and Garhammer 1981) and college football players (Kraemer 1997) demonstrate greater strength gains with a periodized program than with a single-set nonvaried program.

Comparisons of gains in motor performance and local muscular endurance (i.e., the maximal number of repetitions at a percentage of 1RM) are less common than strength comparisons. Periodized programs have shown significantly greater gains in vertical jump ability, short-term cycling ability, and local muscular endurance than nonvaried single-set and multiple-set programs. However, not all studies have shown significantly greater increases with periodized training, and relatively few studies have examined the training effects on motor performance. Therefore, conclusions concerning motor performance must be viewed with caution. However, comparisons to date do favor strength/power periodized models over nonperiodized models in terms of motor performance.

Similar to motor performance, fewer studies have examined body compositional and total-body weight changes from periodized compared to nonvaried training models. Some comparisons

Table 7.4 Undulating Periodization Studies

Reference	Mean age (yr) and sex	Training length	Frequency per week	Sets × reps	Intensity	Exercises trained	Test(s)	Percent increase
Kraemer et al. 2000	19 F	36	2-3	1 × 8-10	Close to 8-10RM	14	Bench press Shoulder press Leg press Wingate power Vertical jump	25* 28a 18a 14a 48a
			2-3	Undulating periodization 3 training zones 2-4 sets 4-6, 8-10, 12-15	Close to RMs	14	Bench press Shoulder press Leg press Wingate power Vertical jump	10a 14a 7a 0 5
Marx et al. 2001	22-23 F	24	3	1 × 8-12	8-12RM	2 alternating groups of 10 exercises	Bench press Leg press Bench press reps at 80% 1RM Leg press reps at 80% 1RM Wingate power Sit-ups in 1 min Vertical jump 40-yd sprint	12* 11* 10* — 19* — 4 13* 10* +1
			4	Undulating periodization 2 sessions/wk used 3 training 3-5, 8-10, 12-15 2 sessions/wk used only 8-10	RMs	Undulating sessions 7 Constant 8-10 rep session 12	Bench press Leg press Bench press reps at 80% 1RM Leg press reps at 80% 1RM Wingate power Sit-ups in 1 min Vertical jump 40-yd sprint	47*a 32*a 24*a — 64*a — 27*a 42*a 40*a -6*a
Hunter et al. 2001	66-67 M and F	25	3	2 × 10	80% of 1RM	10	Bench press Leg press Shoulder press Arm curl	34* 43* 42* 69*
			3	Undulating periodization 3 training zones 50%, 65%, and 80% of 1RM	50%, 65%, and 80% of 1RM	10	Bench press Shoulder press Leg press Arm curl	23* 31* 30* 59*

* = significant change pre- to posttraining; a = significant difference from 1 × 8-12 group.

of a strength/power periodized program to a single-set program (McGee et al. 1992) and to nonvaried multiple-set programs (McGee et al. 1992; O'Bryant, Byrd, and Stone 1988; Schiotz et al. 1998; Stone, O'Bryant, and Garhammer 1981) show neither program causing a significant change in total body weight. Other comparisons show periodized training and multiple-set programs to result in significant, but identical, increases in total body weight (Baker, Wilson, and Carlyon 1994a) and a significantly greater increase in total body weight with a strength/power periodized program compared to a single-set program (Kraemer 1997).

Comparisons of body compositional changes have shown strength/power periodized and multiple-set training programs to result in significant but identical increases in fat-free mass, with neither group showing a change in total body fat (Baker, Wilson, and Carlyon 1994a). Such comparisons have also shown nonsignificant increases in fat-free mass with both types of training, a small nonsignificant decrease with multiple-set training in body fat percentage, a small but significant decrease with periodized training in body fat percentage (Schiotz et al. 1998), and a significantly greater change in fat-free mass and percentage body fat with periodized training compared to a nonvaried multiple-set program (Stone, O'Bryant, and Garhammer 1981). A comparison of a single-set nonvaried program to a strength/power periodized program reported a significantly greater decrease in body fat percentage with periodized training (Kraemer 1997). Although changes in fat-free mass were not reported in this study because periodized training also resulted in a significantly greater gain in total body weight, it can be concluded that periodized training also resulted in a greater increase in lean body mass than the single-set program.

Because of the paucity of studies examining changes in total body weight, fat-free mass, and body fat, and the use of skinfolds to determine body composition in several of the studies, conclusions concerning the superiority of one type of training over the other in bringing about changes in these variables must be viewed with caution. However, as with strength gains and motor performance changes, it is important to note that whenever a significant difference between training programs has been reported, it has always been in favor of the strength/power periodized programs.

Several studies do offer some insight into why strength/power periodized training may result in greater strength gains than nonperiodized train-

ing. One unique aspect of the Willoughby 1993 study was that for the first 8 of 16 weeks of training there was no significant difference in total training volume between the periodized model and two multiple-set training models. After 8 weeks of training the periodized training volume significantly decreased compared to the multiple-set programs. After 8 weeks of training all groups demonstrated significant but identical increases in 1RM strength. Only after week 8, when the training volume in the periodized model was reduced, did significant differences in strength in favor of the periodized model become apparent. This indicates that the decreases in training volume present in strength/power periodized models may in part explain the greater improvement in 1RM strength. Another aspect of this study was that subjects were at least moderately trained (able to squat 150% and bench press 120% or greater of total body weight). So the results also indicate that trained individuals may need up to at least 8 weeks of training for periodized training to demonstrate superior results compared to nonvaried programs.

The conclusion that changes in training volume may in part explain the differences between training programs is supported by another study (Baker, Wilson, and Carlyon 1994a). During a 12-week training period, training volume (total mass lifted) and relative training intensity (percent of 1RM) were equated between a periodized and multiple-set program. This allowed any difference in strength gains between groups to be attributed to the manipulation of training volume and intensity and not to the total training volume or intensity used throughout the training program. Both programs resulted in significant strength increases, with no significant difference shown between groups. This indicated that greater increases in strength with periodized training may be due to greater training volumes, changes in training intensity, or both.

The results of Herrick and Stone (1996) in a comparison of a multiple-set program and a periodized program indicated that total training volume may be more important in strength development than changes in volume brought about by manipulation of sets, repetitions, and/or active rest periods during training. The exact factors related to greater fitness gains from strength/power periodized training compared to nonvaried models (when apparent) remains to be elucidated. However, the majority of studies do favor strength/power periodized models over nonvaried training models.

Undulating Periodization Training Studies

Because undulating periodization is a relatively new training model, relatively few studies have investigated its efficacy. The studies that have, however, indicate that undulating periodization is effective. Three studies have investigated the effect of using a typical undulating model in which three training zones are used successively on a training session basis compared to a single-set nonvaried model (see table 7.4). The earliest of the studies used college football players as subjects and demonstrated that the undulating model resulted in significantly greater gains in strength, local muscular endurance, and motor performance (Kraemer 1997). A second study using athletes as subjects also clearly demonstrated undulating periodization to be more effective than a single-set model (Kraemer et al. 2000). This study trained female collegiate tennis players for 9 months. The undulating model resulted in significantly greater increases in strength and motor performance measures. The motor performance measures included maximal serve velocity, which indicated that the undulating model is effective in bringing about changes in sport-specific activities. These two projects demonstrate that the undulating model is effective in bringing about physiological adaptations in athletes. A 6-month study demonstrated an undulating model to be more effective in bringing about changes in strength, motor performance, and local muscular endurance than a single-set model in previously untrained college-age females (Marx et al. 2001). Interestingly, this study also indicated that differences in the athletes' hormonal response (e.g., increased resting serum testosterone and IGF-I, and decreased cortisol) due to the undulating compared to the single-set model may in part account for the differences in strength and performance measures. The 6-month (Marx et al. 2001) and 9-month (Kraemer et al. 2000) studies also clearly indicate that the undulating model results in more consistent and significant gains throughout the training period than a low-volume nonvaried single-set model (see table 7.1). Collectively, these studies suggest that the undulating model is effective in bringing about physiological adaptations in healthy, young, trained and untrained adults.

A variation of an undulating model employing three training zones has been shown to be as effective as a nonvaried multiple-set model in adults 66 to 77 years old (Hunter et al. 2001). The multiple-set model used a resistance equivalent to 80% of 1RM in all training sessions, whereas the undulating model used training zones equivalent to 80%, 65%, and 50% of 1RM. It is important to note that all training sessions for both training models consisted of two sets of 10 repetitions or reps to concentric failure, whichever occurred first. Thus, the undulating model did not use training RM or near-RM training zones in all training sessions. No significant differences in strength between the two training programs were shown (see table 7.4). However, the nonvaried model showed greater percent strength gains. This indicated that not only is the undulating model as effective as a high-intensity multiple-set model, but also that high intensity (80% of 1RM) is not necessary in all training sessions with this age group. The undulating model did show some advantage over the non-varied model with the undulating model demonstrating a significantly greater decrease in difficulty of performing a carrying task.

A comparison of an undulating periodization model, with training zones varied on a biweekly basis, to a classic strength/power model and a nonvaried multiple-set model showed no significant differences in 1RM strength or vertical jump ability (Baker, Wilson, and Carlyon 1994a). However, the undulating model did demonstrate slightly greater changes in these variables on a percentage basis over the 12-week training program (see table 7.3). However, a comparison of the typical daily undulating model to a variation of the strength/power model (see table 7.3) demonstrated significantly greater strength gains in both the leg press and bench press (Rhea et al. 2002). In this study the absolute gain in bench press ability was not significantly different between the two training models; however, the absolute difference in leg press ability was significantly greater with the undulating model. It is also important to note that in this study the undulating and strength/power periodized models had equal total training volume and intensity. Thus, the difference between the two models cannot be attributed to differences in volume and intensity. It is also important to note that the subjects in this study had been weight training for at least two years before the start of the study using some type of variation of the strength/power periodization training model. These results do indicate that undulating periodization can be effective in individuals with previous weight training experience and that undulating periodization may be an effective training variation after performing strength/power periodization for a period of time. These results indicate that an undulating model with the undulating pattern varied every 2 weeks is at least as effective as a typical strength/power periodized model and a multiple-set nonvaried model, and that the typical daily undulating pattern is more effective than a strength/power model.

Undulating models have also been shown to be effective in bringing about body composition changes. The studies training collegiate football players (Kraemer 1997), female collegiate tennis athletes (Kraemer et al. 2000), and previously untrained college-age females (Marx et al. 2001) all demonstrate the undulating models to bring about greater decreases in percent body fat and greater increases in fat-free mass than single-set nonvaried models. The results of the studies concerning total body weight are mixed, with a significantly greater increase in total body weight reported in subjects using the undulating model and no significant change in total body weight reported from either training model. A variation of the undulating model is also as effective as a multiple-set model in bringing about increases in fat-free mass and decreases in percent body fat in older adults (Hunter et al. 2001). This study also reported no significant change in total body weight in either training group. Undulating on a biweekly basis resulted in significant increases in fat-free mass and total body weight, but those increases were equivalent to those seen in subjects using the multiple-set and strength/power periodized model (Baker, Wilson, and Carlyon 1994a). Body fat levels did not change significantly in any of the training groups in this study. Although data are limited, the undulating model appears to be more effective than nonvaried single-set models and at least as effective as nonvaried multiple-set and strength/power periodized models in bringing about changes in body composition.

The majority of information indicates that both the strength/power and undulating periodized models are more effective in bringing about physiological adaptations than nonvaried models. However, more studies are definitely warranted concerning periodized training models. In particular, studies examining the effects of periodized models in pubescents, seniors, and women are needed. Ideally, future studies should be long term in nature and examine the response of a wide array of variables, including strength, body composition, motor performance, and sport-specific activities, as well as variables such as hormonal responses that will help in explaining any differences in the training adaptations between training models.

Power Development

Power development is intimately related to the performance of most daily life activities (e.g., climbing stairs) as well as sport tasks (e.g., throwing a ball). The relationship of power to force, distance, and the time involved in performing a movement is related by the following power equation:

$$\text{Power} = \frac{\text{Force} \times \text{Distance}}{\text{Time}}$$

Working with this fundamental equation, one can start to see the different ways that power can be improved. The top part of the equation is "work," and the bottom part of the equation implicates the importance of the time used to perform a task. Training programs dedicated to the development of power require both high-force training and high-quality power movements in which time and the rapidity of movements play a vital role in the quality of the exercise. Remember that in the classic concentric force-velocity curve, as the speed of the muscle action increases, the force that can be produced decreases (Knuttgen and Kraemer 1987). However, the power output peaks at an intermediate speed between zero velocity and the maximal velocity of movement. Viewing it from another perspective, starting at very fast velocities, force is very low; this combination of force and velocity results in low power output. As velocity decreases, force increases until force is maximal at the point at which no movement occurs (isometric action). Power, on the other hand, increases to maximal at an intermediate velocity, while power decreases until it is zero at maximal force and no movement. The relationships among force, velocity of movement, and power can be seen in figure 7.2.

Training for power production in various movements should take these concepts into consideration. The success of a power training program will be related to the specificity of the training activity and the ability to target the training session's quality to optimize physiological function for high-power movements at different velocities. For example, Newton, Kraemer,

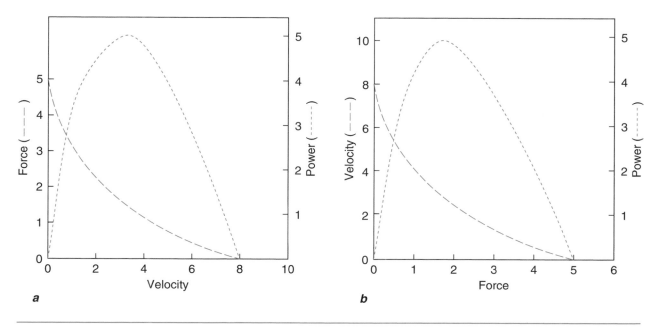

Figure 7.2 *(a)* Relationship of force generation (––––, left ordinate) and power generation (----, right ordinate) to velocity of shortening in maximal concentric actions. *(b)* Relationship of velocity shortening (––––, left ordinate) and power generation (----, right ordinate) to force development in maximal concentric actions. All muscular actions are concentric except those at zero velocity, which are isometric.

Adapted, by permission, from H.G. Knuttgen and W.J. Kraemer, 1987, "Terminology and measurement in exercise performance," *Journal of Applied Sport Science Research* 1: 1-10.

and Häkkinen (1999) showed that with ballistic training, maximal force production and rate of force development are the main contributors to improved vertical jumping during the preseason training of collegiate volleyball players.

Explosive resistance training creates specific increases in muscle activation and rates of force development (Häkkinen and Komi 1985c). The increases in what is called "explosive strength" occur when stretch-shortening cycle exercises (i.e., plyometrics) are used or when lighter loads (30-60% of 1RM) are used in "power-type" exercises (e.g., pulls, cleans) in which inhibitory decelerations and antagonist activation are minimized (Newton et al. 1996). Newton and coworkers (1996) demonstrated that when a "normal" bench press was performed explosively (e.g., speed reps) with a light load (e.g. 30% of 1RM), power decreased during approximately the last 50% of the range of motion because the lifter had to hold on to the bar and reach zero velocity when the bar was at arm's length. When the weight could be released at the end of the range of motion with the use of a specialized testing device, power output and acceleration were enhanced throughout the range of motion. The reduction in power and decreased rate of acceleration when the bar was "held on to" was due to decreased agonist activa-

tion and increased antagonist activation of muscles of the upper back, which actually created a pulling force on the bar to decelerate it because it had to be at zero velocity at arm's length. Figure 7.3 shows the results of the study by Newton and coworkers (1996). The authors theorized that this effect was needed to protect the joints from a sudden deceleration at the end of the range of motion when the weight was not released. This was not observed when the weight could be released at the end of the bench press's range of motion. Such data demonstrate why "speed reps" may be counterproductive to power development in some exercises (e.g., bench press, shoulder press, knee extension) and supports the proper use of resistance training tools that allow release of the weight in such exercises (e.g., medicine ball) or use exercise and equipment in which momentum of a mass is not a problem (e.g., isokinetics, pneumatics, hydraulics, rubber bands, etc.).

The development of power may be one of the most important physiological adaptations for increased physical performance. The ability to exert force earlier in a movement and through a greater portion of a movement plays a vital role in almost all athletic and everyday activities, as most activities are time and force dependent. From an athletic perspective it may be more appropriate

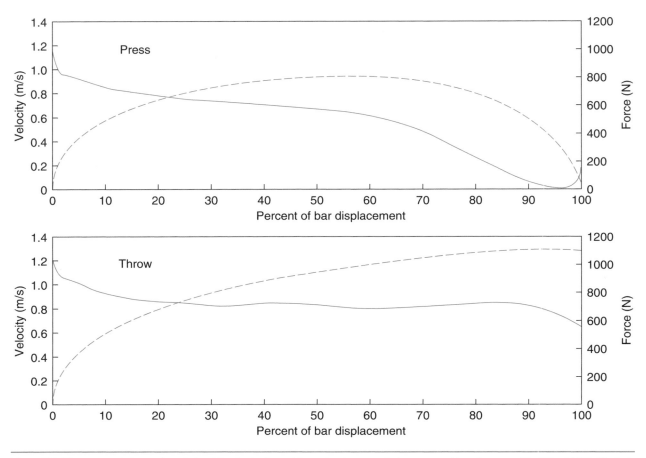

Figure 7.3 The top panel shows the relationship of velocity and force development during a normal bench press with 45% of 1RM. The bottom panel shows the relationship of velocity and force development during a bench press throw with 45% of 1RM.

Solid lines = force development; dashed lines = velocity.

Adapted, by permission, from R.U. Newton, et al., 1996, "Kinematics, kinetics, and muscle activation during explosive upper body movements: Implications for power development," *Journal of Applied Biomechanics* 13: 31-43.

to think of strength as the force capability of the muscle for actions ranging from the fastest eccentric to the slowest concentric actions. The force-velocity relationship for muscle dictates that the faster the velocity of concentric muscle action, the lower the force that can be produced, yet maximal power is produced at intermediate velocities of movement (approximately 30% of maximum shortening velocity) (Knuttgen and Kraemer 1987). Pure 1RM strength is required in the sport of power lifting (thus, the name of the sport is inappropriate) because there is no requirement for maximal or near-maximal power development since lifters must move heavy weights slowly. If an athlete is attempting to lift the maximum amount of weight, movement velocities are just higher than zero. Thus, the athlete exhibits maximal force, but a very low level of power when lifting 1RM resistances in most exercises.

Many strength and conditioning specialists believe that if the athlete's slow velocity strength increases, then power output and dynamic performance will also improve. This is true to a certain extent because maximum strength, even at slow velocities, is a contributing factor to explosive power as this affects the force variable in the power equation. All explosive movements start from zero or slow velocities, and it is at these phases of the movement that slow-velocity strength can contribute to power development. However, as the muscles begin to achieve high velocities of shortening, slow-velocity strength capacity has a reduced impact on the ability to produce high force at rapid shortening velocities (Duchateau and Hainaut 1984; Kanehisa and Miyashita 1983a; Kaneko et al. 1983; Moss et al. 1997). This fact becomes increasingly important as the athlete attempts to train specifically for optimal power development.

In terms of training, several studies have shown improved performance in power activities (e.g., the vertical jump) after a strength training program (Adams et al. 1992; Bauer, Thayer, and Baras 1990; Clutch et al. 1983; Wilson et al. 1993). Research by Häkkinen and Komi (1985a) showed a 7% improvement in vertical jump ability after 24 weeks of intense weight training. In a related study (Häkkinen and Komi 1985b), a group of subjects performed explosive jumps with a lighter resistance and produced a significant 21% improvement in vertical jump ability. The results indicate that trainees may experience specific training adaptations using heavy resistance versus power-type training. Several studies have shown that training for strength is an important part of power training, but when strength plateaus for an individual, specialized power training appears to be even more important to optimize power development (Baker 2001a; Newton, Kraemer, and Häkkinen 1999).

Heavy resistance strength training using high resistance and slow velocities of concentric muscle action leads primarily to improvements in maximal strength (i.e., the high-force/low-velocity portion of the force-velocity curve), and the improvements are reduced at higher velocities. In power training, which uses lighter resistances and higher velocities of muscle action, force output is higher at higher velocities of movement, and the rate of force development improves (e.g., more force at 100 milliseconds). This is important to increased power development in activities in which time to develop power is limited, such as in sprinting (Häkkinen and Komi 1985b).

Resistance- and velocity-specific training adaptations have been shown with training (Kaneko et al. 1983; Moss et al. 1997). Moss and colleagues (1997) trained the elbow flexors with resistances of 90%, 35%, and 15% of 1RM for 9 weeks. All groups trained for maximal power by attempting to move the resistance as fast as possible during each repetition. Power was tested with loads of 2.5 kg (5.5 lb), and 15%, 25%, 35%, 50%, 70%, and 90% of pretraining 1RM. The group training with 15% of 1RM showed significant increases in power at loads equal to or less than 50% of 1RM and no significant increases above loads greater than 50% of 1RM. No significant difference in power increase was shown between groups at loads equal to or less than 50% of 1RM. The 35% and 90% groups showed no significant differences between each other at any load, but did demonstrate significantly greater power increases than the 15% group at loads of 70% and 90% of 1RM. However, the 90% group showed the greatest power increases at the heaviest two loads, and the 35% group showed the most consistent power gains across all loads.

Kaneko and colleagues (1983) also found velocity-specific effects for a task that involved lifting a weight as quickly as possible. Subjects trained with a resistance of either 0%, 30%, 60%, or 100% of maximum isometric strength. The results demonstrated a classic resistance-specific training effect. The groups training with the heavier resistances showed the greatest increases in isometric strength, and the group training with 0% resistance produced the greatest increase in unloaded movement velocity. Perhaps the most interesting finding was that the 30% resistance produced the greatest increase in force and power over the entire concentric velocity range and also resulted in the greatest increase in maximum mechanical power. The results of these studies do demonstrate some training specificity for power.

Performance changes with training are not always consistent with the principle of training specificity. The conflict results from the complex nature of explosive muscle actions and the integration of slow and fast force production requirements within the context of a complete movement. Another confounding influence in observing clear, specific training adaptations is the fact that in untrained people, a wide variety of training interventions will produce increases in strength and power because the force part of the equation may dominate power increases until a stable base of strength is attained (Baker 2001c). Komi and Häkkinen (1988) suggest that, depending on the training status of the individual, the response may not always follow the velocity-specific training principle. Individuals with low levels of strength may show improvements throughout the force-velocity spectrum regardless of the training resistance or style used (Komi and Häkkinen 1988). Specialized types of training appear to cause training adaptations of single factors (i.e., high force, high power) only after a base level of strength and power training has been established. This is supported by the fact that if an athlete already has an adequate level of strength, then increases in explosive power performance in response to traditional strength training will be poor, and more specific power training interventions are required to further improve power output (Baker 2001c; Häkkinen 1989; Newton, Kraemer, and Häkkinen 1999). Thus, improvement of power performance in trained athletes may require complex training strategies (Baker 2001a; Newton, Kraemer, and Häkkinen 1999; Wilson et al. 1993).

Training for Power

Newton and Kraemer (1994) proposed a "mixed model" concept to develop all power development aspects (i.e., power, coordination, strength, and muscle size). The use of solely slow-velocity, heavy resistance training for the development of explosive power is often justified based on the fact that force is a primary factor in power development. However, specialized power training consisting of appropriate exercises and set and repetition schemes is needed for optimal training as a part of a periodized resistance training program (Kraemer and Newton 2000). If power performance is to be maximized, then both the force and the velocity components must be trained. The movement distance is usually fixed by the lifter's joint ranges of motion, so velocity is determined by the time taken to complete the movement. Therefore, if the individual trains using methods that decrease the time to perform a movement, power output increases. Intimately linked to this concept is the rate of force development.

Rate of Force Development

Because time is limited to develop power during muscle actions due to factors such as foot contact time during sprinting, it is advantageous for the muscle to exert as much force as possible in a short period. One factor contributing to this has been termed the **rate of force development** (RFD) or the rate at which strength is developed or increases. This may explain to some extent why heavy resistance training has not always increased power performance, especially during movements requiring very little time (e.g., 100 to 200 milliseconds). Squat training with heavy resistances (70-120% of 1RM) has been shown to improve maximum isometric strength; however, it did not improve the maximum RFD (Häkkinen, Komi, and Tesch 1981) and may even reduce the muscle's ability to develop force rapidly (Häkkinen 1989). On the contrary, activities during which the athlete attempts to develop force rapidly (e.g., explosive jump training with light resistances) increase the athlete's ability to develop force rapidly (Behm and Sale 1993; Häkkinen, Komi, and Tesch 1981). Baker, Nance, and Moore (2001a, 2001b) also observed that trained athletes who have undertaken both strength and power train-

ing may express maximal power outputs at higher percentages of maximal 1RM strength (47-63% of 1RM). Thus, higher percentages of maximum strength may be needed at certain phases of training to optimize power. Specialized power training may result in the use of resistances in the 30 to 45% of 1RM range, which is classically associated with peak mechanical power.

Explosive-type resistance training increases the slope of the early portion of the force-time curve. Figure 7.4 compares the effects of heavy resistance training versus explosive-type training on the isometric RFD curve. Although heavy resistance training increases maximal strength and thus the highest point of the force-time curve, this type of training does not improve power performance appreciably, especially in athletes who have already developed a strength training base (i.e., have had more than 6 months of training). This is because the movement time during explosive activities is typically less than 300 milliseconds, and most of the maximal force increases cannot be realized over such a short period of time. The individual does not have the time to use his developed slow-velocity strength.

Deceleration Phase and Traditional Weight Training

The **deceleration phase** of a repetition occurs when the resistance's movement slows even

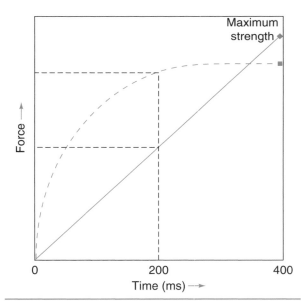

Figure 7.4 With power training, force developed in 200 ms or less is increased compared to training to increase only maximal strength levels.
------ = power training; —— = strength training.

though there is an attempt to increase or maintain movement speed. It is important to understand that deceleration of mass or resistance over the range of motion results in an exercise that will contribute less than optimally to power and high force production. The results of many studies (Berger 1963c; Wilson et al. 1993; Young and Bilby 1993) highlight a problem with traditional weight training and power development. Elliott, Wilson, and Kerr (1989) observed that when an individual lifts a weight, the bar is decelerating for a considerable proportion (24%) of the concentric movement. The deceleration phase increases to 52% when the individual performs the lift with a lighter resistance (e.g., 81% of 1RM) (Elliott, Wilson, and Kerr 1989). In an effort to train at a faster velocity more specific to a sport activity, athletes may attempt to move the bar rapidly during the lift. This also increases the duration of the deceleration phase (Newton and Wilson 1993a), as the athlete must slow the bar to a complete stop at the end of the range of motion.

Plyometric training and weighted jump squats avoid this problem by allowing the individual to accelerate throughout the movement to the point of load projection (e.g., takeoff in jumping, ball release in throwing, or impact in striking activities). It could be argued that traditional weight training promotes development of the deceleration action. The deceleration results from a decreased activation of the agonists during the later phase of the lift and may be accompanied by considerable activation of the antagonists, particularly when using lighter resistances and trying to lift the weight quickly (Kraemer and Newton 2000). This obviously is very undesirable when attempting to maximize power performances. To offset this, a style of lifting must be incorporated that involves "ballistic" resistance training.

The problem of the deceleration phase can be overcome if the athlete actually throws or jumps with the weight. This has been termed "dynamic" or "explosive" resistance training, but is probably best described as "ballistic" resistance training. The term *dynamic* is not really applicable because all training that involves movement (i.e., is not static or isometric) would be classified as dynamic. In addition, the term *explosive* is too general, as one can be explosive from the bottom position of a traditional squat, but reduce the effort near the top of the range of motion and never leave the ground. Ballistic infers acceleration, high velocity, and actual projection into free space. So this type of training is perhaps best described as "ballistic resistance training" (Newton and Wilson 1993b).

A pioneering study by Wilson and colleagues (1993) compared the effects of 10 weeks of training using traditional back squats, loaded jump squats, or plyometric or stretch-shortening cycle training (drop jumps) on vertical jump performance. The loaded jump squats were completed using a resistance of 30% of 1RM. This allowed the subjects to produce the greatest mechanical power output. All training groups showed increases in vertical jump performance; however, the loaded-jump-squats group showed significantly greater increases (18%) than the other two groups (heavy resistance training, 5%; stretch-shortening cycle training, 10%). These results were similar to that obtained by Berger (1963c), who also found that performance of jump squats with a resistance of 30% of maximum resulted in greater vertical jump ability increases compared with traditional weight training, plyometric training, or isometric training.

Studies of muscle fiber contractile characteristics (Faulkner, Claflin, and McCully 1986; Green 1986) seem to suggest that a great range of adaptations exists within the muscle cell, which alters its maximum velocity of shortening and force output at specific velocities. In particular, a considerable difference exists between the power capacity of fast-twitch (type II) muscle fibers and that of slow-twitch (type I) muscle fibers (Faulkner, Claflin, and McCully, 1986). One study by Duchateau and Hainaut (1984) removed the confounding variable of neural innervation and only considered contractile changes within the muscle. Subjects completed 12 weeks of training using either dynamic contractions with a resistance of 30% of maximum voluntary action (MVMA) or isometric training. The dynamically trained group showed increases in maximum shortening velocity, and the isometrically trained group did not. Whether the actual shortening velocity of the muscle fiber or the frequency of neural input is the stimulus to adaptations in force production at specific velocities remains speculative.

Behm and Sale (1993) presented evidence that the intention to move quickly determines the velocity-specific response. This means that heavy resistance weight training may be effective in increasing power if the athlete attempts to move the resistance as quickly as possible. This theory has been tested by Young and Bilby (1993), who compared the effects of slow and fast weight training on vertical jump ability and RFD. This study failed to find a velocity-specific effect on RFD, and the slow weight training was more effective for increasing vertical jump performance.

The subjects had had no prior weight training experience, and this may have influenced the results. Still, more study is needed to determine if "intention" to move a weight is enough to cause adaptations resulting in increased power.

Whether performing traditional or ballistic resistance training, there is considerable controversy over the resistance to be used for the development of explosive power (Wilson et al. 1993; Young 1993). Athletes who are limited to traditional resistance training techniques should use heavy (>80%) resistances because they simply cannot overload the muscle sufficiently using light resistances while stopping the weight at the end of the range of motion (Newton et al. 1996). With ballistic resistance training there is perhaps no one optimal intensity or resistance for use by all individuals. Both heavy (>80%) and light (<60%) resistances have application in the training of muscular power, with each affecting different components of explosive muscle action. If one had to choose a single resistance, the resistance that produces maximal power output (30% maximal voluntary action) has been shown to be optimal (Wilson et al. 1993), and 35% of 1RM has shown the most consistent power increases across varying resistances. However, as previously described, some load/velocity training specificity does exist. For highly trained athletes the resistances used may be increased and still remain effective (45-65% of 1RM). However, the degree to which this increase in power output will transfer to athletic performance may depend on whether the mass being moved is a similar resistance to that used in training. Accelerating the leg to kick a football or throwing a baseball represents a much lighter resistance than 30%, even though this resistance may be the resistance resulting in maximal power. Similarly, performing an Olympic lift can involve a much heavier resistance. In reality there is a wide selection of resistances to use for power or ballistic training. The greatest increase in power or performance may result when training with resistances that span the concentric force-velocity curve.

Although ballistic resistance training is effective for improving power performance, it does present the problem of the high eccentric forces exerted on trainees when they land from a jump or catch a falling weight in some exercises (Newton and Wilson 1993a). However, weight training equipment can be adapted to reduce the eccentric resistance (Newton and Wilson 1993a). In addition, ballistic weight training should progress gradually from the unloaded to loaded conditions with the athlete having completed a prior strength training program. Therefore, preparatory phases designed to develop basic strength are vital in a progression to ballistic training techniques.

Ballistic Training and Neural Protective Mechanisms

Neural protective mechanisms can affect force output. Plyometric or stretch-shortening cycle training results in an increase in the overall neural stimulation of the muscle and thus force output; however, qualitative changes are also apparent. In subjects unaccustomed to intense jumping-type stretch-shortening cycle training, there is a reduction in EMG activity starting 50 to 100 milliseconds before ground contact and lasting for 100 to 200 milliseconds (Schmidtbleicher, Gollhofer, and Frick 1988). Gollhofer (1987) attributed this to a protective mechanism by the Golgi tendon organ reflex acting during sudden, intense stretch loads to reduce the tension in the tendomuscular unit during the peak force of the stretch-shortening cycle. After a period of plyometric training, the inhibitory effects are reduced (this is termed *disinhibition*), and increased stretch-shortening cycle performance results (Schmidtbleicher, Gollhofer, and Frick 1988).

Plyometric training places considerable forces on the musculoskeletal system, and some recommend that the athlete have a preliminary strength training base before commencing a plyometric training program (e.g., squat 1.5 times body weight). Additionally, the potential for injury is thought to be much higher for some types of plyometric training such as drop jumps and should not be attempted by the beginner (Schmidtbleicher, Gollhofer, and Frick 1988).

Importance of the "Quality" of Training Repetitions

It is becoming obvious that the effectiveness of a power training program may in fact be related to the quality of each repetition. In other words, if a repetition does not achieve a high percentage (e.g., 90% or greater) of the maximal power output or maximal velocity possible, its impact on training adaptations may be negligible. Thus, if an athlete is fatigued or not ready to exercise maximally, a truly effective power training session may not be possible. For years the emphasis on quality of effort has been emphasized for plyometric training, and this may also be the case for all types of power training. An exception may be in the area of power development under conditions of extreme fatigue, such as a wrestler performing a throw at the end of a match under physiological conditions in which blood lactate concentrations are high (20 mmol/L). Training power under such conditions may enhance performance. In sports optimal training can be limited by too much sport practice, leaving athletes chronically fatigued and unable to focus on maximal efforts in their conditioning training sessions. Optimal combinations of the number of repetitions used in a set and the amount of rest used between sets needs further study. Our data show that 3 repetition sequences allow trainees to achieve at least 90% of peak power in a jump squat more often than performing 1 repetition at a time (unpublished data from Dr. Kraemer's laboratory).

Figure 7.5 shows the results of our pilot data related to what combination of repetitions allow for at least 1 repetition in each set to achieve a set cutoff point of 90% of maximal power output or greater. The amount of rest between sets also remains a question for the optimal exercise prescription. Fatigue should not be present if maximal power is to be achieved. Yet our example shows that performing 3 repetitions rather than 1 in a set using 3 minutes of rest between sets results in more repetitions achieving at least 90% of maximal power output. How this interacts with shorter rest periods remains to be determined. Nevertheless, the results show that acute or chronic fatigue that inhibits an individual from maximal efforts will reduce the impact of such exercise on power development. Research is moving into new concepts of training design, but similar to plyometrics, weight room exercises demand "quality of effort" to achieve optimal impact on actual training adaptations.

Plyometrics

A type of power training that has been used for a greater period of time than the types of power training described in the previous section, such as weighted jump squats and bench pressing in which the bar is thrown into the air, is **plyometrics**. Plyometric training is typically thought of as performing body weight jumping–type exercises and throwing medicine balls. Synonymous with the term *plyometrics* is the term *stretch-shortening cycle exercise*. However, body weight jumps and medicine ball throws are more accurately described by the term *stretch-shortening cycle exercise* than by the term *plyometrics*.

The **stretch-shortening cycle** refers to a natural part of most movements. As an example, every time a foot hits the ground during walking, the quadriceps go through a stretch-shortening cycle. When the foot hits the ground, the quadriceps first go through an eccentric action, then a brief isometric action, and finally a concentric action. If the reversal of the eccentric action to an isometric and then a concentric action is performed quickly, the muscle is stretched slightly and the resultant concentric action is more powerful than if a slight stretch did not occur. This entire sequence of eccentric, isometric, and concentric actions is called a stretch-shortening cycle.

When the sequence of eccentric to concentric actions is performed quickly, the muscle is stretched slightly before the concentric action. Thus, the term *stretch-shortening cycle* describes what actually happens. The muscle is stretched slightly and then shortens. The slight stretching stores elastic energy. The addition of the elastic energy to the force of a normal concentric action is one of the reasons commonly given to explain

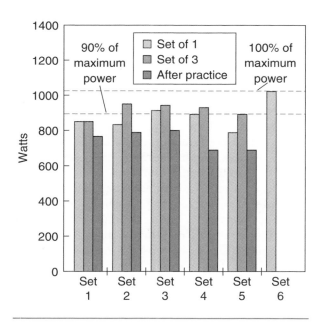

Figure 7.5 Pilot data for the squat jump demonstrating that a greater "quality of repetitions" (i.e., at least 1 repetition per set above 90% of maximal power) may well occur with the use of 3 repetitions in a set compared to 1-repetition attempts when multiple sets are performed. In addition, performing such training (3 reps per set) under conditions of fatigue (e.g., after practice) can diminish the power production and would not contribute to quality training. Resistance equals 30% of 1RM.

Unpublished data, Dr. Kraemer's laboratory.

why a more forcible concentric action results after a stretch-shortening cycle. The other common explanation for the more forcible concentric action is that a neural reflex results in a quicker recruitment of muscle fibers or a recruitment of more muscle fibers.

That the stretch-shortening cycle results in a more powerful concentric action is easy to demonstrate. During a normal vertical jump (a countermovement jump), the jumper bends at the knees and hips (eccentric action of the extensors), quickly reverses direction, and jumps (isometric followed by concentric action). Thus, a countermovement jump involves a stretch-shortening cycle. A jump performed by bending at the knees and hips, stopping for 3 to 5 seconds in the bent-knee and -hip position, and then jumping is termed a noncountermovement jump; it does not involve a stretch-shortening cycle and will result in a lower jump than a countermovement jump (a jump involving a stretch-shortening cycle). It is also possible to demonstrate the effect of a stretch-shortening cycle by throwing a ball for distance. Throwing a ball with a normal overhand throwing motion, which involves a stretch-shortening cycle, will result in a longer throw than throwing a ball without a windup, or starting the throwing motion from the end of the windup position (no stretch-shortening cycle).

Stretch-shortening cycle exercises can be performed with both the upper and lower body. Many medicine ball exercises for the upper body involve a stretch-shortening cycle. The depth jump (stepping off a bench and immediately jumping upon hitting the ground) is the exercise perhaps associated most frequently with the stretch-shortening cycle, but virtually all jumping exercises and throwing motions in which no pause is taken in the movement involve the stretch-shortening cycle.

Mechanisms Causing Greater Force With a Stretch-Shortening Cycle

Several physiological mechanisms may account for increased force with the stretch-shortening cycle. The ability to use stored elastic energy and neural reflexes are the most frequently cited explanations of why stretch-shortening cycle training increases force output. Evidence supports the use of stored elastic energy during a stretch-shortening cycle (Biewener and Roberts 2000;

Bosco et al. 1987; Bosco, Tarkka, and Komi 1982; Farley et al. 1991). Bosco and colleagues (1987) estimated that the elastic energy may account for 20 to 30% of the difference between a countermovement and noncountermovement jump. Elastic energy can be stored in tendons, other connective tissues, and the myosin cross-bridges (Biewener and Roberts 2000). If elastic energy were stored during a prestretch in the myosin cross-bridges, it would be lost as soon as the cross-bridges detached from active sites. Therefore, use of elastic energy stored in this fashion would have to be recovered very quickly. The average attachment time of a cross-bridge to an active site is 30 milliseconds. Since the enhancement of force from a prestretch lasts longer than this, other mechanisms to store elastic energy must also be present. Thus, although it is possible to store elastic energy at the myosin cross-bridge level, the majority of elastic energy is probably stored within connective tissues. An adaptation in connective or muscle tissue may take place with training to enhance storage and therefore the use of more elastic energy; this is implicated in studies showing changes in muscle stiffness as a result of plyometric training (Cornu, Almeida Silveira, and Goubel 1997; Hunter and Marshall 2002).

Another mechanism involved in creating greater force with a stretch-shortening cycle is muscle or fascicle length. During plyometric-type exercise in humans, the vastus lateralis generates more force with a prestretch compared to no prestretch, yet there is no difference in electromyographic activity (Finni, Ikegawa, and Komi 2001). The force enhancement may be related to longer fascicle length before the concentric action in the prestretch condition. This would place the muscle in a more advantageous position on the length-tension diagram to produce force.

Reflex recruitment of additional motor units, or an increased rate of firing by already recruited units, may result in increased force as a result of a stretch-shortening cycle. However, electromyographic activity does not change significantly in muscle that performs an isometric action and is then stretched (Thompson and Chapman 1988). Electromyographic activity has been reported to be not significantly different between a prestretch and a nonprestretch muscle action (Finni, Ikegawa, and Komi 2001). This indicates that reflex activity does not account for the increased force caused by the stretch-shortening cycle. Clearly some type of force potentiation is caused by the stretch-shortening cycle. However, the mechanism responsible is not completely elucidated; in fact, more than a single mechanism may be involved.

Long and Short Stretch-Shortening Cycle Training Exercises

Schmidtbleicher (1994) classified stretch-shortening cycle actions as either long or short based on the ground contact time. A long stretch-shortening cycle action has a ground contact time greater than 250 milliseconds, such as a countermovement jump and block jump in volleyball. A long stretch-shortening cycle action is also characterized by large angular displacement at the hip, knee, and ankle joints. A short stretch-shortening cycle action has a ground contact time less than 250 milliseconds, such as a drop jump in which an attempt is made to minimize ground contact time, sprinting, and takeoff in the high and long jumps. A short stretch-shortening cycle action is also characterized by small angular displacements at the hip, knee, and ankle joints. Correlations between countermovement jump height and drop jump height with minimum ground contact time are low, indicating that these tests are measuring different movement characteristics (Hennessy and Kilty 2001; Schmidtbleicher 1994). Therefore, these two types of stretch-shortening cycle actions should be considered different training modalities, and this difference should be considered when planning a stretch-shortening cycle training program for different activities.

The concept that long and short stretch-shortening cycle actions do affect performance differently is supported by correlation data. For example, in nationally ranked female sprinters and hurdlers, correlations between long and short stretch-shortening cycle tests and sprint ability at varying distances do vary (Hennessy and Kilty 2001). Correlations between 30-m sprint ability and performance in a drop jump with minimal ground contact time and a countermovement jump are −0.79 and −0.60, respectively. Correlations between 100-m sprint ability and performance in a drop jump with minimal ground contact time and a countermovement jump are −0.75 and −0.64, respectively. Correlations between 300-m sprint performance and performance in a drop jump with minimum ground contact time and a countermovement jump are −0.49 and −0.55, respectively. All correlations were significant except for 300-m sprint performance and performance in

a drop jump with minimal ground contact time. The drop jump with minimal ground contact time was the primary variable related to 30-m sprint performance, with this variable and ground contact time explaining 70% of the variance in 30-m sprint performance. For the 100-m sprint, 61% of the variance was explained by countermovement jump height and drop jump height with minimal ground contact time. This suggests that both long and short stretch-shortening cycle actions are related to 100-m sprint performance. Countermovement jump ability explained 30% of the variance in 300-m sprint performance, and drop jump ability with minimal ground contact time was not significantly related to 300-m sprint performance. These results indicate that trainers should consider the differences between short and long stretch-shortening cycle actions when planning a stretch-shortening cycle training program for an athlete in a particular activity or sport.

Efficacy of Stretch-Shortening Cycle Training

Training studies support the contention that performing only stretch-shortening cycle training can improve performance in motor performance tasks such as vertical jumping, sprinting, sprint cycling, and long jumping. Studies ranging in length from 6 to 12 weeks have shown improvements in the motor performance tasks of subjects using only one or two types of plyometric exercise such as depth jumps (Bartholomeu 1985; Blackey and Southard 1987; Gehri et al. 1998; Matavulj et al. 2001; Miller 1982; Scoles 1978; Steben and Steben 1981). Subjects in these studies typically trained two to three times per week, but some trained only once a week. Results showed that a relatively few number of repetitions of plyometric exercises may be needed to bring about significant improvements in motor performance. For example, depth jumps for three sets of 10 repetitions (3 × 10) per session (Matavulj et al. 2001), depth jumps for 2 × 10 to 4 × 10 per session (Blackey and Southard 1987), and countermovement jumps and depth jumps each for 4 × 8 (Gehri et al. 1998) have all brought about significant improvements in motor performance.

The effect of a single type of plyometric exercise on upper-body performance has received less study than the effect on the lower body. However, a study in which subjects used only plyometric push-ups during three sessions per week for 6 weeks did demonstrate significant improvement in upper-body power using a medicine ball throw (Vossen et al. 2000). Plyometric push-ups involve performing a normal push-up except that the trainee propels his body upward so that his hands leave the ground and then he must catch his own body weight upon returning to the ground before performing another plyometric push-up. Training in this study consisted of 3 × 10 to 4 × 11 plyometric push-ups per session. These studies demonstrate that stretch-shortening cycle training using only one or two types of plyometric exercises can improve motor performance in both the upper and lower body.

Studies in which subjects used a variety of plyometric exercises from 6 to 12 weeks have also shown significant improvements in motor performance tasks (Adams et al. 1992; Bartholomeu 1985; Bosco and Pittera 1982; Diallo et al. 2001; Fatouros et al. 2000; Ford et al. 1983; Potteiger et al. 1999; Rimmer and Sleivert 2000; Wagner and Kocak 1997). These studies used combinations of depth jumps, countermovement jumps, alternate-leg bounding, hopping, and other plyometric exercises. Training frequency in these studies was two to three sessions per week. Training programs varied substantially in these studies with as few as 23 to as many as 300 total foot contacts per training session being performed. A foot contact is a typical way of determining training volume in plyometric training. One foot contact consists of a foot or both feet together contacting the ground. Therefore, if an individual performs 2 × 10 depth jumps, 20 total foot contacts are counted. Several studies have also increased the number of foot contacts per session as training progressed. In studies using one or several types of plyometric exercises, a large variation in the number of foot contacts per training session can bring about significant improvements in motor performance.

The majority of studies using only one or two types of plyometric exercises and a combination of plyometric exercises used untrained subjects. A few studies of trained athletes (basketball and soccer players), however, have shown positive improvements in motor performance (Diallo et al. 2001; Matavulj et al. 2001; Wagner and Kocak 1997). Thus, athletes can use plyometric exercises to bring about changes in motor performance.

Height of a Depth Jump

Depth jumps are one of the most popular types of plyometric training, and increases in jumping ability has resulted from the performance

of depth jumps from a wide range of heights. However, the determination of the optimal height has received little attention from the sport science community. Verhoshanski (1967) stated that depth jumps from a height greater than 110 cm (43.3 in.) are counterproductive because the change from eccentric to concentric action takes place too slowly. Schmidtbleicher and Gollhofer (1982) also suggested that the height should not be so great that the athlete cannot prevent her heels from touching the ground. This is in part because of the increased chance of injury from the high-impact forces encountered if the heels do touch the ground.

After 8 weeks of training with depth jumps only, no significant difference in increased vertical jumping has been shown between training from 50 or 80 cm (19.7 or 31.5 in.) (Bartholomeu 1985). After 16 weeks of performing an identical resistance training program with and without depth jump training from 75 or 110 cm (29.5 or 43.3 in.), no significant difference was shown in increased vertical jump ability, 1RM squat strength, or isometric knee-extension strength (Clutch et al. 1983). No significant difference between groups in motor performance or leg strength was also shown when weight training was performed concurrently with depth jumps from either 40 or 110 cm (15.7 or 43.3 in) for 8 weeks (Blackey and Southard 1987). After training 3 days per week for 6 weeks from either 50 or 100 cm (19.7 or 39.4 in.), both groups demonstrated significant increases in countermovement jump ability, hip and knee extensor maximal force, and hip and knee extensor rate of force development, but no significant differences were shown between groups (Matavulj et al. 2001). Presently, information is insufficient to substantiate the optimal height from which to perform depth jumps.

Weighted Lower-Body Plyometric Exercises

The wearing of a weight vest or belt of up to 12% of body weight while performing stretch-shortening cycle exercises has resulted in increased vertical jump ability. This type of exercise is quite similar to the power-type training described in the previous section. Blattner and Noble (1979) and Polhemus and colleagues (1981) reported increases in vertical jump ability in untrained individuals over 6 and 8 weeks with this type of training. However, Bosco and Pittera

(1982) reported a decrease in vertical jump ability of 2.6 cm (1.0 in.) in skilled jumpers. The use of a 1.36-kg (3-lb) weighted jump rope while performing rope jumping exercises has also been shown to increase vertical jump ability and power output during a 30-second stationary bicycle maximal sprint, but it had no significant effect on 50-yd (45.7-m) sprint time (Masterson and Brown 1993). The training in this study was performed three times a week for 10 weeks. These studies generally show positive effects on motor performance ability. These studies and studies described in the previous power training section indicate that additional resistance to stretch-shortening cycle exercise does result in positive effects on performance and strength.

Concurrent Strength and Stretch-Shortening Cycle Training

Performance of both strength and stretch-shortening cycle exercises two to three times per week for 4 to 10 weeks of training results in increased vertical jump ability, countermovement jump ability, and leg strength (Adams et al. 1992; Bauer, Thayer, and Baras 1990; Blackey and Southard 1987; Clutch et al. 1983; Fatouros et al. 2000; Hunter and Marshall 2002). Increases in vertical jump ability have ranged from 3.0 to 10.7 cm (1.2 to 4.2 in.) with this type of training. This type of training has also been shown to significantly increase standing long jump ability in males but not females, to significantly decrease 40-yd (36.6-m) sprint time (Polhemus et al. 1981), and to significantly increase performance in a sprint stair-climbing task (Blackey and Southard 1987). In general, the positive changes in motor performance tests with concurrent strength and stretch-shortening cycle training are greater than with either training type alone (Adams et al. 1992; Bauer, Thayer, and Baras 1990; Fatouros et al. 2000; Polhemus et al. 1981). For example, vertical jump ability improved 3.3, 3.8, and 10.7 cm (1.3, 1.5, and 4.2 in.) with squat-only, plyometric-only, and combination training, respectively (Adams et al. 1992) and 11%, 9%, and 15% with lower-body weight training only, plyometric training only, and combination training, respectively (Fatouros et al. 2000). The combination group improved significantly more than either type of training alone in these studies. These results indicate that both types of training should be included in resistance

training programs when gains in motor performance are desired.

Stretch-Shortening Cycle Training Effect on Strength

The effect of stretch-shortening cycle training on strength has received some study. The isometric force of the knee extensors, but not the knee flexors, is significantly increased by performing only stretch-shortening cycle jump training (Bauer, Thayer, and Baras 1990). Jump rope training with a weighted rope has resulted in significant increases in 1RM leg press and bench press ability (Masterson and Brown 1993). Drop jumps have also been shown to increase hip extensor strength (Matavulj et al. 2001). Plyometric push-up training significantly increases seated 1RM bench press ability, but not to a greater extent than training with normal push-ups (Vossen et al. 2000). As would be expected, the combination of strength and plyometric training also increases strength (Blackey and Southard 1987; Fatouros et al. 2000). Interestingly, one of the studies reports leg press and squat ability to be enhanced significantly more with combination training compared to plyometric or strength training alone (Fatouros et al. 2000). This study reports a 12%, 22%, and 29% increase in 1RM squat ability with plyometric-only, weight-only, and combination training. The increase shown by the weight-only group was significantly greater than that shown by the plyometric-only group, and the increase shown by the combination group was significantly greater than either type of training alone. Although the subjects in this study were not weight trained, they could squat 1.5 times their body weight. Thus, whether plyometric training only will increase 1RM strength in highly weight trained individuals is speculative. Stretch-shortening cycle training can increase strength. Although minimal data are available, strength increases may be greater when strength and plyometric training are performed concurrently.

Effect of Stretch-Shortening Cycle Training on Body Composition

Studies examining the effects of plyometric-only training on body composition and muscle fiber size are inconclusive. The performance of only jump-type stretch-shortening cycle training in females for 10 weeks resulted in no significant change in percent body fat or fat-free mass (Bauer, Thayer, and Baras 1990). In boys aged 12 to 13 years, stretch-shortening cycle training performed along with normal soccer training resulted in a significant decrease in percent body fat (Diallo et al. 2001). Performance of stretch-shortening cycle jump-type training and some normal resistance training for 16 weeks resulted in no significant type I or II muscle fiber hypertrophy or change in percent body fat or fat-free mass (Häkkinen et al. 1990). However, Potteiger and colleagues (1999) reported that stretch-shortening cycle training performed for 8 weeks resulted in a significant increase in both type I and II fiber hypertrophy. As with any type of training the effect on body composition and muscle fiber size may depend on initial training status, the length of training, the volume of training, and whether other types of training were performed concurrently.

Injury Potential of Stretch-Shortening Cycle Training

As with any type of physical training, stretch-shortening cycle training does have inherent injury risks; anecdotal evidence indicates that injuries have occurred as a result of stretch-shortening cycle training. However, some of these injuries appear to be related to such factors as performing depth jumps from too great a height or improper flooring or landing areas. Several authors of stretch-shortening cycle training studies explicitly state that no injuries occurred from performance of the training (Polhemus et al. 1981), even in untrained individuals who had no preparatory resistance training before performing the stretch-shortening cycle training (Bartholomeu 1985; Blattner and Nobel 1979). As an injury prevention measure, some have suggested that any individual performing stretch-shortening cycle lower-body exercises should first be capable of performing a back squat with at least 1.5 to 2 times body weight. This might preclude many individuals from ever performing stretch-shortening cycle training even after a significant amount of normal weight training.

In a 1987 study, Blackey and Southard compared drop jump training combined with normal weight training in subjects of two different initial strength levels. Subjects who initially had a maximal 1RM leg press of less than two times and greater than two times body weight trained for 8 weeks. Training consisted of normal lower-body weight training and performing drop jumps from either 110 or 40 cm (43.3 or 15.7 in.). Initial strength level or height from which drop jumps were performed had no significant impact on either leg press 1RM increases or performance in a sprint stair-climbing task. The authors made no mention of injury in any of the training groups.

Although limited data are available, having to meet certain strength criteria before beginning a strength-shortening cycle training program does not seem warranted. However, because of the stresses encountered during this type of training, stretch-shortening cycle training should be introduced into the program slowly and should begin with a relatively low training volume.

Compatibility of Stretch-Shortening Cycle Training and Other Training Types

Questions concerning the compatibility of stretch-shortening cycle training with other training types have been raised. However, other training types seem quite compatible with stretch-shortening cycle training. As previously discussed, combining stretch-shortening cycle training with normal weight training may actually result in greater motor performance and strength gains compared to either type of training performed alone (Fatouros et al. 2000). Performing stretch-shortening cycle training combined with 20 minutes of aerobic training (70% of maximal heart rate) or performing only stretch-shortening cycle training results in significant gains in vertical jump ability, but no significant difference between groups (Potteiger et al. 1999). It is interesting to note that significant increases in both type I and type II muscle fiber cross-sectional area occurred with both training programs, but no significant difference was noted between programs. Normal weight and stretch-shortening cycle training 2 days per week for the lower body and flexibility training 4 days per week for the lower body show no incompatibility (Hunter and Marshall 2002). Both groups significantly improved in countermovement vertical jump ability as well as drop jump ability from 30, 60, and 90 cm (11.8, 23.6, and 35.4 in.), but no significant difference between groups was noted. Although data are limited, stretch-shortening cycle training shows no incompatibility with normal volumes of strength, aerobic, or flexibility training.

Comparisons With Other Types of Strength Training

Because few studies have compared stretch-shortening cycle to other types of strength training, conclusions must be viewed with caution. Training 2 days per week for 7 weeks results in no significant difference in increasing vertical jump ability between stretch-shortening cycle and normal dynamic constant external resistance training (Adams et al. 1992). The normal weight training consisted of back squats using a variation of the classic strength/power periodized training model, whereas stretch-shortening cycle training consisted of a periodized program of depth jumps, double-leg hops, and split jumps. The squat and stretch-shortening cycle training resulted in similar increases in vertical jump ability of 3.3 and 3.8 cm (1.3 and 1.5 in.), respectively. Training with either a stretch-shortening cycle or dynamic constant external resistance training program for 12 weeks resulted in significant, but similar, gains in vertical jump height in both groups (Fatouros et al. 2000). However, significant differences in favor of the dynamic constant external resistance training program in leg press (9% vs. 15%) and squat (12% vs. 22%) 1RM strength were shown.

Blattner and Noble (1979) performed a comparison of stretch-shortening cycle and isokinetic training. Eight weeks of training with three sessions per week resulted in no significant difference in increases of vertical jump ability between these two training methods. The stretch-shortening cycle and isokinetic training resulted in increased vertical jump ability of 4.8 and 5.1 cm (1.9 and 2.0 in.), respectively.

Other Considerations

Stretch-shortening cycle training is normally associated with training for anaerobic activities such as sprints and jumping. However, this type of training may also play a role in training for longer-duration sport activities. Distance in a plyometric leap test consisting of three consecutive leaps of jumping from one foot to the opposite foot and landing on both feet after the last leap explained 74% of the variance in a 10K race (Sinnett et al. 2001). Subjects in this study were recreationally trained distance runners. The results indicate that some type of stretch-shortening cycle training should be included in the total training program of moderately trained 10K runners.

Typically, the goal of stretch-shortening cycle training is to increase maximal power. Normally, relatively long recovery periods are allowed with this type of training so that near-maximal power can be expressed during each repetition. In some programs this means allowing rest periods between every repetition with some types of stretch-shortening cycle training. A study comparing 15-, 30-, and 60-second rest periods between each depth jump in a set of 10 jumps showed no significant difference in jump height or ground reaction force (Read and Cisar 2001). Although it is generally believed that sufficient recovery must be allowed during a stretch-shortening cycle training session, excessively long rest periods between every repetition do not seem necessary.

Body weight and body composition may be a consideration in the stretch-shortening cycle exercise prescription. The majority of these types of exercises, especially lower-body exercises, use body weight as the resistance to overcome. An individual with a higher percentage of body fat must perform the exercises with greater resistance (body weight) and with a smaller relative fat-free mass. Thus, a heavy individual may need to use a smaller training volume (i.e., total number of foot contacts) than an individual with a lower percentage of body fat.

Two Training Sessions in One Day

Two or more resistance training sessions on the same day are becoming relatively common. Some trainees may have started this practice because of time and schedule constraints. Others may include more than one session per day in an attempt to accumulate a greater total training volume. However, training at a relatively high volume twice a day is not recommended for the beginning trainee. As with all physical training, time must be allowed for the trainee to adapt to increases in intensity or volume.

When elite Olympic-style weightlifters perform a training session in the morning and one in the afternoon on the same day, strength measures decrease after the first training session, but recover by the second session (Häkkinen 1992; Häkkinen, Pakarinen et al. 1988c). Strength measures of Olympic-style weightlifters also recover between training sessions when two training sessions per day are performed on 4 out of 7 days (Häkkinen, Pakarinen et al. 1988b). Thus, well-conditioned resistance-trained athletes appear to be able to tolerate two training sessions per day, at least for short periods of time.

When elite Olympic-style weightlifters performed two training sessions on the same day for 2 days, no significant change in maximal snatch ability occurred (Kauhanen and Häkkinen 1989). However, the angular velocity of the knee in the drop under the bar decreased, and the barbell was pulled to a slightly lower height. After 1 day of rest, angular velocity of the knee increased, and the maximal height of the pull returned to normal. After 1 week of two training sessions per day, maximal leg isometric force production was unchanged in these elite weightlifters (Kauhanen and Häkkinen 1989). However, the time needed to reach maximal isometric force or rate of force development did increase. After 2 weeks of two to three training sessions per day, vertical jump ability decreased in junior elite Olympic-style weightlifters (Warren et al. 1992). Collectively, this information indicates that elite strength-trained athletes can tolerate two sessions per day at least for short periods of time, but that changes in exercise technique and decreased power output can occur. Possible indications that the athlete is not tolerating two training sessions per day may be small changes in exercise or sport technique and decreases in power-oriented tasks such as vertical jump ability.

One reason for performing two training sessions per day is to increase the total training volume. Another reason is to split a training session into two half-sessions to allow almost complete recovery between halves. This allows the athlete to achieve a higher intensity in the second half of the training. This schedule was investigated, and the results indicate that when total training volume is equal, two half-volume training sessions per day are advantageous (Häkkinen and Pakarinen 1991). In a 2-week period trained bodybuilders and power lifters performed one training session per day. In another 2-week period they performed the same training exercises with the same volume, but divided the volume into two training sessions on the same day. Thus, total training volume was equal in the 2-week periods; the only difference was the number of training sessions per day. Each 2-week training period was followed by 1 week at a reduced training volume. Isometric force during a squat-type movement was unchanged after

each 2-week training period. Isometric force was also unchanged after the week of reduced training volume after the one-training-session-per-day period. However, isometric force significantly increased after the week of reduced training volume after the two-training-sessions-per-day period. In a similar study female competitive athletes performed a 2-week training period during which their normal training volume was equally distributed between two training sessions on the same day followed by a 1-week period of reduced training volume (Häkkinen and Kallinen 1994). Compared to subjects in a normal one-session-per-day program over 3 weeks, the subjects in the two-sessions-per-day group demonstrated significant increases in maximal isometric strength and quadriceps cross-sectional area. These results indicate that dividing total training volume into two sessions a day may result in greater strength increases after a short recovery period.

Summary

Advanced training strategies, such as periodization and stretch-shortening cycle training, are necessary to optimize training adaptations in advanced lifters. More research concerning advanced training strategies is needed, especially with advanced lifters or elite athletes. However, information presently available does indicate that advanced training strategies do work and can be more effective than training strategies not including an advanced strategy. Therefore, advanced strategies should be used especially when developing resistance training programs for well-trained individuals and athletes.

Key Terms

classic strength/power periodization
deceleration phase
long stretch-shortening cycle
periodization
plyometrics
power
rate of force development
short stretch-shortening cycle
stretch-shortening cycle
undulating periodization

Selected Readings

Fleck, S.J. 1999. Periodized strength training: A critical review. *Journal of Strength and Conditioning Research* 13: 82-89.

Fleck, S.J. 2002. Periodization of training. In S*trength training for sport*, edited by W.J. Kraemer and K. Häkkinen, 55-68. Oxford, UK: Blackwell Science.

Häkkinen, K. 2002. Training-specific characteristics of neural muscular performance. In *Strength training for sport*, edited by W.J. Kraemer and K. Häkkinen, 20-36. Oxford, UK: Blackwell Science.

Kraemer, W.K. 1997. A series of studies—the physiological basis for strength training in American football. *Journal of Strength and Conditioning Research* 11: 131-142.

Kraemer, W.J., and Newton, R.U. 2000. Training for muscular power. *Physical and Medical Rehabilitation Clinics of North America* 11: 341-368.

Schmidtbleicher, D. 1994. Training for power events. In *Strength and power and sport,* edited by P. V. Komi, 381-395. London: Blackwell Science.

CHAPTER 8

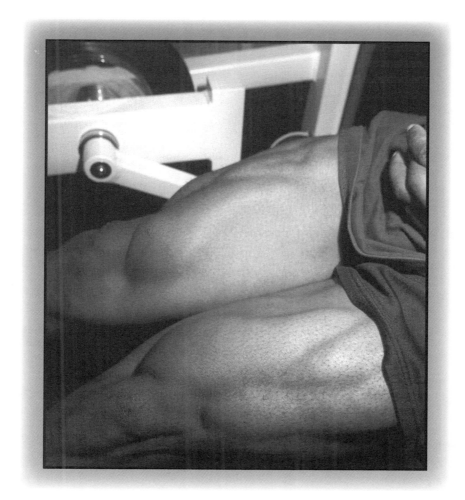

The Detraining Phenomenon

The classic definition of detraining is the "cessation of exercise training." However, detraining may also occur with a planned or unplanned (e.g., an injury) reduced volume or intensity of training. When strength and power performance decrements occur or when muscle mass is lost, some type of "detraining" may have occurred. Detraining can take place after several weeks or after many years (e.g., as a result of no exercise training with aging). Short-term (weeks to months) detraining is typically more relevant to resistance training program design. The goals of many maintenance programs in resistance training are to prevent detraining from occurring while allowing more time to train other fitness components.

Detraining is a deconditioning process that affects performance because of diminished physiological capacity. Detraining can occur in several situations including complete cessation of weight training, decreased volume of weight training such as during an in-season resistance training program, and long periods of no weight training or reduced volume of resistance training such as following completion of an athletic career. The general effects of detraining are depicted in figure 8.1. Cessation or reduction of resistance training may occur from injury or as a planned part of the yearly training cycle, such as may occur during many in-season programs. An understanding of detraining will facilitate the design of optimal resistance training programs for improving performance and maintaining strength and power during periods of training in which resistance training is reduced.

Mujika and Padilla (2001) recently reviewed the time course of detraining responses. From a cardiovascular perspective, detraining has been characterized by decreased capillary density, which may take place after 2 to 3 weeks of inactivity, with arterial-venous oxygen difference declines if training is stopped for 3 to 8 weeks. Rapid declines in oxidative enzymes bring about reduced mitochondrial ATP production. These are related to a reduction in peak oxygen consumption and are important for cardiovascular fitness. Athletes who have greater cardiovascular

fitness levels will have greater reductions in functions related to the transport and use of oxygen for the generation of energy. However, following a period of detraining, athletes still have values for such variables that are higher than those in untrained, sedentary subjects, and their physiological functions return quickly with retraining after a short detraining period. Yet, cardiovascular fitness may be lost more quickly than high force and power production. Strength may be maintained for up to 2 weeks in power athletes (Hortobagyi et al. 1993), and in recreationally trained individuals strength loss has been shown to take longer (i.e., 6 weeks) to occur due to lower initial strength fitness levels than highly trained individuals prior to detraining (Kraemer, Koziris, Ratamess et al. 2002). However, eccentric force and power may be more sensitive to detraining effects over a few weeks, especially in trained athletes (Kraemer, Koziris, Ratamess et al. 2002; Mujika and Padilla 2001). Interestingly, detraining periods of up to 24 weeks in middle-aged and elderly individuals have been shown to induce muscle atrophy and strength loss, whereas explosive jumping and walking actions remained

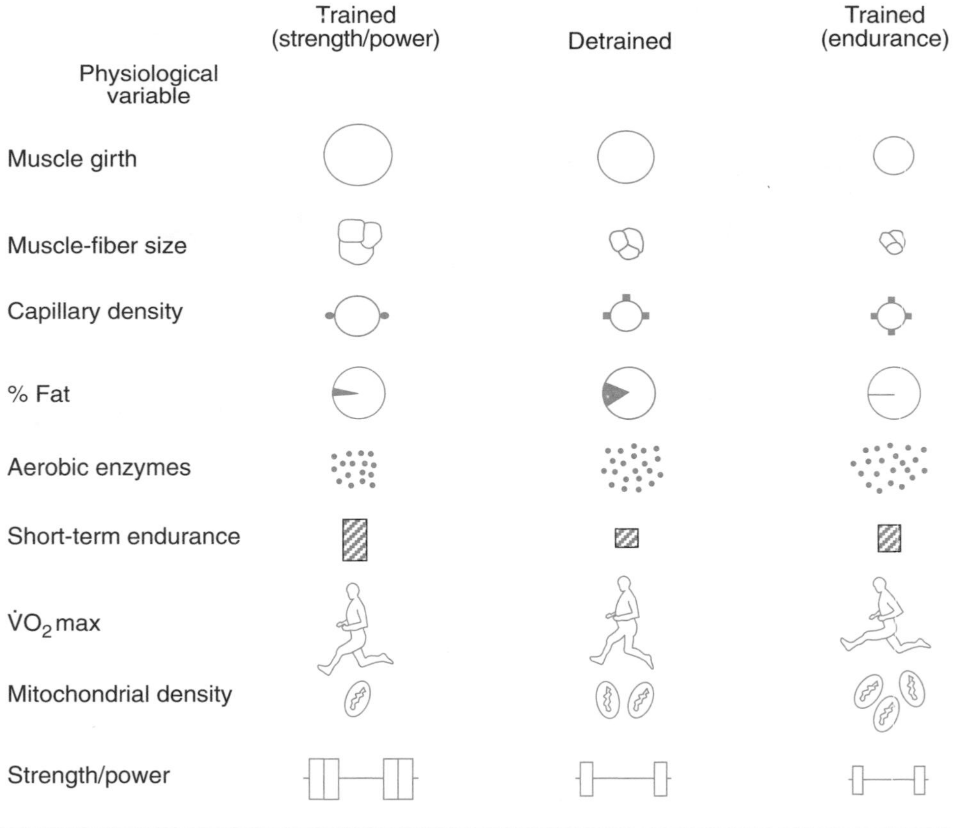

Figure 8.1 General effects of detraining.

elevated above pretraining levels (Häkkinen, Alen et al. 2002). These data indicate that neural retention of such force-production activities may be retained if normal physical activity is more robust during the detraining period. The magnitude of the effect may be due to the greater reliance on neural mechanisms and the level of adaptation attained prior to detraining.

Types of Detraining

Detraining classically occurs in several situations. The first is complete cessation of all types of training. This type of detraining may occur at the end of a season or at the termination of an athletic career. Complete cessation of training is seldom desirable because it has negative physical performance as well as health implications. A reduction in weight training volume after a period of performing weight training can occur in several situations. One is a situation in which only weight training was being performed and the training volume is reduced. This situation might occur as part of a research project or following an injury. Another type of detraining is a planned reduction in weight training volume with continued performance of other types of physical training. This situation occurs in many in-season weight training programs for a sport in which weight training volume is reduced, but other types of training continue.

Cessation of Resistance Training

Early studies indicate that when training ceases completely or is drastically reduced, strength gains decline at a slower rate than the rate at which strength increased due to training (McMorris and Elkins 1954; Morehouse 1967; Rasch 1971; Rasch and Morehouse 1957; Waldman and Stull 1969). In most instances, complete cessation of resistance training results in an immediate decline of strength (see table 8.1). For example, squat ability of Olympic weightlifters (see figure 8.2) shows a decline of approximately 10% in a 4-week period after cessation of weight training. However, active males, after a period of training, showed a slight increase in isometric force during a 2-week detraining period (see figure 8.3). This suggests that the direction and magnitude of strength changes during a short detraining period may vary depending on the initial level of conditioning. However, generally a short detraining period does result in a decrease in strength, but the level of maximal strength after detraining will still be greater than pretrained levels (see table 8.1).

Longer periods of detraining (up to 30 weeks) also result in a significant decrease in strength (see table 8.1), with strength still being greater after the detraining period compared to before beginning resistance training. Generally, relatively quick decreases in strength occur during a detraining period followed by a slower decline in strength (Häkkinen, Alen et al. 2000; Ishida, Moritani, and Itoh 1990; Ivey et al. 2000). Narici and colleagues (1989) reported the average rate of decline (0.3% per day) in maximal isometric force to be the same at which it was gained during isokinetic training.

However, a study by Lemmer and colleagues (2000) shows a slightly different pattern of strength loss due to detraining after 9 weeks of training the knee extensors. Young (20- to 30-year-old) and older (65- to 75-year-old) males and females showed significant increases of 34% and 28%, respectively, in 1RM strength following training. However, the gains made by the younger subjects were significantly greater than those shown by the older subjects. During 31 weeks of detraining, the younger and older subjects showed significant decreases in strength of 8% and 14%, respectively. The loss shown by the older subjects was significantly greater than that of the younger subjects. Interestingly, both the older (13%) and younger (6%) subjects showed the majority of strength loss from weeks 12 to 31. The young men, older men, and older women all showed significant strength decreases from week 1 to week 12 and from week 12 to week 31 of the detraining period. The younger women showed a similar pattern of strength loss, except that the loss from weeks 12 through 31 was not significant. The results indicate that both young and old individuals maintain strength quite well during 12 weeks of detraining, but that older subjects in particular lose strength rapidly after 12 weeks of detraining.

Collectively, the information available on both short (2 to 4 weeks) and long periods of detraining indicates that strength decreases do occur, but the loss is quite variable in magnitude. The rate of strength loss may depend in part on the length of the training period prior to detraining, the type of strength test used (e.g., bench press, eccentric, concentric, etc.), and the specific muscle group examined. In general, these trends also apply for older individuals, with the exception that older women appear to be more susceptible to detraining (Ivey et al. 2000).

Normal resistance training (concentric and eccentric actions) may result in a slower loss of strength during 4 weeks of detraining than

Table 8.1 Strength and Power Changes With Detraining

Reference	Subjects	Length of training (wk)	Type of training	Days/wk	Sets × Reps	Length of detraining (wk)	Type of strength test	% above pretrained Trained	Detrained
Kraemer, Koziris, and Ratamass 2002	Resistance-trained males	2+ years	Total body, periodized	3-4	3-5 × 1-12RM	6	1RM squat 1RM bench press 1RM shoulder press Wingate-power	?	–3.2
Häkkinen, Alen et al. 2000	Males/females—middle aged Males/females—elderly Males/females—middle aged Males/females—elderly	24 24 24 24	Leg press/extension Leg press/extension Leg press/extension Leg press/extension	2 2 2 2	3-4, 8-15 × 50-80% 1RM 3-4, 8-15 × 50-80% 1RM 3-4, 8-15 × 50-80% 1RM 3-4, 8-15 × 50-80% 1RM	3 3 24 24	1RM knee extension 1RM knee extension 1RM knee extension 1RM knee extension	27* 29* 29* 23*	27* 29* 23* 19*
Lemmer et al. 2000	Males/females—young Males/females—elderly	9 9	Knee extension Knee extension	3 3	5 × 5-10 5 × 5-10	31 31	1RM knee extension 1RM knee extension	34* 28*	26* 14*
LeMura et al. 2000	Females	16	Total body weightlifting	3	2 wk 2 × 8-10 × 60-70% 1RM	6	1RM of several upper-body exercises 1RM of several lower-body exercises	29* 38*	19* 24*
Taaffe and Marcus 1997	Males—elderly	24	Upper and lower body	3	3 × 8 75% 1RM (+GH)	12	1RM knee extension	40.4*	10.5*
Faigenbaum et al. 1996	Males/females—children	8	Weightlifting	2	4 wk 2 × 6-8 RM 4 wk 3 × 6-8 RM	8	6RM knee extension 6RM chest press	53* 41*	17 19*

Study	Group		Exercise		Protocol		Test		
Hortobagyi et al. 1993	Power lifters and football players	8.1	Weightlifting	3.4	2-5 × 1-12	2	1RM squat 1RM bench press	? ?	−1.7 −0.9
Dudley et al. 1991	Males	19	Leg press, knee extension	2	4-5 × 6-12	4	3RM leg press 3RM knee extension	26* 29*	20 20
Häkkinen et al. 1989	Male—strength athletes Males Females	10.5 10.5 10.5	Weightlifting Weightlifting Weightlifting	3.5 3.5 3.5	70-100% 1 RM 70-100% 1 RM 70-100% 1 RM	2 2 2	Knee extension, maximal isometric	8* 13* 19*	5 15 18
Narici et al. 1989	Males	8.6	Isokinetic, 120°	4	6/10	5.7	Isometric	21*	3 wk = 10 5.7 wk = 4
Häkkinen and Komi 1983	Males	16	Squat	3	15 reps 80-100% 1RM 5 reps eccentrically 100-120% 1RM	8	Isometric squat	30*	19*
Ishida et al. 1990	Males	8	Calf raises	3	3 × 15 70% 1RM	8	Isometric	32*	4 wk = 20 8 wk = 16
Blimkie et al. 1989	Boys	20	Total body weight training	3	3 × 15 70% 1RM	8	Bench press Leg press Isometric knee extension Isometric elbow flexion	35* 22* 21* 31*	34 17 14 30
Häkkinen, Alen, and Komi 1985	Males	24	Squat	3	18-30 reps 70-100% 1RM 3-5 reps eccentrically 100-120%	12	Isometric squat	27*	12*
Häkkinen, Komi, and Alen 1985	Males	24	Squat	3	18-30 reps 70-100% 1RM 3-5 reps eccentrically 100-120%	12	Squat 1RM	30*	15*

(continued)

Table 8.1 (continued)

Reference	Subjects	Length of training (wk)	Type of training	Days/wk	Sets × Reps	Length of detraining (wk)	Type of strength test	% above pretrained	
								Trained	Detrained
Houston et al. 1983	Males	10	Leg press, knee extension	4	3 × 10 RM	12	Knee extension, 0-270 deg · sec	39-60	4 wk = 29-52 12 wk = 15-29*
Häkkinen et al. 1985	Males	24	Jump training with 10-60% of 1RM squat	3	100-200 jump session	12	Isometric squat	6.9*	2.6*
Staron et al. 1991	Females	20	Leg press, squat, knee extension	2	3 × 6-8 RM one session, 3 × 10-12 RM one session	30-32	Squat 1RM Leg press 1RM Knee extension 1RM	67* 148* 70*	45* 105* 61*

* = significantly different from pretrained.

concentric-only training (Dudley et al. 1991). In this study normal resistance training and concentric-only training consisted of three sets of 10 to 12 repetitions at a 10 to 12RM resistance. Double-volume concentric training consisted of six sets of 10 to 12 repetitions at the normal resistance training 10 to 12RM resistance. Thus, with double-volume concentric training, the total number of concentric-only muscle actions was equal to the total number of concentric and eccentric actions performed during the normal resistance training. Concentric-only

regimes consisted of lifting the weight, but never lowering the weight. Subjects performed only the leg press and knee extension exercises, and trained 3 days per week for 19 weeks. A 3RM leg press and knee extension were used to evaluate strength after the training and detraining periods. Strength increases for both exercises were tested with concentric actions only and using normal weight training (concentric and eccentric actions). All groups improved significantly in concentric-only leg press ability (see figure 8.4).

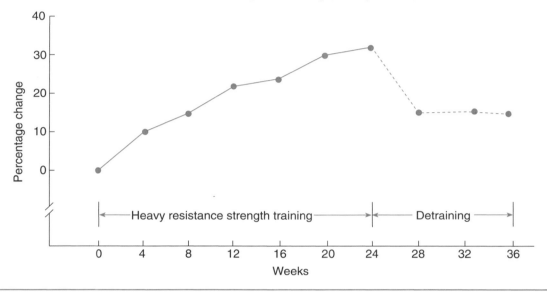

Figure 8.2 Percent changes in 1RM squat of Olympic-style weightlifters with training and detraining.

Adapted, by permission, from K. Häkkinen and P.V. Komi, 1985, "Changes in electrical and mechanical behavior of leg extensor muscles during heavy resistance strength training," *Scandinavian Journal of Sports Science* 7: 55-64.

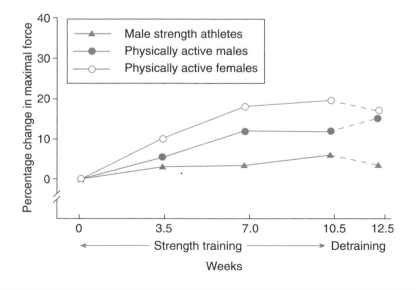

Figure 8.3 Percent changes in maximal isometric force with training and detraining.

Reprinted from *Journal of Biomechanics*, Vol. 8, K. Häkkinen et al., "Neuromuscular adaptations and hormone balance in strength athletes, physically active males, and females, during intensive strength training," pp. 889-894, Copyright 1989, with permission from Elsevier.

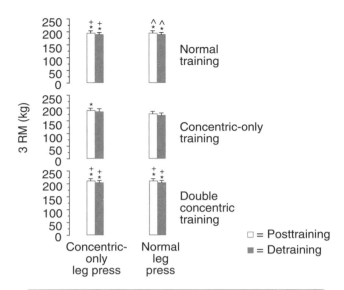

Figure 8.4 Changes in 3RM leg press with normal resistance training, concentric-only training, and double-volume concentric training.

* = increase over pretraining; + = greater increase than concentric-only group; ^ = increase greater than concentric-only and double-volume concentric groups.

Adapted, by permission, from G.A. Dudley et al., 1991, "Importance of eccentric actions in performance adaptations to resistance training," *Aviation, Space, and Environmental Medicine* 62: 543-550.

After the detraining period, the normal resistance and double-volume concentric training resulted in greater retention of strength than the concentric-only training (see figure 8.4). In addition, the normal resistance training resulted in a smaller loss of strength than the double-volume concentric training. The knee-extension strength followed a similar pattern. This information indicates that normal resistance training results in greater strength retention during detraining than

does concentric-only training, even when the volume of concentric-only training is doubled.

Reduction of Training Volume

An early study (Berger 1962a) indicated that strength could be improved over a 6-week detraining period using only one set of 1RM and training only 1 day a week. This study shows that strength can be maintained with a program consisting of reduced training frequency and volume of exercise.

A study using various jumping and stretch-shortening cycle drills three times per week for 16 weeks showed an increase in isometric leg strength of 28% (Häkkinen et al. 1990). After 8 weeks of performing the same type of training session at a reduced frequency of only once a week, isometric strength had decreased to 6% above pretraining levels. This, however, was a nonsignificant decrease, and a great deal of individual variation in response to the detraining period occurred.

Reducing training frequency for 12 weeks after 10 to 18 weeks of training may not have an effect on isometric strength and training weight used (Graves et al. 1988). The training session in this study consisted of one set of 7 to 10 variable resistance knee extensions at 7 to 10RM. Training was performed either two or three times per week and reduced to one, two, or no training sessions per week. All training frequencies significantly increased the isometric and training resistance used (see table 8.2). After the 12 weeks of training at reduced frequencies, no reduced training frequency resulted in a significant decline in strength from pretraining values.

Table 8.2 Changes in Knee Extension Strength After 10-18 Weeks of Training Followed by 12 Weeks of Detraining

	Isometric force % above pretraining		Training weight % above pretraining	
Training/detraining frequency	Trained	Detrained	Trained	Detrained
3/2	27*	23*	64*	65*
3/1	20*	20*	59*	59*
2/1	17*	15*	47*	40*+
3-2/0	18*	6*+	40*	—

* = significantly greater than pretraining; + = significantly less than posttraining.

Data from "Effect of Reduced Training Frequency on Muscular Strength" by J.E. Graves, et al., 1988, *International Journal of Sports Medicine*, 9, 316-319.

In another study, 12 weeks of reduced training after 10 to 12 weeks of variable resistance or isometric training resulted in no change in isometric back strength at seven angles of back extension (Tucci et al. 1992). Training was performed one to three times per week and consisted of either two sets of variable-resistance back extensions of 8 to 12 repetitions at an 8 to 12RM, two sets of isometric back extensions, or one set of each type of exercise. During detraining, frequency was reduced to either one session every 2 weeks, one session every 4 weeks, or no training at all. Training resulted in significant increases in isometric back extension strength at all seven angles tested (8-60%). Detraining frequencies of one session once every 2 or 4 weeks resulted in nonsignificant decreases in isometric strength from posttraining values (+1% to –13%). No training at all during the 12-week detraining period resulted in significant decreases from posttraining values at all seven back angles (6-14%).

In another study investigating the impact of different training frequencies during a detraining period, McCarrick and Kemp (2000) examined 12 weeks of isokinetic training of the rotator cuff musculature. Training significantly improved all measures of torque production. After training, participants were placed in either a two-, one-, or zero-sessions-per-week detraining group. The participants in the one- and two-sessions-per-week groups showed no significant decreases in concentric or eccentric peak or mean torque during the 12 weeks of detraining. Participants who did not train at all during the detraining period experienced significant decreases in the majority of concentric and eccentric internal and external isokinetic tests with greater losses in eccentric strength. These findings show that a training frequency of one or two sessions per week of the rotator cuff musculature can maintain torque, but that eccentric force production may be more susceptible to detraining.

Collectively, these studies indicate that reduced training can maintain strength levels in a variety of muscle groups if training intensity is maintained at a high level, but no training at all does result in loss of strength during detraining.

In-Season Detraining

In-season detraining refers to losses of performance when individuals stop resistance training completely or train at a reduced volume while undertaking other sport-type training. This type of detraining is important to consider, but it has received little attention from the sport science community.

A study by Campbell (1967) showed that isometric elbow-flexion strength increased over spring football practice, but that isometric leg-extension strength significantly decreased with no resistance training program. The amount of both weight-bearing activity and leg stress involved in the sport might have contributed to the impaired isometric leg strength performances.

Koutedakis and colleagues (1992) examined the effects of an alpine ski season on the knee-extension and -flexion strength and power output of elite downhill, freestyle, and speed skiers. Three months into the season isokinetic knee-extension strength at 60 degrees per second decreased significantly by 6% and knee-flexion strength nonsignificantly by 7%. After 7 months knee-extension strength at 60 degrees per second decreased significantly by 14% and knee-flexion strength by 16%. Isokinetic knee-flexion and -extension strength at 180 degrees per second after 3 and 7 months of detraining showed small, nonsignificant decreases. The skiers demonstrated nonsignificant changes in power output during a 30-second maximal cycling test (Wingate test). Thus, skiers may lose strength at very slow velocities, but not intermediate velocities, during a season. However, since no loss of power output occurs, the effect on performance may be minimal.

Rowing requires a high level of strength and aerobic conditioning. After 10 weeks of resistance training three times per week, rowers demonstrate increased strength (see figure 8.5; Bell et al. 1993). Six weeks of resistance training at a reduced frequency of either one or two times per week resulted in either no significant change or an increase in strength (see figure 8.5). All training sessions consisted of approximately three sets of each of the six exercises shown in figure 8.5 at an intensity of approximately 75% of maximal. Rowers performed their normal training other than weight training throughout both the initial and reduced resistance training frequency portions of training. These results indicate that strength can be maintained or increased for a period of 6 weeks in rowers who do not weight train but continue rowing. Rowing, however, in and of itself, does have a high strength component, so the applicability of these results to other sports or activities that do not have a high strength component is questionable.

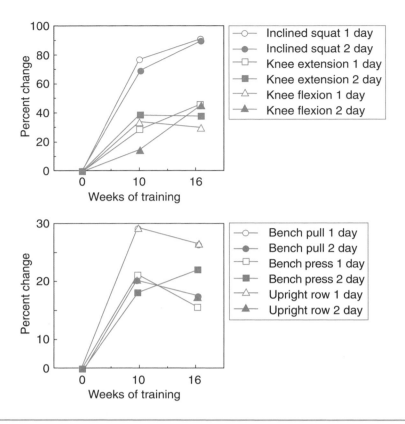

Figure 8.5 Changes in strength during 10 weeks of resistance training 3 days per week followed by 6 weeks of resistance training 1 or 2 days per week in oarswomen.

Data from G.J. Bell et al., 1993.

Another study examined a Division I men's basketball team that performed a 5-week resistance training program immediately prior to a 20-week season (Hoffman et al. 1991). The 5-week program resulted in significant increases in 1RM squat of 18% and nonsignificant changes in 1RM bench press, 27-m (29-yd) sprint time, and vertical jump ability of 4%, 2%, and 0%, respectively. During the 20-week basketball season, subjects performed no resistance training. Nonsignificant changes occurred in 1RM bench press, 1RM squat, and vertical jump ability during the 20-week season (–1 to +5%), and 27-m (29-yd) sprint ability declined significantly (3%). This indicates that most measures of fitness can be maintained during the course of a college basketball season without an in-season resistance training program, and that playing basketball and the associated drills with training may maintain fitness levels. An important consideration in the interpretation of this study is that the preseason training program did not cause a significant change in three of the four tests. A study of female collegiate tennis players indicates that playing tennis and participating in tennis drills does maintain fitness during a 9-month season (Kraemer et al. 2000). However, it is important to note that performance measures, including serve velocity, did not improve during the season.

The majority of these studies indicate that, at least for the sports examined, normal training may maintain the fitness levels of athletes for a short period of time. However, some decrements in performance measures may occur. Another important factor to consider is whether athletes play regularly or sparingly, as playing is a training stimulus.

In-Season Programs

The goal of an **in-season program** is to perform resistance training to further increase or at least maintain strength and power during a competitive season. Unpublished data by Kraemer support the concept that reduced training frequencies can maintain strength levels during a playing season.

Sixty-eight college football players performed a 1RM on three separate occasions: preseason, midseason, and postseason. All athletes trained twice a week during the 14-week season. The in-season program is presented in table 8.3.

Table 8.3 14-Week In-Season Training Program for College Football Players

Exercise	Reps/Set
Bench press	8, 5, 5, 8
Squats	5, 5, 5, 5
Single-leg knee extension	10, 10
Single-leg knee curls	10, 10
Military press	8, 8, 8
Power cleans	8, 8, 8

Note. 2-min rest period between sets and exercises. Training frequency was 2 times per week.

Each player completed winter and summer resistance training programs that involved lifting 4 or 5 days per week with a much larger training volume and more exercises than the in-season program. The entire group exhibited no significant decreases in 1RM for any of the exercises tested between the time periods (see figure 8.6). A separate evaluation of backs and linemen produced similar results.

Another study of American football players shows that some measures of motor performance and fitness decrease significantly while others decrease nonsignificantly in-season even with a maintenance weight training program during a 16-week season (see table 8.4).

During a 22-week basketball season in which female players performed resistance training once or twice a week, vertical jumping ability increased significantly by 6% (Häkkinen 1993). Maximal isometric leg-extension force remained unchanged. The in-season training consisted of one to two lower-extremity exercises per session and 3 to 8 repetitions per set at 30 to 80% of maximal. Subjects performed 20 to 30 total repetitions

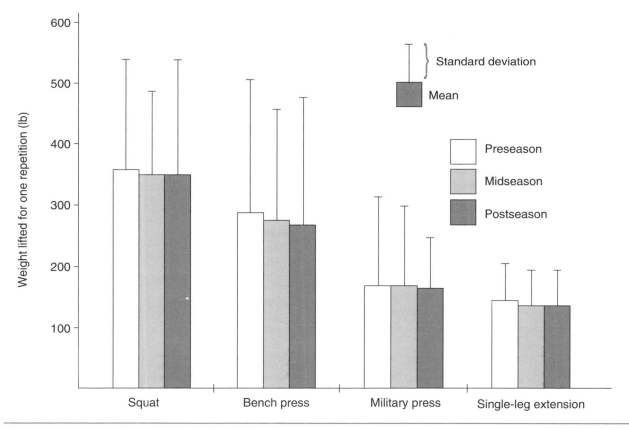

Figure 8.6 Results of in-season resistance program on 1RM lifts in American football players.

Table 8.4 Percent Change in Fitness Tests During a College Football Season

Test	Nonlineman % change	Lineman % change
Bench press	–8.1*	–7.8*
Flexibility	–3.0*	–6.6*
Vertical jump	–4.6*	–2.8
Long jump	–1.1	–0.4
Agility run	–0.2	–1.1

* = significant decrease from start to end of 16-week season.

Data from V. Schneider et al., 1998, "Detraining effects in college football players during the competitive season," *Journal of Strength and Conditioning Research* 12: 42-45.

per training session, and once every two weeks they undertook a jump training session consisting of 100 to 150 total jumps of various horizontal and vertical jumps. This in-season program maintained strength and increased vertical jumping ability.

A comparison of a multiple-set undulating and a single-set program performed by female tennis players for 9 months including the tennis season shows some interesting results (Kraemer et al. 2000) (this study is described in more detail in chapter 7). Both programs were performed two or three times per week for the entire 9 months depending on the match schedule. Generally, the undulating program resulted in consistent and significant gains in fitness measures, including serve velocity, throughout the 9-month period. The single-set program generally resulted in no change in fitness measures or a significant change during the first 3 months and then a plateau in fitness for the remaining 6 months. The single-set program resulted in no significant change in serve velocity throughout the 9 months. Over the 9 months the undulating program generally resulted in greater fitness gains than the single-set program. The results indicate that fitness gains can be made in-season, but the magnitude and whether a gain is achieved depends on the total volume of the program performed.

Collectively, the studies presented in this and the preceding section indicate that in-season programs can maintain or increase strength and power during a season, and that the type of program can influence whether fitness gains are achieved. In addition, athletes in sports that have an inher-

ent high strength component can tolerate periods of no in-season resistance training with little or no decrease in strength or performance.

Long Detraining Periods

Long periods of detraining (i.e., months or years) have received very little attention from the sport science community. However, two case studies have been performed. Table 8.5 depicts the effects of 7 months of detraining and dieting on an elite power lifter. The individual performed no resistance training during this period. The data from this study (Staron, Hagerman, and Hikida 1981) suggest that detraining results in a physiological shift from a strength profile to an improved aerobic profile. Three observations reflected this shift: the improvement of peak oxygen consumption ($\dot{V}O_2$peak), increased mitochondrial density,

Table 8.5 Physiological Changes After Seven Months of Detraining

Variable	Trained	Detrained
Ht (cm)	170.0	170.0
Wt (kg)	121.5	94.0
% body fat	25.2	14.8
Thigh girth (cm)	82.5	66.5
BP (systolic/diastolic)	146/96	137/76
$\dot{V}O_2$peak (ml/kg/min)	32.6	49.1
Max HR	200	198
% volume of mitochondria Type I (slow twitch) Type II (fast twitch)	3.04 1.76	4.41 2.46
Fiber type SO (%) FG (%) FOG (%)	31.2 53.2 15.6	38.1 43.7 27.2
Cross-sectional area (um²) SO FG FOG	5,625 8,539 9,618	3,855 5,075 5,835

BP = blood pressure; HR = heart rate; SO = slow oxidative; FG = fast glycolytic; FOG = fast oxidative glycolytic. SO fibers are smaller than fast-twitch fibers and FOG fibers.

Adapted from *Journal of Neurological Sciences*, 51, R.S. Staron, F.C. Hagerman, and R.S. Hikida, "The effects of detraining on an elite power lifter," 247-257, Copyright 1981, with permission from Elsevier.

and improved oxidative enzyme profile of the muscle fibers. These changes occurred without any aerobic training stimulus during the 7-month detraining period. The large weight loss (27.5 kg or 60.5 lb) and reduction in body fat during this period may have accounted for some of these changes. The decrease in muscle fiber area contributed to the decrease in thigh girth. These observations are consistent with changes normally attributed to muscle atrophy.

A second study examined two men who performed resistance training for 8 weeks and then detrained for 5 months (Thorstensson 1977). The initial training period consisted of various exercises for the leg extensors, and weighted and unweighted jumping exercises. After the initial training period, one individual performed resistance training at a reduced volume 2 or 3 days per week and did not perform any jumping exercises. The other subject performed no training at all for the 5-month detraining period. The individual training at a reduced volume during the detraining period showed increases compared to immediately after the 8-week training period in 1RM squat and isokinetic torque at 60 degrees per second and faster (but not at slower velocities), but decreases in isometric leg-extension force, vertical jump ability, and horizontal jump ability. However, all measures were still above pretraining values. The individual not training showed decreases in all of the measures with only the 1RM squat still being greater than pretraining values after the detraining period. Fat-free mass continued to increase in the individual training at a reduced volume and decreased to slightly below pretrained levels in the individual not training. The type II to type I fiber area ratio decreased in both individuals during the detraining period, but was still above pretraining values for both subjects, indicating a greater loss of type II fiber area compared to type I fiber area.

Thus, after 5 months of detraining, virtually all increases in strength and muscle mass from an 8-week training period are lost if no resistance training is performed. However, resistance training at a reduced volume for 5 months can maintain or even increase gains in strength and muscle mass following an 8-week training program.

Detraining Effects on Motor Performance

The effect of detraining on motor performance has received much less attention than the effect on strength. After 24 weeks of heavy resistance training three times per week, vertical jump ability increased 13% (Häkkinen and Komi 1985c). Training primarily consisted of squat-type movements using 70 to 100% of 1RM. Twelve weeks of detraining resulted in a decrease in vertical jump ability, but it was still 2% above the pretraining value. Another study showed that 24 weeks of stretch-shortening cycle training increased vertical jump ability 17%, and that after 12 weeks of detraining vertical jump ability decreased, but was still 10% above the pretraining value (Häkkinen and Komi 1985a). Training consisted of various jumps with and without added weight. During both of these studies decreases in squat jump ability (jump with no countermovement) during the detraining period also occurred. Two weeks of detraining in strength-trained athletes (power lifters and American football players) resulted in small, nonsignificant increases in vertical jump (2.3%) and squat jump (3.6%) ability (Hortobagyi et al. 1993).

Short-term detraining periods do not seem to affect vertical jump ability significantly, but longer periods of detraining do result in decreased vertical jump ability. Whether the vertical jump results can be generalized to other types of motor performance is unknown, but it is an attractive hypothesis. Data from Thorstensson (1977) suggest that the ability to perform complex skills involving strength components (e.g., the vertical jump) may be lost if not included in the training program. Thus, if the goal of an in-season program is to maintain motor performance, the motor performance task should be included in the training program.

In-season training programs may be sufficient to maintain motor performance, even though small decreases occur. College football players performed an in-season weight training program twice a week during a 16-week season (Schneider et al. 1998). Both linemen and nonlinemen showed either significant decreases or small, nonsignificant decreases in typical measures of motor performance as well as flexibility and strength (see table 8.4).

Physiological Mechanisms of Strength Loss

As with strength gains during training, several mechanisms could result in strength and power changes during periods of detraining. Knowledge of these mechanisms will help the practitioner design better in-season programs.

Electromyographic (EMG) changes during muscular actions after training and detraining indicate changes in motor unit firing rate and motor unit synchronization. EMG changes have been followed during detraining periods ranging from 2 to 12 weeks in length. During short periods of detraining, decreases and no change in strength and power measures were not accompanied by changes in EMG activity (Häkkinen et al. 1990; Häkkinen and Komi 1985c; Hortobagyi et al. 1993). However, decreases in EMG activity due to short periods of detraining have also been shown (Häkkinen and Komi 1986; Häkkinen, Komi, and Alen 1985; Narici et al. 1989). The decreases in EMG have shown significant correlations to decreases in strength (Häkkinen, Alen, and Komi 1985; Häkkinen and Komi 1985a; Häkkinen and Komi 1986). However, decreases in EMG activity of some muscles (vastus lateralis), but not others (vastus medialis, rectus femoris) have also been shown (Häkkinen, Alen, and Komi 1985). This EMG information indicates that the initial strength loss, when it does occur during the first several weeks of detraining, is due to neural mechanisms, with muscle atrophy contributing to further strength loss as the detraining duration increases (Häkkinen and Komi 1983).

Training adaptations of the muscle fiber were discussed extensively in chapter 3. However, few studies have examined the effects of detraining on cellular-level variables (see table 8.6). During periods of detraining, most positive adaptations that occurred due to training regress toward the untrained or pretrained state. During short periods (2 to 8 weeks) of detraining in men, type I and type II fiber area (Häkkinen, Komi, and Alen 1985; Häkkinen, Komi, and Tesch 1981; Hather et al. 1992; Hortobagyi et al. 1993) may decrease compared to the trained state. However, no change also has been reported (Hather et al. 1992; Hortobagyi et al. 1993). In older individuals (65 to 77 years) the return to pretraining cross-sectional area muscle fiber sizes in both type I and type II muscle fibers may be more rapid than in younger individuals even when accompanied with hGH recombinant therapy (Taafe and Marcus 1997). This may be due in part to differences in spontaneous activity and lifestyle in younger and older individuals. Interestingly, training resulted in a 40% increase in strength, of which 30% was lost despite muscle fiber areas returning to pretraining levels, thereby suggesting that neural mechanisms account for part of the strength retention (Taafe and Marcus 1997). After 8 weeks of retraining, strength returned to posttraining values with only modest improvements in muscle size.

Several authors (Häkkinen, Komi, and Tesch 1981; Hather et al. 1992) reported that the type I to type II fiber area ratio decreased during periods of detraining in men (indicating a selective atrophy of type II fibers) or remained unchanged compared to the trained state (Hather et al. 1992). In women, small but nonsignificant decreases in type I fiber area accompanied by a significant decrease in the combined areas of type IIAB and B fibers has been shown (Staron et al. 1991). No change in either type I or type II fiber area has also been reported during 8 weeks of detraining; however, this study showed no increase in fiber area due to the stretch-shortening cycle-type (plyometric) training performed prior to the detraining period (Häkkinen et al. 1990).

Collectively, this information indicates that type II fibers may atrophy to a greater extent than type I fibers during short periods of detraining in both men and women. This, of course, can only occur if the training induced an increase in fiber area.

During short periods of detraining, fat-free mass and percent body fat show small, nonsignificant changes (Häkkinen et al. 1990; Häkkinen, Komi, and Alen 1985; Häkkinen, Komi, and Tesch 1981; Hortobagyi et al. 1993; Staron et al. 1991). Although muscle cross-sectional areas show either nonsignificant (Häkkinen et al. 1989) or significant decreases (Narici et al. 1989), the lack of a significant change in fat-free mass is probable due to the gross nature of this measurement and the short duration of the detraining period. However, changes in fat-free mass and percent body fat do occur in short-term detraining periods in the direction that would negatively affect performance. For example, after 16 weeks of weight training, fat-free mass increased 1.3 kg (48.1 to 50.3 kg) and percent fat decreased 2.6% (24.8 to 22.2%) in young women. During 6 weeks of detraining, fat-free mass decreased (48.5 kg) and percent fat increased (23%) back toward pretraining values. None of the changes in body composition were significant at any point in the training or detraining period, but the changes are in the direction that would negatively affect performance during the detraining period.

Andersen and Aagaard (2000) showed that after 3 months of detraining, myosin heavy chain IIX (IIB) content significantly increased while myosin heavy chain IIA content decreased. The detraining effect produced myosin heavy chain IIX values that were higher than they were before resistance training. This study was the first to show that after a resistance training program,

Table 8.6 Fiber Changes With Detraining

Reference	Length of training (wk)	Length of detraining (wk)	Type of training	Type of detraining	Fiber μm² atrophy	Type I/type II ratio	Fiber transformation
Häkkinen, Komi, and Tesch 1981	16	8	Squats, concentric 1-6 reps/set at 100-120% 1RM	No training	Type I *, Type II*	*	FT%*
Houston et al. 1983	10	12	Knee extension, leg press 8RM, 4/wk 3 sets		Type IIB*	—	None
Staron, Hagerman, and Hikida 1981	3 yr	7 mo	6-5/wk, power lifter, case study	No training	FOG*, FG*, SO*	—	FG to FOG
Thorstensson 1977	8	5 mo		3-2 sessions/wk, weights and jumping / No activity	Type II*, Type II*	*	FT only
Hather et al. 1991	19	4	Leg press, knee extension 4-5 sets, 6-12 reps	Con/ecc; Con/con; Con	Type I none; Type II * but still above pre after training; Type II * but above pre after detraining	*	None; None; None; Type IIA to type IIB
Staron et al. 1991	20	30-32	Squats, knee extension, leg press	No activity	Type IIA* + type IIB	*	—
Anderson and Aagaard 2000	12	12	Heavy load lower body	No activity	Type I* and type II	*	Type IIA to type IIB

1RM = one repetition maximum; RM = repetition maximum; * = p ≤ 0.05 significant reductions or decreases; FT = fast twitch glycolytic fiber type; FG = fast twitch glycolytic fiber type; FOG = fast oxidative glycolytic fiber type; SO = slow oxidative fiber type; FOG = fast oxidative glycolytic fiber type; LBM = lean body mass.

detraining resulted in an "overshoot" in the myosin heavy chain IIX values to a level higher than what was observed before training.

Kraemer and colleagues (Kraemer, Dudley, Tesch et al. 2001) showed that the pituitary gland is especially sensitive to detraining and most likely interacts with the changes in the motor cortex. In this study groups trained with concentric repetitions alone, double concentric repetitions, or the typical concentric-eccentric repetitions. Growth hormone responded differently when an eccentric repetition phase was included in training compared to the other groups, and after 4 weeks of detraining, all of the groups responded the same to both concentric and eccentric exercise protocols. Conversely, testosterone and cortisol showed no differential responses with training or detraining, indicating that not all hormonal systems respond similarly (see chapter 3). Thus, the effects of detraining may vary dramatically. This was shown in a recent study by Kraemer and colleagues (Kraemer, Koziris, Ratamess et al. 2002) in which no changes were observed in testosterone or cortisol concentrations during 6 weeks of detraining in recreationally trained men. Some of the changes in muscle and neurological function may in fact be due to differential responses of the endocrine system during detraining.

Changes in the blood hormonal profile during detraining could have an impact on strength, body composition, and muscle fiber hypertrophy. During 12 weeks of detraining, decreases in the testosterone/cortisol and testosterone/sex hormone binding globulin ratios are significantly related to leg-extensor isometric strength decreases (Häkkinen et al. 1985). Short periods of detraining have also not resulted in significant changes in testosterone and free testosterone concentrations in men and women (Häkkinen et al. 1989, 1990). During 2 weeks of detraining, growth hormone, testosterone, and the testosterone/cortisol ratio increased significantly while cortisol decreased significantly in strength-trained athletes (American football players and power lifters) (Hortobagyi et al. 1993). The authors suggested that this might be an initial compensatory response to combat muscle atrophy (Hortobagyi et al. 1993). After 2 weeks of daily training followed by a 1-week period of reduced training volume, no significant changes in testosterone, free testosterone, cortisol, or the testosterone/cortisol ratio occurred (Häkkinen and Pakarinen 1991). However, when the same training volume was performed but divided into two training sessions per day for 1 week followed by a 1-week period of reduced training volume, testosterone and the testosterone/cortisol ratio significantly decreased while cortisol significantly increased after the 1 week of reduced training (Häkkinen and Pakarinen 1991). No significant changes during short periods of detraining have been shown in follicle stimulating hormone, luteinizing hormone, progesterone, and estradiol (Häkkinen and Pakarinen 1991; Häkkinen et al. 1985, 1990). Thus, the hormone response to detraining periods may be quite varied and is probably dependent on the volume, intensity, and duration of training prior to the detraining period as well as the training history of the individual.

Effect of Muscle Action Type

The previously described studies by Dudley and colleagues (1991) and Hather and colleagues (1992) indicate that normal resistance training and double-volume concentric-only training result in greater retention of training adaptations during a short (4-week) detraining period than concentric-only training (see figure 8.4). In addition, when using concentric-only repetitions, detraining may demonstrate greater losses in maximal isometric strength when compared to that of dynamic 1RM strength changes over 8 weeks of detraining (Weir et al. 1997). In another study, Housh and colleagues (1996) demonstrated that 8 weeks of unilateral eccentric-only training (three to five sets of 6 repetitions at 80% of the eccentric 1RM) increased strength in both limbs (29% in trained and 17% in nontrained limbs for dynamic strength), but not in isokinetic concentric strength across different velocities (indicating specificity of training effects). With 8 weeks of detraining, the eccentric 1RM strength for both limbs was maintained, which again points to the potential importance of the eccentric component of the repetition.

In the study by Dudley and colleagues (1991), all three types of training resulted in an increase in the percentage of type IIA fibers and a corresponding decrease in type IIB fibers. These changes were maintained during the detraining period. This could be interpreted to indicate that the concentric portion of resistance training is responsible for the type II subtype transformations. Alternatively, it could mean that any type of high-intensity resistance training will cause this subtype transformation. The normal resistance training and the double-volume concentric training resulted in an increase in mean fiber area, but only the normal resistance training resulted in maintenance of this increase after the detraining period. The concentric-only training resulted in no increase in mean fiber area. Only the normal resistance training resulted in an increased fiber area and maintenance of this increase during the detraining period of both type I and II fibers. The double-volume concentric training resulted in an increased size of only the type II fibers and maintenance of this increase after detraining. The concentric-only training resulted in no significant size increase of either the type I or type II fibers. This could be interpreted to indicate that normal resistance training and high-volume training result in the greatest maintenance of fiber size during a short detraining period.

The number of capillaries per fiber increased following all three types of training and remained above pretraining values after the detraining period. However, only the double-volume concentric and concentric-only training resulted in an increase due to training and maintenance of capillaries per cross-sectional area. This was due in part to a slightly greater fiber size increase following normal resistance training and a slightly greater increase in capillaries per fiber following double-volume concentric and concentric-only training. This change could be interpreted to indicate that concentric-only training may be appropriate for athletes needing to maintain aerobic fitness capabilities.

Detraining Effects on Bone

Very little is known about the effects of detraining on bone even though this has potentially important implications, especially if the normal sedentary lifestyle of many individuals is viewed as detraining. The short-term effects of weight training may be viewed as an adaptation that combats the long-term effects of a sedentary lifestyle on bone.

Studies have shown bone metabolism, structure, and status to be very sensitive to the loading with weight training and unloading with detraining. The neuromuscular system appears to mediate much of what happens in bone, and this may also be due to the resultant hormonal changes that occur with resistance exercise and training.

It has now become obvious that bone may be affected by the cessation of resistance training. The time course of changes in bone and the influence of the different types of resistance training programs on the detraining period remain unclear. In addition, the length of the detraining period may be important, as changes in some bone parameters may not be observable on the same time line as changes in muscle force production.

In a study by Winters and Snow (2000), women 30 to 45 years old who completed a 12-month program of lower-body resistance training and maximal unloaded and loaded (10-13% of body mass) jumps showed dramatic increases in strength and power (13-15% above controls) along with increases in bone mineral density (1-3% above controls). After 6 months of detraining, bone mineral density, muscle strength, and power all decreased significantly toward baseline values, whereas those of the control subjects did not change. Such data indicate the importance of maintaining a training program to keep not only muscle force performance elevated but bone mineral density as well. Conversely, Heinonen and colleagues (1996) examined flexion and extension resistance training of the arms in younger women (23.8 $\pm$ 5 years). The authors observed an increase in strength in arm flexion and extension movements but no dramatic changes in bone mineral density or geometry. With detraining of 8 months, both arms showed decreases in strength, but no changes occurred in bone. Thus, the type of resistance training program used, the inherent normal activity, and the limbs involved may all play a role in the responses of bone to periods of detraining. In many situations in which unloading or detraining may occur (e.g., space, bed rest, inactivity), resistance training may be an important intervention to improve physiological status and protect against bone mineral loss.

Detraining the Bulked-Up Athlete

Little attention has been given to detraining the bulked-up athlete. A bulked-up athlete is an athlete who through resistance training and dietary practices has gained substantial amounts of body weight. These weight gains are related to the increased muscle mass and total body weight necessary for successful participation in sports such as American football, throwing events, and power lifting. Chronic detraining may lead to potential health problems following an athletic career. Obesity and a sedentary lifestyle, for example, often contribute to an increased risk of cardiovascular disease (Kraemer 1983a).

Many athletes who exercise to increase muscle mass and strength do not know how to exercise for health and recreation using other types of training (e.g., aerobic training, circuit weight training). The retired athlete needs to start training again with new objectives and to examine dietary habits in order to avoid large weight gains. This is especially true for strength- and power-type athletes, as an aptitude for these types of athletic events, including weightlifting, does not offer protection against cardiovascular disease after retirement from competitive sport. However, an aptitude for athletic events requiring endurance and the continuation of vigorous physical activity after retirement from competitive sport does offer protection against cardiovascular disease (Kujala et al. 2000).

Some studies have shown that, compared to nonathletes, former athletes have an advantage in cardiovascular fitness (Fardy et al. 1976). This advantage did not exist in a comparison of former athletes with nonathletes who engaged in strenuous leisure-time activities. One study (Paffenbarger et al. 1984) concluded that postcollege physical activity is more important than participation in college athletics in predicting low coronary artery disease. Few data exist with regard to specific athletic subgroups and lifelong health. However, a survey of former Finnish world-class athletes concluded that athletes do have a longer-than-normal life expectancy and hypothesized that recreational aerobic activity and infrequent smoking after athletic retirement may explain the longer life expectancy (Fogelholm, Kaprio, and Sarna 1994). On the other hand, athletes who require substantial body weight gains for success during their sport careers may be at the greatest risk for cardiovascular diseases. To reduce this risk, retired athletes require the proper prescription of exercise, along with diet and weight control.

Retired strength-trained athletes should feel that they can still enjoy resistance training. Periodization of training and the development of new training goals will be important to facilitate this feeling. More than anything, the continuation of training is of paramount importance, as many athletes "drop out" from their exercise routine. Healthy detraining of the resistance-trained athlete necessitates a reexamination of the training goals to improving health and fitness by including aerobic exercise programs for improving cardiovascular function and reduc-

ing body weight as well as resistance training to maintain muscular fitness. In addition, nutritional counseling may be important to deal with aberrant calorie intake behaviors (e.g., American football training tables have shown that football players ingest from 5,000 to 10,000 calories a day) over an athletic career to gain body mass (e.g., American football linemen). As an ex-competitive athlete ages, the goal should be consistent with anyone else: to improve health and fitness and reduce pathological risk factors for chronic diseases (e.g., cardiovascular disease, cancer, diabetes).

When individuals have all four primary risk factors for cardiovascular disease (see table 8.7), the danger of heart attack is five times greater than when none are present (Fox and Mathews 1981). Management of these risk factors helps to reduce the risk of cardiovascular disease. It is easy to perform a risk factor analysis; this procedure has been described extensively in Kraemer (1983a) and Wilmore and Costill (1994).

Former athletes, like anyone else, should continue an active lifestyle with new goals for their training programs. The role of teachers and coaches is to educate students and athletes about lifelong health and fitness, exposing them to exercise other than heavy resistance training only. Frequently, trainers can suggest different programs either during certain periods of the training cycle or as a supplement to the regular exercise prescription. This adds variation to the program and also contributes to a healthy transition for athletes whose careers end after high school, college, or professional participation in sports. It is up to the conditioning professionals to help athletes make a transition from competitive sports to lifetime sports and exercise for health.

Table 8.7 Cardiovascular Disease Risk Factors

Primary risk factors	Secondary risk factors
Smoking	**Changeable** Obesity Diabetes Stress
Blood lipids High LDL-cholesterol Low HDL-cholesterol High triglycerides	**Unchangeable** Heredity (family history) Male gender Advancing age
High blood pressure	
Physical inactivity	

Summary

Detraining can occur in several situations including complete cessation of weight training, decreased volume of weight training such as during an in-season resistance training program, and long periods of no weight training or reduced volume of resistance training such as following completion of an athletic career. Research has not yet indicated the exact resistance, volume, and frequency of resistance training or the type of program needed to maintain the training gains achieved by an individual. In-season programs are probably as specific for maintaining different fitness gains as the strength development prescription was for initially creating the fitness gains. Studies do indicate, however, that to maintain strength gains or slow strength loss during a detraining period, the intensity should be maintained, but the volume and frequency of training can be reduced.

Key Terms

bulked-up athlete
detraining
in-season detraining
in-season program
long periods of detraining

Selected Readings

Bell, G.J., Syrotuik, D.G., Attwood, K., and Quinney, H.A. 1993. Maintenance of strength gains while performing endurance training in oarswomen. *Journal of Applied Physiology* 18: 104-115.

Häkkinen K. 1993. Changes in physical fitness profile in female basketball players during the competitive season including explosive type strength training. *Journal of Sports Medicine and Physical Fitness* 33: 19-26.

Häkkinen, K., Pakarinen, A., Komi, P.V., Ryushi, T., and Kauhanen, H. 1989. Neuromuscular adaptations and hormone balance in strength athletes, physically active males and females during intensive strength training. In *XII International Congress of Biomechanics Congress Proceedings*, edited by R.J. Gregor, R.F. Zernicke, and W.C. Whiting, 889-894. Champaign, IL: Human Kinetics.

Hather, B.M., Tesch, P.A., Buchanan, P., and Dudley, G.A. 1992. Influence of eccentric actions on skeletal muscle adaptations to resistance training. *Acta Physiologica Scandinavica* 143: 177-185.

Hoffman, J.R., Fry, A.C., Howard, R., Maresh, C.M., and Kraemer, W.J. 1991. Strength, speed and endurance changes during the course of a division I basketball season. *Journal of Applied Sport Science Research* 3: 144-149.

Hortobagyi, T., Houmard, J.A., Stevenson, J.R., Fraser, D.D., Johns, R.A., and Israel, R.G. 1993. The effects of detraining on power athletes. *Medicine and Science in Sports and Exercise* 25: 929-935.

Koutedakis, Y., Boreham, C., Kabitsis, C., and Sharp, N.C.C. 1992. Seasonal deterioration of selected physiological variables in elite male skiers. *International Journal of Sports Medicine* 13: 548-551.

Lemmer, J.T., Ivey, F.M., Ryan, A.S., Martel, G.F., Hurlbut, D.E., Metter, J.E., Fozard, J.L., Fleg, J.L., and Hurley, B.F. 2001. Effect of strength training on resting metabolic rate and physical activity: Age and gender comparisons. *Medicine and Science in Sports and Exercise* 33: 532-541.

LeMura, L.M., Von Duvillard, S.P., Andreacci, J.A., Klebez, J.M., Chelland, S.A., and Russo, J. 2000. Lipid and lipoprotein profiles, cardiovascular fitness, body composition, and diet during and after resistance, aerobic and combination training in young women. *European Journal of Applied Physiology* 82: 451-458.

Mujika, I., and Padilla, S. 2000a. Detraining loss of training-induced physiological and performance adaptations. Part I. Short term insufficient training stimulus. *Sports Medicine* 30: 79-87.

Mujika, I., and Padilla, S. 2000b. Detraining loss of training-induced physiological and performance adaptations. Part II. Long term insufficient training stimulus. *Sports Medicine* 30: 79-87.

Mujika, I., and Padilla, S. 2001. Muscular characteristics of detraining in humans. *Medicine and Science in Sports and Exercise* 33: 1297-1303.

Staron, R.S., Leonardi, M.J., Karapondo, D.L., Malicky, E.S., Falkel, J.E., Hagerman, F.C., Hikda, R.S. 1991. Strength and skeletal muscle adaptations in heavy-resistance-trained women after detraining and retraining. *Journal of Applied Physiology* 70: 631-640.

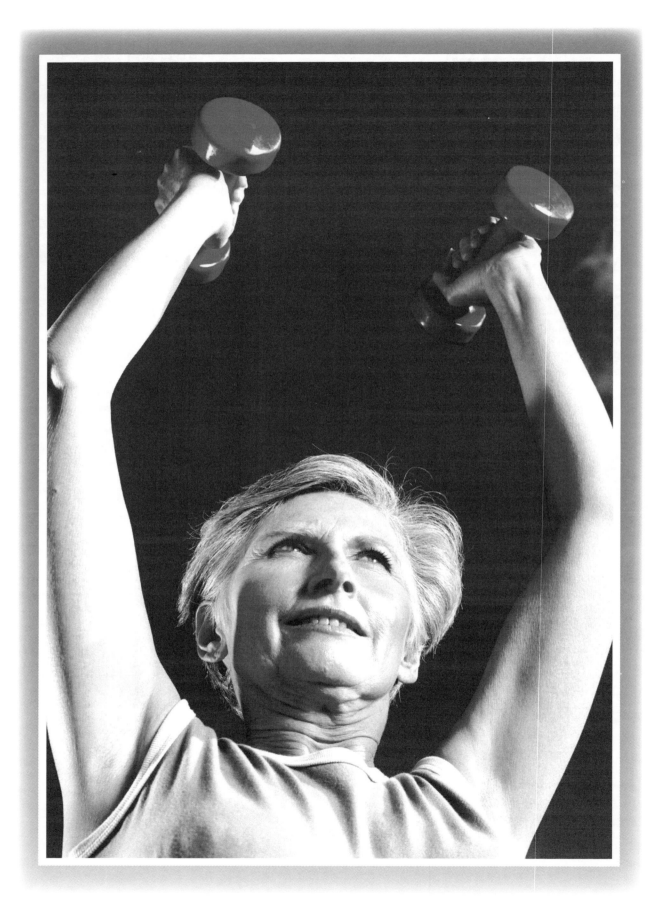

PART III

Women, Children, and Seniors and Resistance Training

Young male athletes are not the only people who resistance train; women, children, and seniors are all discovering the benefits of resistance training. Chapter 9 discusses research on gender differences and examines special considerations for female athletes and women in general who engage in resistance training. Chapter 10 explores resistance training for children and discusses program design and safety issues unique to younger resistance trainers. Chapter 11 examines issues relevant to seniors who perform resistance training, such as loss of strength and power with aging and the benefits of resistance training to the senior population. The information in these chapters is important for anyone designing resistance training programs for these populations.

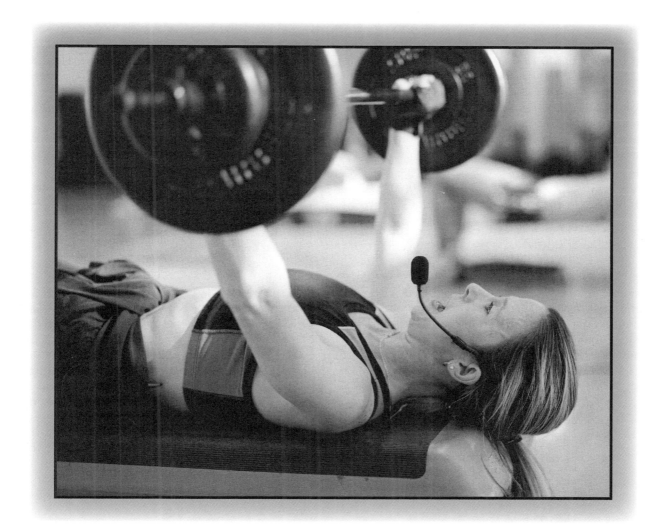

Women and Resistance Training

More and more women are performing resistance training as part of their total physical conditioning programs. Increasingly, female athletes also are using resistance training to improve sport performance. This is evident by the great number of resistance training facilities available to women; the number of female high school and college athletes performing resistance training; and the increasing popularity of bodybuilding, power lifting, and Olympic-style weightlifting contests for women. This chapter examines issues concerning women and resistance training and addresses some common misconceptions about women and resistance training.

Gender Absolute Strength Differences

Absolute strength refers to the maximal amount of strength or force (i.e., 1RM) generated in a movement or exercise. A woman's average maximal mean whole-body strength is 60.0 to 63.5% of the average man's (Laubach 1976; Shephard 2000a). A woman's upper-body strength averages 55% of a man's, and her lower-body strength averages 72% of a man's (Bishop, Cureton, and Collins 1987; Knapik et al. 1980; Laubach 1976; Sharp 1994; Wilmore et al. 1978). This large variation in strength between the genders (see figure 9.1) is a result of several factors including the large number of single-joint (e.g., elbow flexion, shoulder extension, hip extension) and multijoint (e.g., bench press, squat, shoulder press) movements possible with both the upper and lower body. Also contributing to this large variation is the difference between the genders in total muscle mass and its distribution in various parts of the body. Generally men have a greater skeletal muscle mass than women, and regional differences in skeletal muscle mass between the genders are greatest in the upper body (Janssen et al. 2000; Nindl et al. 2000). Other comparisons (see tables 9.1 and 9.2) of strength differences

between the genders support that large variations in a woman's strength compared to a man's do exist and that generally a woman's lower-body strength is closer to a man's than her upper-body strength. Contributing in part to the large variation shown in table 9.1 is the use of different types of maximal strength tests, such as 1RM, concentric isokinetic, eccentric isokinetic, and isometric tests. For example, the knee-extension strength of women (as determined by 1RM on a machine), maximal isometric, and concentric isokinetic peak torque at 150 degrees per second have been reported to be 50%, 68%, and 60% of men's, respectively.

Gender differences in maximal strength and large variations in these differences are still apparent in young male and female adults after 24 weeks of weight training 3 days per week (Lemmer et al. 2001) and after women perform a total-body weight training program for 6 months, 3 days per week (Kraemer, Mazzetti et al. 2001) compared to untrained males (see table 9.2). These gender differences are even apparent in highly trained athletes. For example, the 2000 world records in power lifting of the International Powerlifting Federation for the 114-lb (52-kg) body weight class for women were 402 lb (182.5 kg) for the squat, 236 lb (107.5 kg) for the bench press, and 435 lb (197.5 kg) for the deadlift. The men's world records in the 114-lb weight class were 611 lb (277.5 kg) for the squat, 391 lb (177.5 kg) for the bench press, and 564 lb (256 kg) for the deadlift. Thus, women's world records for the squat, bench press, and deadlift were 65.7%, 60.4% and 77.1% of the men's. Similarly, isokinetic peak torque of national-caliber male volleyball players is generally higher than that of female players (Puhl et al. 1982). This gender difference is greatly reduced when expressed relative to total body weight, but men can still show greater strength relative to total body weight. Generally the difference between the male and female volleyball players in peak torque is also reduced as the isokinetic velocity of movement increases, especially when expressed relative to total body weight.

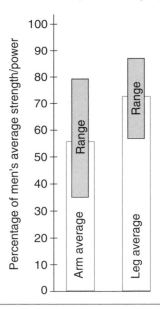

Figure 9.1 Range and average of various dynamic strength measurements of the average woman compared with those of the average man.

Adapted, by permission, from L.L Laubach, 1976, "Comparative muscular strength of men and women: A review of the literature," *Aviation, Space and Environmental Medicine* 47: 534-542.

Gender Relative Strength Differences

Total body weight and fat-free mass may explain in part the gender differences in absolute strength. Relative strength refers to absolute strength divided by or expressed relative to total body weight or fat-free mass. In a classic study,

Table 9.1 Representative Absolute Strength Differences by Gender

Reference	Movement or exercise	Type of test	Female (% of male)
Kraemer, Mazzetti et al. 2001	Squat	1RM with free weights	51
Kraemer, Mazzetti et al. 2001	Bench press	1RM with free weights	41
Kraemer, Mazzetti et al. 2001	High-pull	1RM with free weights	54
Cureton et al. 1988	Elbow extension	1RM with free weight	42
Cureton et al. 1988	Elbow flexion	1RM with machine	53
Cureton et al. 1988	Knee flexion	1RM with machine	54
Cureton et al. 1988	Knee extension	1RM with machine	50
Wilmore 1974	Leg press	Maximal isometric	73
Wilmore 1974	Elbow flexion	1 RM with machine	52
Wilmore 1974	Bench press	1RM with machine	37
Wilmore 1974	Grip	Maximal isometric	57
Maughan et al. 1986	Knee extension	Maximal isometric	68
Maughan et al. 1986	Elbow flexion	1RM with machine	46
Ryushi et al. 1988	Knee extension	1RM with machine	58
Ryushi et al. 1988	Knee extension	Maximal isometric	73
Miller et al. 1992	Elbow flexion	1RM with machine	69
Miller et al. 1992	Elbow extension	1RM with machine	52
Davies, Greenwood, and Jones 1988	Grip	Maximal isometric	60
Clarke 1986	Grip	Maximal isometric	62
Neder et al. 1999	Knee extension	Concentric peak torque: 60 deg/s	54
Kanehisa et al. 1996	Knee extension	Concentric isokinetic peak torque: 180 deg/s	66
Kanehisa et al. 1994	Knee extension	Concentric isokinetic peak torque: 60 deg/s 180 deg/s 300 deg/s	65 66 63

(continued)

Table 9.1 *(continued)*

Reference	Movement or exercise	Type of test	Female (% of male)
Alway, Sale, and MacDougall 1990	Elbow flexion	Concentric isokinetic peak torque: 60 deg/s 120 deg/s 180 deg/s 240 deg/s 300 deg/s	 45 50 44 40 36
Colliander and Tesch 1989	Knee extension	Concentric isokinetic peak torque: 60 deg/s 90 deg/s 150 deg/s	 64 62 60
Colliander and Tesch 1989	Knee flexion	Concentric isokinetic peak torque: 60 deg/s 90 deg/s 150 deg/s	 64 62 62
Colliander and Tesch 1989	Knee extension	Eccentric isokinetic peak torque: 60 deg/s 90 deg/s 150 deg/s	 69 78 76
Colliander and Tesch 1989	Knee flexion	Eccentric isokinetic peak torque: 60 deg/s 90 deg/s 150 deg/s	 64 73 71
Borges and Essen-Gustavsson 1989	Knee extension	Concentric isokinetic peak torque: 12 deg/s 90 deg/s 150 deg/s	 78 78 72
Borges and Essen-Gustavsson 1989	Knee extension	Maximal isometric	70
Hayward, Johannes Ellis, and Romer 1986	Shoulder flexion	Concentric isokinetic peak torque: 60 deg/s	 64
Hayward, Johannes Ellis, and Romer 1986	Knee extension	Concentric isokinetic peak torque: 60 deg/s	 68

Table 9.1 *(continued)*

Reference	Movement or exercise	Type of test	Female (% of male)
Falkel et al. 1985	Elbow flexion	Concentric isokinetic peak torque: 30 deg/s	56
Falkel et al. 1985	Elbow extension	Concentric isokinetic peak torque: 30 deg/s	63
Falkel et al. 1985	Knee extension	Concentric isokinetic peak torque: 30 deg/s	68
Falkel et al. 1985	Knee flexion	Concentric isokinetic peak torque: 30 deg/s	66

Table 9.2 Gender Percent Differences in 1RM Before and After Resistance Training for 24 Weeks

Exercise	Pretraining female (% of male)	Posttraining female (% of male)
Both sexes train for 24 weeks	Pretraining females compared to pretraining males	Posttraining females compared to posttraining males
Chest press	50	53
Lat pull-down	48	49
Shoulder press	58	52
Triceps push-down	54	53
Biceps curl	40	51
Leg extension	91	92
Leg press	63	69
Only women train for 24 weeks	Pretraining females compared to untrained males	Posttraining females compared to untrained males
Squat	52	70
Bench press	44	56
Clean high-pull	54	66

women's 1RM bench press was 37% that of men's (Wilmore 1974). If expressed relative to total body weight and fat-free mass, women's 1RM bench press was 46% and 55%, respectively, that of men's. Similarly, women's maximal isometric force in a leg press movement was 73% that of men's. However, if expressed relative to total body weight and fat-free mass, women's isometric leg press strength was 92% and 106%, respectively, that of men's. Thus, women's lower-body strength was more equivalent to men's when expressed relative to total body weight or fat-free mass than was upper-body strength.

The equivalency of lower-body but not upper-body strength between the genders when expressed relative to total body weight or fat-free mass is supported by other data (Shephard 2000a). For example, women's maximal absolute isokinetic bench press and leg press strength is 50% and 74% that of men's, respectively (Hoffman, Stauffer, and Jackson 1979). When adjusted for height and fat-free mass, women's bench press strength is 74% that of men's, but women's leg press strength is 104% that of men's.

However, Morrow and Hostler (1981) reported that the maximal isokinetic peak torque of female basketball and volleyball players' bench press and leg press, both absolute and relative to fat-free mass, was less than the average male's (bench press: absolute 50%, relative to fat-free mass 56%; leg press: absolute 71%, relative to fat-free mass 75%).

Some maximal strength isokinetic data at various velocities of movement indicate that both upper- and lower-body strength are equivalent between the genders when expressed relative to fat-free mass. Shoulder-flexion and knee-extension peak torque at 60 degrees per second is equivalent between the genders when expressed relative to fat-free mass (Hayward, Johannes Ellis, and Romer 1986). Similarly, women's maximal concentric isokinetic peak torque at 30 degrees per second for elbow extension, knee extension, and knee flexion, but not elbow flexion, is equal to men's when expressed relative to fat-free mass (Falkel et al. 1985). This study matched the genders for absolute (L/min) peak oxygen consumption. Thus, the women in this study possibly were above average in total fitness, whereas the men were average in total fitness. This may explain in part the parity in three out of four strength measures in this study.

Generally, data indicate that women's upper-body strength is less than that of men's in absolute terms and relative to total body weight or fat-free

mass. Women's absolute lower-body strength is less than that of men's, but may be equivalent relative to fat-free mass. This may indicate that women's weight training programs for many sports and activities should emphasize upper-body training in an attempt to improve performance.

Eccentric isokinetic peak torque relative to fat-free mass may be more similar between the genders than concentric isokinetic peak torque (Colliander and Tesch 1989; Shephard 2000a). Women's concentric isokinetic peak torque relative to fat-free mass of the quadriceps and hamstrings at 60 degrees per second, 90 degrees per second, and 150 degrees per second averaged 81% of men's (see table 9.3). Women's eccentric isokinetic peak torque relative to fat-free mass at the same velocities averaged 93% of men's. This indicates that women's lower-body eccentric strength relative to fat-free mass is almost equal to men's, whereas concentric strength is not. The reason for this difference is not clear, but it may be that women are able to store elastic energy to a greater extent than men (Aura and Komi, 1986) or because women are not able to recruit as many of their motor units during concentric muscle actions as during eccentric muscle actions compared to their male counterparts. Whatever the reason, women may be better at performing eccentric than concentric muscle actions.

Some of the discrepancies in the previously cited studies concerning whether upper-body and lower-body maximal strength when expressed relative to fat-free mass is equivalent between the genders may be related to fat-free mass distribution differences between the genders. Generally men do have a larger fat-free mass with the greatest regional difference in fat-free mass being in the upper body (Janssen et al. 2000). Thus, when strength is expressed relative to fat-free mass, women's values are overcorrected for the lower body and undercorrected for the upper body. This means that upper-body strength relative to fat-free mass will not be equivalent between the genders, but lower-body strength relative to fat-free mass will be higher in females compared to males.

Strength Relative to Muscle Cross-Sectional Area

Perhaps relative strength is best expressed relative to muscle cross-sectional area. Strength relative to muscle cross-sectional area (see figure 9.2) has shown significant correlations to maximal

Table 9.3 Women's and Men's Quadriceps and Hamstrings Eccentric and Concentric Isokinetic Peak Torque

	Percentage of women's strength to men's relative to body mass	
	Eccentric	Concentric
Quadriceps		
60 deg/s	90	83
90 deg/s	102	81
150 deg/s	99	77
Hamstrings		
60 deg/s	84	84
90 deg/s	90	80
150 deg/s	92	81

Adapted, by permission, from E.B. Colliander and P.A. Tesch, 1989, "Bilateral eccentric and concentric torque of quadriceps and hamstring muscles in females and males," *European Journal of Applied Physiology* 59: 230.

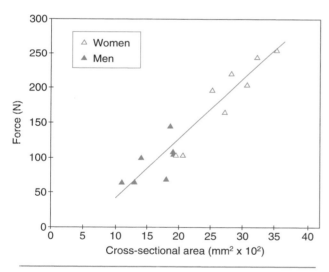

Figure 9.2 Elbow flexor strength is significantly correlated to the cross-sectional area of the elbow flexors (*r* = 0.95) in a group composed of both genders.

Adapted, by permission, from A.E.J. Miller et al., 1992, "Gender differences in strength and muscle fiber characteristics," *European Journal of Applied Physiology* 66: 254-264. © Springer-Verlag.

strength (Castro et al. 1995; Miller et al. 1992; Neder et al. 1999). Women's 1RM knee extension and elbow flexion has been reported to be 80% and 70% of men's when expressed relative to fat-free mass (Miller et al. 1992). However, when expressed relative to the muscle's cross-sectional area, no significant difference is demostrated between the genders (Miller et al. 1992). The ef-

fect of normalizing maximal strength relative to total body weight, fat-free mass, and muscle size is clearly shown by several studies. The percent difference between men and women in concentric isokinetic knee extension torque (60 degrees per second) is gradually reduced when expressed in absolute terms (54% difference), relative to body weight (30% difference), relative to fat-free mass (13% difference), and relative to bone-free lean leg mass (7% difference). The difference between the genders is statistically significant until peak torque is expressed relative to bone-free lean leg mass (Neder et al. 1999). In the upper arms (elbow flexor plus elbow extensor divided by total muscle cross-sectional area) and thighs (knee flexor plus knee extensor divided by total muscle cross-sectional area) of both trained and untrained individuals, maximal isometric force shows a similar pattern when expressed in absolute terms, relative to body weight, relative to fat-free mass, and relative to muscle cross-sectional area (see table 9.4).

Even when strength is normalized relative to muscle size, however, Kanehisa and colleagues (1994, 1996) reported no significant differences between the genders. For example, the authors showed an average 11% difference in concentric isokinetic peak torque relative to muscle cross-sectional area across three velocities (60, 180, and 300 degrees per second) between young men and women (Kanehisa et al. 1994). Even though the

Table 9.4 Relationship of Maximal Isokinetic Torque at 30 deg/s Relative to Body Weight, Lean Body Mass, and Muscle Cross-Sectional Area

	Absolute torque		Torque/BW		Torque/FFM		Torque/CSA	
	Elbow flexors	Knee flexors	Elbow flexors	Knee flexors	Elbow flexors	Knee flexors	Elbow flexors	Knee flexors
Untrained females (% of males)	52	73	68	97	74	105	95	101
Trained females (% of males)	66	79	84	102	92	112	98	98

BW = body weight; FFM = free-fat mass; CSA = cross-sectional area.

Data from M.J. Castro et al., 1995, "Peak torque per unit cross-sectional area differs between strength-trained and untrained young adults," *Medicine and Science in Sports and Exercise* 27: 391-403.

difference between the sexes is still significant, it is substantially below the absolute difference in maximal torque of 65% shown by the same study. Despite the significant difference in maximal force expressed relative to muscle size in both of these studies, they both showed a significant relationship between maximal force and muscle size. It is interesting to note that both of these studies determined muscle cross-sectional area using ultrasound techniques. When a difference in force per muscle cross-sectional area is noted between the sexes, it may be related to females having lower integrated electromyographic activity during maximal voluntary muscular actions, a longer electrical-mechanical delay time, or both (Kanehisa et al. 1994). Any difference in maximal force relative to muscle size is unlikely to be related to a difference between the sexes in noncontractile tissue within a muscle, as nonsignificant differences in noncontractile tissue between the sexes in young adults (6%) and competitive bodybuilders (10%) in a muscle cross-section have been shown (Alway, Grumbt et al. 1989; Kent-Braun, Ng, and Young 2000).

Pennation Angle

Muscle fiber pennation angle and length are associated with muscle fiber force and velocity shortening capabilities. **Pennation angle** refers to the angle of the muscle fiber's direction of pull relative to the direction of pull of the entire muscle or the direction of pull needed to produce movement at a joint (see figure 9.3). Larger pennation angles may permit a greater degree of muscle fiber packing, which results in a greater force exerted on a tendon for the same muscle volume (see figure 9.3). Longer muscle fibers

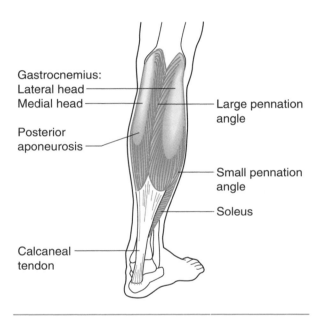

Figure 9.3 Pennation angle is determined by the angle at which muscle fibers attach to their tendon.

have more sarcomeres arranged in series, thus permitting greater muscle excursion and contraction velocity. Only a few studies have examined the effect of gender on muscle fiber characteristics. In the gastrocnemius (medialis and lateralis) and soleus muscles, females have been reported to have greater average muscle fiber length and greater variation in fiber length (Chow et al. 2000), whereas males had greater pennation angles in these same muscles. Conversely, fascicle length of the triceps (long head), vastus lateralis, and gastrocnemius (medialis) have been reported to be not significantly different between the genders (Abe et al. 1998). Pennation angle in these same muscles, however, is greater in males.

Significant positive correlations (pennation angle increases as muscle thickness increases) have been shown between pennation angle and muscle thickness (Abe et al. 1998; Ichinose et al. 1998). The greater muscle thickness in males (Abe et al. 1998; Chow et al. 2000) may account for their greater pennation angle. Because relatively few studies have examined these characteristics, no firm conclusions concerning gender differences in muscle fiber length and pennation angles can be reached. In both genders, however, it would likely be found that the increases in muscle size due to weight training would yield increases in pennation angle.

Number of Muscle Fibers

Total muscle cross-sectional area is a product of muscle fiber cross-sectional area and the number of muscle fibers. It is generally accepted that women have smaller muscle fiber areas than men (see figure 9.4). However, comparisons of the estimated number of fibers in various muscles are inconclusive. The number of muscle fibers in the average woman's biceps brachii has been reported to be less than (Sale et al. 1987) or the same as (Miller et al. 1992) the average man's. Female bodybuilders have been reported to have the same number of muscle fibers in the biceps brachii as male bodybuilders (Alway, Grumbt et al. 1989). Women's tibialis anterior has been reported to have fewer muscle fibers than men's (Henriksson-Larsen 1985), whereas women's triceps brachii and vastus lateralis have the same number of muscle fibers as men's (Schantz et al. 1983, 1981). Thus, whether differences in the number of muscle fibers in a muscle between the genders contributes to differences in total muscle cross-sectional area and so differences in absolute and relative strength is unclear.

In summary, the majority of evidence indicates that the average woman's absolute upper- and lower-body strength is not as great as the average man's. However, a large range exists when comparing absolute strength (see figure 9.1, table 9.1, and table 9.2). This large range is caused in part by the large number of movements possible with both the upper and the lower body and by different testing methods of maximal force (e.g., isometric, 1RM, isokinetic). When expressed

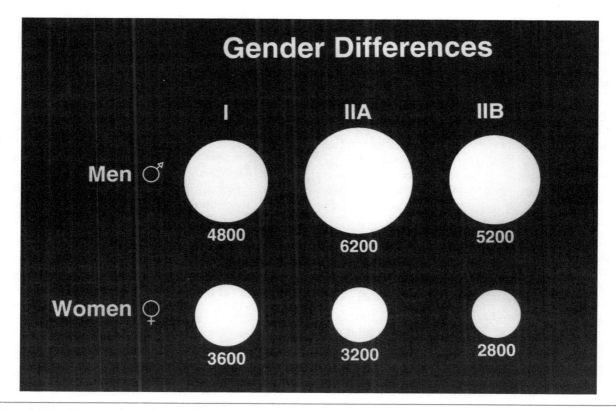

Figure 9.4 Graphic comparisons of woman's and man's muscle fiber size (um²) relationships for the different muscle fiber types. Note the greater cross-sectional area of the man's compared to the woman's fibers in their size relationships among the fibers.

Courtesy of Dr. Robert S. Staron's laboratory. © and property of OU-COM ED&R Photographic Resources, Irvine Hall, Athens, Ohio, 45701.

relative to total body weight, fat-free mass, and finally muscle size, the difference in maximal strength between the genders is gradually reduced and is often nonexistent when expressed relative to muscle size. However, lower-body strength is more likely to be equivalent between the genders than upper-body strength when expressed relative to fat-free mass or muscle size.

Gender Power Output Differences

Power output in many sports and activities is a major determinant of success. One such event is the snatch lift in Olympic weightlifting. Comparisons of international-caliber Olympic weightlifters indicate that for the complete pull phase of the snatch lift, women's power output relative to total body weight is 65% of men's (Garhammer 1989). The untrained average woman's clean high-pull is 54% of the average man's, whereas after 24 weeks of weight training, the average woman's high-pull increases to 66% of the average untrained man's (see table 9.2). Maximal vertical jump and standing long jump ability are also in large part determined by power output. The average woman has been reported to have 54 to 79% of the maximal vertical jump and 75% of the maximal standing long jump of the average male (Colliander and Tesch 1990b; Davies, Greenwood, and Jones 1988; Maud and Shultz 1986; Mayhew and Salm 1990). For the standing long jump this translates to the average woman generating approximately 63% of the power generated by the average man (Davies, Greenwood, and Jones 1988). However, women have also shown only small decrements (–5%) compared to men in vertical jump power (Sayers, Harackiewicz et al. 1999).

This gender difference in power exists even in the world of competitive Olympic weightlifting (Kraemer and Koziris 1994). For example, in the open age category of Olympic weightlifting for the 62-kg (136.4-lb) weight class for men and the 63-kg (138.6-lb) weight class for women, the 2000 world records for women were 132.5 kg (292 lb) in the clean and jerk and 110 kg (242 lb) in the snatch, whereas for men the records were 180.5 kg (397 lb) in the clean and jerk and 152.5 kg (336 lb) in the snatch. The women's world records were 73% and 72% of the men's in the clean and jerk and snatch lift, respectively. Thus, a woman's maximal power output in absolute terms as well as relative to total body weight is less than that of her male counterpart.

Vertical jump ability when expressed relative to fat-free mass shows only small (0-5.5%) differences between the genders (Maud and Shultz 1986; Mayhew and Salm 1990). Likewise, cycling short-sprint ability (30-second Wingate test) is not significantly different (2.5% difference) between the genders if expressed relative to fat-free mass (Maud and Shultz 1986). Women's concentric isokinetic knee-extension power (300 degrees per second) when expressed in absolute terms, relative to body weight, relative to fat-free mass, and relative to bone-free lean leg mass is 62%, 34%, 18%, and 13% lower than men's, respectively (Neder et al. 1999). This difference is statistically significant until expressed relative to bone-free lean leg mass. Thus, similar to maximal strength, differences in muscle size may account for differences in maximal power output between the genders.

The power generated by women during the standing long jump per unit of lean leg volume is significantly less than that generated by men (Davies, Greenwood, and Jones 1988). If fat-free mass is accounted for, women's short-sprint running and maximal stair-climbing ability (Margaria-Kalamen test) are 77% and 84% to 87%, respectively, of men's (Maud and Shultz 1986; Mayhew and Salm 1990). As discussed in the section on gender relative strength differences, normalizing by fat-free mass tends to overcorrect for the lower-body measures. This means that relative to fat-free mass the normalized measure would be higher in females than in males. Despite this overcorrection for lower-body measures, females in the previously cited measures do not demonstrate equivalent power to their male counterparts. Accounting for differences in fat-free mass or muscle size between the genders does appear to explain differences in power output to a greater extent in some tasks than in others.

Muscle Fiber Types and Power

Although the data are not consistent, in some tasks the question is raised of why women may generate less power per unit volume of muscle. One possible reason is a difference in muscle fiber type; however, there is no consistent evidence that percent muscle fiber type varies by gender within a particular muscle (Drinkwater 1984; Staron, Hagerman et al. 2001). Women's type I (slow-twitch) and type II (fast-twitch) muscle fibers both have a smaller cross-sectional area than males (Alway, Grumbt et al. 1989; Alway et al. 1992; Miller et al. 1992; Ryushi et al. 1988; Staron et al. 2000), with the type I muscle fibers having a smaller cross-sectional area relative to males than do the type II muscle fibers (Alway, Grumbt et al. 1989; Alway et al. 1992). For example, female bodybuilders' average type I fiber cross-sectional area is 64% that of male bodybuilders, whereas their average type II fiber cross-sectional area is 46% that of male bodybuilders (Alway et al. 1992). Thus, females' type I fibers are closer to their male counterparts in cross-section than are females' type II fibers. In fact, females' type I fibers can be equivalent or even larger in cross-sectional area than their type II fibers (Alway, Grumbt et al. 1989; Staron et al. 1989, 2000). This results in a smaller type II/type I muscle fiber area in females than in males, which may result in females' lower power output per muscle cross-sectional area than males'.

The total area occupied by specific muscle fiber types is different between the genders as well. In order from the greatest area to smallest area occupied, the order of muscle fiber types in males is type IIA, I, and IIB, whereas in females the order is type I, IIA, and IIB. This may also explain in part the differences in power between the genders, when apparent. The smaller type II/type I muscle fiber area in females may also explain their slower fatigue rate in some high-intensity types of exercise (Kanehisa et al. 1996; Pincivero et al. 2000). For example, fatigue rate during 50 consecutive isokinetic knee-extension actions is significantly less in females than in males (48% vs. 52%) (Kanehisa et al. 1996).

Power at faster velocities of movement would be affected if women's force-velocity curve were different from men's. However, it appears that the drop-off in force as the concentric velocity of movement increases is similar in both genders (Alway, Sale, and MacDougall 1990; Griffin et al. 1993) and that peak velocity during knee extension is not different between the genders (Houston, Norman, and Froese 1988).

Rate of force development could also affect power output. It appears that the skeletal muscles' rate of force development is slower for the average woman than for the average man (Komi and Karlsson 1978; Ryushi et al. 1988). Brown and colleagues (1998) have also reported that during isokinetic knee extension women require a greater portion of the range of motion than men

to achieve maximal velocity. Either of these differences between the sexes could result in a lower power output in women. A slower rate of force development in women may be attributed in part to differences between the genders in type I and type II muscle fibers as discussed earlier. This difference may also be related to some neural difference between the genders that affects muscle fiber recruitment.

Although the reasons are not entirely clear, women's maximal power output in absolute terms as well as relative to muscle size is lower than men's in some physical tasks. Reasons for this gender difference may be related to differences in type I and type II muscle fiber cross-sectional area and differences in rate of force development between the sexes.

Training Effects

Does resistance training produce the same effects in women as it does in men? Some people believe that women's adaptations to resistance training are less than men's, and therefore that women benefit less from resistance training than do men. However, research to date indicates that resistance training is generally at least as beneficial, if not more so, for women as for men.

Peak Oxygen Consumption

Women's relative peak oxygen consumption (ml/kg/min) increases 8% on average as a result of 8 to 20 weeks of circuit weight training, and men's increases an average of 5% over the same time period (Gettman and Pollock 1981). The average woman's cardiovascular endurance capabilities therefore increase more than those of the average man after circuit weight training. The reason women's peak oxygen consumption increases more than men's is unclear, but it may be related to the average man's higher cardiovascular fitness level before beginning the circuit weight training program. Women can realize even greater gains in relative peak oxygen consumption if they perform an aerobic circuit weight training program, which consists of resistance training exercises interspersed with short periods of aerobic training. This type of program, when performed using five groups of five resistance and calisthenic exercises separated by five 3-minute periods of aerobic exercise, results in a 22% increase in peak oxygen consumption in previously untrained women over 12 weeks of training (Mosher et al. 1994).

Body Composition

Body compositional changes are a goal of many women and men performing resistance training. Increases in fat-free mass and decreases in percent body fat from short-term (8 to 20 weeks) resistance training programs are of the same magnitude in both genders (see table 3.3 on page 92). Men and women performing identical short-term weight training programs have both shown significant decreases in percent body fat with no significant difference shown between the genders (Staron et al. 2000). Lemmer and colleagues (2001) also reported that both genders show a significant increase in fat-free mass and no change in percent body fat when performing the identical weight training program for 24 weeks. In this study only men showed a significant reduction in fat mass, indicating that women may have a more difficult time losing body fat during resistance training.

Body composition changes in different regions of the body after training may also be an important consideration in women (Nindl et al. 2000). After 6 months of performing a periodized weight training program and endurance training exercise, women showed a 31% loss in fat mass with no change in lean mass in the arms. They also showed a 5.5% gain in lean mass in the legs, but no change in fat mass. These results indicate that it may be more difficult to increase lean mass in the upper body of women compared to the lower body. However, other data contradict this assertion. After performing several weight training programs for 6 months, untrained women demonstrated upper-arm muscle cross-sectional area increases from approximately 15% to 19% and increases in thigh muscle cross-sectional area from approximately 5% to 9% (Kraemer, Koziris, Ratamess et al. 2002). This indicates that the upper-arm musculature undergoes greater hypertrophy than the thigh.

Differences in regional body compositional changes have also been shown during 13 weeks of endurance training (Abe et al. 1997). Female subjects who performed aerobic training 1 to 2 days per week with caloric restriction and females who performed three to four aerobic training sessions per week without caloric restriction both demonstrated significant decreases in body fat percentage and total fat mass. However, only the group that performed aerobic training 3 to 4 days a week showed a significant reduction in subcutaneous fat, whereas both groups showed a significant and equivalent loss in visceral fat. The loss in subcutaneous fat showed a significant negative correlation ($r = -0.65$) to training frequency. This suggests that for women to lose subcutaneous fat, they may need higher exercise frequencies in addition to caloric restriction.

Hypertrophy

Increased muscle cross-sectional area determined by computerized tomography after isometric (Davies, Greenwood, and Jones 1988) and dynamic constant external resistance training (Cureton et al. 1988; O'Hagen et al. 1995b) are of the same magnitude in both genders. Muscle fiber hypertrophy of type I (slow-twitch) and two major type II (fast-twitch, types IIA and IIB) can occur in women performing resistance training (Staron et al. 1989, 1991). After 8 weeks of resistance training, all fiber types in both genders showed similiar gradual nonsignificant increases in cross-sectional area (Staron et al. 1994). This information indicates that changes in whole muscle and fiber cross-sectional area during an initial short-term training period are similar between the genders.

Some women do not perform heavy resistance training because they believe their muscles will hypertrophy excessively and that they may look less feminine. The average woman's muscles do not, however, hypertrophy excessively. This is encouraging for a woman who wants to perform resistance training but does not want an excessive increase in muscle size. It is discouraging, however, for a woman who does want an increase in muscles size, such as a woman bodybuilder. The greatest increase in various body circumferences in women after 10 weeks (Wilmore 1974), 12 weeks (Boyer 1990), or 20 weeks (Staron et al. 1991) of resistance training was 0.6, 0.4, and 0.6 cm (0.2, 0.16, and 0.2 in.), respectively. With the 10-week program hip, thigh, and abdomen circumferences actually decreased 0.2 to 0.7 cm (0.08 to 0.3 in.). During three different 12-week programs abdomen circumference decreased 0.2 to 1.1 cm (0.08 to 0.4 in.) (Boyer 1990). The finding that resistance training in women results in no change or small changes in body circumferences is supported by other studies (Capen, Bright, and Line 1961; Häkkinen et al. 1989; Staron et al. 1994; Wells, Jokl, and Bohanen 1973). Body circumferences do not change because of small increases in muscle mass (see table 3.3 on page 92) and decreases in adipose tissue in the limb or body part, which conceal any circumference gain due to increased muscle mass (Mayhew and Gross 1974). Previously discussed changes in upper-arm and thigh muscle cross-sectional area after 6 months of weight training support limb circumference data that indicate that women generally experience significant yet small increases in muscle size (Kraemer, Koziris, Ratamess et al. 2002; Nindl et al. 2000).

Because muscle tissue is denser than adipose tissue, an increase in muscle mass accompanied by a decrease in adipose tissue equaling the gain in muscle mass will result in a slight decrease in body circumferences. The 10-, 12-, and 16-week training studies discussed earlier all demonstrated decreases in skinfold thicknesses, indicating a decrease in subcutaneous fat. There may, however, be regional body differences in the ability to lose adipose tissue and gain muscle mass (Nindl et al. 2000). After 6 months performing a periodized weight training program and endurance training, women showed a significant loss in fat mass with no change in lean mass in the arms and trunk.

This would result in a reduction in arm and trunk circumferences. The legs showed a small but significant gain in lean mass but no change in fat mass. This would result in a small increase in leg circumference (see figure 9.5). The lack of increases or even small decreases in body circumferences are encouraging for woman who want increased strength or the fit-firm look of trained muscle without increased body circumferences.

Some women do develop larger-than-average amounts of hypertrophy from resistance training. One outcome of large gains in muscle hypertrophy can be increased body circumferences. After a 6-month resistance training program a group of female athletes exhibited increases of 3.5, 1.1, and 0.9 cm (1.4, 0.4, and 0.35 in.) (5%, 4%, and 2%) in shoulder, upper-arm, and thigh circumferences, respectively (Brown and Wilmore 1974). Larger-than-average increases in fat-free mass and limb circumferences in some women are probably related to several factors, including the following:

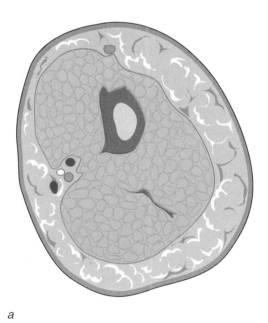 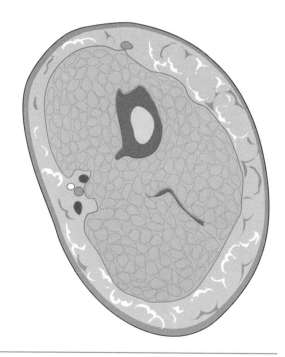

a
b

Figure 9.5 Magnetic resonance image of a woman's upper thigh musculature *(a)* before and *(b)* after performing a weight training program.

Courtesy of Dr. William Kraemer's laboratory, University of Connecticut, Storrs, Connecticut.

- Higher-than-normal resting testosterone, growth hormone, or other hormone concentrations
- Greater hormonal response than normal to the performance of resistance training
- Lower-than-normal estrogen-to-testosterone ratio
- Genetic disposition to develop a large muscle mass
- Ability to perform a more intense or higher-volume resistance training program

Muscle Fiber Types

One difference between the genders is the fact that the transformation of myosin heavy chains from type IIB to type IIAB to type IIA takes place at a faster rate in women than in men (Staron et al. 1994). As discussed in the previous section on gender power output differences, women's type I muscle fibers have a closer cross-sectional area relative to men's than do the type II muscle fibers (Alway, Grumbt et al. 1989; Alway et al. 1992). This difference in untrained muscle fiber cross-sectional area between the genders may result in a greater potential for type II fiber hypertrophy in women. Such a tendency has been shown in women performing weight training for the lower body (Staron et al. 1994), with women demonstrating muscle fiber hypertrophy (vastus lateralis) of 25%, 23%, and 11% in type IIA, IIB, and I fibers, respectively.

Men demonstrated a less dramatic difference in fiber type hypertrophy of 19%, 20%, and 17% in type IIA, IIB, and I fiber types, respectively, after performing the identical resistance training program (Staron et al. 1994). O'Hagen and colleagues (1995b), however, reported relative increases in type II fiber cross-sectional area in the upper body (biceps) to be similar between the genders. Thus, some differences between the genders may exist in the hypertrophy response of muscle fibers to weight training.

Rate of Strength Gain

When performing the identical resistance training program, women generally gain strength at the same rate or faster than men (Cureton et al. 1988; Lemmer et al. 2000; Wilmore 1974; Wilmore et al. 1978). Over the course of a 24-week (see figure 9.6) and a 16-week (see figure 9.7) resistance training program, women generally gained strength at a rate equal to or greater than men. Men may demonstrate greater absolute increases in strength than women, but women generally demonstrate the same or greater relative increases (percent increases) than men. Despite the substantial increases in maximal strength apparent in women after 6 months of resistance training, however, the average woman's maximal strength (1RM back squat, bench press, clean high-pull) is still significantly lower than the average untrained man's (Kraemer, Mazzetti et al. 2001).

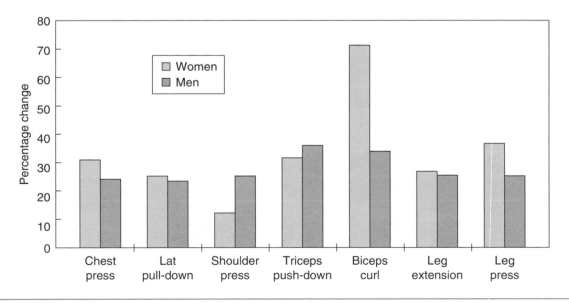

Figure 9.6 Male and female strength changes after a 24-week resistance training program.

Data from J.T. Lemmer et al., 2001, "Effect of strength training on resting metabolic rate and physical activity: age and gender comparisons," *Medicine and Science in Sports and Exercise* 33: 532-541.

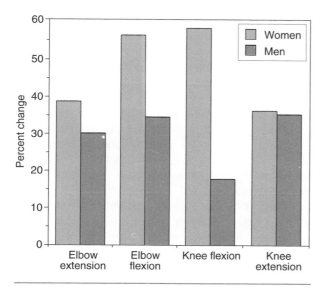

Figure 9.7 Male and female strength changes after a 16-week resistance training program.

Data from K.J. Cureton, M.A. Collins, D.W. Hill, and McElhannon, 1988, "Muscle hypertrophy in men and women," *Medicine and Science in Sports and Exercise* 20: 338-344.

Some data indicate that women's strength gains may plateau after 3 to 5 months of training and may not progress as quickly as men's after this point (Häkkinen 1993; Häkkinen et al. 1989). When apparent, such a plateau may be related to the type of training program performed. Periodized multiple-set programs have not shown plateaus in strength, power, and body composition during 6 to 9 months of training (Kraemer et al. 2000; Kraemer, Mazzetti et al. 2001; Marx et al. 2001), whereas nonvaried single-set programs have shown plateaus in strength, power, and body composition after 3 months of training (Kraemer et al. 2000; Marx et al. 2001). This suggests that either periodized programs or higher-volume programs may help women avoid training plateaus.

Women's Hormonal Response to Resistance Training

The acute hormonal response (i.e., to a training session) and chronic hormonal response (i.e., long-term training response at rest or to a training session) to resistance training affects the anabolic/catabolic environment to which muscle tissue is exposed. This is true for both genders and may partly explain gains in muscle size and strength from resistance training. When interpreting a woman's hormonal response to training, the potential effects of the menstrual cycle must be considered. It must also be remembered that a low concentration of a hormone does not necessarily mean that the hormone does not have an active role in controlling a bodily function or process, such as tissue growth. Hormones at low concentrations may still affect a bodily function due to increased interaction with receptors, higher rates of utilization, or both.

Testosterone

At rest, men normally have 10 times the serum testosterone concentration of women (Kraemer et al. 1991; Wright 1980). This may account in part for the larger muscle mass of men compared to women. Even though the testosterone concentration of women is low compared to men, small changes in its concentration may affect muscle tissue growth. Women's serum testosterone has been reported to increase significantly in response to one session of resistance training (Cummings et al. 1987; Nindl, Kraemer, Gotshalk et al. 2001). However, Kraemer and colleagues (Kraemer et al. 1991; Kraemer, Fleck et al. 1993) reported a nonsignificant acute response of women's testosterone concentration to one training session (see figure 9.8). They also noted that the concentration

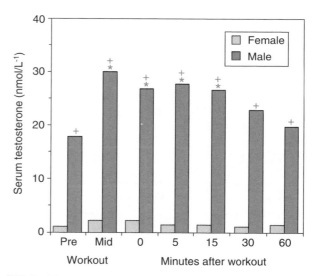

Figure 9.8 Serum testosterone concentrations in men and women caused by performing the same resistance training session of three sets of eight exercises at 10RM with 1-minute rests between sets and exercises.

* = significantly different from preexercise value of same gender; + = significantly different from female value at the same time point.

Adapted, by permission, from W.J. Kraemer et al., 1991, "Endogenous anabolic hormonal and growth factor responses to heavy resistance exercise in males and females," *International Journal of Sports Medicine* 12: 231.

of testosterone was not affected by the total volume of the training session (the number of sets of an exercise performed). Men's serum testosterone concentrations consistently increase in response to the identical resistance training session.

Resting serum testosterone concentrations are not significantly different between untrained and highly competitive female Olympic weightlifters (Stoessel et al. 1991). Eight weeks of resistance training (Staron et al. 1994) and 16 weeks of power training (Häkkinen et al. 1990) have both been reported not to alter resting serum testosterone concentrations in women. Kraemer, Staron, and colleagues (1998), however, reported that 8 weeks of resistance training by women does significantly increase resting testosterone concentrations as well as the immediate postexercise response compared to the exercise response in the untrained state. None of the aforementioned studies, however, controlled for menstrual cycle phase. When menstrual cycle phase was controlled (serum obtained in early follicular phase), increases in resting testosterone concentrations from 6 months of resistance training occurred (Marx et al. 2001). Additionally, training volume did affect the resting testosterone concentration response. Women performing a multiple-set periodized program demonstrated a small but significantly greater increase in resting testosterone concentration after 3 and 6 months of training than women performing a nonvaried single-set program (Marx et al. 2001). Nindl, Kraemer, Gotshalk, and colleagues (2001) demonstrated that the testosterone response of women is related to regional body fat distribution, with women having a higher degree of upper-body fat showing an accentuated response.

Cortisol

Cortisol plays several regulatory roles in metabolism and negatively affects protein metabolism. Women's serum cortisol concentrations, when menstrual cycle phase is controlled, can increase in response to a resistance training session (Cummings et al. 1987; Kraemer, Fleck et al. 1993; Mulligan et al. 1996); the same can occur when menstrual cycle phase is not controlled (Kraemer, Staron et al. 1998). Additionally, higher training volumes (one vs. three sets of exercises) result in an increased cortisol response in women (Kraemer, Fleck et al. 1993; Mulligan et al. 1996). Similarly, the cortisol response of men also depends in part on training volume. Resting serum

cortisol concentrations have been reported to not change after 8 weeks of resistance training (Staron et al. 1994) or 16 weeks of power-type resistance training (Häkkinen et al. 1990) when menstrual cycle phase is not controlled. When menstrual cycle phase is not controlled, resting cortisol concentrations have also decreased after 8 weeks of resistance training, and the response immediately after a resistance training session is decreased after 8 weeks of resistance training compared to the untrained state (Kraemer, Staron et al. 1998). Training volume may be an important factor in determining whether resting cortisol concentrations will decrease. After 6 months of a multiple-set periodized resistance training program in which menstrual cycle phase was controlled, resting concentrations of cortisol decreased significantly, whereas no significant change occurred following a 6-month single-set program (Marx et al. 2001).

Testosterone/Cortisol Ratio

The testosterone/cortisol ratio has been used as a general marker of anabolic status (Häkkinen et al. 1990), with an increase in this ratio indicating an increased theoretical anabolic environment. Women's resting testosterone/cortisol ratio has been reported to increase after 6 months of resistance training in which menstrual cycle phase is controlled (Marx et al. 2001). The magnitude of the resting testosterone/cortisol ratio response appears to be related to training volume. During 6 months of resistance training, a nonvaried single-set program resulted in a significant increase in the testosterone/cortisol ratio at 3 months, but no further change occurred from 3 to 6 months (Marx et al. 2001). During 6 months of resistance training, a periodized multiple-set program resulted in a significant increase after 3 months and a further significant increase from 3 to 6 months (Marx et al. 2001). This indicates an advantage of the periodized multple-set program in increasing the theoretical anabolic environment represented by the testosterone/cortisone ratio.

Growth Hormone

Similar to men, women respond to a resistance training session (see figure 9.9) with an increase in serum human growth hormone (22 kD isoform) (Kraemer et al. 1991; Kraemer, Fleck et al. 1993; Kraemer, Staron et al. 1998; Mulligan et al. 1996). Also, similar to men, the acute increase in growth hormone in women is responsive to the total volume of a session, with a significantly higher response to sessions of greater volume compared (one vs. three sets of each exercise) to sessions of lower volume (Kraemer et al. 1991; Kraemer, Fleck et al. 1993; Mulligan et al. 1996). Higher-volume sessions are especially effective at increasing the human growth hormone response in both genders when short rest periods (approximately 1 minute) are used between sets and exercises.

Training status may also affect women's acute human growth hormone response. Women with at least 1 year of weight training experience exhibited a longer time period of growth hormone elevation above resting values resulting in a greater magnitude of growth hormone response compared to women with no regular weight training experience (Taylor et al. 2000). Women's resting serum human growth hormone concentration is unaffected by 8 weeks (Kraemer, Staron et al. 1998) and 6 months (Marx et al. 2001) of resistance training. However, Taylor and colleagues (2000) reported that women with at least 1 year of weight training experience had a lower resting serum growth hormone concentration immediately before a resistance training session than women with no regular weight training experience. Several isoforms of growth hormone exist, and the decrease could be related to a shift in the molecu-

lar isoform of growth hormone produced by the pituitary gland. However, to date the acute growth hormone response and the resting chronic response appear to be quite similar between the genders.

The acute and chronic response to resistance training of various hormones creates the anabolic environment to which skeletal muscle, bone, and other tissues are exposed. The hormonal response to resistance training is responsible in part for both genders' strength and muscle hypertrophy increases following resistance training. Although women's testosterone response to resistance training appears to be lower than that of their male counterparts, the growth hormone response to resistance training is quite similar between the genders. Although not discussed here, other hormones (IGF-I, luteinizing hormone, follicle-stimulating hormone) may also be responsive to resistance training and so affect women's long-term adaptations to resistance training.

Menstrual Cycle Phase Effects on Strength and Weight Training

Little information is available on the effect of menstrual cycle phase on maximal strength, and the information available is contradictory. Lebrun (1994) reported increases in measures of maximal strength during the follicular phase (menstrual flow to approximately 14 days after menstrual flow) compared to the luteal phase (approximately 14 days after the menstrual flow to the beginning of the next menstrual flow) but no difference in maximal strength between these phases. There are, however, possibly large individual variations of the effect of menstrual cycle phase on maximal strength.

The explanation of why strength or physical performance may vary during different phases of the menstrual cycle are normally explained by hormonal variations. For example, progesterone is supposed to have a catabolic effect on muscle and reaches its highest blood concentrations during the luteal phase. Cortisol, which also has catabolic effects, also reaches higher concentrations during the luteal compared to the follicular phase. Testosterone remains at a relatively constant concentration throughout the entire menstrual cycle, except for an increase during ovulation. Such increases in catabolic hormones can be offset by a disinhibition of receptors to anabolic hormones. Thus, receptors may not interact with catabolic hormones even though their concentrations have increased.

These hormonal changes with different phases of the menstrual cycle have led some to postulate

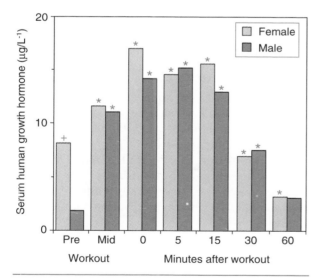

Figure 9.9 Serum growth hormone concentrations in men and women caused by performing the same resistance training session of three sets of eight exercises and a 10RM with 1-minute rests between sets and exercises.

* = significantly different from preexercise value of same gender; + = significantly different from female value at the same time point.

Adapted, by permission, from W.J. Kraemer et al., 1991, "Endogenous anabolic hormonal and growth factor responses to heavy resistance exercise in males and females," *International Journal of Sports Medicine* 12: 232.

that strength training should be varied during the different menstrual cycle phases. The varying hormone concentrations result in conditions for muscle growth and repair being better in the follicular compared to the luteal phase (Reis, Frick, and Schmidtbleicher, 1995). Thus, resistance training intensity or volume should be reduced during the luteal phase and increased during the follicular phase (Reis, Frick, and Schmidtbleicher 1995). Reis, Frick, and Schmidtbleicher (1995) compared such a training plan to a more normal resistance training plan over two consecutive menstrual cycles (approximately 8 weeks). Normal training consisted of performing resistance training every third day throughout the menstrual cycle. "Menstrual cycle–triggered training" consisted of performing training every second day during the follicular phase and about once a week during the luteal phase. Maximal isometric leg strength increased 33% following menstrual cycle–triggered training and 13% with the normal training. Muscle cross-sectional area increases of the quadriceps femoris were equivalent (approximately 4%) between the two groups; however, maximal strength per muscle cross-sectional area was significantly greater with the menstrual cycle–triggered training (27% vs. 10%). Significant correlations between hormones and strength and muscle cross-sectional area increases were shown. For example, estradiol in the training period correlated with increased muscle cross-sectional area ($r = 0.85$), and changes in progesterone concentrations between the first and second luteal phases in the training period correlated with maximal strength increases ($r = 0.77$).

Not all information supports the rationale of the menstrual cycle–triggered training plan that hormonal conditions during the follicular phase are more conducive to muscle tissue growth and repair. In untrained women a higher acute growth hormone response to resistance training is apparent in the luteal phase compared to the follicular phase (Kraemer, Fleck, Dziados et al. 1993). Thus, although varying training with the different phases of the menstrual cycle is an attractive hypothesis, more study of this subject is needed.

Menstrual Cycle Alterations Due to Physical Training

Some women engaged in physical training, including resistance training, experience variations in their menstrual cycles. Common irregularities include shortening of the luteal (postovulatory) phase to less than 10 days; lack of ovulation (release of an egg); **oligomenorrhea,** an irregular menstrual cycle in women who previously had a normal menstrual pattern or a cycle with more than 36 days between menstrual flows; **secondary amenorrhea,** the absence of menstruation for 180 days or more in women who previously menstruated regularly; and **dysmenorrhea,** pain during menstruation. Research concerning the frequency of these irregularities in women who perform resistance training is limited. The physiological mechanisms responsible for development of menstrual irregularities are currently not fully defined. Because differences in menstrual cycle patterns among women can be considerable, it can be difficult to determine what constitutes a regular, as opposed to an irregular, menstrual cycle for a particular woman. The majority of menstrual irregularities return to normal with reduction or cessation of training, so there is no long-term negative effect from physical training on women's reproductive systems.

Oligomenorrhea and Secondary Amenorrhea

Oligomenorrhea and secondary amenorrhea have been reported to be more common in women engaged in vigorous physical activity (DeSouza and Metzger 1991; Gray and Dale 1984; Loucks and Horvath 1985; Prior, Vigna, and McKay 1992; Shepard 2000b; Williams et al. 1999). However, a wide range in the prevalence of menstrual cycle disorders exists. For example, amenorrhea in an athletic population occurs with a prevalence of 3.4 to 66% compared to 2 to 5% in the general female population (Nattiv et al. 1994). This wide range is due in part to differences in the definition of amenorrhea and possibly athlete caliber, as well as differences in training volume and intensity.

Out of 199 Olympic-style weightlifters of an average age of 16 years, 25% reported having irregular menses; only three of these athletes aged 13 to 15 had not yet begun to menstruate (Liu, Liu, and Qin 1987). The prevalence of oligomenorrhea and secondary amenorrhea in women not taking oral contraceptives was 20% and 2%, respectively, in a group of recreational resistance trainers; 71% and 14%, respectively, in a group of women who had competed in at least one bodybuilding contest; and 9% and 4% in a group of sedentary women (Walberg and Johnston 1991). Thirty-three percent of women who competed in a bodybuilding contest and did not take oral contraceptives reported oligomenorrhea or secondary amenorrhea (Elliot and Goldberg 1983). The data available indicate that, similar to other forms of vigorous physical activity, resistance training may put women at greater risk than normal of experiencing menstrual cycle irregularities.

In distance runners, greater training volume, intensity, frequency, and training session duration have all been implicated as factors that increase the risk of menstrual irregularities (Cameron, Wark, and Telford 1992; Gray and Dale 1984; Loucks and Horvath 1985). Athletes who train for long periods of time (daily or over years) at high intensities appear to be at greater risk of experiencing oligomenorrhea and secondary amenorrhea. In female recreational resistance trainers who do not use oral contraceptives, the incidence of either oligomenorrhea or amenorrhea is 22%, whereas it is 85% in competitive bodybuilders (Walberg and Johnston 1991). Thus, greater resistance training intensity or volume seems to result in a greater risk of menstrual irregularities. However, not all athletes performing high-volume, high-intensity training will experience menstrual irregularities.

Aspects of reproductive history and maturity have been associated with menstrual irregularities. The incidence of amenorrhea is higher in younger than in older women. For example, 85% of runners experiencing secondary amenorrhea were reported to be under 30 years of age (Speroff and Redwine 1980). Several researchers have also proposed that physical training at an early age delays menarche and that late menarche is associated with a greater chance of experiencing amenorrhea (Gray and Dale 1984; Loucks and Horvath 1985; Nattiv et al. 1994). A previous pregnancy has been associated with a decreased risk of amenorrhea (Loucks and Horvath 1985). Insufficient caloric intake, psychological stress, abrupt changes in body composition, and previous menstrual irregularities have all been associated with increased risk of menstrual irregularities (Lebenstedt, Platte, and Pirke 1999; Loucks and Horvath 1985; Nattiv et al. 1994; Shepard 2000b). Although not completely elucidated, all of these factors may be associated with hormonal disturbances resulting in menstrual irregularities. For example, insufficient caloric intake while performing physical training may predispose women to hormonal disturbances (luteinizing hormone secretion) associated with menstrual cycle disturbances (Williams et al. 1995), whereas sufficient caloric intake may prevent these changes.

Premenstrual Symptoms and Dysmenorrhea

One of the first adaptations to an exercise program is a decrease in normal premenstrual symptoms (Prior, Vigna, and McKay 1992), such as breast enlargement, appetite cravings, bloating, and mood changes. Active, athletic women have fewer difficulties with premenstrual symptoms than sedentary women (Prior, Vigna, and McKay 1992). If training is decreased, however, premenstrual symptoms may increase, especially if weight gain is concurrent with a decrease in training (Prior, Vigna, and McKay 1992). Thus, athletes with excessive premenstrual symptoms who are decreasing training should not decrease training abruptly. They should also try to avoid large weight gains.

Dysmenorrhea, or abdominal pain with menstruation, may increase with an increase in premenstrual symptoms (Prior, Vigna, and McKay 1992). Dysmenorrhea is reported by 60 to 70% of adult women, and increases with chronological and gynecological age (Brooks-Gunn and Rubb 1983; Widholm 1979). Like premenstrual symptoms, dysmenorrhea occurs less frequently and is less severe in athletes than in the general population (Dale, Gerlach, and Wilhite 1979; Timonen and Procope 1971). Although the effect of controlling premenstrual symptoms and dysmenorrhea with oral contraceptives is unclear, some anecdotal and retrospective studies have reported increases in performance with the use of oral contraceptives (Lebrun 1994). Lebrun (1994) hypothesized that controlling dysmenorrhea with oral contraceptives may be related to decreased traumatic injury rates in athletes (soccer players) because of the effects of dysmenorrhea on coordination.

Increased production of the hormone prostaglandin is associated with uterine cramping and is thought to be the cause of dysmenorrhea (Dawood 1983). The reduced frequency and severity of premenstrual and dysmenorrhea symptoms in athletes could be caused by differences in hormonal concentrations or a higher pain threshold in athletes. In either case physical training appears to decrease the incidence of premenstrual symptoms and dysmenorrhea. Prior, Vigna, and McKay (1992) reviewed treatment strategies for athletes with premenstrual symptoms and dysmenorrhea.

Performance During the Menstrual Cycle and Menstrual Problems

Lebrun (1994) noted little or no difference in aerobic or anaerobic performance at various times during the menstrual cycle. However, decrements in performance during the premenstrual or menstrual phase have been shown, with the best performances occurring during the immediate postmenstrual period and the 15th day of the menstrual cycle (Allsen, Parsons, and Bryce 1977; Doolittle and Engebretsen 1972; Lebrun 1994). Likewise, Masterson (1999) showed peak power, anaerobic capacity, and fatigue rate (Wingate test) to be negatively affected during the follicular phase compared to the luteal phase. Individual variations in the effects of menstrual cycle phase on performance can be substantial, with some athletes even noticing an improvement in performance during menstruation (Lebrun 1994).

Reasons for decreased performance during the premenstrual or menstrual phase may be associated with many factors, including self-expectancies, negative attitudes toward menstruation, and weight gain. The possible detrimental effect on athletic performance of premenstrual symptoms or dysmenorrhea has led some researchers to recommend the use of oral contraceptives or progesterone injections to ensure that menses do not occur during major competitions (Liu, Liu, and Qin 1987). However, Olympic medal–winning performances have taken place during all phases of the menstrual cycle. The effect of the menstrual cycle on performance is therefore unclear and is probably very specific to the individual. Oligomenorrhea and amenorrhea, although having potential long-term health effects such as bone loss, should have no effect on performance. Participation in physical training and athletic events during menstruation or any other phase of the menstrual cycle should not be discouraged and has no detrimental effect on health.

Bone Density

Physical activity (Chilibeck, Sale, and Webber 1995; Dalsky et al. 1988; DeCree, Vermeulen, and Ostyn 1991; Jacobson et al. 1984), including weight training (Chilibeck, Sale, and Webber 1995), in women can result in increased bone density. In women the possibility of increasing bone density due to weight training appears to

cover a wide range of ages, with increased bone density shown in women aged 20 to 23 (Hawkins et al. 1999) and 40 to 50 (Dornemann et al. 1997). Significant correlations of fat-free mass, regional lean tissue, and strength to bone density support the contention that weight training can increase bone density (Aloia et al. 1995; Hughes et al. 1995; Nichols et al. 1995). However, no significant change in bone mineral density in a wide age range of women has also been shown. No change in bone density in women 28 years of age (Nindl et al. 2000) and 54 years of age (Pruit et al. 1992) has also been shown. Many factors, including the weight training program design, duration of training, and site where bone density is measured may affect whether bone density changes occur after weight training. However, weight training does appear to offer a good possibility of increasing bone density in women, or at least slowing bone density loss as women age.

Menstrual Cycle Dysfunction and Bone Density

Menstrual dysfunction can result in decreased bone density and an increased risk of osteoporosis (Cameron, Wark, and Telford 1992; Constantini 1994; DeCree, Vermeulen, and Ostyn 1991; Nyburgh et al. 1993; Shepard 2000b; Tomten et al. 1998). The effect of menstrual dysfunction on bone density may be dramatic. Women who have never had regular menstrual cycles show on average a 17% deficit in bone density compared to their normally menstruating peers (Shephard 2000b). The loss of bone mass may occur predominantly during the first 3 to 4 years of amenorrhea (Cann et al. 1984). Age at menarche, age at menarche with subsequent amenorrhea, duration of oligomenorrhea, and duration of menstrual dysfunction have all been correlated with reduced bone density compared to normal values (Cameron, Wark, and Telford 1992; Drinkwater, Bruemner, and Chestnut 1990; Lloyd et al. 1987; Nyburgh et al. 1993). Athletes who were amenorrheic and then regained menses for 15 months showed an increase in bone density, whereas athletes who did not regain menses showed no change or a continued loss of bone density (Cameron, Wark, and Telford 1992). How readily a normal bone density can or may be restored in amenorrheic individuals once a normal menstrual cycle resumes is yet to be determined (Drinkwater, Bruemner, and Chestnut 1990). Young amenorrheic women may therefore be losing bone mass at a point in their lives when bone mass should be increasing. Cameron, Wark, and Telford (1992) reported that amenorrheic athletes have greater bone density than amenorrheic nonathletes. This indicates that amenorrhea is associated with a decrease in bone density and mass, but that physical activity may partially slow the loss of bone mass caused by amenorrhea.

Highly trained women, including weight trainers, however, appear to have a greater-than-normal risk for menstrual problems (as previously discussed) and therefore may also be at risk for osteoporosis. This may be especially true for women using oral contraceptives. Women performing recreational activity, including weight training, over 2 years showed a positive effect on total body bone mineral content. However, oral contraceptives had a negative impact on total-body bone mineral content even when exercise was performed (Weaver et al. 2001).

Types of Bone

Whether bone mass or density changes is a complex issue that is made more complex by the existence of two major types of bone. Cancellous or trabecular bone has a high turnover rate and responds to changes in hormonal concentrations to a greater extent than to exercise. Cortical bone has a slower turnover rate and is influenced more by mechanical strain than cancellous bone (Rico et al. 1994; Young et al. 1994). Decreased bone density and mass can occur both in the lumbar spine, composed predominantly of cancellous bone (Cameron, Wark, and Telford 1992; Prior, Vigna, and McKay 1992; Tomten et al. 1998), and in the axial skeleton or vetebral column, composed primarily of cortical bone (Nyburgh et al. 1993; Tomten et al 1998). Thus, the entire skeleton of amenorrheic women, including amenorrheic athletes (Nyburgh et al. 1993), can experience a decrease in bone density.

The many possible interactions and small differences that may bring about an increase or decrease in bone density is made apparent by a comparison of normally menstruating female runners (Petit, Prior, and Barr 1999). Over 1 year, runners with an average luteal phase greater than 11 days showed no significant change in lumbar cancellous bone mineral density, whereas runners with an average luteal phase less than 10 days showed a significant 3.6% lumbar cancellous bone mineral density loss. Even though this is a complex issue, it does appear that physical activity, including weight training, can positively affect bone mineral density in women.

Hormonal Mechanisms of Menstrual Cycle Disturbances and Bone Density Loss

The hormonal mechanisms that result in menstrual cycle irregularities and bone loss are not completely defined. Stressors such as physical stress from training, psychological stress, inadequate caloric intake, and other dietary deficiencies may result in menstrual cycle disturbances (Chilibeck, Sale, and Webber 1995; Prior, Vigna, and McKay 1992). The stressors cause an increase in corticotropin-releasing hormone from the hypothalamus (see figure 9.10), causing a decrease in gonadotropin-releasing hormone, which in turn results in a decrease in the pituitary hormones, luteinizing hormone and follicle-stimulating hormone. The decrease in the pituitary hormones results in menstrual cycle disturbances. Menstrual cycle disturbances result in decreases in the ovarian hormones progesterone and estrogen, which in turn eventually affect osteoclasts, which resorb bone, and osteblasts, which form bone, resulting in a net decrease in bone mass or density.

The interactions of hormones are complicated. Whether bone mass or density increases or decreases due to physical training and menstrual cycle disturbances is related to the factors stimulating bone resorption (bone loss) and formation. Decreased concentrations of the ovarian hormones estrogen and progesterone are the hormonal factors most frequently associated with osteoporosis and bone loss. Some have suggested that estrogen may reduce bone reabsorption, but that it has little impact on bone formation, resulting in a net loss of bone (Cameron, Wark, and Telford 1992; DeCree, Vermeulen, and Ostyn 1991). Receptors in bone for some hormones (estrogens, androgens, progesterone, corticosteroids) have been found, and their effect on bone formation or resorption is generally understood (Bland 2000; Quaedackers et al. 2001). It is also possible that a hormone such as estrogen has an indirect effect on bone by acting through another hormone (DeCree, Vermeulen, and Ostyn 1991).

Corticotropin released from the anterior pituitary stimulates cortisol release from the adrenal cortex and may result in bone loss and be related to menstrual cycle disturbances (DeSouza and Metzger 1991; Prior, Vigna, and McKay 1992). Increased beta-endorphin may also be associated

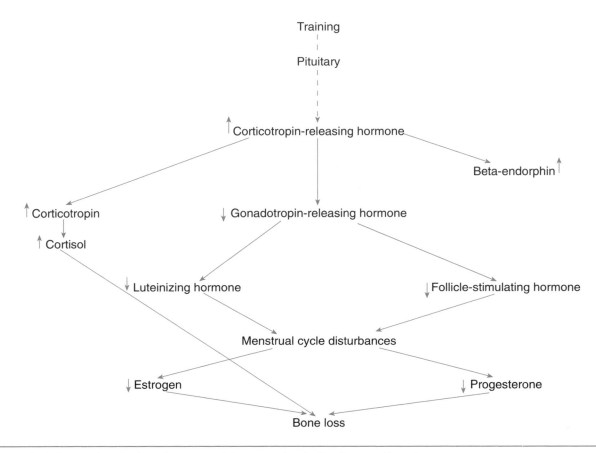

Figure 9.10 Hormonal mechanisms that may result in menstrual cycle disturbance and bone loss.

with menstrual cycle disturbances (Cameron, Wark, and Telford 1992; DeCree, Vermeulen, and Ostyn 1991; Prior, Vigna, and McKay 1992). Increases in beta-endorphin have been shown to occur in women in response to resistance training, especially when accompanied by a negative caloric balance, and this could be responsible in part for menstrual cycle disturbances in these women (Walberg-Rankin, Franke, and Gwazdauskas 1992). Many other hormones, such as growth hormone, testosterone, estradiol, progesterone, corticosteroids, insulin, and calcitonin, are also probably involved to varying degrees with menstrual cycle disturbances and bone loss in active women (Bland 2000; Cameron, Wark, and Telford 1992; Prior, Vigna, and McKay 1992).

Other local factors are also involved in bone resorption and formation. Prostaglandin, which stimulates osteoblasts, released from bone itself is implicated in the early response of bone formation due to mechanical loading (Chilibeck, Sale, and Webber 1995; Chow 2000). Insulin-like growth factor I, which stimulates bone forma-

tion, is produced by many cells in response to growth hormone and may be released from bone itself in response to mechanical loading from exercise and prostaglandin stimulation (Chow 2000; Snow, Rosen, and Robinson 2000). Similar to the hormonal factors that affect bone formation and resorption, local factors are also complicated and interrelated.

Knee Injuries

Female athletes in jumping and sports where cutting is needed are four to six times more likely to sustain a serious knee injury than their male counterparts in the same sports (Hewett 2000). There are four major hypotheses for why this is so. One anatomical theory is related to the Q-angle. Generally women's wider pelvic structure and lower-extremity alignment results in a greater Q-angle than men's. **Q-angle** is defined as the angle between a line connecting the anterior superior iliac crest and the midpoint of the patella, and a line connecting the midpoint of the patella to the tibia tubercle. Researchers have reported Q-angle to be associated and not associated with increased incidence of knee injury (Hewett 2000; Lathinghouse and Trimble 2000). A second anatomical theory is that women have smaller femoral notch widths relative to the anterior cruciate ligament than men. Evidence for a difference in femoral notch width explaining differences in injury rates between the genders is inconclusive (Hewett 2000). Note that no conditioning program could reduce the knee injury rate in women if the femoral notch width theory were valid.

Neuromuscular differences between the genders have also been proposed to explain the differential knee injury rate between the genders. This theory hypothesizes that differences in muscle recruitment patterns and longer reaction times or longer time to generate maximum force during cutting or landing predisposes women to knee injury. Differences in recruitment patterns, such as female athletes relying more on their quadriceps muscle in response to anterior tibial translation compared to males, have been shown (Huston and Wojtys 1996). Likewise, longer reaction times and longer times to generate maximum force have also been shown in females compared to males (Hewett 2000; Huston and Wojtys 1996). However, other studies have reported no difference between the genders in these measures.

Hormonal variations throughout the menstrual cycle have also been theorized to predispose women to knee injury (Hewett 2000). The hormones estrogen, progesterone, and relaxin have been reported to increase joint laxity, slow muscle relaxation, affect tendon and ligament strength, and decrease motor skills (Hewett 2000). These factors could predispose women to knee injury at various phases within the menstrual cycle.

The greater knee injury rate in women compared to men is likely to be multifactorial. However, physical conditioning programs, including plyometric and weight training, have been shown to drastically reduce the knee injury rate in women (Hewett 2000). For example, high school female athletes who participated in a 6-week conditioning program had a knee injury rate 1.3 times higher than that of a control group of high school male athletes (Hewett et al. 1999), whereas female athletes who did not participate in the conditioning program had a knee injury rate 4.8 times higher than that of the male athletes and 3.6 times higher than that of the female athletes participating in the conditioning program. These studies do not address the mechanism by which

injury rate is reduced. However, they do demonstrate that physical conditioning programs can reduce the knee injury rates in women.

General Needs Analysis

The needs analysis for a woman in a particular sport or activity or for general strength fitness is conducted using the outline presented in chapter 5. What it takes to be successful in a particular sport is generally dictated by the sport or activity and not by the gender of the participant. The training program for the particular sport is based on the requirements for successful participation in that sport and the athlete's individual weaknesses, training history, and injury history. The process of designing a resistance training program for a sport or activity is essentially the same for both genders. The absolute strength differences between the genders make it apparent that one difference between programs for men and for women is the total amount of resistance used for particular exercises.

The higher incidence of knee injuries in women should be considered in the program design. A preseason conditioning program, including lower-body plyometrics and weight training, should be performed to help decrease the knee injury rate. It may also be advisable to continue an in-season conditioning program so that any physiological adaptation resulting in a decreased incidence of knee injury is maintained throughout the season.

For sports or activities that require upper-body strength and power, the needs analysis must take into account women's weaker upper body in absolute as well as relative terms compared with men's. Women's generally smaller upper-body muscle mass may limit their performance in sports requiring upper-body strength or power. The training program for such sports or activities therefore should stress upper-body exercises in an attempt to increase total upper-body strength and power. This can be accomplished in several ways. If the program is relatively low in total training volume, one or two upper-body exercises may be added to the program. Perhaps the most effective way to address this need is to lengthen the preseason weight training program to provide additional time for physiological adaptations.

Women's weaker upper-body musculature can also cause difficulties in the performance of structural exercises, such as power cleans and squats. In these types of exercises women may find it very difficult or impossible for their upper bodies to support the resistances their lower bodies can tolerate. Pratictioners should not tolerate lifters using incorrect technique in order to lift slightly greater resistances. Sacrificing exercise technique can cause injury to lifters. Instead, the program should stress exercises to strengthen the upper-body musculature over time.

Summary

Although women's absolute strength is less than men's, the difference is greatly reduced or nonexistent if expressed relative to fat-free mass or muscle cross-sectional area. Women's lower-body strength relative to fat-free mass is more equivalent to men's than upper-body strength due to a greater relative distribution of women's fat-free mass in the lower body. Women's adaptations to resistance training programs are generally of the same magnitude or even slightly greater than men's for some variables. This emphasizes that, in general, resistance training programs for women do not need to be different from those for men, except that the absolute resistance used by women will be less. Menstrual irregularities may be more prevalent in women performing strenuous resistance activity, as compared to the normal population. However, menstrual irregularities normally cease once strenuous training is reduced or stopped. Resistance training can result in many of the fitness characteristics desired by many women including a fit appearance and increased strength and power for daily life and sport activities.

Key Terms

absolute strength
dysmenorrhea
oligomenorrhea
pennation angle
Q-angle
relative strength
secondary amenorrhea

Selected Readings

Chow, J.W.M. 2000. Role of nitrate oxide and prostaglandins in the bone formation response to mechanical loading. *Exercise and Sport Sciences Reviews* 28: 185-188.

DeCree, C., Vermeulen, A., and Ostyn, M. 1991. Are high-performance young women athletes doomed to become low-performance old wives? A reconsideration of the increased risk of osteoporosis in amenorrheic women. *Journal of Sports Medicine and Physical Fitness* 31: 108-114.

Drinkwater, B.L. 1984. Women and exercise: Physiological aspects. In *Exercise and sport science reviews*, edited by R.L. Terjung, 21-52. Lexington, KY: MAL Callamore Press.

Häkkinen, K., Pakarinen, A., Komi, P.V., Ryushi, T., and Kauhanen, H. 1989. Neuromuscular adaptations and hormone balance in strength athletes, physically active males and females during intensive strength training. In *Proceedings of the XII International Congress of Biomechanics* no. 8, edited by R.J. Gregor, R.F. Zernicke, and W.C. Whiting, 889-894. Champaign, IL: Human Kinetics.

Hewett, T.E. 2000. Neuromuscular and hormonal factors associated with knee injuries in female athletes: strategies for intervention. *Sports Medicine* 29: 313-327.

Kraemer, W.J., Fleck, S.J., Dziados, J.E, Harman, E.A., Marchitelli, L.J., Gordon, S.E., Mello, R., Frykman, P.N., Koziris, L.P., and Triplett, N.T. 1993. Changes in hormonal concentrations following different heavy resistance exercise protocols in women. *Journal of Applied Physiology* 75: 594-604.

Laubach, L.L. 1976. Comparative muscular strength of men and women: A review of the literature. *Aviation, Space and Environmental Medicine* 47: 534-542.

Lebrun, C.M. 1994. The effect of the phase of the menstrual cycle and the birth control pill on athletic performance. *Clinics in Sports Medicine* 13: 419-441.

Mayhew, J.L., and Salm, P.C. 1990. Gender differences in anaerobic power tests. *European Journal of Applied Physiology* 60: 133-138.

Miller, A.E.J., MacDougall, J.D., Tarnopolsky, M.A., and Sale, D.G. 1992. Gender differences in strength and muscle fiber characteristics. *European Journal Applied Physiology* 66: 254-262.

Nattiv, A., Agonstini, R., Drinkwater, B., and Yeager, K.K. 1994. The female athlete triad: The inter-relatedness of disorder eating, amenorrhea, and osteoporosis. *Clinics in Sports Medicine* 13: 405-418.

Nyburgh, K.H., Bachrach, L.K., Lewis, B., Kent, K., and Marcus, R. 1993. Low bone mineral density at axial and appendicular sites in amenorrheic athletes. *Medicine and Science in Sports and Exercise* 25: 1197-1202.

Prior, J.C., Vigna, Y.M., and McKay, D.W. 1992. Reproduction for the athletic female: New understandings of physiology and management. *Sports Medicine* 14: 190-199.

Shephard, R.J. 2000a. Exercise and training in women, part I: Influence of gender on exercise and training responses. *Canadian Journal of Applied Physiology* 25: 19-34.

Shephard, R.J. 2000b. Exercise and training in women, part II: Influence of menstrual cycle and pregnancy on exercise responses. *Canadian Journal of Applied Physiology* 25: 35-54.

Staron, R.S., Karapondo, D.L., Kraemer, W.J., Fry, A.C., Gordon, S.E., Falkel, J.E., Hagerman, F.C., and Hikida, R.S. 1994. Skeletal muscle adaptations during the early phase of heavy-resistance training in men and women. *Journal of Applied Physiology* 76: 1247-1255.

Walberg, J.L., and Johnston, C.S. 1991. Menstrual function and eating behavior in female recreational weight lifters and competitive body builders. *Medicine and Science in Sports and Exercise* 23: 30-36.

Walberg-Rankin, J., Franke, W.D., and Gwazdauskas, F.C. 1992. Response of beta-endorphin and estradiol to resistance exercise in females during energy balance and energy restriction. *International Journal of Sports Medicine* 13: 542-547.

CHAPTER 10

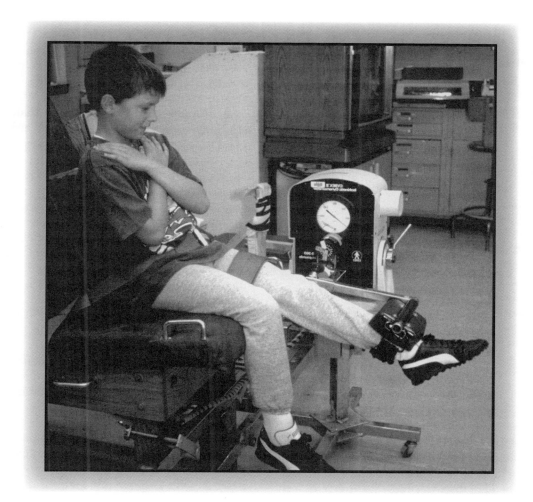

Children and Resistance Training

The popularity of resistance training among prepubescents and adolescents has increased dramatically over the last decade. Acceptance of youth resistance training is becoming universal from qualified professional organizations. The following organizations have all produced statements indicating that youth resistance training is both effective and safe when properly supervised: the American Academy of Pediatrics (1990), the American College of Sports Medicine (1993), the American Orthopedic Society for Sports Medicine

(1988), and the National Strength and Conditioning Association (1996), which is endorsed by the American College of Sports Medicine. Despite these statements, youth resistance training still raises some important issues and concerns. Can resistance training harm a child's skeletal system? What type of weight training program is appropriate for prepubescent males (prior to growth spurt) and females (prior to first menstruation)? What type of weight training program is appropriate for a pubescent, and how should this program differ from a prepubescent program? How can resistance training be safely adapted for youth? All of these questions have more scientifically based answers than previously. However, many misconceptions and misunderstandings still exist about resistance training, its dangers, and how it can be adapted for young people.

The information in this chapter, especially that concerning some types of injuries such as skeletal injuries, stresses the difference between resistance training and the sports of Olympic weightlifting, power lifting, and bodybuilding. Resistance training involves individualized exercise prescription to make a youth stronger and more powerful. Resistance training does not have to involve the use of maximal or near-maximal resistances. On the other hand, Olympic weightlifting and power lifting, by their very nature, involve lifting maximal resistances (1RM weights), and bodybuilding typically involves greater training volumes than would be recommended for young individuals.

As with all physical activity, injuries due to resistance training will occur. However, the risk to children of injury from weightlifting may not be as dramatic as perceived (Hamil 1994). Paradoxically, many of the competitive sporting activities children participate in carry much greater risk of injury than resistance training. The benefits from a properly designed and supervised resistance training program for children outweigh the risks.

Training Adaptations

Statements from the National Strength and Conditioning Association, the American Orthopedic Society for Sports Medicine, and the American Academy of Pediatrics all indicate that children can benefit from participation in a properly prescribed and supervised resistance training program. The major benefits include the following:

- Increased muscular strength, power, and local muscular endurance (i.e., the ability of a muscle or muscles to perform multiple repetitions against a given resistance)
- Decreased injuries in sports and recreational activities
- Improved performance in sports and recreational activities

To confer these benefits, however, resistance training programs for youth must be properly designed, properly progressed, correctly taught, and competently supervised. All of these areas are paramount for safe and effective youth resistance training programs. Although greater understanding has diminished the unrealistic fears about youth and resistance training, further research is needed concerning all aspects of youth resistance training.

Strength Gains

Research clearly demonstrates that resistance training brings about significant increases in strength in children (table 10.1; National Strength and Conditioning Association 1996). Meta-analysis demonstrates that boys younger than 13 years and older than 16 years as well as girls younger than 11 years and older than 14 years (Payne et al. 1997) and boys and girls under the ages of 12 and 13, respectively, demonstrate significant strength gains following resistance training (Falk and Tenenbaum 1996). Strength gains as great as 74% have been shown after 8 weeks of progressive resistance training (Faigenbaum et al. 1993), although more typically gains of 30 to 50% are found after short-term resistance training programs (8 to 20 weeks) in children (National Strength and Conditioning Association 1996). Relative (percent improvement) strength gains in prepubescents are equal to or greater than relative gains shown by adolescents (National Strength and Conditioning Association 1996). Adolescents' absolute strength gains are greater than prepubescents' gains and generally less than adults' gains (National Strength and Conditioning Association 1996). It is important to note that many of the studies report that no injuries occurred in preadolescents or adolescents from performing resistance training.

In the late 1970s many believed that resistance training of prepubescents would result in little if any gains in strength or muscle hypertrophy beyond that caused by normal growth because of their immature hormonal systems (Legwold 1982). Some early studies reporting no strength gains in children due to resistance training seemed to support this immature hormonal system hypothesis (Vrijens 1978). In untrained individuals resting testosterone and growth hormone levels increase from age 11 to 18 in boys, but not in girls (Ramos et al. 1998). Despite this gender difference, a significant positive correlation ($r = 0.64$, boys; $r = 0.46$, girls) in both genders is found between testosterone concentration and absolute muscle strength. This indicates that hormonal changes are in part responsible for increased strength from age 11 to 18 in both genders. Tsolakis and

Table 10.1 Strength Training Studies in Prepubescent Children

Reference	Age or grade	Sex	Training mode	Testing mode	Duration (wks)	Training description	Frequency (per wk)	Control group	Strength increase
Hetherington 1976	Grade 5	M	Isometric	Isometric	6-8	3×3, each 6 s	2-5	Yes	No
Vrijens 1978	10.4	M	Weights	Isometric	8	1×8-12RM	3	No	No
Nielson et al. 1980	7-19	F	Isometric	Isometric	5	24 maximal actions	3	Yes	Yes
Blanksby and Gregory 1981	10-14	M, F	Weights		3	2×8-12RM			
Baumgartner and Wood 1984	Grades 3-6	M, F	Calisthenics	Calisthenics	12	$1 \times$ to fatigue	3	Yes	Yes
Pfeiffer and Francis 1986	8-11	M	Weights	Isokinetic	8	3×10, at 50%, 75%, and 100% 10RM	3	Yes	Yes
Sewall and Micheli 1986	10-11	M, F	Weight machines	Isometric	9	3×10-12, at 50%, 80%, and 100% 10-12RM	3	Yes	Yes
Weltman et al. 1986	6-11	M	Isokinetic	Isokinetic	14	3×30 sec	3	Yes	Yes
Docherty et al. 1987	12.6	M	Isokinetic		4-6	2×20 sec	3	No	No
Rains et al. 1987	8.3	M	Hydraulic concentric	Hydraulic concentric	14	Max number reps in 30 sec	3	Yes	Yes
Sailors and Berg 1987	12.6	M	Free weights	Free weights	8	3×5, at 65%, 80%, and 100% 5RM	3	Yes	Yes
Siegal, Camaione, and Manfredi, 1989	8.4	M, F	Weights, calisthenics	Isometric, calisthenics	12	30-45 sec exercise, 15 rest	3	Yes	Yes
Ramsay et al. 1990	9-11	M	Free weights, machines	Weights, isokinetic, isometric	20	3×10-12RM, $1 \times$ to fatigue	3	Yes	Yes
Fukunaga, Funato, and Ikegawa 1992	Grades 1, 3, 5	M,F	Isometric	Isometric, isokinetic	12	3×10 sec max isometric action, 2 times/day	3	Yes	Yes
Faigenbaum et al. 1993	10.8	M, F	Weights	Weights	8	3×10-15	2	Yes	Yes
Ozmun, Mikesky, and Surburg 1994	9.8-11.6	M, F	Free weights	Free weights, isokinetic	8	3×7-10RM	3	Yes	Yes
Falk and Mor 1996	6-8	M	Calisthenics and body-weight exercises	Body-weight exercises	12	3×1-15	2	Yes	Yes
Faigenbaum et al. 1996	7-12	M, F	DCER machines	DCER machines	8	4 wks 1×10 and 2×6; 4 wks 3×6	2	Yes	Yes
Faigenbaum et al. 2001	8.1	M, F	DCER machines	DCER machines	8	1×6-8RM	2	Yes	No
Faigenbaum et al. 2001	8.1	M, F	DCER machines	DCER machines	8	1×13-15RM	2	Yes	Yes

DCER = dynamic constant external resistance.

Adapted, by permission, from A. Faigenbaum, 1993, "Strength training: A guide for teachers and coaches," *National Strength and Conditioning Association Journal* 15(5): 20-29.

colleagues (2000) reported that resting blood concentrations of hormones (testosterone, growth hormone) indicative of a more anabolic environment can occur due to resistance training in prepubertal boys (11 to 13 years) and pubertal boys (14 to 16 years). Thus, although more research is definitely needed, changes in resting hormonal concentrations may in part explain increased strength due to resistance training in prepubertal and pubertal individuals.

Training history may also play a part in hormonal changes and therefore strength hypertrophy increases over time in young individuals. Male Olympic weightlifters 14 to 17 years old with less than 2 years of training experience did not show an increase in serum testosterone after a training session. However, lifters with more than 2 years of training experience did show an increase in serum testosterone after a training session (Kraemer et al. 1992), indicating that past training experience affects the response to training.

Similar to women, prepubescent children do not show an increase in serum testosterone concentration after an exercise bout (see figure 10.1). Yet both women and prepubescent children clearly can experience strength increases from resistance training. Neural factors and other hormonal changes are in part responsible for increased strength and hypertrophy in women (see chapter

9) and may also play a role in strength increases in prepubescent boys and girls. Although the exact mechanisms resulting in strength increases in prepubescent and pubescent individuals are not completely elucidated, resistance training clearly increases strength in both boys and girls.

Muscle Hypertrophy

Weight training in adults brings about strength increases in part as a result of neural adaptations and hypertrophy. However, the vast majority of evidence indicates that strength gains in prepubescents are related much more to neural mechanisms than to hypertrophy (Blimkie 1993; National Strength and Conditioning Association 1996). Lack of muscle hypertrophy in prepubescent studies less than 8 weeks in length is not surprising. However, lack of muscle hypertrophy in prepubescent studies greater than 8 weeks in length (Blimkie 1993) and up to 20 weeks in length (Ramsay et al. 1990) is surprising because hypertrophy is typically found in adults over this time frame (Blimkie 1993). Lack of significant hypertrophy accompanied by significant increases in strength indicates that neural adaptations are responsible for the majority of strength gains in prepubescents and that hypertrophy is more difficult to achieve in children (especially prepubescents) than in adults.

Enhanced growth of muscle in response to resistance training may begin after adolescence, when male and female adult hormonal profiles start to emerge (Kraemer and Fleck 1993). Starting at puberty in males, the influence of testosterone on muscle size and strength is dramatic without any training. After puberty, resistance training has the ability to enhance muscular hypertrophy beyond normal growth. Limited data does indicate, however, that significant hypertrophy can occur in children. In a study by Fukunaga, Funato, and Ikegawa (1992), first-, third-, and fifth-grade students trained using isometric contractions twice a day, 3 days a week for 12 weeks. After the resistance training program, the authors observed a significant increase in muscle and bone cross-sectional area in the training group. A control group demonstrated only an increase in fat cross-sectional area.

Figure 10.2 presents a group of physiological variables that ultimately contribute to the ability to exhibit strength. Dramatic progress in each of the variables is observed during adolescence, indicating that physiological age will affect the magnitude of strength increases from resistance training in prepubescents and adolescents.

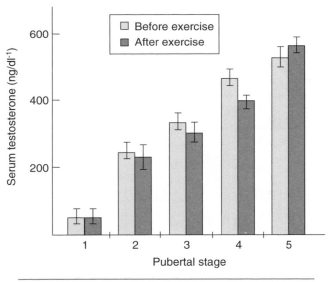

Figure 10.1 Serum testosterone levels before and after an exercise bout in pubescent children. Pubertal stages 1 through 5 refer to the maturity of the individual, with 1 being immature and 5 being fully mature.

Adapted, by permission, from T.D. Fahey et al., 1989, "Pubertal stage difference in hormonal and hematological responses to maximal exercise in males," *Journal of Applied Physiology* 46: 825.

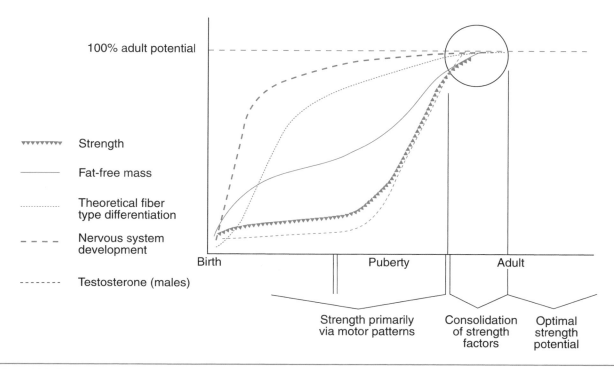

Figure 10.2 Theoretical model of strength development factors in males.

Adapted, by permission, from W.J. Kraemer et al., 1993, "Resistance training and youth," *Pediatric Exercise Science* 1(4): 336-350.

Although increases in muscle hypertrophy may not occur in young children, many other adaptations in the muscle, nerve, and connective tissue of children may still be occurring. Such adaptations include changes in muscle protein (i.e., myosin isoforms), recruitment patterns, and connective tissue, all of which could contribute to improved strength, sport performance, and injury prevention.

Younger boys sometimes envy the better-defined, larger muscles of older boys (16- to 17-year-olds) and believe that merely by lifting weights they can have the muscle size and physique they desire in a few months. Since increases in muscle mass beyond normal growth are not possible in younger children, however, muscle hypertrophy should not be a goal of their training programs. Only after a child has entered adolescence do muscle size gains become a realistic training goal. However, because of differences in maturation rates among children, care must be taken to evaluate this goal individually, especially for girls and boys 14 to 15 years of age.

Bone Development

Resistance training can have a favorable effect on bone mineral density in prepubescents and adolescents of both sexes (National Strength and Conditioning Association 1996; Naughton et al. 2000). However, not all studies report an effect on bone mineral density in children. Twisk (2001) hypothesized that mechanical loading of bone has a threshold that must be met to have a positive effect on factors related to bone health, such as bone mineral density. Thus, studies that report no effect on bone mineral density due to resistance training may not have reached the threshold of mechanical loading needed to affect bone mineral density. The mechanical loading caused by resistance training is a result of exercise choice, sets, repetitions per set, resistance used, and training duration. Unfortunately, the minimal mechanical loading necessary to bring about changes in bone health is not known.

Increased bone density from resistance training may be one of the primary mediating factors involved in empirical observations that resistance training prevents injury in young athletes (Hejna et al. 1982). Additionally, although data is limited, the prepubertal trainee may be in the best position to increase bone mineral density and periosteal expansion of cortical bone through physical activity (Bass 2000; Khan et al. 2000). This is an important consideration for long-term bone health, as studies of retired athletes and detraining indicate that athletes who increase bone mineral density in adolescence may suffer less bone loss in later years despite reduced physical activity (Khan et al. 2000). Thus, any increase in bone mineral density above normal growth during the prepubertal and adolescent years may help prevent osteoporosis later in life.

Detraining

Examination of detraining in adolescents and prepubescents is complicated by the fact that natural growth processes result in increased strength even without resistance training. Moreover, few studies have examined detraining in children. However, as in adults, detraining in children results in strength loss so that strength regresses toward untrained control values (National Strength and Conditioning Association 1996). For example, complete detraining (performance of no resistance training) for 8 weeks in children who previously completed 20 weeks of weight training results in strength loss such that after the detraining period no significant strength differences between the previously weight-trained children and untrained children exist (Blimkie 1993). Differences in how quickly strength loss occurs with complete detraining may vary slightly by muscle group (Faigenbaum et al. 1996). During an 8-week detraining period children (mean age 10.8 years) showed a decrease of 28% in leg-extension strength and 19% in bench press strength. Leg-extension strength after the detraining period was not significantly different from that of a control group of children who performed no weight training, whereas bench press strength was still significantly greater than the control group.

The training frequency necessary to maintain strength gains during a short-term reduced-volume detraining period appears to be similar between prepubescents and adults (DeRenne et al. 1996). A training frequency of one session per week was just as effective as two sessions per week in maintaining previously made strength gains in prepubescents (mean age 13.25 years) during 12 weeks of a reduced-volume detraining period. Both training frequencies showed no significant decrease in strength, with no significant difference between the two training frequencies shown. This indicates that one session per week is sufficient to maintain strength gains during a short-term detraining period. Although information is limited, the response of children to complete detraining and reduced-volume detraining appears to be similar to that of adults.

Interestingly, the advantage of resistance training in children is only maintained with continuous training. With such rapid growth during youth, cessation of training over a three-month period can equalize strength levels between a training group and controls (Blimkie 1992, 1993). Thus, any advantage is only maintained with continued training two to three days per week.

Concerns About Injury

Resistance training appears to help prevent injuries in adults. Evidence also suggests that resistance training helps prevent injuries in adolescent athletes (Hejna et al. 1982; National Strength and Conditioning Association 1996), and that stronger athletes may be less susceptible to certain types of injury (Moskwa and Nicholas 1989). For example, high school male and female athletes who performed resistance training had an injury rate of 26% compared to 72% in athletes who did not perform resistance training (Hejna et al. 1982). Additionally, the rehabilitation time required for those who were injured was only 2 days for the athletes performing resistance training compared to 4.8 days for athletes who did not perform resistance training. Thus, one goal of a resistance training program for child athletes should be to prepare them physically for their sport or activity.

Despite the possible positive effects of resistance training on injury prevention, the possibility of acute and chronic injuries to children is a valid concern (Dalton 1992; Markiewitz and Andrish 1992; Naughton et al. 2000). A resistance training program for children therefore should not focus primarily on lifting maximal or near-maximal resistances. Children's resistance training programs should focus on proper exercise technique because most injuries in resistance exercise are related to improper technique. In fact, many weight training injuries in children are related to poorly designed equipment, equipment that does not fit children, use of excessive resistance, free access to the equipment, or lack of qualified adult supervision.

Like adults, children need time to adapt to the stress of resistance training; thus, training progression should be gradual. Children who find training difficult or do not enjoy resistance training at a particular age should not be forced to participate. Interest, growth, physical maturity, psychological maturity, and understanding all influence children's views of exercise training and proper safety precautions. All of these factors need to be considered on an individual basis to ensure a safe and effective resistance training program.

Acute Injuries

Acute injury refers to a single trauma that causes an injury. Acute injuries to the skeletal system, such as growth cartilage damage or bone fractures, are rarely caused by weight training.

Muscle Strains and Sprains

The most common acute injuries in prepubescent weight trainees, as in adults, are muscle strains and sprains (National Strength and Conditioning Association 1996). Strains and sprains can be the result of not warming up properly before a training session. Trainees should perform several sets of exercise before beginning the actual training sets of a workout. Another common cause of muscle strain or sprain is attempting to lift too much weight for a given number of repetitions. Children should understand that the suggested number of repetitions is merely a guideline, and that they can perform more or less repetitions and this will allow them to learn what resistances produce what repetition number. The incidence of this type of injury, as with all injury types, can be reduced by taking proper safety precautions.

Growth Cartilage Damage

In addition to the possibility of the types of injury that occur in adults, the prepubescent child is subject to possible growth cartilage injury. **Growth cartilage** is located at three sites: the **epiphyseal plate,** or growth plate; the **epiphysis,** or joint surface; and the **apophyseal** insertion, or tendon insertion (see figure 10.3). The long bones of the body grow in length from the epiphyseal plates located at each end of the long bones. Normally, because of hormonal changes, the epiphyseal plates ossify after puberty. Once ossified, growth of long bones, and therefore increased height, is no longer possible. Cartilage of the epiphyseal plate may be at its weakest during the most intensive phases of growth in adolescence (Collins and Evarts 1971) and is weaker than bone (Bright, Burstein, and Elmore 1974). The cartilage of the epiphysis acts as a shock absorber between the bones that form a joint. Damage to this cartilage may lead to a rough articular surface and subsequent pain during joint movement. The growth cartilage at apophyseal insertions of major tendons ensures a solid connection between the tendon and bone. Damage to apophyseal insertions may cause pain and also increase the chance of separation between the tendon and bone, result-

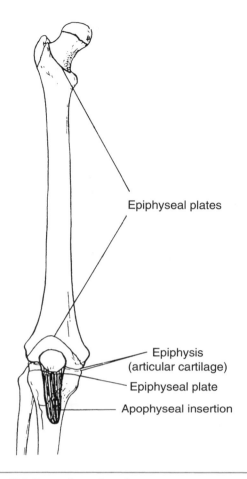

Figure 10.3 Types of growth cartilage.

ing in an avulsion fracture. All three growth cartilage sites are more susceptible to injury during the adolescent growth spurt because of other factors as well, such as increased muscle tightness across joints.

Epiphyseal Plate Fractures

Several researchers have reported cases of epiphyseal plate fractures in adolescent weight trainees (Grumbs et al. 1982; Jenkins and Mintowt-Czyz 1986; Rowe 1979). The epiphyseal plate is prone to fractures in children because it is not yet ossified and is weaker than bone (Bright, Burstein, and Elmore 1974). The majority of epiphyseal plate fracture cases involve overhead lifts, such as the overhead press and jerk, with near-maximal resistances. These cases demonstrate the need for two precautions for prepubescent and adolescent programs: First, maximal or near-maximal lifts (1RM) should be discouraged, especially in unsupervised settings. Second, because improper form is a contributing factor to many injuries, proper technique in all exercises, especially in overhead lifts, should be emphasized to young resistance trainees.

Fractures

Because the metaphysis or shaft of the long bones is more elastic in children and adolescents than in adults, fractures of the shaft occur more readily in children and adolescents (Naughton et al. 2000). Peak fracture incidence in boys occurs between the ages of 12 and 14 and precedes the age of peak height increase, or growth spurt (Blimkie 1993). The increased fracture rate appears to be caused by a lag in cortical bone thickness and mineralization in relation to linear growth (Blimkie 1993). Therefore, controlling the resistance used during weight training by boys between the ages of 12 and 14 may be important. The same line of reasoning may apply to girls between the ages of 10 and 13.

Lumbar Back Problems

Acute trauma can cause lumbar back problems in adults as well as prepubescents and adolescents. In resistance training, such problems may be caused by lifting maximal or near-maximal resistances or attempting to perform too many repetitions with a given resistance. In many cases back pain is associated with improper form, especially in the squat or deadlift exercises. When performing these exercises, as well as other exercises, trainees should use proper exercise technique, which involves maintaining as upright a position as possible to minimize the stress on the low back.

Chronic Injuries

The terms *chronic injury* and *overuse injury* refer to injury caused by repeated microtraumas. Shinsplints and stress fractures are common examples of these injuries. Using improper exercise technique over long periods of time can result in overuse injuries (e.g., improper bench press technique can cause shoulder problems and pain).

Growth Cartilage

Repeated physical stress can cause damage to all three growth cartilage sites. As an example, repeated mechanical stresses to the shoulder and elbow from baseball pitching results in inflammation and irritated ossification centers in the elbow and epiphyseal plate of the humerus. This causes pain with shoulder and elbow movement and is a probable cause of shoulder and elbow pain in prepubescent and adolescent baseball pitchers (Barnett 1985; Lyman et al. 2001).

The growth cartilage on the articular surface of prepubescent joints, especially at the ankle, knee, and elbow, may be more prone to injury than that of adult joints. Repeated microtrauma from pitching appears to be responsible in part for elbow and shoulder pain in young (9- to 12-year-old) pitchers (Lyman et al. 2001) and ankle pain in young runners (Conale and Belding 1980). In many cases joint pain in adolescents and prepubescents is caused by osteochondritis (inflammation of growth cartilage) or osteochondritis dissecans (separation of a portion of the joint surface from the bone). Tiny avulsions of the growth cartilage at the site of the patellar tendon insertion onto bone may be related to the pain associated with Osgood-Schlatter disease (Micheli 1983). Although damage to growth cartilage is a concern, incidences of this type of injury as a result of weight training appear to be very rare (Blimkie 1993; National Strength and Conditioning Association 1996).

Low Back Problems

As in adults, low back problems may be one of the most common types of injury in adolescents and prepubescents performing weight training. Low back problems constituted 50% of the total number of injuries reported in adolescent power lifters who presumably trained with maximal or near-maximal resistances (Brady, Cahill, and Bodnar 1982). Although this report involved adolescents, the potential for similar injury in prepubescents needs to be recognized. Adolescents may be at a greater risk than adults for spondylitis (inflammation of one or more vertebrae) and stress related pain. The incidence of this abnormality in adolescents is 47% percent, whereas in adults it is only 5% (Micheli and Wood 1995).

Lordosis is an anterior bending of the spine, usually accompanied by flexion of the pelvis. Many children during the growth spurt have a tendency to develop lordosis of the lumbar spine. Several factors contribute to lordosis, including enhanced growth in the anterior portion of the vetebral bodies and tight hamstrings that cause the hips to assume a flexed position (Micheli 1983). Lordosis may contribute to low back pain. However, low back soft-tissue injuries are also often associated with low back pain in adolescents (Blimkie 1993).

Back pain from resistance training can be minimized by performing exercises that strengthen the abdominal and low back musculature. Strengthening these areas will help maintain proper exercise technique, thus reducing the stress on the low back. Light to moderate resistances that allow a performance of at least 10 repetitions can be helpful in reducing the incidence of low back pain.

Programs for Children

The development of a prepubescent or adolescent resistance training program should follow the same steps as that of an adult program. However, the following questions also need to be considered before a child begins a resistance training program:

- Is the child psychologically and physically ready to participate in a resistance exercise training program?
- What type of resistance training program should the child follow?
- Does the child understand the proper lifting techniques for each exercise in the program?
- Do spotters understand the safety spotting techniques for each exercise in the program?
- Does the child understand the safety concerns for each piece of equipment used in the program?
- Does the resistance training equipment fit the child properly?
- Does the child's exercise training program include aerobic and flexibility training to address total fitness needs?
- Does the child participate in other sports or activities in addition to resistance training?

These last two questions need to be considered in the context of the total training stress to which the child is exposed. For example, in young baseball pitchers weight training during the season is associated with elbow but not shoulder pain (Lyman et al. 2001). However, the total number of pitches thrown and pitching arm fatigue are also associated with elbow and shoulder pain. These results do not necessarily indicate that young pitchers should not perform weight training during the season, but that the total training stress placed on children may be associated with some types of injuries.

A well-organized and well-supervised basic training program for children can be as short as 20 minutes per training session. During the initial training period a frequency of two sessions per week in children (8 to 10.8 years old) does bring about significant strength gains and changes in body composition (Faigenbaum et al. 1993, 1999). Also, during the initial training period higher numbers of repetitions (13 to 15) per set may produce greater gains in strength and local muscular endurance than lower numbers (6 to 8) of repetitions per set (Faigenbaum et al. 1999, 2001). Like adults, children can realize significant changes in strength and body composition from low-volume single-set programs. Thus, a program for children may be composed initially of one set of approximately 13 to 15 repetitions per set with at least one exercise for all the major muscle groups of the body. As a child gets older, more advanced programs that resemble adult programs can be introduced gradually. However, the NSCA recommends that the heaviest resistance lifted be controlled by having preadolescents not lift a resistance heavier than a 5 to 6RM weight (National Strength and Conditioning Association 1996).

Table 10.2 depicts a program progression from age 5 to 18. The resistance training program should be conducted in an atmosphere conducive to both the child's safety and enjoyment. The training environment should reflect the proper psychological mind set with any posters, goal charts, and pictures reflecting the proper goals and expectations of a youth resistance training program.

Exercise Tolerance

The importance of the child's ability to tolerate the exercise stress cannot be overemphasized. For individualized exercise prescription, proper supervision, and program monitoring to work optimally, parents, teachers, and coaches need to communicate with the prepubescents and adolescents performing the program. Adults should encourage discussion and feedback of the children's concerns and fears. Most important, adults must take steps to address the concerns expressed by the children. Trainers need to use common sense in providing exercise variation, active recovery periods, and total rest from training in individualized resistance training programs for children. They must also be careful not to fall into the trap that more training is always better.

The general guidelines for program design offered in this chapter are only suggestions. No single optimal program exists. Prepubescents

Table 10.2 Basic Guidelines for Resistance Exercise Progression for Children

Age (yr)	Considerations
5-7	Introduce child to basic exercises with little or no resistance; develop the concept of a training session; teach exercise techniques; progress from body-weight calisthenics, partner exercises, and lightly resisted exercises; keep volume low.
8-10	Gradually increase the number of exercises; practice exercise technique for all lifts; start gradual progress of loading of exercises; keep exercises simple; increase volume slowly; carefully monitor tolerance to exercise stress.
11-13	Teach all basic exercise techniques; continue progressive loading of each exercise; emphasize exercise technique; introduce more advanced exercises with little or no resistance.
14-15	Progress to more advanced resistance exercise programs; add sport-specific components; emphasize exercise techniques; increase volume gradually.
16 or older	Entry level into adult programs after all background experience has been gained.

If a child at a particular age level has no previous weight training experience, progression must start at previous levels and move to more advanced levels as exercise tolerance, exercise technique, and understanding permit.

Adapted, by permission, from W.J. Kraemer and S.J. Fleck, 1993, *Strength training for young athletes* (Champaign, IL: Human Kinetics Publishers), p. 5.

and adolescents should start with a program that is individually tolerable, but becomes more aggressive as they grow older. Dramatic changes in the tolerance to resistance training programs can reflect the increased maturity of the individual. Trainers should be careful, however, not to overestimate the child's ability to tolerate the total amount of physical activity being performed, which may include resistance training, aerobic training, and a sport program. It is better to start the child out conservatively than to overestimate exercise tolerance and reduce his or her enjoyment of participation. Using the proper resistance training principles, the designer can create a program that reflects the child's developmental stage. All adults associated with a program must remember that they are not the ones for whom the program is developed; their job is to provide a positive environment that protects and serves the children participating. Children, for their part, should be free to participate or not participate in any exercise or sport program.

Needs Analysis

The needs of each child, like those of adults, are unique. Prepubescents and adolescents need to develop their total health and fitness including cardiovascular fitness, flexibility, body composition changes, and motor skills as well as strength. A resistance training program should not be so time consuming as to ignore these other aspects of total fitness or interfere with a child's play time. Prepubescents as well as many adolescents should not be expected to perform an adult training program. To ensure compliance with the training program, adults should allow children to set their own goals and monitor their physical and psychological tolerance of the program. Children's comments such as, "I don't want to do this," "This program is too hard," "Some of these exercises are hurting me," "I am just too tired after a workout," or "What other exercises can I learn?" may indicate that the program needs to be evaluated and appropriate alterations made.

Most of the dangers of resistance training are related to inappropriate exercise demands being placed on the prepubescent or adolescent. Although general guidelines can be offered and should be followed, sensitivity to the special needs that arise with each individual is necessary. The program must be designed for each child's needs, and proper exercise techniques and safety considerations must be employed. A properly designed and supervised resistance training program provides many positive physical and psychological benefits for the child. Perhaps the most important outcome is the behavioral development of an active lifestyle in the prepubescent or adolescent. Good exercise behaviors contribute to better health and well-being over a lifetime.

With the increasing popularity of youth sports, from football and gymnastics to soccer and T-ball, children need better physical preparation to prevent sport-related injuries. The American College of Sports Medicine (1993) estimated that over 50% of the overuse injuries diagnosed in adolescents are preventable. A total fitness training program including resistance training to prepare the individual for the stresses of sport competition along with preparticipation screening and regular visits to sports medicine health professionals has great potential to reduce the number of athletic and overuse injuries.

Another consideration for all children is upper-body strength. The recent declines in upper-body strength in boys and girls (Hass, Feigenbaum, and Franklin 2001) represents a significant weakness in prepubescent and adolescent fitness profiles. Upper-body strength limits many sport-specific tasks even at the recreational level. The general lack of upper-body strength in many prepubescent and pubescent children indicates the need for exercises for the upper body in resistance training programs for these groups.

After considering the general needs discussed previously, the needs analysis is further developed by determining the major goals of the program. Some common goals for a resistance training program include the following:

- Increased strength and power of specific muscle groups
- Increased local muscular endurance of specific muscle groups
- Increased motor performance (e.g., increased ability to jump, run, or throw)
- Increased total body weight (age dependent)
- Increased muscle hypertrophy (age dependent)
- Decreased body fat

Developmental Differences

Preadolescents and adolescents differ from each other physically and psychologically. Some children are tall for their chronological age and others are short, some are fast sprinters and others are slow, and some become upset when they make a poor play in a game while others seem unconcerned. Physical and psychological differences are the result of different genetic potentials and growth rates. Adults must realize that children are not miniature adults. Furthermore, all preadolescents and adolescents of the same chronologi-

cal age are not equal physically or emotionally. Understanding some of the basic principles of growth and development will help adults have more realistic expectations of children. This understanding will also help when developing goals and exercise progressions for resistance training programs. Every exercise program must manage the physical and psychological level of each individual child.

There are many aspects of children's growth and development besides height. These include fitness gains, genetic potential, nutrition, and sleep patterns. Also included in discussions of children's development is maturation, which has been defined as progress toward adulthood. Maturation of children involves several areas, including the following:

- Physical size
- Bone maturity
- Reproductive maturity
- Psychological maturity

Each of these areas can be evaluated clinically, generally by the family physician. Physicians recognize that each individual has a chronological age as well as a physiological age for each of the areas listed. Since physiological age determines the functional capabilities and performance for the individual, it is the most important factor to consider when developing a resistance training program.

Resistance training programs for preadolescent and adolescent boys and girls are generally quite similar. However, some developmental differences should be considered when developing goals for boys and girls. In prepubescent males the velocity of strength gain appears to peak following peak height velocity or the growth spurt (Naughton et al. 2000), whereas many girls peak in strength before or during peak height velocity. Whatever the developmental stage at which peak strength gain occurs, it is consistently greater in boys than in girls.

Individualized Resistance Training Programs

The design of the total conditioning program as well as of the resistance program should incorporate the following elements to address the needs of all children:

- Conditioning of all fitness components (aerobic, flexibility, strength)
- Generally balanced choice of exercises for upper- and lower-body development (although as the child ages, some sport-specific exercises may be added)
- Balanced choice of exercises for muscles on both sides of each joint (exercises for both agonists and antagonists)
- Incorporation of body-part (single-joint) as well as structural (multijoint) exercises

After the needs analysis, but before beginning a resistance training program, children, like adults, should be examined by a physician to ensure awareness of any physical problems that need to be considered in the program's design. For example, if a child has Osgood-Schatter disease, exercises involving extreme bending of the knees may be contraindicated. All children should begin with the basic resistance training program that exercises all of the major muscle groups of the body and the agonists and antagonists at all major joints. A warm-up, a cool-down, and flexibility exercises should be a part of each session. Sport-specific exercises and exercises based on individual need can be added to the program after the child has learned basic lifting techniques and demonstrates the emotional maturity to perform advanced exercises safely. Individualizing the program requires considering the physical strengths and weaknesses as well as the goals of each individual. Sport performance is not dependent on the child's gender, but on the strength and power of particular muscle groups. Therefore, sport-specific programs for boys and girls generally include the same exercises.

Sample Programs

Two sample programs are outlined in this section. One involves the use of no weight training equipment, and the second requires resistance training equipment in the form of free weights or typical weight training machines. Both programs can be modified to provide exercise variation and increases or decreases in the difficulty of an exercise, and to use existing equipment. The programs are meant to be performed using the existing resistance training guidelines for children: two to three training sessions per week, a minimum of one set of each exercise, 6 to 15 repetitions per set, and a variety of upper- and lower-body exercises to train all the major muscle groups (National Strength and Conditioning Association 1996).

Program Using Little Equipment

This program uses either the child's body weight, self-resistance using one muscle group against another muscle group, resistance provided by another child, or another child's body weight as resistance (see table 10.3). This program can be performed as a circuit, moving from one exercise to the next, or in a set-repetition manner, performing all three sets of an exercise with a rest between sets before moving on to the next exercise. The resistance used in all of the exercises can be increased or decreased in some manner. For example, the difficulty of push-ups can be decreased by doing knee push-ups and increased by placing the feet on a chair. The self-resistance and partner-resisted exercises are meant to be performed in a dynamic manner with each concentric and eccentric repetition phase taking approximately 6 seconds to complete for a total of 12 seconds per repetition. Exercises can also be modified. For example, self-resisted arm curls could be replaced by partner-resisted arm curls using a towel. The goal is to provide some form of resistance training for all of the major muscle groups using little or no equipment.

Program Using Equipment

This program can be performed with a variety of either free weights or typical weight training machine exercises using either a circuit or a set-repetition protocol (see table 10.4). Several weight training companies manufacture resistance training machines specifically designed to fit children to ensure proper exercise technique. If adult-size machines are used, trainers should make sure that each individual child is properly fitted to the machine to ensure proper exercise technique. Initially, the resistance used for each exercise should be such that the trainee can perform the minimum recommended number of repetitions with correct technique. When the maximum recommended number of repetitions can be performed, the resistance is increased so that the trainee can perform the minimum number of repetitions per set. Children should perform all exercises in a controlled manner to prevent injury, learn proper exercise technique, and prevent damage to equipment. Trainers should continually stress the importance of correct exercise and spotting techniques for all exercises.

Table 10.3 Resistance Training Program for Children Using Body Weight and Self-Resistance

Exercise	Sets and repetitions
Push-ups	1-3 × 10-20
Bent-leg sit-ups	1-3 × 15-20
Parallel squats	1-3 × 10-20
Self-resistance arm curls using opposite arm as resistance	1-3 × 10 actions 6-s in duration
Toe raises	1-3 × 20-30
Partner-resisted lateral arm raises	1-10 reps of 12-s duration
Lying-back extensions	1-3 × 10-15

Table 10.4 Resistance Training Program for Children Using Equipment

Exercise	Sets and repetitions
Squat or leg press	1-3 × 10-15
Bench press	1-3 × 10-15
Knee curl	1-3 × 10-15
Arm curl	1-3 × 10-15
Knee extension	1-3 × 10-15
Overhead press	1-3 × 10-15
Crunches	1-3 × 15-20
Back extension	1-3 × 10-15

Copying Elite Athlete Programs

Prepubescents or pubescents should not perform programs designed for collegiate or professional athletes. The ability of older athletes to improve strength and power using these programs is in part a result of their years of resistance training experience. Often these programs involve lifting very heavy resistances (1-3RM), which, as previously discussed, may result in injury to prepubescents. Lifting such heavy resistance is also contrary to the guidelines established for children. Forcing prepubescents or pubescents to perform programs designed for mature, gifted athletes can overstress them and may result in injury.

Program Periodization

Periodization, which is discussed in more detail in chapter 7, is a popular way of varying the training volume and intensity of workouts in adult athletes and fitness enthusiasts. Periodization and its effects on prepubescents and adolescents have received little study. Stone, O'Bryant, and Garhammer (1981) demonstrated that the use of the traditional strength and power periodization model with a high school football team led to greater gains in 1RM strength and vertical jumping ability than nonperiodized resistance training. This model, however, requires trainees to perform with near-maximal and maximal resistances and therefore may not be applicable for prepubescents. Variation in training volume and intensity can, however, be accomplished within the guidelines of a program for prepubescent individuals (see table 10.5). Training variation leads to greater and faster gains in strength and power and local muscular endurance and helps keep the program interesting to the trainee.

Resistance training for prepubescents can be varied in several ways, including any or all of the following:

- Increasing the resistance for a particular RM
- Varying the RM used (6-20RM)
- Varying the number of sets per exercise (one to three)
- Varying the exercises for the same muscle groups

Table 10.5 Strength and Power Periodization Model for Prepubescents

Training phase	Repetitions (RM range)	Sets
Base	1-3	10-15
Strength	1-3	6-10
Power	2-3	6-8
Peaking	1-2	6-8
Active rest	Physical activity (not necessarily resistance training)	

Adapted, by permission, from W.J. Kraemer and S. J. Fleck, 1993, *Strength training for young athletes* (Champaign, IL: Human Kinetics), 40.

Program Philosophy

Formal programs, such as those in schools or health clubs, should express their philosophies openly and clearly in the environment. Signs, wall charts, and handouts can reflect a positive attitude about weight training to prepubescents and adolescents. This is especially important when both adults and children are training in the same facility. The program philosophy can be promoted using the following methods:

1. Posting of age-related instructions for children next to the adult instructions. This can include both program and exercise instructions.

2. Use of posters and pictures that depict prepubescents and adolescents of both genders using proper resistance training techniques.

3. Use of charts, contests, and awards to promote the principles that prepubescents and adolescents need to concentrate on. This can include consistency charts and awards, exercise technique contests and awards, "total conditioning and fitness" awards focusing on progress in other aspects of total fitness (e.g., cardiovascular endurance, flexibility), fitness preparation awards prior to sports seasons, and in-season program awards during sports seasons.

The environment, exercise programs, and awards should all reflect the program philosophy. Because prepubescents and adolescents learn and retain information in different ways than adults, the weight training program should communicate the correct expectations and philosophy in all forms of communication, including oral, written, audio, video, and pictorial media. All forms of communication need to be clear and appropriate for prepubescents and adolescents so that intimidation, confusion, or misunderstanding do not occur in any aspect of the program.

Equipment Modification and Organizational Difficulties

Children require more individualized help than do adults. Moreover, trainers often encounter organizational problems with children that are not present with adults. For example, exercise stations may need pads or blocks to modify the equipment to fit the smaller bodies of children, or equipment such as dumbbells of the correct weights may be needed to provide an alternate exercise when a machine does not fit or cannot provide the proper resistance for some children in a group. Trainers must also be aware of the fact that equipment may need to be modified as the child grows. Some trainers check equipment for proper fit as frequently as every month, especially during the growth spurt of the child.

The organizational problems created by having to accommodate children need not be difficult to solve. Two solutions are to mark needed modifications on each child's workout card to help adults keep track, or to teach children to make their own equipment modifications. However, adults need to carefully check that equipment modifications are done properly, and as growth occurs these modifications need to be modified to refit size changes. Although effective, these solutions may be impractical with a large group of children. With timed workouts (specific exercise periods and rest periods), the time needed for equipment modifications must be considered, especially when a group of children are training and modifications are needed on an individual basis.

Trainers sometimes find it helpful to perform the training session to find out how long a particular equipment modification takes. They may then choose to alter rest periods to account for the time needed for equipment modifications. Although they may prefer 1-minute rest periods in a particular training session, organizational problems such as equipment modification may make this impossible. In such cases, the safety of the children and correct exercise technique are the priority rather than maintaining the desired rest period. Typically, exercise machines made for adults require more modifications than free weight exercises. Organizational problems must be resolved without sacrificing safety or correct exercise technique, and without making the training session ineffective.

The most important equipment consideration when training children is whether the resistance training equipment fits each child properly. With free weights, body-weight exercises, or partner-resisted exercises, fit is typically not a concern. With resistance training weight machines, however, fit can be critical. Although several companies now manufacture machines specifically designed for children, most resistance training machines are designed to fit adults. Most prepubescents lack the height and arm and leg length to properly fit many resistance training machines. If the machine does not fit the child properly, correct technique and full exercise range of motion are impossible. A critical problem of an ill-fitting machine is the chance that a body part may slip off its point contact, such as a foot or arm pad, resulting in injury.

Another common problem of poor fit is that the bench for machine or free weight exercise is too wide to allow free movement of the shoulder during the exercise. When children perform exercises with inappropriate technique because of ill-fitting equipment, their joints and musculature can become stressed, resulting in an injury.

Children should not use equipment that cannot be safely adapted to fit properly. Simple alterations of some machines, such as additional seat pads, can allow a trainee to use the machine safely. However, just adjusting the seat is often not enough. Although the seat adjustment may be appropriate, adjustments may also be needed to allow proper positioning of the arms or legs on the contact points of the machine. In addition, raising the seat height may make it impossible for the child's feet to reach the floor, compromising balance. Placing blocks under the feet can help in such cases.

Altering a piece of equipment to fit one child does not guarantee that the equipment will fit another child. Proper fit must be checked before the equipment is used by each child. Care must be taken to ensure that additional padding or blocks do not slide during the exercise, which could result in injury. Sliding can be avoided in some alterations by attaching nonskid mats to the top and bottom of blocks and the backs of additional pads. The safety of the lifter must always be the top priority when making any equipment adjustments.

Appropriate Resistance Increases

Another potential problem when prepubescents use many resistance machines is that the resistance increments are too large to allow smooth resistance progression as the child becomes stronger. Many machines' weight stacks increase in increments of 10 to 20 lb (4.5 to 29.1 kg). If a child can bench press 30 lb (13.6 kg), a weight stack increment of 10 lb (4.5 kg) represents a 30% increase in resistance, which is too large for a safe and smooth progression in resistance. This problem is remedied on some machines by built-in small resistance increases. On other machines this can be remedied by using weights, usually 2.5 lb (1.1 kg) and 5 lb (2.3 kg), that are specially designed to be easily added and removed from the machine's weight stack. Use of such small increases in resistance will not hinder strength gains. In adults resistance increases of 0.5 lb (0.22 kg) with 7 or 8 repetitions and 1 lb (0.44 kg) with 9 or more repetitions per set result in the equivalent strength gains as larger increases in resistance (Hostler, Crill et al. 2001).

On some machines the starting resistance will be too great for a prepubescent to perform even 1 repetition. In this case the child will have to perform an alternate exercise for the same muscle group using either a free weight, body-weight, or partner-resisted exercise until he or she is strong enough to perform the desired number of repetitions using the machine. For example, if the child cannot perform leg presses on a machine because the starting resistance is too great, the child could perform body-weight squats and then squats holding light dumbbells in each hand until he or she is strong enough to perform leg presses at the starting resistance on the machine.

Summary

Resistance training for prepubescents and adolescents has gained acceptance and popularity primarily because strength gains can occur, bone development may be enhanced, and injuries may be prevented in other sport activities with developmentally appropriate programs. Designers should consider the developmental and physical differences among children, exercise tolerance, and safety issues so that acute and chronic injuries are minimized and the benefits of participation are maximized.

Key Terms

apophyseal
epiphyseal plate
epiphysis
growth cartilage
lordosis
osteochondritis
osteochondritis dissecans

Selected Readings

Bar-Or, O. 1989. Trainability of the prepubescent child. *Physician and Sportsmedicine* 17: 65-82.

Bass, S.L. 2000. The prepubertal years a uniquely opportune stage of growth when the skeleton is most responsive to exercise? *Sports Medicine* 30: 73-70.

Blimkie, C.J.R. 1993. Resistance training during preadolescence. *Sports Medicine* 15: 389-407.

Falk, B, and Tenenbaum, G. 1996. The effectiveness of resistance training in children: A meta-analysis. *Sports Medicine* 22: 176-186.

Freddson, P.S., Ward, A., and Rippe, J.M. 1990. Resistance training for youth. *Advances in Sports Medicine and Fitness* 3: 57-65.

Hass, C.J., Feigenbaum, M.S., and Franklin, B.A. 2001. Prescription of resistance training for healthy populations. *Sports Medicine* 31: 9539-9564.

Kraemer, W.J., and Fleck, S.J. 1993. *Strength training for young athletes.* Champaign, IL: Human Kinetics.

National Strength and Conditioning Association. 1996. Youth resistance training: Position statement paper and literature review. Colorado Springs, CO: NSCA.

Naughton, G., Farpour-Lambert, N.J., Carlson, J., Bradney, M., and Van Praagh, E. 2000. Physiological issues surrounding the performance of adolescent athletes. *Sports Medicine* 30: 309-325.

Payne, V.G., Morrow, J.R. Jr., Johnson, L., and Dalton, S.N. 1997. Resistance training in children and youth: A meta-analysis. *Research Quarterly for Exercise and Sport* 68: 80-88.

Ramsey, J.A.. Blimkie, C.J.R., Smith, K., Garner, S., MacDougall, J.D., and Sale, D.G. 1990. Strength training effects in pubescent boys. *Medicine and Science in Sports and Exercise* 22: 605-614.

Twisk, J.W.R. 2001. Physical activity guidelines for children and adolescents: A critical review. *Sports Medicine* 31: 617-627.

CHAPTER 11

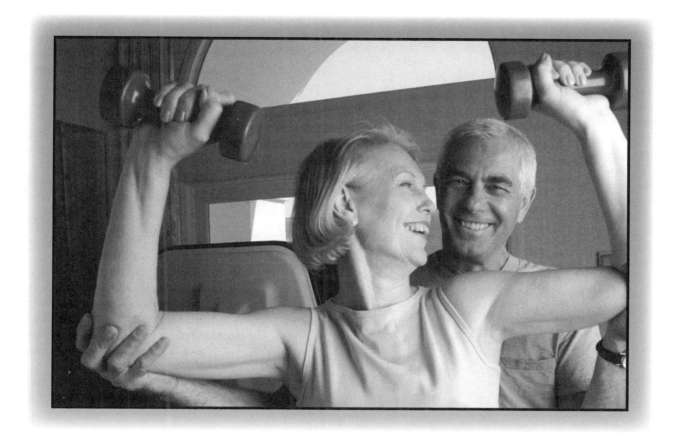

Resistance Training for Seniors

eniors can demonstrate substantial strength. For example, master power lifters over the age of 65 weighing about 180 lb (81 kg) have squatted in excess of 450 lb (204.5 kg) and bench pressed over 350 lb (159.1 kg) (Harder 2000). These older lifters demonstrate that seniors can maintain substantial strength with training, and this conclusion is supported by research. Over a decade ago, Fiatarone and coworkers (1990) demonstrated that individuals over the age of 90 can make strength gains over just an 8-week training period. This finding brought great attention to the concept of strength training for older adults. The benefits of weight training to seniors—even those with chronic illnesses—are related to improved health, improved functional abilities (e.g., mobility), and a better quality of life.

A key finding that promoted resistance training in seniors was that older individuals are capable of performing heavy resistance training (80% of 1RM or higher) and tolerating the stress. Later direct findings demonstrated that the use of very light wrist weights did not stimulate strength increases in the elderly (Engels et al. 1998), which indirectly supported the need for heavy resistance training. This does not imply that moderate resistances do not result in significant fitness gains in middle-aged or elderly individuals. Significant increases in strength and muscle cross-sectional area in females 45 years old have been shown following training with three sets at approximately 50% of 1RM (Takarada and Ishii 2002). Heavy resistances need not be used in every training session, either. Training 3 days per week with either 80% of 1RM every session or 80%, 65%, and 59% of 1RM one session per week both resulted in significant and similar increases in strength and fat-free mass in senior men and women (61-77 years old) (Hunter et al. 2001). The group training with varied resistances, however, showed a significant decrease in the difficulty of a carrying task compared to a group training with only 80% of 1RM. These results indicate that heavy resistances may only be necessary during one out of three training sessions per week to bring about optimal strength increases, and that a varied type of resistance use is effective with seniors.

An individualized strength training program is one way to diminish the age-related declines in strength and muscle mass, which in turn results in improved health and quality of life. However, as one ages, care must be taken to optimize the training effects while reducing the potential for injury.

Age-Related Loss of Muscular Strength and Power

The earlier one becomes involved with physical activity, the greater the positive health benefits will be over time (Kell, Bell, and Quinney 2001). Strength is an important factor in maintaining functional abilities (Brill et al. 2000). Muscle weakness can advance to the stage at which an elderly individual cannot do common activities of daily living, such as getting out of a chair, sweeping the floor, or taking out the trash. Reduced functional ability increases the chance of nursing home placement. The loss in strength and power is mediated by a loss of muscle mass in men and women. This appears to be most problematic for women as they pass the age of 60 because their absolute starting point for muscle tissue mass is lower than that of men (Carmeli, Coleman, and Reznick 2002; Roubenoff 2001; Vandervoot and Symons 2001). Thus, muscle mass as well as strength and power are important to maintain as we age.

Strength Loss

Under normal conditions strength appears to peak between the ages of 20 and 30, after which it remains relatively stable or slightly decreases over the next 20 years (Häkkinen, Kallinen, and Komi 1994). In the sixth decade of life, a more dramatic decrease occurs in both men and women, with this decrease perhaps being more dramatic in women. However, loss of muscles' functional ability does start at earlier ages. In women, cross-sectional data indicate a loss of maximal voluntary and speed of contraction by the age of 40, while speed of relaxation is decreased by the age of 50 (Paasuke et al. 2000). Conflicting reports concerning the magnitude of strength loss exist. This may be due in part to the use of cross-sectional and longitudinal data. Cross-sectional studies may seriously underestimate the magnitude of strength loss with age (Bassey and Harries 1993). For example, the cross-sectional data of Bassey and Harries (1993) show a 2% loss of grip strength per year in the elderly. However, when individuals were followed longitudinally, the loss of hand grip strength was 3% per year for men and nearly 5% per year for women over a 4-year period. Additionally, longitudinal rates of leg strength loss per decade are about 60% of estimates of strength loss from cross-sectional data (Hughes et al. 2001).

Figure 11.1 depicts a general theoretical aging curve for muscle strength in trained and untrained individuals. However, the magnitude of strength decrease varies by gender and individual muscles and muscle groups. For example, Hughes and colleagues (2001) found that the decline in the isokinetic strength of knee extensors averages about 14% and 16% for knee flexors per decade in both sexes. However, women demonstrated slower rates of decline in elbow extensor and flexor strength (about 2% per decade) than men (about 12% per decade). The strength loss in the lower extremities has been shown to be greater than that of the upper extremities in both sexes (Häkkinen, Kallinen, and Komi 1994; Lynch et al. 1999). The strength decline with aging may be related to different factors in different muscle groups. For example, Landers and colleagues (2001) demonstrated that for leg tasks, factors other than lean tissue are involved in the force production loss, whereas in the arm flexors, the loss of lean tissue explains the functional decline in strength. Lynch and colleagues (1999) reported

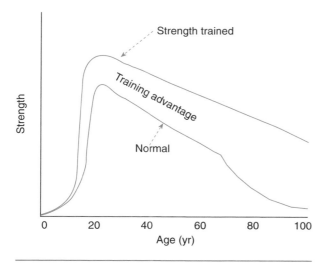

Figure 11.1 A theoretical aging curve for muscle strength. The magnitude of change will vary by muscle group and gender.

that concentric and eccentric peak torque per cross-sectional area of both the arm and leg musculature declines with age, but that differences exist between muscle groups and muscle action types.

Muscle strength loss appears to be most dramatic after the age of 70. For example, knee-extensor strength of a group of healthy 80-year-old men and women studied in the Copenhagen City Heart Study (Danneskoild-Samsoe et al. 1984) was found to be 30% lower than that reported in a previous population study (Aniansson and Gustavsson 1981) of 70-year-old men and women. Cross-sectional as well as longitudinal data indicate that muscle strength declines by approximately 15% per decade in the sixth and seventh decade and about 30% thereafter (Danneskoild-Samsoe et al. 1984; Harries and Bassey 1990; Larsson 1978; Murray et al. 1985). Long-term involvement with strength training appears to offset the magnitude of strength loss and enhances the actual absolute strength capabilities of an individual, but declines do occur even in competitive weightlifters (Kraemer 1992a; Meltzer 1994). Interestingly, the aging curve of fitness parameters of "master athletes" indicated that the decline with aging of peak oxygen consumption was not different from that of sedentary populations, but that strength losses are not linear and exhibit plateaus at various ages (Wiswell et al. 2001). It is important to note that maintenance of higher physiological and functional abilities appears to be mediated only with maintenance of training, as strength and aerobic abilities decline when training ceases.

One important cautionary note concerning strength testing and study interpretation is that adequate familiarization in strength testing is necessary to gain accurate information for assessing 1RM strength (Ploutz-Snyder and Giamis 2001). In the study by Ploutz-Snyder and Giamis, older (66 ± 5 years) and younger (23 ± 4 years) individuals were tested repetitively for knee extension 1RM strength (a relatively simple single-joint exercise). Older women required more practice and familiarization despite having the same experience with lifting as younger women. The older women required eight to nine sessions compared to the three to four sessions required by the younger women to gain a stable and reliable baseline strength measure. Dudley and colleagues (1991) demonstrated younger men's need for several familiarization sessions over 2 weeks to gain adequate reliability. Thus, strength assessment does have an age-related need for greater familiarization, and some of the dramatically high percentage gains in strength with training must be viewed with caution if such test reliability is not assured. Conversely, one may also hypothesize that over the first several training sessions neural adaptations resulting in strength gains are taking place (i.e., a "training effect") at a slower rate in older individuals.

Power Loss

In addition to the loss in muscle strength, a decrease in the muscle's ability to exert force rapidly (power development), especially in explosive type movements and speed of relaxation, also appear to diminish with age (Häkkinen, Kraemer, and Newton 1997; Paasuke et al. 2000). This is likely due to the atrophy of muscle resulting in muscle mass loss and decreases in the rate of voluntary activation of the muscles. However, other factors related to the quality of muscle may preferentially affect power. Myosin heavy chains (MHC) shift to slower types with aging, which could affect the speed of myosin and actin cross-bridge cycling during muscle actions (Sugiura et al. 1992). Weight training in seniors (65 years old), however, does produce a similar change in MHC transformation (MHC IIb to MHC IIa) as in younger individuals (Sharman et al. 2001). It has also been known for some time that myosin ATPase activity decreases with aging (Syrovy and Gutmann 1970). The loss of type II muscle fibers with aging also means a loss of fast MHC proteins (Fry, Allemeier, and Staron 1994). Thus, the loss of both quantity and quality of proteins in the contractile units of muscle provide a structural biochemical basis for the loss of both strength and power with aging.

The ability of muscles to produce force rapidly is vital, and may serve as a protective mechanism when falling. Falls in the elderly have been shown to be one of the top causes of injury, may lead to death, and are a major public health problem (Wolinsky and Fitzgerald 1994). Muscle power and its trainability in seniors has not received a great deal of study, but it may be even more important for the functional abilities of the individual, as many everyday activities (walking, climbing stairs, lifting objects) require rapid force development or a certain degree of power. In a study by Bassey and colleagues (1992) elderly men's (88.5 ± 6 years) and women's (86.5 ± 6 years) leg-extensor power was significantly correlated with chair-rising speed, stair-climbing speed and power, and walking speed (see table 11.1). Correlations between power and functional ability were greater in women than men. However, for both genders the data indicate that power is important for the performance of daily activities. If power decreases, so does the ability to perform daily activities.

Earles, Judge, and Gunnarsson (2001) examined high-velocity resistance training in the elderly (mean age of 77) and reported significant improvements in muscle power. Interestingly, the greatest power improvements were observed during the leg press exercise with a relatively high percent of body mass (60-70%), demonstrating weight or velocity-specific power improvements in the elderly. The large power improvements were accompanied by a significant improvement in walking ability but only small, nonsignificant improvements in chair rise time and balance. Twelve weeks of training at 80% of 1RM with two sets of 8 repetitions and a third set to volitional fatigue did show power increases, but the increases were not specific to the resistance used in training (Campbell et al. 1999). Arm pull power increased significantly at 20%, but not at 40%, 60%, or 80% of 1RM. Knee extension power significantly increased at 20%, 40%, and 60%, but not at 80% of 1RM. Thus, power increases can occur, but may be different from muscle group to muscle group and may not show training resistance or velocity specificity. The effect of training on power needs further study in older individuals.

Examining the force-time curve characteristics of younger and older men and women, Häkkinen and Häkkinen (1991) suggested that the ability to produce force early in the force-time curve (0 to 200 msec) may be compromised by the aging process. The time needed to produce maximal isometric force was significantly longer in older women (70 years) when compared to middle-aged women (50 years) and younger women (30 years). The ability to produce force rapidly may decrease even more than maximal strength, especially at older ages. It has been estimated from cross-sectional studies that lower limb power capabilities may be lost at a rate of 3.5% a year from the ages of 65 to 84 (Young and Skelton 1994). Grassi and colleagues (1991) observed that peak anaerobic power in master endurance and power athletes, when expressed in watts per kilogram of body mass, decreased linearly as a function of age at a rate of about 1% a year. This means that a 75-year-old has only 50% of the anaerobic power of a 20-year-old.

In 1980, Bosco and Komi identified that aging (18 to 73 years) resulted in reduced vertical jump heights. Performing drop jumps from various heights so that the stretch-shortening cycle could be used resulted in even greater decreases in vertical jump ability due to aging. This indicates that the underlying effects on the elastic contractile components in the muscle are affected by age and may affect power performance.

Table 11.1 Overview of Correlations Between Leg Extensor Power and Functional Performances

	Men	Women	Both genders
Chair-rising speed	0.45	0.83*	0.65*
Stair-climbing speed	0.76*	0.85*	0.81*
Walking speed	0.58*	0.93*	0.80*
Stair-climbing power	0.91*	0.86*	0.88*

* = $p < 0.05$.

Reproduced, with permission, from E.J. Bassey et al., 1992, *Clinical Science*, 82, 321-327. © The Biochemical Society and the Medical Research Society.

Decreased power may be one of the primary factors contributing to a loss of functional abilities and to injury from falls in older adults. For this reason, improvement in muscular power should be a primary training goal in older populations. Figures 11.2 and 11.3 depict the difference in rate of force development between older and younger individuals in bilateral (two limbs working together) and unilateral (single-limb) strength. The ability to produce force in a short period of time is dramatically reduced by age in both men and women.

Aging Mechanisms and Adaptations to Resistance Training

A number of factors potentially contribute to the loss of muscle strength and power with age. How

these factors interact with each other and what exact mechanisms predominate under certain conditions or at certain ages remains speculative. The following are some of the primary factors associated with muscle weakness with aging (Fiatarone and Evans 1993; Kraemer 1992b):

- Senescent musculoskeletal changes
- Accumulation of chronic diseases
- Medications needed to treat diseases
- Disuse atrophy
- Undernourishment
- Reductions in hormonal secretions
- Nervous system changes

Muscle Mass Loss

Decreased muscle mass has been suggested as the primary reason for the reduction in force production capabilities with age. This age-associated reduction in muscle mass has been termed **sarcopenia** (Evans and Campbell 1993). Researchers have noted the reduction in muscle mass as people age (Evans and Campbell 1993; Frontera et al. 1991; Häkkinen, Kallinen, and Komi 1994; Häkkinen and Häkkinen 1991; Janssen et al. 2000). This decrease begins to be apparent by age 30, but is most pronounced starting at age 50 (Janssen et al. 2000). Frontera and colleagues (1991) reported that this effect on muscle mass is independent of muscle location (upper versus lower extremities) and function (extension versus flexion), and Janseen and colleagues noted a greater decrease in lower-body compared to upper-body muscle mass. In women, Young, Stokes, and Crowe (1984) demonstrated that the quadriceps cross-sectional area of women in their 70s was 77% of that of women in their 20s. However, not only is there a decrease in cross-sectional area of muscles, but there is also an increase of intramuscular fat, which is most pronounced in women (Imamura et al. 1983.) Seniors also have a twofold increase in noncontractile tissue in muscle compared to younger individuals (Kent-Braun, Ng, and Young 2000). Izquierdo and colleagues (2001) compared middle-aged men (42 years) to older men (65 years) and demonstrated that older men had a 14% reduction in the 1RM squat, a 24% reduction in maximal isometric force, a 13% reduction in the quadriceps femoris muscle mass, and a lower concentration of free testosterone. Thus, the continued reduction in strength as people age is related to many physiological factors.

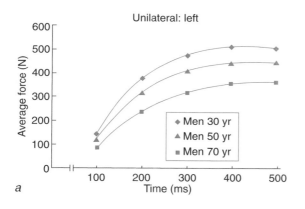

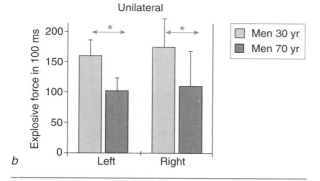

Figure 11.2 Unilateral force development curves.

Figure 11.2a is adapted, by permission, from E.B. Colliander and P.A. Tesch, 1995, "Neuromuscular performance in voluntary bilateral and unilateral contraction and during electrical stimulation in men at different ages," *European Journal of Applied Physiology* 70: 518-527. © Springer-Verlag; figure 11.2b is adapted, by permission, from K. Häkkinen, W.J. Kraemer, and R. Newton, 1991, "Muscled activation and force production during bilateral and unilateral concentric and isometric contractions of the knee extensors in men and women at different ages," *Electromyography Clinical Neurophysiology* 37: 131-142.

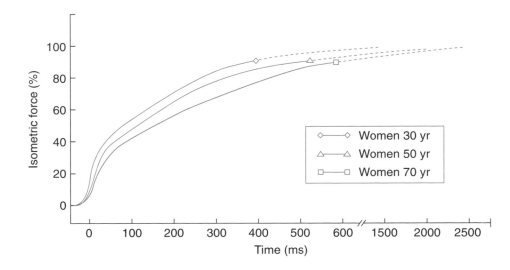

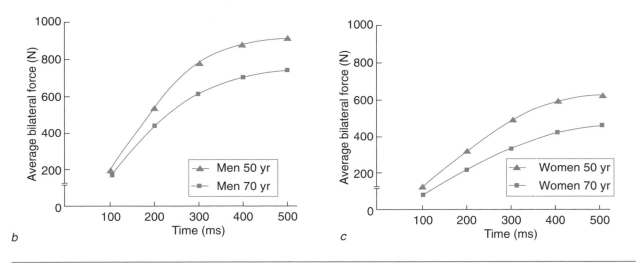

Figure 11.3 Bilateral force development curves.

Figure 11.3a adapted, by permission, from K. Häkkinen and A. Häkkinen, 1991, "Muscle cross-sectional area, force production and relaxation characteristics in women at different ages," *European Journal of Applied Physiology* 62: 410-414. © Springer-Verlag. Figures 11.3 b and c adapted, by permission, from Häkkinen, W.J. Kraemer, and M. Kallinen et al., 1996, "Bilateral and unilateral neuromuscular function and muscle cross-sectional area in middle–aged and elderly men and women," *Journal of Gerontology and Biological Science* 51A: B21-B29. Copyright © The Gerontological Society of America.

The decline in muscle mass appears to be due to the reduction in the size of the individual muscle fibers, the loss of individual muscle fibers, or both (Frontera et al. 1988; Larsson 1982; Lexell et al. 1983; Lexell, Taylor, and Sjostrom 1988). There also appears to be a preferential loss of type II (fast-twitch) muscle fibers with aging, which would negatively affect power capabilities. Additionally, there may also be a loss of force per cross-sectional area with aging due to some unknown intrinsic defect in con-

tractile proteins with aging (Frontera et al. 2000). Figure 11.4 overviews the basic muscle fiber changes with aging. For example, the number of muscle fibers in the midsection of the vastus lateralis of autopsy specimens is lower by about 23% in elderly men (age 70-73) compared to young men (age 19-37) (Lexell et al. 1983). The decline is more marked in type II muscle fibers, which fall from an average of 60% in sedentary young men to below 30% of total fibers after the age of 80 (Larsson 1983).

Mechanisms of Muscle Mass Loss

The reasons for loss of muscle fibers with aging is not completely elucidated, but a possible explanation is as follows. Each cell in the body has a minimum size, which is set by genetic predisposition. When a cell shrinks below this size, cell death might occur. The loss of muscle fibers with aging may be a result of muscle cell death or of the loss of contact with the nervous system resulting in a denervation process (Häkkinen, Kallinen, and Komi 1994). Some muscle fibers are lost with age, but other fibers may undergo a reinnervation process as a result of maintained or increased activity and so are not lost. Muscle fibers that are lost are subsequently replaced with fat or fibrous connective tissue. The loss of muscle fibers compromises the individual motor unit's functional ability to produce force and affects basic metabolic functions of the entire muscle (such as reduced caloric expenditure due to reduced muscle mass).

Motor Unit Loss

Loss of motor units or other neurological changes may contribute to strength loss with aging. Using single motor unit EMG procedures, Nelson, Soderberg, and Urbscheit (1984) observed that large motor units were used in older individuals (79 years) where typically smaller motor units would be used in younger individuals, indicating a loss of smaller motor units. Later work by Doherty and colleagues (1993) indicated that the loss of motor units, even in healthy, active individuals, is a primary factor underlying the age-associated reductions in strength. Using computerized EMG single motor unit analyses, researchers estimated a 47% reduction in the number of motor units in older individuals (60-81 years). So, loss of motor units is in part responsible for strength loss with aging.

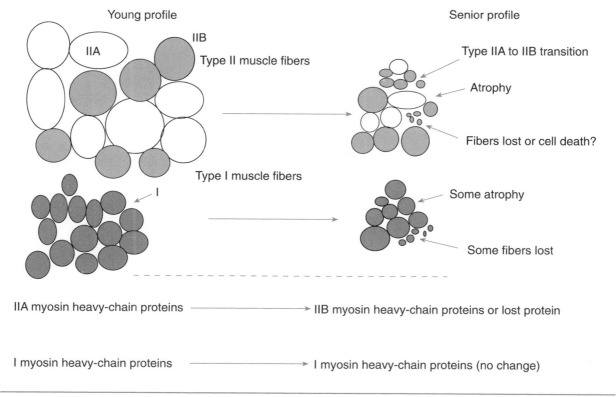

Figure 11.4 Theoretical muscle fiber and myosin heavy chain alterations with aging.

Muscle Fiber Recruitment Changes

Some have questioned whether older individuals can activate their muscles maximally (i.e., recruit all muscle fibers maximally). Twitch interpolation data from Phillips and coworkers (1992) indicate that both old and young individuals can fully activate their muscles. Therefore, muscle weakness that occurs with aging may not be caused by a failure in muscle activation. Brown, McCartney, and Sale (1990) also concluded that older individuals are able to fully activate their muscles, but activation for dynamic activities may differ from activation for isometric muscle actions. Thus, the extent to which central voluntary neural drive decreases with increasing age remains speculative. If aging does result in an inability to activate muscle, the factors primarily responsible may be peripheral neuromuscular mechanisms (e.g., neuromuscular junction) (Häkkinen, Kallinen, and Komi 1994) rather than decreased neural voluntary ability.

Many older individuals experience a decrease in steadiness during muscular actions. This decreased steadiness is caused in part by increased coactivation of antagonistic muscles and increased variability in the discharge rate of motor units. Four weeks of weight training of the hand muscles (first dorsal interosseus) resulted in improved steadiness of both concentric and eccentric actions, but especially during eccentric actions (Laidlaw et al. 1999). This was true during both a constant resistance and a constant percent of 1RM task. The increased steadiness was associated with a decrease in muscle activation. So in older individuals resistance training may also offer the possibility of increasing steadiness of muscular actions.

Prevention of Strength and Muscle Mass Loss

A great deal of attention has focused on strategies for preventing or reversing age-associated losses of muscle mass and strength. Resistance training has been shown to be an effective means of increasing strength and improving functional status in the elderly. Aniansson and Gustavsson (1981) demonstrated that a low-intensity resistance training regimen can produce limited results. This led to the conclusion that the elderly have a

lower capacity to respond to strengthening exercises than younger individuals.

Moritani and DeVries (1980) examined a higher-intensity training program (two sets of 10 repetitions using 66% of the 1RM or maximal voluntary contraction [MVC] for elbow flexors, 3 days per week for 8 weeks) in 72-year-old men and concluded that the capacity to increase strength is preserved in the elderly. They were unable to detect any evidence of muscle hypertrophy, which suggests that neural mechanisms predominate in the expression of strength improvements in older individuals. The methods used in the Moritani and DeVries study, however, were indirect, consisting of limb circumferences and skinfold determinations to estimate muscle size. In addition, the authors used only a short-term training program of 8 weeks.

Häkkinen, Newton, and colleagues (1998) demonstrated that with 10 weeks of training, both younger and older men can increase the average maximum integrated electromyography (IEMGs) of the vastus lateralis. In addition, MRI cross-sectional area increased with training, but differences existed in the absolute volume of muscle gain between young men (29 years) and older men (61 years). This study demonstrated that with short-term training both neural and training-induced hypertrophy mediate strength, yet isometric rate of force production was not altered, indicating power may not be altered.

In 1990 Fiatarone and colleagues examined a group of very old (87-96 years) men and women who trained the knee extensors for 8 weeks. This study was the first to demonstrate that the capacity for muscle strength improvement is preserved even in the very old. This study also demonstrated a significant increase in muscle size using CAT scans. This group of investigators (Fiatarone et al. 1994) then trained a larger group of very old, frail men and women and demonstrated that high-intensity resistance training (80% of 1RM for 10 weeks) is safe for this population and produced significant increases in strength, but no significant increase in muscle size. It is important to note that the increase in strength was associated with an increase in gait speed, stair-climbing power, balance, and overall spontaneous activity. The heavier loading in the later studies and the differences in age may have contributed to the differences in findings compared to the earlier studies.

Additional studies further indicated the importance of loading in optimizing training adaptations. Hostler and colleagues (Hostler, Schwirian et al. 2001) using light elastic cords for training were unable to demonstrate the same magnitude of changes as observed with free weights in muscle strength and muscle fiber training-related adaptations even in younger men and women. This was supported in a prior study by Engles and colleagues (1998) in which older individuals (68 years) using light hand weights demonstrated no beneficial effects in the measured training outcomes. Thus, loading is important for optimal activation of muscle tissue and adaptations to resistance exercise.

In 1988 Frontera and coworkers trained a group of sedentary older men (60-72 years) using a high-intensity resistance training regimen (three sets of 8 repetitions at 80% of 1RM, 3 days per week for 12 weeks). The men demonstrated substantial strength gains (up to a 200% increase in 1RM) and showed evidence of muscle hypertrophy from computerized tomography scans and muscle biopsy analyses. The capacity for high-intensity resistance training to increase muscle fiber size has also been demonstrated in older women. Charette and coworkers (1991) and Campbell and coworkers (1999) examined muscle biopsies taken before and after 12 weeks of high-intensity resistance training; subjects had an increase in type II fiber area, but no significant change in type I area. The results of these studies showing increases in fiber size and individual muscles are supported by a 12-week study (Campbell et al. 1999), a 21-week study (Häkkinen, Pakarinen et al. 2001), a 24-week study (Lemmer et al. 2001), and a 36-week study (Hunter et al. 2001), all of which showed significant increases in fat-free mass in older individuals. However, the increase in fat-free mass is less in seniors than in younger individuals (Lemmer et al. 2001).

Aniansson, Grimby, and Hedberg (1992) suggested that in men between 76 and 80 years of age who maintain physical activity, a compensatory hypertrophy of type I and type II muscle fibers is an adaptation for the loss of muscle fibers and motor units. The percentage of type I and II muscle fibers do not change between the ages of 76 to 80, but there is a significant reduction in the type IIB fibers. This could be interpreted as a loss of muscle fibers or more likely a transition of type IIB to type IIA muscle fibers as a result of maintaining physical activity (Hikida et al. 2000). Following resistance training, the type I,

type IIA, and type IIB fibers of seniors were all hypertrophied. Myosin heavy chains along with fiber types made the same transitions (see chapter 3) in the elderly as in younger individuals. This shift in the myosin heavy chain transition was correlated to the change in fiber type (i.e., type IIB to IIA). These observations have been supported by other work (Häkkinen, Kraemer et al. 2001; Sharman et al. 2001). There was a trend (p = 0.07) for the cytoplasm-to-myonucleus ratio to increase with resistance training. As pointed out in chapter 3, the number of nuclei must increase as the muscle hypertrophies (to maintain nuclear domains), as this is a limiting factor in the size change of muscle and it has been feared to be less responsive in older individuals.

Seniors appear to be able to increase strength in a manner similar to younger individuals as a result of improvements in neurological function (Brown, McCartney, and Sale 1990; Moritani and DeVries 1980). Moritani and DeVries (1980) observed increases in strength, with no significant changes in muscle circumferences, but significant changes in maximal IEMG. This indicated that in older men neural factors were the primary mechanism mediating strength gains during an initial 8-week period of strength training. Given the time course of muscle fiber changes, it is not surprising that no hypertrophy was observed (Staron et al. 1994). IEMG of the vastus lateralis muscle was found to dramatically increase over a 6-month heavy resistance training period for middle-aged and older men and women (40 and 70 years), which mirrored increases in strength (Häkkinen, Pakarinen et al. 2000). Taaffe and Marcus (1997) offered further indications of neurological function affecting strength in seniors when they demonstrated that resistance training increased muscle fiber size and detraining caused muscle size to revert to pretraining values. Strength increased with retraining, but the muscle fiber did not respond as dramatically, indicting that neural factors appear to mediate the rapid return of force production with retraining. Thus, as in younger individuals, neural factors appear to contribute considerably to the improvements in strength in both middle-aged and older adults.

Although many resistance training studies have examined short-term adaptations in the elderly, only a few have examined strength and body composition changes during long training periods of 52 weeks or more. Morganti and colleagues (1995) examined 39 healthy women (59 ± 0.9 years) who were randomized to either a control group or a progressive resistance training group (three sets of 8 reps, 80% of 1RM, upper- and lower-body exercises) that trained twice weekly for 12 months. Strength continually improved in the training group, with no evidence of plateauing during the 12 months of the study. In the lat pull-down, knee extension, and leg press, the greatest changes in strength were seen in the first 3 months of the study. However, smaller but statistically significant increases were seen in the second 6-month period of the study. These data demonstrate that seniors experience a reduction in the rate of strength gains over long-term training similar to that found in younger individuals.

Power and Training

Häkkinen, Newton, and colleagues (1998) identified a deficit in power development with training in older men (61 ± 4 years) compared to younger men (29 ± 5 years). Ten weeks of training resulted in significant improvements in 1RM strength in both groups using a nonlinear periodization training program (i.e., 3 days per week with each day dedicated to one of the trainable characteristics of muscle—strength, power, or local muscular endurance). Power did not improve in the older men despite similar percentage changes in cross-sectional area of the thigh and strength as in the younger men. Such data indicate either that a greater frequency of power training may be needed in older individuals over a short-term training program or that older individuals may not have the physiological mechanisms required to adapt optimally to power training.

A study by Jozsi and colleagues (1999) in which participants trained 2 days a week for 12 weeks with 80% of 1RM using pneumatic resistance (which allowed higher speeds of movement during each training session without negative deceleration effects associated with rapid movements) did show some increases in power. Both older (56-66 years) and younger (21-30 years) participants had similar increases in power at 40% and 60% of 1RM with no changes in power at the training velocity of 80% of 1RM. Men increased strength and power more than women except for the double-legged leg press. Thus, power at lighter loads can be improved, although a gender-specific difference may exist in certain lifts.

A study by Häkkinen, Alen, and colleagues (2000), in which older (63-78 years) and middle-aged (37-44 years) men and women strength trained twice weekly for 24 weeks and also performed explosive power exercises, investigated the effects on strength and power performances. Strength (1RM), as well as jump performance and walking speed, increased in both younger and older groups. In older women (64 years) a 21-week strength training program also showed significant increases in maximal strength and rate of force development (Häkkinen, Pakarinen et al. 2001). The use of a longer training period and possible combination training of strength and supplemental explosive exercises (e.g., maximal jumps) appears to be important for positive training effects of power in older individuals.

Many factors contribute to the loss of strength and muscle mass with aging. Resistance training has been shown to maintain or increase strength, power, and muscle mass in seniors, thus slowing or even reversing the process of strength loss with aging. Table 11.2 overviews some of the responses with resistance exercise training.

Acute Muscle Damage With Exercise

Recovery after a resistance exercise workout is important, especially in older individuals. As in all age groups, proper nutritional intake and rest are needed for recovery. However, we might speculate that the muscles of older adults require longer periods of time to recover between exercise sessions. Therefore, workouts for seniors should be varied in intensity and volume to ensure recovery, especially after workouts in which significant muscle damage has occurred because of heavy loads or high volumes.

Roth and colleagues (1999) examined older men (65-75 years) after a unilateral 9-week training program to determine the effect of five sets of 5 to 20 repetitions at near-maximal resistance on the thigh musculature. Prior to training, 0 to 3% of the muscle fibers exhibited damage in both young and older men (65-75 years), whereas after training 7% and 6% of the fibers exhibited damage in the younger and older men, respectively. The authors concluded that muscle damage as a result of weight training is very similar in younger and older men. In a follow-up study on women, Roth and colleagues (2000) used a similar experimental approach, but found that older women exhibited higher levels of muscle damage than younger women after a short-term resistance training program. Fano and colleagues (2001) evaluated markers of oxidative damage to DNA in younger and older men and women. The authors observed significant oxidative damage in

Table 11.2 Basic Resistance Training Adaptations in Older Adults (60 years and older)

Experimental variable	Response
Muscle strength (1RM)	Increased
Muscle power (W)	Increased
Muscle fiber size	Increased (both major types)

Isokinetic peak torque
    60 deg/sec^{-1}
    240 deg/sec^{-1}
	Increased
	Increased but less than 60 degrees

Isometric peak torque (Nm)	Increased
Local muscle endurance	Increased
Cross-sectional thigh muscle size	Increased
Regional bone mineral density	Increased
Total bone mineral density (men)	No change
Pain levels	Decreased
Intra-abdominal and subcutaneous fat	Decreased
Percent fat	Decreased
Daily tasks	Improved
Gastrointestinal motility	Improved
Flexibility	Increased
Resting metabolic rate	Increased
Balance	Increased
Walking ability	Increased
Functional performance Rising from chair, stairs	Increased
Risk factors for falling	Reduced
Back strength	Increased
Peak oxygen consumption	Increased
Blood pressure/CV demand	Decreased
Capillary density	May increase
Blood lipid profiles	May improve
Insulin resistance	Reduced
Submaximal aerobic capacity	Increased
Psychological factors	Positive effects

Neural factors
    Integrated EMG
    Twitch half relaxation time
    Rate of force development
	Enhanced
	Increased
	Increased
	No changes to increased

the older groups of individuals, with more oxidative damage observed in older men. In a study examining muscle damage in older women before and after a resistance training program, Ploutz-Snyder, Giamis, and Rosenbaum (2001) showed that resistance training provided a protective mechanism, reducing the amount of muscle damage from an eccentric work bout in older women, such that after training older women showed no significant difference in muscle damage compared to younger untrained women.

Resistance training does result in muscle damage in older individuals. However, the damage appears to be similar to that observed in younger individuals. Moreover, older muscle tissue still exhibits the development of protective mechanisms to combat damage due to physical activity.

Hormonal Changes With Aging and Resistance Training

The endocrine system and its many hormones provide important regulatory signals for a variety of metabolic functions in the body (see the discussion of endocrine system responses and adaptations in chapter 3). Of particular interest in resistance training are the anabolic hormones such as testosterone, growth hormones, insulin, and growth factors, which help to stimulate development of the muscle and nerve tissues (Kraemer 1992a, 1992b). Anabolic hormonal concentrations in serum increase above normal resting values during and after an effective resistance exercise workout (Kraemer et al. 1990, 1991; Kraemer, Noble et al. 1987; Kraemer, Dziados et al. 1993), which helps to mediate muscle remodeling and growth. As we age, the endocrine system loses it ability to alter hormonal concentrations with exercise, and reductions in resting concentrations of anabolic hormones have been observed with aging.

Certain hormonal systems may be better maintained than others. In a case study of a 51-year-old male competitive lifter, Fry, Kraemer, and colleagues (1995) demonstrated that reductions in some hormonal responses to an exercise session took place despite over 35 years of training. This older lifter had lower resting serum testosterone concentrations than young controls, but a similar acute increase from exercise. However, growth hormone did not change acutely in response to resistance exercise. This study showed that despite long-term training, the exercise-induced endocrine response was modified with age.

This concept of a compromised endocrine system is supported by early studies of the testosterone and growth hormone response to resistance exercise in older adults (Chakravati and Collins 1976; Häkkinen and Pakarinen 1993; Hammond et al. 1974; Vermeulen, Rubens, and Verdonck 1972). It is interesting to note that although growth hormone (GH) administration has been suggested as an anabolic agent (Rudman et al. 1990), when GH administration is combined with resistance training, it does not cause any greater increase in muscle mass than training alone (Yaresheski et al. 1992). This suggests that the hormonal system in older individuals still functions to the extent necessary to adapt to resistance training.

Other more recent studies also support the hypothesis that the response of the endocrine system to resistance exercise is compromised in middle-aged and older individuals. Häkkinen and Pakarinen (1995) reported that no changes took place in the circulating testosterone concentrations in older men (70 years) after a heavy resistance exercise protocol (i.e., five sets of 10RM with 3 minutes of rest between sets and exercises), whereas in younger men (30 years) and middle-aged men (50 years), increases occurred. This same pattern of change with aging was observed for growth hormone. Similar to men, older women also demonstrated a lack of growth hormone response to resistance training. Häkkinen, Pakarinen, and colleagues (1998) examined the acute responses of growth hormone, total and free testosterone, and cortisol to several different resistance exercise protocols. Serum growth hormone increased in both young men (26.5 years) and older men (70 years), but the increase was greater in the young men. Total testosterone increased for all protocols in the young men, but the older men demonstrated only an increase in response to a leg-extension protocol. Free testosterone increased for all exercise protocols in the young men and in only one protocol for the older men. Concentrations of testosterone were always higher in young men. No changes were observed in cortisol concentrations with exercise. These data show that some acute resistance exercise protocols can produce increases in anabolic hormones in older men, but the absolute concentrations are lower and the magnitude of response are less than in young men.

A study by Kraemer, Häkkinen, and colleagues (1998) examined the hormonal responses to four sets of 10RM of the squat exercise with 90 seconds of rest between sets in young men (30 years) and older men (62 years) who were matched for prior activity patterns. The only differences between groups preexercise was a higher free testosterone concentration in the younger men. The acute postexercise response of the younger men was higher than that of the older men for testosterone, ACTH, and growth hormone. The acute response of lactate and cortisol were not significantly different between groups. This study indicates that the endocrine status of older men is diminished in comparison to younger men even when matched for activity patterns. Figure 11.5 overviews the hormonal changes to resistance exercise with aging.

Kraemer, Häkkinen, and colleagues (1999) examined a 10-week, 3-days-per-week training program using a nonlinear periodization training protocol in young men (30 years) and older men (62 years) who were matched for similar activity profiles. Following training, increases in strength and MRI cross-sectional area of the thigh were observed, with the younger men having higher absolute values at all times. The younger group

demonstrated higher total and free testosterone and insulin-like growth factor I (IGF-I) than the older men at all time points measured pre- and posttraining. The short-term training program resulted in higher free testosterone and IGF-I binding protein-3 at rest and in response to an acute exercise stress in the younger men. In the older men training resulted in a significant increase in total testosterone along with a reduction in resting cortisol concentrations. Thus, the early phase response to short-term training appears to be different between younger and older men, but positive alterations did occur in the older group of men.

Häkkinen, Pakarinen, and colleagues (2000) examined a longer training period of 6 months in middle-aged (42 years) and older (70 years) men and women. Strength dramatically improved in the middle-aged men as well as in the older men and women. However, only the men were able to stimulate increased free and total testosterone concentrations in response to acute exercise, and this increased with training. Greater acute increases in growth hormone occurred in both groups of men in response to resistance exercise stress after training, but not in the older women. This study demonstrated that, especially in older women, a lower testosterone concentration along with the inability to increase growth hormone may compromise the ability to adapt to resistance training.

Häkkinen, Pakarinen, and colleagues (2001) also examined the response of older women (64 years) to 21 weeks of resistance training and found that 1RM leg extension strength increased 21% and maximal force production increased 37%. This was accompanied by a significant increase in the rate of force development. In addition, IEMG and cross-sectional area of the total quadriceps femoris also increased with training. Type I, IIB, and IIA muscle fiber areas also significantly increased. However, with all of these adaptations occurring, no differences pre- to posttraining were observed in resting concentrations of testosterone, growth hormone, cortisol, or IGF-I. No direct comparison to younger women was made in this study. Nevertheless, these results indicate that resting concentrations of these hormones are not recoverable to the values observed in younger individuals. Interestingly, the changes in testosterone concentrations correlated with the changes in cross-sectional area in the quadriceps femoris ($r = 0.64$), indicating that in women testosterone may play a role in adaptations to resistance exercise.

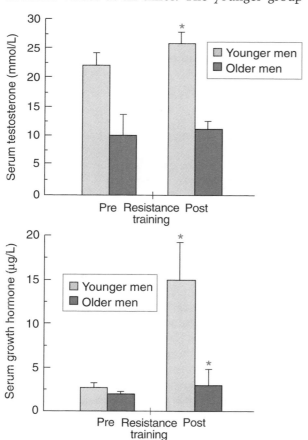

Figure 11.5 Hormonal alterations with aging.
* = significant difference from preexercise value.

Data courtesy of Dr. William Kraemer, University of Connecticut.

Examining middle-aged men (46 years) and older men (64 years), Izquierdo and colleagues (2001) found no changes in free or total testosterone following 16 weeks of training twice a week. The authors observed strength and power increases in both groups. However, the absolute concentrations of testosterone were higher in the middle-aged men. Chronic resistance training does not appear to return hormonal concentrations of older individuals to that of younger individuals. Nevertheless, many hormonal changes beyond the untrained state do occur that may well benefit the body's metabolic and repair processes. The development of strength and muscle size appears to be, in part, related to the response of the anabolic hormones. Of particular concern are older women who seem to show a much more dramatic decrease in muscle tissue mass and a lack of hormonal responses to exercise stress compared to younger women and similar-aged men.

The roles of insulin and insulin-like growth factors (IGF) have been of interest in the aging population. Insulin is one of the pulsatile hormones and typically declines with acute resistance exercise stress even in older individuals (Kraemer, Häkkinen et al. 1998). However, despite an acute decrease with resistance training, 6 months of training have been shown to improve insulin's action in older individuals (64-74 years) who are insulin resistant as a result of physical inactivity and obesity. This is a potentially important benefit of resistance training especially because most individuals with various pathological conditions can perform resistance training.

The effect of resistance training on IGF has received considerable study. Singh and colleagues (1999) observed that even in frail elderly individuals increases in IGF-I staining in muscle after resistance training appeared to be related to increased type II muscle hypertrophy. The authors believed that this may be related to a remodeling stress of muscle. Bermon and colleagues (1999) reported that older men (67-80 years) performing two sets of 12RM and four sets of 5RM demonstrated increases in total and free IGF-I immediately after and 6 hours after a workout, yet no changes were observed in the binding proteins. With training, IGF-I and binding proteins showed no significant changes, indicating that the acute response of IGF-I may be more important in the adaptations related to IGF-I. Borst and colleagues (2001) and Marx and colleagues (2001) reported increases in resting IGF-I concentrations in younger men and women, which suggests that

differences in older individuals may exist. In a study by Parkhouse and colleagues (2000), older women (68 years) with low bone mineral density performed a resistance training program. Before training, concentrations of IGF-I, along with the binding proteins, were all significantly lower than those in an age-matched healthy group of women. Resistance training increased the resting IGF-I hormonal concentrations, but no changes took place in the binding proteins. The authors theorized that in women with low bone mineral density, the stimulation of IGF-I with training may contribute to improved physiological function.

Although poorly understood, autocrine and paracrine mechanisms are important for muscle regeneration after mechanical damage in younger men (Bamman et al. 2001) and may also be important in older individuals. Ultimately, anabolic mechanisms related to tissue growth are affected by aging. Furthermore, evidence to date does not indicate that chronic performance of a resistance training program can maintain endocrine function or cause the same acute response as in younger individuals. However, the acute responses to resistance training protocols, though modest, may contribute in part to the strength and muscle fiber changes observed in older individuals.

Protein Synthesis

Research efforts have also focused on the effects of resistance training on muscle protein metabolism. Campbell and coworkers (1995) examined nitrogen balance before and after 12 weeks of high-intensity resistance training (three sets of 8 repetitions, 80% of 1RM, upper- and lower-body exercises) in a group of older men and women. They found that resistance training increases nitrogen retention. In addition, constant infusion of 13C-leucine revealed that the training resulted in a significant increase in the rate of whole-body protein synthesis.

In another study, Yarasheski, Zachwieja, and Bier (1993) determined the rate of quadriceps muscle protein synthesis using the in vivo incorporation rate of intravenously infused 13C-leucine into mixed-muscle protein in both young (24 years) and older (63-66 years) men and women before and after 2 weeks of resistance exercise training (two to four sets of 4 to 10 repetitions at 60 to 90% of 1RM, 5 days per week). They observed that, although the older individuals had a lower rate of muscle protein synthesis before the training, the resistance exercise resulted in a significant increase in muscle protein synthesis in the young as well as the old individuals.

Bone Health and Resistance Training

Bone may also benefit from resistance training in seniors. However, the use of resistance training to affect bone is difficult to understand as any effect involves multiple factors including the amount of activity each day, the type and length of resistance training program that can be tolerated by the older individual, training status, and genetics (see chapter 3). Training a population of older women, Nelson and colleagues (1994) demonstrated that high-intensity resistance training had significant effects on bone health with increases reported in femoral and lumbar spine density after one year of training. In addition, the resistance training group demonstrated an improvement in balance, total level of physical activity, and muscle mass. Thus, resistance training may have an effect on most of the major risk factors for an osteoporotic bone fracture.

Although resistance training appears to benefit bone, resistance training prescription may be important. A resistance training program in older women (45-65 years) demonstrated no changes in bone after a 24-week program despite increases in muscular strength, suggesting that a longer period of training may be necessary to affect bone (Humphries et al. 2000). Maddalozzo and Snow (2000) examined resistance training for 24 weeks and concluded that an advantage was given to men for changes in bone when compared to women. The investigators suggested that although resistance training of moderate to high intensity produced similar changes in muscle strength in older adults, a higher intensity was necessary to stimulate osteogenesis in the spine, and men appeared to be capable of higher training intensities. In this study, men showed increases in bone mineral density of the spine, but women did not. Both groups demonstrated increases in bone mineral density of the greater trochanter, but no changes in IGF-I or the binding proteins. It is important to note that these studies did not use the theoretical optimal programs for developing bone density (Conroy and Earle 2000).

The capacity to adapt to increased levels of physical activity is clearly preserved even in the very old. Regular exercise has been shown to result in a remarkable number of positive changes in elderly men and women. Because sarcopenia and weakness may be an almost universal characteristic of advancing age, strategies for preserving or increasing muscle mass in the elderly should be implemented. With greater muscle strength, increased levels of spontaneous activity have been seen in both healthy, free-living older individuals and very old, frail men and women. Resistance training, in addition to its positive effects on bone density, energy metabolism, and functional status, may also be an important modality to increase levels of physical activity in the elderly. Resistance training may be one of the most effective and least costly ways to preserve independent living in a wide segment of the population (Rogers and Evans 1993).

Nutrition and Aging

As individuals age, excessive kilocalorie intake can increase fat stores, which increases cardiovascular risk and negatively affects physical performance. Increased fat stores in seniors is in part the result of fat-free mass loss, which has a significant correlation to resting metabolic rate in both young (18-35 years) and older (50-77 years) individuals (i.e., the higher the fat-free mass, the higher the resting metabolic rate) (Piers et al. 1998). Weight training for 24 weeks did increase resting metabolic rate in young as well as older men by 9% (Lemmer et al. 2001). However, young and older women showed no significant increase in resting metabolic rate from performing the same weight training program. Since weight training may be less effective at increasing resting metabolic rate in women, it will be less effective in helping them combat increased fat stores.

Resistance training over 26 weeks appears to be valuable for increasing total energy expenditure in older adults (61-77 years) and does contribute to greater oxidation of lipids (Hunter et al. 2000). The ability to increase total energy expenditure, including spontaneous activity, in seniors may be related to an increase in aerobic ability from performing resistance training (Jubrias et al. 2001). After 6 months of resistance training, seniors showed an increase in muscle oxidative ability of 57%, as well as an increase in muscle size (10%) and mitochondrial volume density (31%). This suggests that resistance training does increase oxidative ability in previously sedentary seniors. Thus, weight training can be of value in helping to control total body weight as well as fat weight with aging, but this may be more difficult to accomplish in older women.

Inadequate energy intake can be a problem with aging and may reduce the body's ability to remodel tissues. Positive energy balance and lack of activity are two of the major factors contributing to an increase in percent body fat and a decrease in muscle mass with aging. Meredith and colleagues (1992) supplemented a group of individuals with extra protein, carbohydrate, vitamins, minerals, and some fat, accounting for an additional 8 kilocalories and 0.33 grams of protein per kilogram of ideal body mass per day. Another group did not receive the additional nutrients. Both groups performed a resistance training program for 12 weeks. The supplemented group showed a dramatic increase in muscle tissue, and the subsequent changes in muscle size were proportional to caloric intake. Improved nutrition and better dietary management should enhance the effects of resistance training on muscle mass in older individuals as it can in younger individuals.

Adequate protein is also vital for muscle hypertrophy in elderly individuals. The necessary protein for hypertrophy may exceed the recommended RDA value of 0.8 g/kg/day (Campbell and Evans 1996; Campbell et al. 2001). Esmark and colleagues (2001) showed that the timing of protein intake should be immediately after the workout to optimize the hypertrophic response of elderly men to resistance training. This may be related to the response of a host of hormonal interfaces that may be active during the recovery period immediately following resistance exercise. Without the necessary protein and other nutrients, increases in fat-free mass will be compromised.

Resistance training in the frail elderly (72-98 years) has been shown to improve muscle fiber structure, and the greatest strength increases were observed in those individuals with the greatest increases in myosin protein, IGF-I, damage, and caloric intake during the weight training period, indicating that multiple factors may mediate the effect of training on muscle (Singh et al. 1999). Although beyond the scope of this text, adequate intake of vitamins, minerals, micronutrients, and macronutrients are vital for optimal function in the recovery and remodeling process of tissues with resistance exercise and training.

Developing a Resistance Training Program

The fundamentals and principles of resistance training program design are the same no matter what the trainee's age. Because of variations in the functional capacity of many older individuals, the best program is individualized to meet the needs and medical concerns of each person. At present, periodized training has been used in several situations when training older adults, and more information on training variation is needed to optimize training for this population (Hunter, Wetzstein et al. 2001; Newton et al. 1995). In addition, the inclusion of functional resistance training (i.e., the use of exercises in an unstable environment) appears to significantly improve muscle balance, strength, and functional capacity (Heitkamp et al. 2001), especially when incorporated into a weight training program.

Elderly people can tolerate high-intensity resistance exercise (i.e., 80% of 1RM), which results in positive adaptations. Some data indicate that the application of the intensity must be carefully applied so as not to initiate an overtraining syndrome in older adults (Hunter and Treuth 1995). It is quite possible that recovery from a training session takes longer in older people, and the use of varied intensities in a periodized format may allow for more optimal adaptation. The types of resistance training programs used in most studies have been quite fundamental in design and have shown positive results. Thus, in the early phases of training, advanced program design is not required. Furthermore, many middle-aged and older adults may require a period of time for conditioning so they can train at the level needed to make training adaptations. A basic overview of programs that have been used for older adults is shown in figure 11.6.

The starting level of strength fitness may be minimal in the frail elderly, with a maximal force capability of only a few pounds. Thus, a progressive resistance training program initially may require that an older individual lift only 0.5 lb (0.2 kg) during a set. Trainers and program designers should use care in choosing the proper equipment to allow manipulations of such low resistance increments.

Needs Analysis

The process of developing a strength training program in older adults consists of pretesting and evaluation, setting individualized goals, designing a program, and developing evaluation methods. In older adults, resistance training should be part of a lifelong fitness lifestyle, so continual re-evaluation of program goals and program design

Choice of Exercise

The primary exercises focus on large muscle groups: 4 to 6 large muscle group exercises, 3 to 5 supplemental small muscle group exercises are usually added. Free weights, isokinetic machines, pneumatic machines, and stack plate machines have all been commonly used. It has been recommended that machine-based exercises be used initially with progression to free weights when applicable.

Order of Exercise

A warm-up is usually followed by exercising large muscle groups. This is followed by smaller muscle group exercise and cool-down activities. For total-body workouts, exercises may be rotated between upper and lower body, and between opposing muscle groups.

Resistance Used

The most common percentage range examined is 50 to 85% of 1RM for 8 to 12 repetitions. Lighter loads are recommended initially. Various loading schemes have been recommended for progression including light, moderate, and moderately heavy loads.

Lifting Velocity

Slow-to-moderate lifting velocities have been recommended for strength and hypertrophy training. When power is a training goal, light loads with faster lifting velocities have been recommended.

Number of Sets

The recommended minimal initial starting point consists of at least 1 set per exercise for 8 to 10 exercises. Progression may ensue from 1 to 3 sets over time (depending on the number of exercises performed) where toleration of 3 sets has been shown by even the frail elderly.

Rest Between Sets and Exercises

Typically 1 to 2 minutes have been used. Shorter rest periods have been associated with very light resistances where recovery is quicker.

Frequency

Resistance training of 2 to 3 days per week has been recommended.

Figure 11.6 General characteristics of resistance training programs for older adults; includes recommendations from the American College of Sports Medicine (ACSM) (2002).

is necessary for optimal results and adherence. The American College of Sports Medicine (ACSM 2001) has advised that people who start an exercise program be classified into one of three risk categories:

I. Apparently healthy, less than one coronary risk factor (hypertension, smoking) or cardiopulmonary or metabolic disease

II. At higher risk, more than two coronary risk factors or cardiopulmonary or metabolic disease symptoms

III. Previously diagnosed with diseases such as cardiovascular, pulmonary, or metabolic disease

Consultation and consent of a physician is recommended in all cases, with additional functional exercise testing for category III recommended by the ACSM. For individuals using resistance training in a fitness program, a strength test or exercise protocol is recommended for evaluating symptoms specific to the exercise modality. Strength testing and resistance exercise workouts using as much as 75% of the 1RM have been shown to have fewer cardiopulmonary symptoms than graded treadmill exercise tests in cardiac patients with good left ventricular function (Faigenbaum et al. 1990). In addition, 1RM testing has been shown to be a safe and effective means of evaluating the elderly provided they are adequately familiar with the protocol (Shaw, McCully, and Posner 1995). Thus, resistance exercise that is not performed with a Valsalva maneuver is considered safe, but should be specifically evaluated in each case. The needs analysis and development of program goals should follow the steps previously outlined. The following fundamental principles of training, previously discussed in this text (chapters 1, 4, and 5), must be considered in the design and progression of a program for an older individual.

Those determining the training progress of an older person should evaluate strength (on the equipment used in training if possible), body composition, functional ability (e.g., the person's ability to lift a chair, get out of chair, etc.), muscle size changes, nutrition, and preexisting medical conditions.

The major concern for older adults is proper progression without injury or acute overuse. Since these people require longer periods to recover from a training session, care is needed not to "overshoot" the physiological ability to repair tissues after a workout. The American College of Sports Medicine presented an overview of progression in its 2002 position stand.

In brief, an overview of the position stand recommends chronically manipulating the acute program variables for long-term progression during resistance training in healthy older adults. Caution must be taken with the elderly population in the rate of progression as too much too soon can cause injury. Further, each individual will respond differently to a given resistance training program based on current training status, past training experience, and response to the training stress. A resistance training program for the older adult should attempt to improve the quality of life by enhancing several components of muscular fitness including muscle hypertrophy, strength, power, and local muscular endurance. The American College of Sports Medicine (2002) recommends that programs include variation, gradual progressive overload, specificity, and careful attention to recovery.

Muscular strength and hypertrophy are crucial components for quality of life. Additionally, resistance training to improve muscle hypertrophy is instrumental in limiting sarcopenia. The basic health and fitness resistance training program recommended by the ACSM for the healthy adult is an effective starting point in the elderly population. When the older adult's long-term resistance training goal is progression toward higher levels of muscular strength and hypertrophy, evidence supports the use of variation in the resistance training program. However, it is important that progression be introduced into this population at a very gradual pace to avoid acute injury and to allow time for adaptation to the program. The ACSM position stand states, "Recommendations for improving muscular strength and hypertrophy in older adults support the use of both multiple- and single-joint exercises (perhaps machines initially with progression to free weights with training experience) with slow-to-moderate lifting velocity, for 1-3 sets per exercise with 60-80% of 1RM for 8-12 repetitions with 1-2 minutes of rest in between sets."

The ability to develop muscular power diminishes with age. An increase in power enables the older adult to improve performance in tasks that require a rapid rate of force development, and reduces the risk of accidental falls. There is support for the inclusion of resistance training specific for power development for the healthy older adult. Muscle atrophy, especially in type II fibers, is most likely the result of a combination of aging and very low physical activity levels and is associated with considerable decreases in muscle strength and power. The decreases in maximal power have been shown to exceed those of maximal muscle strength. Power development programs for the elderly may help optimize functional abilities as well as have secondary effects on other physiological systems, such as connective tissue. Based on available evidence it appears prudent to include high-velocity (nonballistic), low-intensity movements to maintain the structure and function of the neuromuscular system. The ACSM position stand states, "The recommendations for increasing power in healthy older adults include: 1) training to improve muscular strength as previously discussed, and 2) the performance of both single- and multiple-joint exercises (machine-based initially progressing to free weights) for 1-3 sets per exercise using light-to-moderate loading (40-60% of 1RM) for 6-10 repetitions with high repetition velocity."

Improvements in local muscular endurance in the older adult may lead to an enhanced ability to perform submaximal work and recreational activities. Studies examining the development of local muscular endurance in the older adult are limited, but suggest that it may be enhanced by circuit weight training; strength training; and high-repetition, moderate-load programs in younger populations. "Considering that local muscular endurance improvements are attained with low-to-moderate loading," the ACSM position stand states, "it appears that similar recommendations may apply to the aged as well, e.g. low-to-moderate loads performed for moderate-to-high repetitions (10-15 or more) with short rest intervals."

Effect of Aging on the Acute Program Variable Choices

Manipulation of the acute program choices is just as important in individualizing the resistance training program for seniors as this process is for any other population. There are, however, some considerations of acute program choices unique to the older adult population.

Choice of Exercise

The choice of exercise varies when working with older adults. The program should include at least one exercise for all the major muscle groups. The equipment used has to fit the individual, and the resistance used must accommodate his or her functional capacity. At some point in the program, exercise should be added that optimally stimulates the majority of the muscle tissue (e.g., total-body exercises such as squats). In addition, different exercise modes (machines and free weights) will help to activate the muscle tissue differently for specificity of the training stimulus (e.g., free weights for balance, machines for isolated loading, beginning plyometrics for power, etc.).

As the program progresses, the progression of exercises should activate as much of the skeletal muscle mass as possible to facilitate adaptation. Furthermore, use of only linear lines of movement may not address some of the more common movement patterns in everyday life (e.g., twisting, turning, etc.).

On some machines even the minimal resistance is too great for some older adults who may have difficulty producing the initial force to start the exercise movement. Also, on some machines the resistance increments are too large, especially at the lighter resistances, to allow a smooth progression in resistance. Some modalities such as isokinetics, pneumatics, or hydraulics allow for easier initiations of the exercise movement and for a smooth resistance progression.

Programs have used all types of resistance tools from free weights, food cans of different sizes, rubber tubing, water-filled milk cartons, and more recently functional devices such as medicine and stability balls. With any of these types of equipment, care needs to be taken to help the individual attain proper range of motion and safely control the resistance throughout the full range of motion. Older adults may need to supplement full range of motion resistance exercise training with specific flexibility exercise training (Hurley

1995). The key is to reach the maximal range of motion and in some movements use resistance to help extend and hold a static stretch (e.g., using light hand weights in the movements or having a partner help with the stretch).

Order of Exercise

Large-muscle group exercises are typically placed in the beginning of the workout. This minimizes fatigue and enables individuals to use higher intensities or greater resistances in these exercises. Optimal stimulation of large-muscle groups in the lower extremities (e.g., with the leg press) and the upper body (e.g., with the bench press or seated row) should be a top priority in programs for older adults.

Rest Between Sets and Exercises

The rest between sets will determine the metabolic demands of the resistance training workout. Rest periods that are too short can also produce a drastic reduction in the resistance used in successive sets if recovery is not sufficient before the next set or exercise is initiated. Short rest intervals are used to enhance local muscular endurance and improve acid-base status, which has been shown to be compromised with aging. Because activation of muscle tissue is related to the resistance and the total amount of work performed, rest period lengths should be consistent with the program goals. Short rest periods can be used with circuit programs. The rest periods should be longer if heavier resistances are being used and can be shortened as exercise toleration is enhanced. The amount of rest may also be dictated by the medical or physical condition of the individual. In some older adults (e.g., those with type I diabetes), gains in strength are the major goal, so care must be taken to properly control the length of rest between sets and exercises so as not to create severe metabolic stress.

Number of Sets

The number of sets is related to the exercise volume. Initially, since older people generally can tolerate only a low volume of exercise, single-set programs are the simplest starting point. Using the principle of progressive resistance training, the volume can be increased by increasing the number of sets or exercises, so that the muscle starts to tolerate a higher volume of exercise. Programs for older adults usually do not involve more than three sets of a given exercise. If the muscle group needs more stimulation, another exercise for that muscle group can be added to the program. In addition, many programs for older adults use a warm-up set at a low percentage of the RM prior to the working sets that are closer to a true RM or RM zone of resistance.

Resistance (Intensity)

The work done in the 1980s and early 1990s demonstrated that older men and women can tolerate and positively adapt to heavier weight training programs (Fiatarone and Evans 1993). The amount of resistance that can be tolerated by frail elderly adults in their 90s is at least 80% of the 1RM. However, heavy resistances, when used, may not have to be lifted every training session because training 3 days per week with either 80% of 1RM every session or 80%, 65%, and 59% of 1RM one session per week both result in significant and similar increases in strength and fat-free mass in senior men and women (61-77 years) (Hunter et al. 2001). The ACSM position stand (ACSM 2002) offers resistance recommendations for beginning programs and program progressions for seniors. The resistance needs to be carefully evaluated so that an overtraining syndrome doesn't develop. Hunter and Treuth (1995) found that progression with lighter resistances (50-60% of the 1RM) may result in greater increases in the 1RM in older women. Also, some research has shown program periodization to be beneficial in resistance training programs for older adults (Hunter et al. 2001; Newton et al. 1995).

Number of Repetitions

As in all populations, the resistance used and the number of repetitions performed by seniors does have an effect on the training adaptations. However, because of the high prevalence of cardiovascular problems and risks in older adults, these factors must also be carefully considered for safety reasons. Performing a set to concentric failure does result in higher blood pressures and heart rates compared to a set not performed to failure. In addition, performing sets to concentric failure using resistances in the 70 to 90% of 1RM range results in blood pressures that are slightly higher than those resulting from sets to failure below and above this range. The highest blood

pressures and heart rates normally occur in the last few repetitions of a set. Therefore, for safety reasons, it is recommended that older adults, especially those with cardiovascular problems or risks, not perform sets to concentric failure, especially in the 70 to 90% of 1RM range. This recommendation is perhaps most important when beginning a program. Performance of a Valsalva maneuver, which increases blood pressure, should also be discouraged in this population.

Designing a resistance program for older adults should follow the same careful planning guidelines used for younger individuals. The program design does, however, need to consider the medical aspects of older adults such as cardiovascular problems and arthritis. An example of a total-body workout for an older adult is described in figure 11.7.

Summary

We have discussed the positive and negative aspects of older adults participating in a resistance training program. The benefits are increased strength, endurance, and muscle capacity; increased flexibility; and more energy. The negative aspects include some pain or stiffness and other nonspecific problems. Thus, the positive and negative aspects of resistance training are very similar to those in younger populations. Scientific investigations have demonstrated that resistance training can be safely and successfully implemented in older populations. Even the frail and very sick elderly can gain benefits that will positively affect their quality of life. Individuals up to 100 years of age have been shown to positively adapt to a resistance exercise training program. The muscle strengthening carries over into enhancement of everyday activities and quality of life. It even enhances the cardiovascular endurance capabilities by placing less stress on the heart and circulatory system, as endurance activities are performed at a significantly lower percent of the maximal voluntary muscle action. The enhancement of muscle and bone mass has important benefits for the health profile of the individual. Proper design and progression of a resistance training program for the older adult is vital to optimizing its benefits.

Beginning Home Program
- For upper-body exercises, use soup cans or light resistance (2- to 5-pound hand dumbbells)
- Perform 1 to 3 sets of 8 to 10 repetitions
- Take 1 to 2 minutes of rest between sets and exercises
- Concentrate on full range of motion movement and balance. A wall or solid chair can be used for help with balance in the beginning. Keep head up.
- Exercises: Front shoulder raise, wall push-up, standing single knee lift, toe raise, arm curl, good morning exercise, side bend, standing knee curls, single arm shoulder press, 1/4 squat, single bent-over arm row, side shoulder raise, triceps extension

Program note: This is a light-resistance, calisthenic-type of program to gain basic movement and range of motion abilities. Progression to heavier resistances, especially for the lower-body musculature, is vital for optimal progression.

Beginning Program in the Weight Room
- Exercises: leg press, knee extension, knee curl, calf raise, chest press, seated row or lat pull-down, upright row, arm curl, trunk curl, triceps extension
- Order of exercises: Large to small muscle group exercises, upper to lower or opposing muscle groups
- Resistance used: 80% of 1RM or 10 to 15RM
- Number of sets: Start out with 1 and progress to 3 over a 12-week program
- Rest between sets and exercises: 1 to 3 minutes or until recovered

Periodized Program for Weight Room and Long-Term Use
- Use a 12-week cycle (e.g., Monday, Wednesday, Friday) followed by an active rest of 2 weeks and then repeat the cycle with appropriate variation in the program variables based on individual training goals and needs.
- Exercises: Leg press or squat, knee extension, knee curl, calf raise, chest press, seated row, upright row, arm curl
- Order of exercises: Large to small muscle group exercises
- Resistance used: 8 to 10RM (M), 6 to 8RM (W), 12 to 15RM (F)
- Number of sets: Start out with 1 and progress to 3 over the 12-week cycle
- Rest between sets and exercises: 1 to 2 minutes (M), 2 to 3 minutes (W), 1 to 2 minutes (F)

Figure 11.7 Example resistance training programs for seniors.

Key Terms

activities of daily living

functional abilities

functional resistance training

sarcopenia

Selected Readings

Brown, A.B., McCartney, N., and Sale, D.G. 1990. Positive adaptations to weight-lifting training in the elderly. *Journal of Applied Physiology* 69: 1725-1733.

Carmeli, E., Coleman, R., and Reznick, A.Z. 2002. The biochemistry of aging muscle. *Experimental Gerontology* 37: 477-489.

Doherty, T.J., Vandervoot, A.A., Taylor, A.W., and Brown, W.F. 1993. Effects of motor unit losses on strength in older men and women. *Journal of Applied Physiology* 74: 868-874.

Evans, W.J., and Campbell, W.W. 1993. Sarcopenia and age-related changes in body composition and functional capacity. In Symposium: Aging and body composition: Technological advances and physiological interrelationships. *Journal of Nutrition* 123: 465-468.

Fiatarone, M.A., O'Neill, E.F., Ryan, N.D., Clements, K.M., Solares, G.R., Nelson, M.E., Roberts, S.B., Kehayias, J.J., Lipsitz, L.A., and Evans, W.J. 1994. Exercise training and nutritional supplementation for physical frailty in very elderly people. *The New England Journal of Medicine* 330: 1769-1775.

Gavrilov, L.A., and Gavrilova, N.S. 2001. The reliability theory of aging and longevity. *Journal of Theoretical Biology* 213: 527-545.

Häkkinen, K., Pastinen, U.M., Karsikas, R., and Linnamo, V. 1995. Neuromuscular performance in voluntary bilateral and unilateral contraction and during electrical stimulation in men at different ages. *European Journal of Applied Physiology* 70: 518-527.

Hurley, B. 1995. Strength training in the elderly to enhance health status. *Medicine, Exercise, Nutrition, and Health* 4: 217-229.

Meredith, C.N., Frontera, W.R., O'Reilly, K.P., and Evans, W.J. 1992. Body composition in elderly men: Effect of dietary modification during strength training. *Journal of American Geriatric Society* 40: 155-162.

Nelson, M.E., Fiatarone, M.A., Morganti, C.M., Trice, I., Greenberg, R.A., and Evans, W.J. 1994. Effects of high-intensity strength training on multiple risk factors for osteoporotic fractures. *Journal of the American Medical Association* 272: 1909-1914.

Ratzin-Jackson, C.G., ed. 2001. *Nutrition and the strength athlete,* pp. 1-307. Boca Raton, FL: CRC Press.

Rogers, M.A., and Evans, W.J. 1993. Changes in skeletal muscle with aging: Effects of exercise training. In *Exercise and sport sciences reviews,* edited by J.O. Holloszy. Baltimore: Williams & Wilkins.

Roubenoff, R. 2001. Origins and clinical relevance of sarcopenia. *Canadian Journal of Applied Physiology* 26: 78-89.

Vandervoot, A.A., and Symons, T.B. 2001. Functional and metabolic consequences of sarcopenia. *Canadian Journal of Applied Physiology* 26: 90-101.

References

Aagaard, P., Andersen, J.L., Poulsen, P.D., Leffers, A.M., Wagner, A., Magnusson, S.P., Kristensen, J.H., and Simonsen, J. 2001. A mechanism for increased contractile strength of human pennate muscles in response to strength training: Changes in muscle architecture. *Journal of Physiology* 534: 613-623.

Abe, T., Bechue, W.F., Fujita, S., and Brown, J.R. 1998. Gender differences in FFM accumulation and architectural characteristics of muscle. *Medicine and Science in Sports and Exercise* 30: 1066-1070.

Abe, T., Brown, J.B., and Brechue, W.F. 1999. Architectural characteristics of skeletal muscle in black and white college football players. *Medicine and Science in Sports and Exercise* 31: 1448-1452.

Abe, T., Kawakami, Y., Sugita, M., and Fukunaga, T. 1997. Relationship between training frequency and subcutaneous and visceral fat in women. *Medicine and Science in Sports and Exercise* 29: 1549-1553.

Adams, G. 1998. Role of insulin-like growth factor-I in the regulation of skeletal muscle adaptation to increased loading. *Exercise and Sports Science Reviews* 26: 31-60.

Adams, G., Hather, B.M., Baldwin, K.M., and Dudley, G.A. 1993. Skeletal muscle myosin heavy chain composition and resistance training. *Journal of Applied Physiology* 74: 911-915.

Adams, G., and McCue, S. 1998. Localized infusion of IGF-I results in skeletal muscle hypertrophy in rats. *Journal of Applied Physiology* 84: 1716-1722.

Adams, K., O'Shea, J.P., O'Shea, K.L., and Climstein, M. 1992. The effect of six weeks of squat, plyometric and squat-plyometric training on power production. *Journal of Applied Sport Science Research* 6: 36-41.

Akima, H., Takahashi, H., Kuno, S., Masuda, K., Masuda, T., Shimojo, H., Anno, I., Ital, Y., and Katsuta, S. 1999. Early phase adaptations of muscle use and strength to isokinetic training. *Medicine and Science in Sports and Exercise* 31: 588-594.

Alen, M., Pakarinen, A., Häkkinen, K., and Komi, P.B. 1988. Responses of serum androgenic-anabolic and catabolic hormones to prolonged strength training. *International Journal of Sports Medicine* 9: 229-233.

Aloia, J.F., Vaswani, A., Ma, R., and Flaster, E. 1995. To what extent is bone mass determined by fat-free for fat mass? *American Journal of Clinical Nutrition* 61: 1110-1114.

Allen, T.E., Byrd, R.J., and Smith, D.P. 1976. Hemodynamic consequences of circuit weight training. *Research Quarterly* 47: 299-307.

Allsen, P.E., Parsons, P., and Bryce, G.R. 1977. Effect of menstrual cycle on maximum oxygen uptake. *The Physician and Sportsmedicine* 5: 52-55.

Alway, S.E. 1994. Characteristics of the elbow flexors in women bodybuilders using androgenic-anabolic steroids. *Journal of Strength and Conditioning Research* 8: 161-169.

Alway, S.E., Grumbt, W.H., Gonyea, W.J, and Stary-Gundersen, J. 1989. Contrast in muscle and myofibers of elite male and female bodybuilders. *Journal of Applied Physiology* 67: 24-31.

Alway, S.E., Grumbt, W.H., Stary-Gundersen, J., and Gonyea, W.J. 1992. Effects of resistance training on elbow flexors of highly competitive bodybuilders. *Journal of Applied Physiology* 72: 1512-1521.

Alway, S.E., MacDougall, J.D., and Sale, D.G. 1989. Contractile adaptations in the human triceps surae after isometric exercise. *Journal of Applied Physiology* 66: 2725-2732.

Alway, S.E., MacDougall, J.D., Sale, D.G., Sutton, J.R., and McComas, A.J. 1988. Functional and structural adaptations in skeletal muscle of trained athletes. *Journal of Applied Physiology* 64: 1114-1120.

Alway, S.E., Sale, D.G., and MacDougall, J.D. 1990. Twitch contractile adaptations are not dependent on the intensity of isometric exercise in the human triceps surae. *European Journal of Applied Physiology* 60:346-352.

Alway, S.E., Winchester, P.K., Davies, M.E., and Gonyea, W.J. 1989. Regionalized adaptations and muscle fiber proliferation in stretch-induced enlargement. *Journal of Applied Physiology* 66: 771-781.

American Academy of Pediatrics. 1990. Strength training, weight and power lifting and bodybuilding by children and adolescents. *Pediatrics* 86: 801-803.

American College of Sports Medicine. 1993. The prevention of sport injuries of children and adolescents. *Medicine and Science in Sports and Exercise* 25 (8 Supplement): 1-7.

American College of Sports Medicine. 1998. The recommended quantity and quality of exercise for developing and maintaining cardiorespiratory and muscular fitness, and flexibility in healthy adults. *Medicine and Science in Sports and Exercise* 30: 975-991.

American College of Sports Medicine. 2000. Chapter 11. Exercise testing and prescription for children, the elderly, and pregnant women. *ACSM's Guidelines for Exercise Testing and Prescription*, 6th ed. Baltimore: Lippincott Williams & Wilkins.

American College of Sports Medicine. 2001. Resource manual. *Guidelines for exercise testing and prescription*, 4th ed. Baltimore: Lippincott Williams & Wilkins.

American College of Sports Medicine. 2002. Position stand. Progression models in resistance training for healthy adults. *Medicine and Science in Sports and Exercise* 34: 364-380.

American Orthopedic Society for Sports Medicine.1988. *Proceedings of the conference on strength training and the prepubescent.* Chicago: American Orthopedic Society for Sports Medicine.

Amusa, L.O., and Obajuluwa, V.A. 1986. Static versus dynamic training programs for muscular strength using the knee-extensors in healthy young men. *Journal of Orthopaedic and Sports Physical Therapy* 8: 243-247.

Andersen, J.L., and Aagaard, P. 2000. Myosin heavy chain IIX overshoot in human skeletal muscle. *Muscle and Nerve* 23: 1095-1104.

Anderson, T. and Kearney, J.T. 1982. Muscular strength and absolute and relative endurance. *Research Quarterly for Exercise and Sport* 53: 1-7.

Aniansson, A., Grimby, G., and Hedberg, M. 1992. Compensatory muscle fiber hypertrophy in elderly men. *Journal of Applied Physiology* 73: 812-816.

Aniansson, A., and Gustavsson, E. 1981. Physical training in elderly men with specific reference to quadriceps muscle strength and morphology. *Clinical Physiology* 1: 87-98.

Ariel, G. 1977. Barbell vs. dynamic variable resistance. *U.S. Sports Association News* 1: 7.

Atha, J. 1981. Strengthening muscle. *Exercise and Sport Sciences Reviews* 9: 1-73.

Atonio, J., and Gonyea, W.J. 1994. Muscle fiber splitting in stretch-enlarged avian muscle. *Medicine and Science in Sports and Exercise* 26: 970-977.

Augustsson, J., Esko, A., Thomee, R., and Svantesson, U. 1998. Weight training of the thigh muscles using closed vs. open kinetic chain exercises: A comparison of performance enhancement. *Journal of Orthopedic and Sports Physical Therapy* 27: 3-8.

Aura, O., and Komi, P.V. 1986. The mechanical efficiency of locomotion in men and women with special emphasis on stretch-shortening exercises. *European Journal of Applied Physiology* 55: 37-43.

Baar, K., and Esser K. 1999. Phosphorylation of $p70^{S6k}$ correlates with increased skeletal muscle mass following resistance exercise. *American Journal of Physiology (Cell Physiology)* 276: C120-C127.

Baechle, T.R., Earle, R.W., and Wathen, D. 2000. Resistance training. In *Essentials of strength training and conditioning,* edited by Baechle, T.R. and Earle, R.W., 2nd ed., 395-425. Champaign, IL: Human Kinetics.

Baker, D. 2001a. A series of studies on the training of high-intensity muscle power and rugby league football players. *Journal of Strength and Conditioning Research* 15: 198-209.

Baker, D. 2001b. Acute and long-term power responses to power training: Observations on the training of an elite power athlete. *Strength and Conditioning Journal* 23: 47-56.

Baker, D. 2001c. Comparison of upper-body strength and power between professional and college-aged rugby league players. *Journal of Strength and Conditioning Research* 15: 30-35.

Baker, D., Nance, S., and Moore M. 2001a. The load that maximizes the average mechanical power output during explosive bench press throws in highly trained athletes. *Journal of Strength and Conditioning Research* 15: 20-24.

Baker, D., Nance, S., and Moore M. 2001b. The load that maximizes the average mechanical power output during jump squats in power-trained athletes. *Journal of Strength and Conditioning Research* 15: 92-97.

Baker, D., Wilson, G., and Carlyon, R. 1994a. Generality versus specificity: A comparison of dynamic and isometric measures of strength and speed-strength. *European Journal of Applied Physiology* 68: 350-355.

Baker, D., Wilson, G., and Carlyon, R. 1994b. Periodization: The effect on strength of manipulating volume and intensity. *Journal of Strength and Conditioning Research* 8: 235-242.

Ballantyne, C.S., Phillips, S.M., MacDonald, J.R., Tarnopolsky, M.A., and MacDougall, J.D. 2000. The acute effects of androstenedione supplementation in healthy young males. *Canadian Journal of Applied Physiology* 25: 68-78.

Ballor, D.L., Becque, M.D., and Katch, V.L. 1987. Metabolic responses during hydraulic resistance exercise. *Medicine and Science in Sports and Exercise* 19: 363-367.

Bamman, M.M., Hunger, G.R., Newton, L.E., Roney, R.K., and Khaled, M.A. 1993. Changes in body composition, diet, and strength of body builders during the 12 weeks prior to competition. *Journal of Sports Medicine and Physical Fitness* 33: 383-391.

Bamman, M.M., Shipp, J.R., Jiang, J., Gower, B.A., Hunter, G.R., Goodman, A., McLafferty, C.L. Jr., and Urban, R.J. 2001. Mechanical load increases muscle IGF-I and androgen receptor mRNA concentrations in humans. *American Journal of Physiology: Endocrinology and Metabolism* 280: E383-E390.

Barbosa, A.R., Santarem, J.M., Filho, W.J., Marucci, M.D.N. 2002. Effects of resistance training on the sit-and-reach test in elderly women. *Journal of Strength and Conditioning Research* 16: 14-18.

Barker, M., Wyatt, T.J., Johnson, R.L., Stone, M.H., O'Bryant, H.S., Poe, C., and Kent, M. 1993. Performance factors, psychological assessment, physical characteristics, and football playing ability. *Journal of Strength and Conditioning Research* 7: 224-233.

Barnett, L.S. 1985. Little league shoulder syndrome: Proximal humeral epiphyseolysis in adolescent baseball pictures. *Journal of Bone and Joint Surgery* 7A: 495-496.

Bartholomeu, S.A. 1985. Plyometrics and vertical jump training. Master's thesis, University of North Carolina, Chapel Hill.

Bass, A., Mackova, E., and Vitek, V. 1973. Activity of some enzymes of energy supplying metabolism in rat soleus after tenotomy of synergistic muscles and in contralateral control muscle. *Physiologica Bohemoslovaca* 22: 613-621.

Bass, S.L. 2000. The prepubertal years: A unique opportune stage of growth when the skeleton is most responsive to exercise? *Sports Medicine* 30: 73-70.

Bassey, E.J., Fiatarone, M.A., O'Neil, E.F., Kelly, M., Evans, W.J., and Lipsitz, L.A. 1992. Leg extensor power and functional performance in very old men and women. *Clinical Science* 82: 321-327.

Bassey, E.J., and Harries, U.J. 1993. Normal values for hand-grip strength in 920 men and women aged over 65 years, and longitudinal changes over 4 years in 620 survivors. *Clinical Science* 84: 331-337.

Bastiaans, J.J., van Diemen, A.B., Veneberg, T., and Jeukendrup, A.E. 2001. The effects of replacing a portion of endurance training by explosive strength training on performance in trained cyclists. *European Journal of Applied Physiology* 86: 79-84.

Bauer, T., Thayer, R.E., and Baras, G. 1990. Comparison of training modalities for power development in the lower extremity. *Journal of Applied Sport Science Research* 4: 115-121.

Baumann, G. 1991a. Growth hormone heterogeneity: Genes, isohormones, variants, and binding proteins. *Endocrine Reviews* 12: 424-443.

Baumann, G. 1991b. Metabolism of growth hormone (GH) and different molecular forms of GH in biological fluids. *Hormone Research Supplement* 36: 5-10.

Baumgartner, T., and Wood, S. 1984. Development of shoulder-girdle strength-endurance in elementary children. *Research Quarterly for Exercise and Sport* 55: 169-171.

Beedle, B., Jesse, C., and Stone, M.H. 1991. Flexibility characteristics among athletes who weight train. *Journal of Applied Sport Science Research* 5: 150-154.

Behm, D.G., Button, D.C., and Butt, J.C. 2001. Factors affecting force loss with prolonged stretching. *Canadian Journal of Applied Physiology* 26: 261-272.

Behm, D.G., and Sale, D.G. 1993. Velocity specificity of resistance training. *Sports Medicine* 15: 374-388.

Belanger, A., and McComas, A.J. 1981. Extent of motor unit activation during effort. *Journal of Applied Physiology* 51: 1131-1135.

Bell, G.J., Petersen, S.R., Maclean I., Reid, D.C., and Quinney, H.A. 1992. Effect of high velocity resistance training on peak torque, cross sectional area and myofibrillar ATPase activity. *Journal of Sports Medicine and Physical Fitness* 32: 10-17.

Bell, G.J., Petersen, S.R., Wessel, J., Bagnall, K., and Quinney, H.A. 1991a. Adaptations to endurance and low velocity resistance training performed in a sequence. *Canadian Journal of Sport Science* 16: 186-192.

Bell, G.J., Petersen, S.R., Wessel, J., Bagnall, K., and Quinney, H.A. 1991b. Physiological adaptations to concurrent endurance training and low velocity resistance training. *International Journal of Sports Medicine* 12: 384-390.

Bell, G.J., Snydmiller, G.D., Neary, J.P., and Quinney, H.A. 1989. The effect of high and low velocity resistance training on anaerobic power output in cyclists. *Journal of Human Movement Studies* 16: 173-181.

Bell, G.J., Syrotuik, D.G., Attwood, K., and Quinney, H.A. 1993. Maintenance of strength gains while performing endurance training in oarswomen. *Journal of Applied Physiology* 18: 104-115.

Bell, G.J., Syrotuik, D., Martin, T.P., Burnham, R., and Quinney, H.A. 2000. Effect of concurrent strength and endurance training on skeletal muscle properties and hormone concentrations in humans. *European Journal of Applied Physiology* 81: 418-427.

Bemben, D.A., Fetters, N.L., Bemben, M.G., Nabavi, N., and Koh, E.T. 2000. Musculoskeletal responses to high-and low-intensity resistance training in early postmenopausal women. *Medicine and Science in Sports and Exercise* 32: 1949-1957.

Bender, J., and Kaplan, H. 1963. The multiple angle testing method for the evaluation of muscle strength. *Journal of Bone and Joint Surgery* 45A: 135-140.

Berg, A., Ringwald, G., and Keul, J. 1980. Lipoprotein-cholesterol in well-trained athletes. A preliminary communication: Reduced HDL-cholesterol in power athletes. *International Journal of Sports Medicine* 1: 137-138.

Berger, R.A. 1962a. Effect of varied weight training programs on strength. *Research Quarterly* 33: 168-181.

Berger, R.A. 1962b. Optimum repetitions for the development of strength. *Research Quarterly* 33: 334-338.

Berger, R.A. 1962c. Comparison of static and dynamic strength increases. *Research Quarterly* 33: 329-333.

Berger, R.A. 1963a. Comparative effects of three weight training programs. *Research Quarterly* 34: 396-398.

Berger, R.A. 1963b. Comparison between static training and various dynamic training programs. *Research Quarterly* 34: 131-135.

Berger, R.A. 1963c. Effects of dynamic and static training on vertical jump ability. *Research Quarterly* 34: 419-424.

Berger, R.A. 1963d. Comparison of the effect of various weight training loads on strength. *Research Quarterly* 36: 141-146.

Berger, R.A., and Hardage, B. 1967. Effect of maximum loads for each of ten repetitions on strength improvement. *Research Quarterly* 38: 715-718.

Bermon, S., Ferrari, P., Bernard, P., Altare, S., and Dolisi, C. 1999. Responses of total and free insulin-like growth factor-1 and insulin-like growth factor binding protein-3 after resistance exercise and training in elderly subjects. *Acta Physiologica Scandinavica* 165: 51-56.

Biewener, A.A., and Roberts, T.J. 2000. Muscle and tendon contributions to force, work, and elastic energy savings: A comparative perspective. *Exercise and Sport Sciences Reviews* 28: 99-107.

Binoux, M., and Hossenlopp, P. 1988. Insulin-like growth factor (IGF) and IGF-binding proteins: Comparison of human serum and lymph. *Journal of Clinical Endocrinology and Metabolism* 67: 509-514.

Biolo, G., Fleming, R.Y.D., and Wolfe, R.R. 1995. Physiologic hyperinsulinemia stimulates protein synthesis and enhances transport of selected amino acids in human skeletal muscle. *Journal of Clinical Investigation* 95: 811-819.

Biolo, G., Maggi S.P., Williams B.D., Tipton K.D., and Wolfe R.R. 1995. Increased rates of muscle protein turnover and amino acid transport after resistance exercise in humans. *American Journal of Physiology* 268: E514-E520.

Biolo, G., Tipton, K.D., Klein, S., and Wolfe, R.R. 1997. An abundant supply of amino acids enhances the metabolic effect of exercise on muscle protein. *American Journal of Physiology* 36:E122-E129.

Biolo, G., Williams B.D., Fleming R.Y., and Wolfe R.R. 1999. Insulin action on muscle protein kinetics and amino acid transport during recovery after resistance exercise. *Diabetes* 48: 949-957.

Bishop, P., Cureton, K., and Collins, M. 1987. Sex difference in muscular strength in equally trained men and women. *Ergonomics* 30: 675-687.

Blackey, J.B., and Southard, D. 1987. The combined effects of weight training and plyometrics on dynamic leg strength and leg power. *Journal of Applied Sport Science Research* 1: 14-16.

Bland, R. 2000. Steroid hormone receptor expression and action in bone. *Clinical Science* 98: 217-240.

Blanksby, B., and Gregory, J. 1981. Anthropometric, strength and physiological changes in male and female swimmers with progressive resistance training. *Australian Journal of Sport Science* 1: 3-6.

Blattner, S.E., and Noble, L. 1979. Relative effects of isokinetic and plyometric training on vertical jumping performance. *Research Quarterly* 50: 583-588.

Blessing, D., Stone, M., Byrd, R., Wilson, D., Rozenek, R., Pushparani, D., and Lipner, H. 1987. Blood lipid and hormonal changes from jogging and weight training in middle-aged men. *Journal of Applied Sport Science Research* 1: 25-29.

Blimkie, C.J.R. 1992. Resistance training during pre- and early puberty: Efficacy, trainability, mechanisms, and persistence. *Canadian Journal of Sport Sciences* 17: 264-279.

Blimkie, C.J.R. 1993. Resistance training during preadolescence issues and controversies. *Sports Medicine* 15: 389-407.

Blimkie, C.J.R., Ramsay, J., Sale, D., MacDougall, D., Smith, K., and Garner, S. 1989. Effects of 10 weeks resistance training on strength development in pre-pubertal boys. In *Children and exercise XIII*, edited by S. Oseid and K.H. Carlsen, 183-197. Champaign, IL: Human Kinetics.

Blimkie, C.J.R., Rice, S., Webber, C.E., Martin, J., Levy, D., and Gordon, C.L. 1996. Effects of resistance training on bone mineral content and density in adolescent females. *Canadian Journal of Physiology and Pharmacology* 74: 1025-1033.

Bond, V. Jr., Wang, P., Adams, R.G., Johnson, A.T., Vaccaro, P., Tearney, R.J., Millis, R.M., Franks, B.D., and Bassett, D.R. Jr. 1996. Lower leg high-intensity resistance training and peripheral hemodynamic adaptations. *Canadian Journal of Physiology* 21: 209-217.

Bonde-Peterson, F. 1960. Muscle training by static, concentric and eccentric contractions. *Acta Physiologica Scandinavica* 48: 406-416.

Bonde-Peterson, F., and Knuttgen, H.G. 1971. Effect of training with eccentric muscle contractions on human skeletal muscle metabolites. *Acta Physiologica Scandinavica* 80: 16A-17A.

Bonde-Peterson, F., Knuttgen, H.G., and Henriksson, J. 1972. Muscle metabolism during exercise with concentric and eccentric contractions. *Journal of Applied Physiology* 33: 792-795.

Bonde-Peterson, F., Mork, A.L., and Nielsen, E. 1975. Local muscle blood flow and sustained contractions of human arms and back muscles. *European Journal of Applied Physiology and Occupational Physiology* 34: 43-50.

Borges, O., and Essen-Gustavsson, B. 1989. Enzyme activities and Type I and II muscle fibers of human skeletal muscle in relation to age and torque development. *Acta Physiologica Scandinavica* 136: 29-36.

Borst, S.E., De Hoyos, D.V., Garzarella, L., Vincent, K., Pollock, B.H., Lowenthal, D.T., and Pollock, M.L. 2001. Effects of resistance training on insulin-like growth factor-I and IGF binding proteins. *Medicine and Science in Sports and Exercise* 33: 648-653.

Bosco, C., Colli, R., Bonomi, R., von Duvillard, S.P., and Viru, A. 2000. Monitoring strength training: Neuromuscular and hormonal profile. *Medicine and Science in Sports and Exercise* 32: 202-208.

Bosco, C., and Komi, P.V. 1980. Influence of aging on the mechanical behavior of leg extensor muscles. *European Journal of Applied Physiology* 45: 209-219.

Bosco, C., Montanari, G., Ribacchi, R., Giovenali, P., Latteri, F., Iachelli, G., Faina, M., Coli, R., Dal Monte, A., La Rosa, M., Cortili, G., and Saibene, F. 1987. Relationship between the efficiency of muscular work during jumping and the energetics of running. *European Journal of Applied Physiology* 56: 138-143.

Bosco, C., and Pittera, C. 1982. Zur trainings Wirkung neuentwicker Sprungubungen auf die Explosivkraft. *Leistungssport* 12: 36-39.

Bosco, C., Tarkka, I., and Komi, P.V. 1982. Effects of elastic energy and myoelectrical potentiation of triceps surae during stretch-shortening cycle exercises. *Sports Medicine* 3: 137-140.

Boyer, B.T. 1990. A comparison of the effects of three strength training programs on women. *Journal of Applied Sport Science Research* 4: 88-94.

Brady, T., Cahill, B., and Bodnar, L. 1982. Weight training related injuries in the high school athlete. *American Journal of Sports Medicine* 10: 1-5.

Brahm, H., Piehl-Aulin, K., Saltin, B., and Ljunghall, S. 1997. Net fluxes over working thigh of hormones, growth factors and biomarkers of bone metabolism during short lasting dynamic exercise. *Calcified Tissue International* 60: 175-180.

Braith, R.W., Graves, J.E., Leggett, S.H., and Pollock, M.L. 1993. Effect of training on the relationship between maximal and submaximal strength. *Medicine and Science in Sports and Exercise* 25: 132-138.

Brandonburg, J.P., and Docherty, D. 2002. The effects of accentuated eccentric loading on strength, muscle hypertrophy, and neural adaptations in trained individuals. *Journal of Strength and Conditioning Research* 16: 25-32.

Brandy, W.D., Irion, J.M., and Briggler, M. 1997. The effect of time and frequency of static stretching on flexibility of the hamstring muscles. *Physical Therapy* 77: 1090-1096.

Brandy, W.D., Irion, J.M., and Briggler, M. 1998. The effect of static stretch and dynamic range of motion training on the flexibility of the hamstring muscles. *Journal of Orthopedic Sports Physical Therapy* 27: 295-300.

Brazell-Roberts, J.V., and Thomas, L.E. 1989. Effects of weight training frequency on the self-concept of college females. *Journal of Applied Sports Science Research* 3: 40-43.

Brechue, W.F., and Abe, T. 2002. The role of FFM accumulation and skeletal muscle architecture in powerlifting performance. *European Journal of Applied Physiology* 84(4): 327-336.

Bricourt, V.A., Germain, P.S., Serrurier, B.D., and Guezeennec, C.Y. 1994. Changes in testosterone muscle receptors: Effects of an androgen treatment on physically trained rats. *Cellular and Molecular Biology* 40: 291-294.

Bright, R., Burstein, A., and Elmore, S. 1974. Epiphyseal-plate cartilage. *Journal of Bone and Joint Surgery* 56-A: 688-703.

Brill, P.A., Macera, C.A., Davis, D.R., Blair, S.N., and Gordon, N. 2000. Muscular strength and physical function. *Medicine and Science in Sports and Exercise* 32: 412-416.

Brockett, C.L., Morgan, D.L., and Proske, U. 2001. Human hamstring muscles adapt to eccentric exercise by changing optimal length. *Medicine and Science in Sports and Exercise* 33: 783-790.

Brooks, G.A., Butterfield, G.E., Wolfe, R.R., Groves, B.M., Mazzeo, R.S., Sutton, J.R., Wolfel, E.E., and Reeves, J.T. 1991. Decreased reliance on lactate during exercise after acclimatization to 4,300 m. *Journal of Applied Physiology* 71: 333-341.

Brooks, G.A., and Fahey, T.D. 1984. *Exercise physiology: Human bioenergetics and its applications.* New York: Wiley & Son.

Brooks, S., Nevill, M.E., Gaitanos, G., and Williams C. 1993. Metabolic responses to sprint training. In *Intermittent intensity exercise*, edited by D.A.D. Macleod, R.J. Maughan, C. Williams, C.R. Madeley, J.C.M. Sharp, and R.W. Nutton, 33-48. London: Taylor and Francis Group.

Brooks-Gunn, J., and Rubb, D.N. 1983. The experience of menarche from a developmental perspective. In *Girls at puberty: Biological and psychosocial perspectives,* edited by J. Brooks-Gunn and A.C. Peterson, 155-177. New York: Plenum Press.

Brose, D.E., and Hanson, D.L. 1967. Effects of overload training on velocity and accuracy of throwing. *Research Quarterly* 38: 528-533.

Brown, A.B., McCartney, N., and Sale, D.G. 1990. Positive adaptations to weight-lifting training in the elderly. *Journal of Applied Physiology* 69: 1725-1733.

Brown, B.S., Gorman, D.R., DiBrezzom, R., and Fort, I. 1988. Anaerobic power changes following short term, task specific, dynamic and static overload training. *Journal of Applied Sport Science Research* 2: 35-38.

Brown, C.H., and Wilmore, J.H. 1974. The effects of maximal resistance training on the strength and body composition of women athletes. *Medicine and Science in Sports* 6: 174-177.

Brown, G.A., Martini, E.R., Roberts, B.S., Vukovich, M.D., and King, D.S. 2002. Acute hormonal response to sublingual androstenediol intake in young men. *Journal of Applied Physiology* 92: 142-146.

Brown, L.E., Whitehurst, M., Findley, B.W., Gilbert, R., Groo, D.R., and Jimenez, J.A. 1998. Effect of repetitions and gender on acceleration range of motion during knee extension on an isokinetic device. *Journal of Strength and Conditioning Research* 12: 222-225.

Brown, S., Byrd, R., Jayasinghe, M.D., and Jones, D. 1983. Echocardiographic characteristics of competitive and recreational weight lifters. *Journal of Cardiovascular Ultrasonography* 2: 163-165.

Burke, J., Thayer, R., and Belcamino, M. 1994. Comparison of effects of two interval-training programmes on lactate and ventilatory thresholds. *British Journal of Sports Medicine* 28: 18-21.

Burst, S.E., De Hoyos, D.V., Garzarella, L., Vincent, K., Pollock, B.H., Lowenthal, D.T., and Pollock, M.L. 2001. Effect of resistance training on insulin-like growth factor-I and IGF binding proteins. *Medicine and Science in Sports and Exercise* 33: 648-653.

Bush, J.A., Kraemer, W.J., Mastro, A.M., Triplett-McBride, N.T., Volek, J.S., Putukian, M., Sebastianelli, W.J., and Knuttgen, H.G. 1999. Exercise and recovery responses of adrenal medullary neurohormones to heavy resistance exercise. *Medicine and Science in Sports and Exercise* 31: 554-559.

Butts, N.K., and Price, S. 1994. Effects of a 12-week weight training program on the body composition of women over 30 years of age. *Journal of Strength and Conditioning Research* 8: 265-269.

Byrd, S.K. 1992. Alterations in the sarcoplasmic reticulum: A possible link to exercise-induced muscle damage. *Medicine and Science in Sports and Exercise* 24: 531-536.

Byrne, H.K., and Wilmore, J.H. 2000. The effects of resistance training on resting blood pressure in women. *Journal of Strength and Conditioning Research* 14: 411-418.

Cabell, L., and Zebras, C.J. 1999. Resistive torque validation of the Nautilus multi-biceps machine. *Journal of Strength and Conditioning Research* 13: 20-23.

Caiozzo, V.J., Laird, T., Chow, K., Prietto, C.A., and McMaster, W.C. 1983. The use of precontractions to enhance the in-vivo force velocity relationship. *Medicine and Science in Sports and Exercise* 14: 162.

Caiozzo, V.J., Perrine, J.J., and Edgerton, V.R. 1981. Training-induced alterations of the in vivo force-velocity relationship of human muscle. *Journal of Applied Physiology: Respiratory, Environmental and Exercise Physiology* 51: 750-754.

Calder, A.W., Chilibeck, P.D., Webber, C.E., and Sale, D.G. 1994. Comparison of whole and split weight training routines in young women. *Canadian Journal of Applied Physiology* 19: 185-199.

Callister, R., Shealy, M.J., Fleck, S.J., and Dudley, G.A. 1988. Performance adaptations to sprint, endurance and both modes of training. *Journal of Applied Physiology* 2: 46-51.

Cameron, K.R., Wark, J.D., and Telford, R.D. 1992. Stress fractures and bone loss: The skeletal cost of intense athleticism. *Excel* 8: 39-55.

Campbell, D.E. 1967. Maintenance of strength during a season of sports participation. *American Corrective Therapy Journal* 21: 193-195.

Campbell, R.C. 1962. Effects of supplemental weight training on the physical fitness of athletic squads. *Research Quarterly* 33: 343-348.

Campbell, W.W., Crim, M.C., Young, V.R., Joseph, L.J., and Evans, W.J. 1995. Effects of resistance training and dietary protein intake on protein metabolism in older adults. *American Journal of Applied Physiology* 268: E1143-E1153.

Campbell, W.W., and Evans, W.J. 1996. Protein requirements of elderly people. *European Journal of Clinical Nutrition* 50 (Suppl): S180-S183.

Campbell, W.W., Joseph, L.J.O., Davey, S.L., Cyr-Campbell, D., Anderson, R.A., and Evans, W.J. 1999. Effects of resistance training and chromium picolinate on body composition and skeletal muscle in older men. *Journal of Applied Physiology* 86: 29-39.

Campbell, W.W., Trappe, T.A., Wolfe, R.R., and Evans, W.J. 2001. The recommended dietary allowance for protein may not be adequate for older people to maintain skeletal muscle. *Journal of Gerontology: Biological Medical Sciences* 56: M373-M380.

Cann, C.E., Martin, M.C., Genant, H.K., and Jaffe, R. 1984. Decreased spinal mineral content in amenorrheic females. *Journal of the American Medical Association* 251: 626-629.

Cannon, R., and Cafarelli, E. 1987. Neuromuscular adaptations to training. *Journal of Applied Physiology* 63: 2396-2402.

Capen, E.K. 1950. The effect of systematic weight training on power, strength and endurance. *Research Quarterly* 21: 83-93.

Capen, E.K., Bright, J.A., and Line, P.Q. 1961. The effects of weight training on strength, power, musclar endurance and anthropometric measurements on a select group of college women. *Journal of the Assocation for Physical and Mental Rehabilitation* 15: 169-173.

Carmeli, E., Coleman, R., and Reznick, A.Z. 2002. The biochemistry of aging muscle. *Experimental Gerontology* 37: 477-489.

Carolyn, B., and Cafarelli, E.1992. Adaptations in coactivation after isometric resistance training. *Journal of Applied Physiology* 73: 911-917.

Carpinelli, R.N., and Gutin, B. 1991. Effects of miometric and pliometric muscle actions on delayed muscle soreness. *Journal of Applied Sport Science Research* 5: 66-70.

Carroll, T.J., Riek, S., and Carson, R.G. 2001. Neural adaptations to resistance training implications for movement control. *Sports Medicine* 31: 829-840.

Caruso, J.F., Signorile, J.F., Perry, A.C., Clark, M., and Bamman, M.M. 1997. Time course changes in contractile strength resulting from isokinetic exercise and b2 agonist administration. *Journal of Strength and Conditioning Research* 11: 8-113.

Castro, M.J., McCann, D.J., Shaffrath, J.D., and Adams, W.C. 1995. Peak torque per unit cross-sectional area differs between strength-trained and untrained young adults. *Medicine and Science in Sports and Exercise* 27: 397-403.

Chakravati, S., and Collins, W. 1976. Hormonal profiles after menopause. *British Medical Journal* 2: 782-787.

Chandler, R.M., Byrne, H.K., Patterson, J.G., and Ivy, J.L. 1994. Dietary supplements affect the anabolic hormones after weight-training exercise. *Journal of Applied Physiology* 76: 839-845.

Chang, D.E., Buschbacker, L.P., and Edlich, R.F. 1988. Limited mobility in power lifters. *The American Journal of Sports Medicine* 16: 280-284.

Charette, S.L., McEvoy, L., Pyka,G., Snow-Harter, C., Guido, D., Wiswell, R.A., and Marcus, R. 1991. Muscle hypertrophy response to resistance training in older women. *Journal of Applied Physiology* 70: 1912-1916.

Chesley, A., MacDougall, J.D., Tarnopolsky, M.A., Atkinson, S.A., and Smith, K. 1992. Changes in human muscle protein synthesis after resistance exercise. *Journal of Applied Physiology* 73: 1383-1388.

Chilibeck, P.D., Calder, A.W., Sale, D.G., and Webber, C.E. 1998. A comparison of strength and muscle mass increases during resistance training in young women. *European Journal of Applied Physiology* 77: 170-175.

Chilibeck, P.D., Sale, D.G., and Webber, C.E. 1995. Exercise and bone mineral density. *Sports Medicine* 19: 103-122.

Chilibeck, P.D., Syrotuik, D.G., and Bell, G.J. 1999. The effect of strength training on estimates of mitochondrial density and distribution throughout muscle fibers. *European Journal of Applied Physiology* 80: 604-609.

Chilibeck, P.D., Syrotuik, D.G., and Bell, G.J. 2002. The effect of concurrent endurance and strength training on quantitative estimates of subsarcolemmal and intermyofibrillar mitochondria. *International Journal of Sports Medicine* 23: 33-39.

Chow, J.C., Ling, P.R., Qu, Z., Laviola, L., Ciccarone, A., Bistrian, B.R., and Smith, R.J. 1996. Growth hormone stimulates tyrosine phosphorylation of JAK2 and STAT5, but not IRS-1 or SHC proteins in liver and skeletal muscle of normal rats *in vivo*. *Endocrinology* 137: 2880-2886.

Chow, J.W.M. 2000. Role of nitrate oxide and prostaglandins in the bone formation response to mechanical loading. *Exercise and Sport Sciences Reviews* 28: 185-188.

Chow, R.S., Medri, M.K., Martin, D.C., Leekam, R.N., Agur, A.M., and McKee, N.H. 2000. Sonographic studies of human soleus and gastrocnemius muscle architecture: Gender variability. *European Journal of Applied Physiology* 82: 236-244.

Chromiak, J.A., and Mulvaney, D.R. 1990. A review: The effects of combined strength and endurance training on strength development. *Journal of Applied Sport Science Research* 4: 55-60.

Chu, E. 1950. The effect of systematic weight training on athletic power. *Research Quarterly* 21: 188-194.

Church, J.B., Wiggins, M.S., Moode, F.M., and Crist, R. 2001. Effect of warm-up and flexibility treatments on vertical jump performance. *Journal of Strength and Conditioning Research* 15: 332-336.

Cirello, V.M., Holden, W.C., and Evans, W.J. 1983. The effects of two isokinetic training regimens on muscle strength and fiber composition. In *Biochemistry of exercise*, edited by H.G. Knuttgen, J.A. Vogel, and S. Poortmans, 787-793. Champaign, IL: Human Kinetics.

Claassen, H., Gerber, C., Hoppeler, H., Luthi, J.M., and Vock, P. 1989. Muscle filament spacing and short-term heavy-resistance exercise in humans. *Journal of Physiology* 409: 491-495.

Clark, S., Christiansen, A., Hellman, H.F., Hugunin, J.W., and Hurst, K.M. 1999. Effects of ipsilateral anterior thigh soft tissue stretching on passive unilateral and straight-leg raise. *Journal of Orthopedic Sports Physical Therapy* 29: 4-9.

Clarke, D.H. 1973. Adaptations in strength and muscular endurance resulting from exercise. *Exercise and Sport Sciences Reviews* 1: 73-102.

Clarke, D.H. 1986. Sex differences in strength and fatigability. *Research Quarterly* 571: 44-49.

Clarkson, P.M., Nosaka, K., and Braun, B. 1992. Muscle function after exercise-induced muscle damage and rapid adaptation. *Medicine and Science in Sports and Exercise* 24: 512-520.

Clarkson, P.M., and Tremblay, I. 1988. Exercise-induced muscle damage, repair and adaptation in humans. *Journal of Applied Physiology* 65: 1-6.

Clutch, D., Wilson, C., McGown, C., and Bryce, G.R. 1983. The effect of depth jumps and weight training on leg strength and vertical jump. *Research Quarterly* 54: 5-10.

Colan, S., Sanders, S.P., and Borrow, K.M. 1987. Physiologic hypertrophy: Effects on left ventricular systolic mechanisms in athletes. *Journal of the American College of Cardiology* 9: 776-783.

Colan, S., Sanders, S.P., McPherson, D., and Borrow, K.M. 1985. Left ventricular diastolic function in elite athletes with physiologic cardiac hypertrophy. *Journal of the American College of Cardiology* 6: 545-549.

Colduck, C.T., and Abernathy, P.J. 1997. Changes and surface EMG of biceps brachii with increasing velocity of eccentric contraction in women. *Journal of Strength and Conditioning Research* 11: 50-56.

Coleman, A.E. 1977. Nautilus vs. Universal gym strength training in adult males. *American Corrective Therapy Journal* 31: 103-107.

Collett-Solberg, P.F., and Cohen, P. 1996. The role of the insulin-like growth factor binding proteins and the IGFBP proteases in modulating IGF action. *Endocrinology and Metabolism Clinics of North America* 25: 591-614.

Colliander, E.B., and Tesch, P. 1988. Blood pressure in resistance-trained athletes. *Canadian Journal of Sports Science* 13: 31-34.

Colliander, E.B., and Tesch, P.A. 1989. Bilateral eccentric and concentric torque of quadriceps and hamstring in females and males. *European Journal of Applied Physiology* 59: 227-232.

Colliander, E.B., and Tesch, P.A. 1990a. Effects of eccentric and concentric muscle actions in resistance training. *Acta Physiologica Scandinavica* 140: 31-39.

Colliander, E.B., and Tesch, P.A. 1990b. Responses to eccentric and concentric resistance training and females and males. *Acta Physiologica Scandinavica* 141: 149-156.

Collins, H.R., and Evarts, C.M. 1971. Injuries to the adolescent athlete. *Post-graduate Medicine* 49: 72-70.

Collins, M.A., Cureton, K.J., Hill, D.W., and Ray, C.A. 1989. Relation of plasma volume change to intensity of weight lifting. *Medicine and Science in Sports and Exercise* 21: 178-185.

Conale, S.T., and Belding, R.H. 1980. Osteochondral lesions of the talus. *Journal of Bone and Joint Surgery* 62A: 97-102.

Conley, M.S., Stone, M.H., Nimmons, M., and Dudley, G.A. 1997. Resistance training and human cervical muscle recruitment plasticity. *Journal of Applied Physiology* 83: 2105-2111.

Conroy, B., and Earle, R.W. 2000. Bone, muscle, and connective tissue adaptations to physical activity. In *Essentials of strength training and conditioning, second edition*, edited by T. Baechle and R.W. Earle. Champaign, IL: Human Kinetics.

Conroy, B.P., Kraemer, W.J., Maresh, C.M., and Dalsky, G.P. 1992. Adaptive responses of bone to physical activity. *Medicine, Exercise, Nutrition, and Health* 1: 64-74.

Conroy, B.P., Kraemer, W.J., Maresh, C.M., Dalsky, G.P., Fleck, S.J., Stone, M.H., Miller, P., and Fry, A.C. 1993. Bone mineral density in elite junior weightlifters. *Medicine and Science in Sports and Exercise* 25: 1103-1109.

Consitt, L.A., Copeland, J.L., and Tremblay, M.S. 2001. Hormone responses to resistance vs. endurance exercise in premenopausal females. *Canadian Journal of Applied Physiology* 26: 574-587.

Constantini, N.W. 1994. Clinical consequences of athletic amenorrheic. *Sports Medicine* 17: 213-223.

Copeland, K.C., Underwood, L.E., and Van Wyk, J.J. 1980. Induction of immunoreactive somatomedin-C in human serum by growth hormone: Dose response relationships and effect on chromatographic profiles. *Journal of Clinical Endocrinology and Metabolism* 50: 690-697.

Corder, K.P., Potteiger, J.A., Nau, K.L., Feigoni, S.E., and Hershberger, S.L. 2000. Effects of active and passive recovery conditions on blood lactate, rating of perceived exertion, and performance during resistance exercise. *Journal of Strength and Conditioning Research* 14: 151-156.

Cordova, M.L., Ingersoll, C.D., Kovaleski, J.E., and Knight, K.l. 1995. A comparison of isokinetic and isotonic predictions of a functional task. *Journal of Athletic Training* 30: 319-322.

Cornelius, W.L. 1985. Flexibility: The effective way. *National Strength and Conditioning Association Journal* 7: 62-64.

Cornelius, W.L., Ebrahim, K., Watson, J., and Hill, D.W. 1992. The effects of cold application and modified PNF stretching techniques on hip joint flexibility in college males. *Research Quarterly for Exercise and Sport* 63: 311-314.

Cornu, C., Almeida Silveira, M.I., and Goubel, F. 1997. Influence of plyometric training on the mechanical impedance of the human ankle joint. *European Journal of Applied Physiology* 76: 282-288.

Costill, D.L., Coyle, E.F., Fink, W.F., Lesmes, G.R., and Witzmann, F.A. 1979. Adaptations in skeletal muscle following strength training. *Journal of Applied Physiology: Respiratory, Environmental and Exercise Physiology* 46: 96-99.

Cote, C., Simoneau, J.A., Lagasse, P., Boulay, M., Thibault, M.C., Marcotte, M., and Bouchard, C. 1988. Isokinetic strength training protocols: Do they induce skeletal muscle fiber hypertrophy? *Archives of Physical Medicine and Rehabilitation* 69: 281-285.

Coyle, E.F., Feiring, D.C., Rotkis, T.C., Cote, R.W., Roby, F.B., Lee, W., and Wilmore, J.H. 1981. Specificity of power improvements through slow and fast isokinetic training. *Journal of Applied Physiology* 51: 1437-1442.

Craig, B.W., Brown, R., and Everhart, J. 1989. Effects of progressive resistance training on growth hormone and testosterone levels in young and elderly subjects. *Mechanisms of Ageing and Development* 49: 159-169.

Craig, B.W., and Kang, H. 1994. Growth hormone release following single versus multiple sets of back squats: Total work versus power. *Journal of Strength and Conditioning Research* 8: 270-275.

Crist, D.M., Peake, G.T., Egan, P.A., and Waters, D.L. 1988. Body composition responses to exogenous GH during training in highly conditioned adults. *Journal of Applied Physiology* 65: 579-584.

Crowley, M.A., and Matt, K.S. 1996. Hormonal regulation of skeletal muscle hypertrophy in rats: The testosterone to cortisol ratio. *European Journal of Applied Physiology* 73: 66-72.

Cumming, D.C., Wall, S.R., Galbraith, M.A., and Belcastro, A.N. 1987. Reproductive hormone responses to resistance training. *Medicine and Science in Sports and Exercise* 19: 234-238.

Cuneo, R.C., Salomon, F., Wiles, C.M., Hesp, R., and Sonksen, P.H. 1991. Growth hormone treatment in growth hormone-deficient adults. I. Effects on muscle mass and strength. *Journal of Applied Physiology* 70: 688-694.

Cureton, K.J., Collins, M.A., Hill, D.W., and McElhannon, F.M. 1988. Muscle hypertrophy in men and women. *Medicine and Science in Sports and Exercise* 20: 338-344.

Dale, E., Gerlach, D., and Wilhite, A. 1979. Menstrual dysfunction in distance runners. *Obstetrics and Gynecology* 54: 47-53.

Dalton, S.E. 1992. Overuse injuries and adolescent athletes. *Sports Medicine* 13: 58-70.

Dalsky, G.P., Stocke, K.S., Ehasani, A.A., Slatpolsky, E., Lee, W.C., and Birge, S. 1988. Weight-bearing exercise training and lumbar bone mineral content in post menopausal female. *Annuals of Internal Medicine* 108: 824-828.

Damon, S.E., Haugk, K.L., Birnbaum, R.S., and Quinn, L.S. 1998. Retrovirally mediated overexpression of insulin-like growth factor binding protein 4: Evidence that insulin-like growth factor is required for skeletal muscle differentiation. *Journal of Cell Physiology* 175: 109-120.

Danneskoild-Samsoe, B., Kofod, V., Munter, J., Grimby, G., and Schnohr, P. 1984. Muscle strength and functional capacity in 77-81 year old men and women. *European Journal of Applied Physiology* 52: 123-135.

Darden, E. 1973. Weight training systems in the U.S.A. *Journal of Physical Education* 44: 72-80.

Davies, A.H. 1977. Chronic effects of isokinetic and allokinetic training on muscle force, endurance, and muscular hypertrophy. *Dissertation Abstracts International* 38: 153A.

Davies, B.N., Greenwood, E.J., and Jones, S.R. 1988. Gender differences in the relationship of performance in the handgrip and standing long jump tests to lean limb volume in young adults. *European Journal of Applied Physiology* 58: 315-320.

Davies, C.T.M., and Young, K. 1983. Effects of training at 30 and 100% maximal isometric force on the contractile properties of the triceps surae of man. *Journal of Physiology* 36: 22-23.

Davies, J., Parker, D.F., Rutherford, O.M., and Jones, D.A. 1988. Changes in strength and cross sectional area of the elbow flexors as a result of isometric strength training. *European Journal of Applied Physiology* 57: 667-670.

Dawood, M.Y. 1983. Dysmenorrhea. *Clinical Obstetrics and Gynecology* 26: 719-727.

Dawson, B., Goodman, C., Lawrence, S., Preen, D., Polglaze, T., Fitzsimons, M., and Fourier, P. 1997. Muscle phosphocreatine repletion following single and repeated short sprint efforts. *Scandinavian Journal of Medicine and Science in Sports* 7: 206-213.

DeCree, C., Vermeulen, A., and Ostyn, M. 1991. Are high-performance young women athletes doomed to become low-performance old wives? A reconsideration of the increased risk of osteoporosis in amenorrheic women. *Journal of Sports Medicine and Physical Fitness* 31: 108-114.

DeKoning, F.L., Binkhorst, R.A., Vissers, A.C.A., and Vos, J.A. 1982. Influence of static strength training on the force-velocity relationship of the arm flexors. *International Journal of Sports Medicine* 3: 25-28.

Deligiannis, A., Zahopoulou, E., and Mandroukas, K. 1988. Echocardiographic study of cardiac dimensions and function in weight lifters and body builders. *International Journal of Sports Cardiology* 5: 24-32.

Delorme, T.L., Ferris, B.G., and Gallagher, J.R. 1952. Effect of progressive exercise on muscular contraction time. *Archives of Physical Medicine* 33: 86-97.

Delorme, T.L., and Watkins, A.L. 1948. Techniques of progressive resistance exercise. *Archives of Physical Medicine* 29: 263-273.

DeLuca, C.J., Lefever, R.S., McCue, M.P., and Xenakis, A.P. 1982. Behavior of human motor units in different muscles during linearly varying contractions. *Journal of Physiology* 329: 113-128.

DeMeyts, P., Wallach, B., Christoffersen, C.T., Ursø, B., Grønskov, K., Latus, L.J., Yakushiji, F., Ilondo, M.M., and Shymko, R.M. 1994. The insulin-like growth factor-I receptor. *Hormone Research* 42: 152-169.

DeMichele, P.D., Pollock, M.L., Graves, J.E., Foster, D.N., Carpenter, D., Garzarella, L., Brehue, W., and Fulton, M. 1997. Isometric dorsal rotations strength: Effective training frequency on its development. *Archives of Physiology and Medical Rehabilitation* 78: 64-69.

DeRenne, C., Hetzler, R.K., Buxton, B.P., and Ho, K.W. 1996. Effects of training frequency on strength maintenance in pubescent baseball players. *Journal of Strength and Conditioning Research* 10: 8-14.

DeRenne, C., Ho, K., and Blitzblau, A. 1990. Effects of weighted implement training on throwing velocity. *Journal of Sport Science Research* 4: 16-19.

Deschenes, M.R., Judelson, D.A., Kraemer, W.J., Meskaitis, V.J., Volek, J.S., Nindl, B.C., Harman, F.S., and Deaver, D.R. 2000. Effects of resistance training on neuromuscular junction morphology. *Muscle Nerve* 10: 1576-1581.

Deschenes, M.R., Maresh, C.M., Armstrong, L.E., Covault, J., Kraemer, W.J., and Crivello J.F. 1994. Endurance and resistance exercise induce muscle fiber type specific responses in androgen binding capacity. *Journal of Steroid Biochemistry and Molecular Biology* 50: 175-179.

Deschenes, M.R., Maresh, C.M., Crivello, J.F., Armstrong, L.E., Kraemer, W.J., and Covault, J. 1993. The effects of exercise training of different intensities on neuromuscular junction morphology. *Journal of Neurocytology* 22: 603-615.

Desmedt, J.E. 1981. The size principle of motorneuron recruitment in ballistic or ramp-voluntary contractions in man. In *Progress in clinical neurophysiology*. Vol. 9, *Motor unit types, recruitment and plasticity in health and disease*, edited by J.E. Desmedt, 250-304. Basel: Karger.

Desmedt, J.E., and Godaux, E. 1977. Ballistic contractions in man: Characteristic recruitment pattern of single motor units of the tibialis muscle. *Journal of Physiology* 264: 673-694.

DeSouza, M.J., and Metzger, D.A. 1991. Reproductive dysfunction in amenorrheic athletes and anorexia patients: A review. *Medicine and Science in Sports and Exercise* 23: 995-1007.

DeVries, H.A. 1980. *Physiology of exercise for physical education and athletics*. Dubuque: Brown.

Diallo, O., Dore, E., Duche, P., and Van Praagh, E. 2001. Effects of plyometric training followed by a reduced training programme on physical performance in prepubescent soccer players. *Journal of Sports Medicine and Physical Fitness* 41: 342-348.

Dickerman, R.D., Pertusi, R., and Smith, G.H. 2000. The upper range of lumber spine bench bone mineral density? An examination of the current world record holder in the squat lift. *International Journal of Sports Medicine* 21: 469-470.

Dickhuth, H.H., Simon, G., Kindermann, W., Wildberg, A., and Keul, J. 1979. Echocardiographic studies on athletes of various sport-types and non-athletic persons. *Zeitschrift fur Kardiologie* 68: 449-453.

DiPrampero, P.E., and Margaria, R. 1978. Relationship between O_2 consumption, high energy phosphates and the kinetics of the O_2 debt in exercise. *Pflugers Archives* 304: 11-19.

Doan, B.K., Newton, R.U., Marsit, J.L., Triplett-McBride, N.T., Kozaris, L.P., Fry, A.C., and Kraemer, W.J. 2002. The effects of increased eccentric loading on bench press. *Journal of Strength and Conditioning Research* 16: 9-13.

Docherty, D., Wenger, H.A., Collis, M.L., and Quinney, H.A. 1987. The effects of variable speed resistance training on strength development in prepubertal boys. *Journal of Human Movement Studies* 13: 377-382.

Doherty, T.J., Vandervoort, A.A., Taylor, A.W., and Brown, W.F. 1993. Effects of motor unit losses on strength in older men and women. *Journal of Applied Physiology* 74: 868-874.

Dohm, G.L., Williams, R.T., Kasperek, G.J., and Van, R.J. 1982. Increased excretion of urea and N tanmethylhistidine by rats and humans after a bout of exercise. *Journal of Applied Physiology* 64: 350-353.

Donnelly, A.E., Clarkson, P.M., and Maughan, R.J. 1992. Exercise-induced muscle damage: Effects of light exercise on damaged muscle. *European Journal of Applied Physiology* 64: 350-353.

Doolittle, R.L., and Engebretsen, J. 1972. Performance variations during the menstrual cycle. *Journal of Sports Medicine and Physical Fitness* 12:54-58.

Dornemann, T.M., McMurray, R.G., Renner, J.B., and Anderson, J.J.B. 1997. Effects of high-intensity resistance exercise on bone mineral density and muscle strength of 40-50-year-old women. *Journal of Sports Medicine and Physical Fitness* 37: 246-251.

Drinkwater, B.L. 1984. Women and exercise: physiological aspects. In *Exercise and sport science reviews*, edited by R.L. Terjung, 21-52. Lexington, KY: MAL Callamore Press.

Drinkwater, B.L., Bruemmer, B., and Chestnut, III., C.H. 1990. Menstrual history as determinant of current bone density in young athletes. *Journal of the American Medical Association* 263: 545-548.

Duchateau, J., and Hainaut, K. 1984. Isometric and dynamic training: Differential effects on mechanical properties of a human muscle. *Journal of Applied Physiology* 56: 296-301.

Dudley, G.A., and Djamil, R. 1985. Incompatibility of endurance and strength training modes of exercise. *Journal of Applied Physiology* 59: 1446-1451.

Dudley, G.A., and Fleck, S.J. 1987. Strength and endurance training: Are they mutually exclusive? *Sports Medicine* 4: 79-85.

Dudley, G.A., and Harris, R.T. 1992. Use of electrical stimulation in strength and power training. In *Strength and power in sport*, edited by P.V. Komi, 329-337. Oxford: Blackwell Scientific.

Dudley, G.A., Harris, R.T., Duvoisin, M.R., Hather, B.M., and Buchanan, P. 1990. Effect of voluntary vs. artificial activation on the relationship of muscle torque to speed. *Journal of Applied Physiology* 69: 2215-2221.

Dudley, G.A., Tesch, P.A., Miller, B.J., and Buchannan, P. 1991. Importance of eccentric actions in performance adaptations to resistance training. *Aviation, Space, and Environmental Medicine* 62: 543-550.

Earles, D.R., Judge, J.O., and Gunnarsson, O.T. 2001. Velocity training induces power-specific adaptations in highly functioning older adults. *Archives of Physical Medicine and Rehabilitation* 82: 872-878.

Ebben, W.P., and Blackard, D.O. 2001. Strength and conditioning practices of national football league strength and conditioning coaches. *Journal of Strength and Conditioning Research* 15: 48-58.

Ebbling, C.B., and Clarkson, P.M. 1989. Exercise-induced muscle damage and adaptation. *Sports Medicine* 7: 207-234.

Ebbling, C.B., and Clarkson, P.M. 1990. Muscle adaptation prior to recovery following eccentric exercise. *European Journal of Applied Physiology* 60: 26-31.

Edgerton, V.R. 1978. Mammalian muscle fiber types and their adaptability. *American Physiology* 60: 26-31.

Edwards, R.H.T., Hill, D.K., and McDonnell, M.N. 1972. Monothermal and intramuscular pressure measurements during isometric contractions of the human quadriceps muscle. *Journal of Physiology* 224: 58-59.

Effron, M.B. 1989. Effects of resistance training on left ventricular function. *Medicine and Science in Sports and Exercise* 21: 694-697.

Elkins, R. 1990. Measurement of free hormones in blood. *Endocrine Reviews* 11: 5-45.

Ellenbecker, T.S., Davies, G.J., and Rowinski, M.J. 1988. Concentric versus eccentric isokinetic strengthening of the rotator cuff. *The American Journal of Sports Medicine* 16: 64-69.

Ellias, B.A., Berg, K.E., Latin, R.W., Mellion, M.B., and Hofschire, P.J. 1991. Cardiac structure and function in weight trainers, runners, and runner/weight trainers. *Research Quarterly for Exercise and Sport* 62: 326-332.

Elliot, B.C., Wilson, G.J., and Kerr, G.K. 1989. A biomechanical analysis of the sticking region in the bench press. *Medicine and Science in Sports and Exercise* 21: 450-462.

Elliot, D.L., and Goldberg, L. 1983. Weight lifting and amenorrhea. *Journal of the American Medical Association* 249: 354.

Elliot, D.L., Goldberg, L., Kuehl, K.S., and Katlin, D.H. 1987. Characteristics of anabolic-androgenic steroid-free, competitive male and female body builders. *Physician in Sportsmedicine* 15: 169-179.

Eloranta, V., and Komi, P.V. 1980. Function of the quadriceps femoris muscle under maximal concentric and eccentric contraction. *EMG and Clinical Neurophysiology* 20: 159-174.

Engels, H.J., Drouin, J., Zhu, W., and Kazmierski, J.F. 1998. Effects of low-impact, moderate-intensity exercise training with and without wrist weights on functional capacities and mood states in older adults. *Gerontology* 44: 239-244.

Escamilla, R.F., Fleisig, G.S., Zheng, N., Lander, J.E., Barrentine, S.W., Andrews, J.R., Bergemann, B.W., and Moorman, C.T. III. 2001. Effects of technique variations on knee biomechanics during the squat and leg press. *Medicine and Science in Sports and Exercise* 33: 1552-1566.

Esmarck, B., Andersen, J.L., Olsen, S., Richter, E.A., Mizuno, M., and Kjaer, M. 2001. Timing of postexercise protein intake is important for muscle hypertrophy with resistance exercise in elderly humans. *Journal of Physiology* 535: 301-311.

Essen, B., Jansson, E., Henriksson, J., Taylor, A.W., and Saltin, B. 1975. Metabolic characteristics of fiber types in human skeletal muscle. *Acta Physiologica Scandinavica* 95: 153-165.

Etnyre, B.R., and Lee, E.J. 1987. Comments on proprioceptive neuromuscular facilitation. *Research Quarterly for Exercise and Sport* 58: 184-188.

Etnyre, B.R., and Lee, E.J. 1988. Chronic and acute flexibility of men and women using three different stretching techniques. *Research Quarterly for Exercise and Sport* 59: 222-228.

Evans, W.J., and Campbell, W.W. 1993. Sarcopenia and age-related changes in body composition and functional capacity. In: Symposium: Aging and body composition: Technological advances and physiological interrelationships. *Journal of Nutrition* 123: 465-468.

Ewing, J.L., Wolfe, D.R., Rogers, M.A., Amundson, M.L., and Stull, G.A. 1990. Effects of velocity of isokinetic training on strength, power, and quadriceps muscle fibre characteristics. *European Journal of Applied Physiology* 61: 159-162.

Exner, G.U., Staudte, H.W., and Pette, D. 1973. Isometric training of rats: Effects upon fats and slow muscle and modification by an anabolic hormone in female rats. *Pflugers Archives* 345: 1-4.

Fahey, T.D., Akka, L., and Rolph, R. 1975. Body composition and VO_2max of exceptional weight trained athletes. *Journal of Applied Physiology* 39: 559-561.

Fahey, T.D., and Brown, H. 1973. The effects of an anabolic steroid on the strength, body composition, and endurance of college males when accompanied by a weight training program. *Medicine and Science in Sports* 5: 272-276.

Fahey, T.D., Rolph, R., Moungmee, P., Nagel, J., and Mortara, S. 1976. Serum testosterone, body composition and strength of young adults. *Medicine and Science in Sports* 8: 31-34.

Faigenbaum, A.D., Larosa Loud, R., O'Connell, J., Glover, S., O'Connell, J., and Westscott, W.L. 2001. Effects of different resistance training protocols on upper-body strength and endurance development in children. *Journal of Strength and Conditioning Research* 15: 459-465.

Faigenbaum, A.D., Skrinar, G.S., Cesare, W.F., Kraemer, W.J., and Thomas, H.E. 1990. Physiologic and symptomatic responses of cardiac patients to resistance exercise. *Archives of Physical Medicine and Rehabilitation* 71: 395-398.

Faigenbaum, A.D., Westcott, W.L., Larosa Loud, R., and Long, C. 1999. The effects of different resistance training protocols on muscular strength and endurance development in children. *Pediatrics* 104: 1-7.

Faigenbaum, A.D., Westcott, W.L., Micheli, L.J., Outerbridge, A.R., Long, C.J., LaRosa-Loud, R., and Zaichkowsky, L.D. 1996. The effects of strength training and detraining on children. *Journal of Strength and Conditioning Research* 10: 109-114.

Faigenbaum, A.D., Zaichowsky, L., Westcott, W., Micheli, L., and Fehandt, A. 1993. The effects of a twice per week strength training program on children. *Pediatrics Exercise Science* 5: 339-346.

Faigenbaum, M.S., and Pollock, M.L. 1997. Strength training: Rationale for current guidelines for adult fitness programs. *Physician and Sportsmedicine* 25: 44-64.

Falk, B., and Mor, G. 1996. The effects of resistance and martial arts training in total 6- to 8-year-old-boys. *Pediatrics Exercise Science* 8: 48-56.

Falk, B., and Tenenbaum, G. 1996. The effectiveness of resistance training in children: A meta-analysis. *Sports Medicine* 22: 176-186.

Falkel, J.E., Fleck, S.J., and Murray, T.F. 1992. Comparison of central hemodynamics between powerlifters and body builders during exercise. *Journal of Applied Sport Science Research* 6: 24-35.

Falkel, J.E., Sawka, M.N., Levine, L., and Pandolf, K.B. 1985. Upper to lower body muscular strength and endurance ratios for women and men. *Ergonomics* 28: 1661-1670.

Fano, G., Mecocci, P., Vecchiet, J., Belia, S., Fulle, S., Polidori, M.C., Felzani, G., Senin, U., Vecchiet, L., and Beal M.F. 2001. Age and sex influence on oxidative damage and functional status in human skeletal muscle. *Journal of Muscle Research Cell Motility* 22: 345-351.

Fardy, P.S. 1977. *Toward an understanding of human performance*, edited by E.J. Burke, 10-14. Ithaca: Movement Press.

Fardy, P.S., Maresh, C.M., Abbott, R., and Kristiansen, T. 1976. An assessment of the influence of habitual physical activity, prior sport participation, smoking habits and aging upon indices of cardiovascular fitness: Preliminary report of a cross-section and retrospective study. *Journal of Sports Medicine and Physical Fitness* 16: 77-90.

Farley, C.T., Blickhan, R., Saito, J., and Taylor, C.R. 1991. Hopping frequency in humans: A test of how springs set stride frequency in bouncing gaits. *Journal of Applied Physiology* 71: 2127-2132.

Farrell, P.A., Hernandez, J.M., Fedele, M.J., Vary, T.C., Kimball, S.R., and Jefferson, L.S. 2000. Eukaryotic initiation factors and protein synthesis after resistance exercise in rats. *Journal of Applied Physiology* 88: 1036-1042.

Fatouros, I.G., Jamurtas, A.Z., Leontsini, D., Taxildaris, K., Kostopoulos, N., and Buckenmeyer, P. 2000. Evaluation of plyometric exercise training, weight training, and their combination on vertical jump in performance and leg strength. *Journal of Strength and Conditioning Research* 14: 470-476.

Fatouros, I.G., Taxildaris, K., Tokmakidis, S.P., Kalapotharakos, V., Aggelousis, N., Athanasopoulos, S., Zeeris, I., and Katrabasas, I. 2002. The effects of strength training, cardiovascular training and their combination on flexibility of inactive older adults. *International Journal of Sports Medicine* 23: 112-119.

Faulkner, J.A., Claflin, D.R., and McCully, K.K. 1986. Power output of fast and slow fibers from human skeletal muscles. In *Human muscle power*, edited by N.L. Jones, N. McCartney, and A.J. McComas, 88. Champaign, IL: Human Kinetics.

Felici, F., Rosponi, A., Sbriccoli, P., Filligoi, G.C., Fattorini, L., and Marchetti, M. 2001. Linear and non-linear analysis of surface electromyograms in weightlifters. *European Journal of Applied Physiology* 84: 337-342.

Fiatrone, M.A., and Evans, W.J. 1993. The etiology and reversibility of muscle function in the aged. *Journal of Gerontology* 48: 77-83.

Fiatarone, M.A., Marks, E.C., Ryan, N.D., Meredith, C.N., Lipsitz, L.A., and Evans, W.J. 1990. High-intensity strength training in nonagenarians. Effects on skeletal muscle. *Journal of the American Medical Association* 263: 3029-3034.

Fiatarone, M.A., O'Neill, E.F., Ryan, N.D., Clements, K.M., Solares, G.R., Nelson, M.E., Roberts, S.B., Kehayias, J.J., Lipsitz, L.A., and Evans, W.J. 1994. Exercise training and nutritional supplementation for physical frailty in very elderly people. *The New England Journal of Medicine* 330: 1769-1775.

Finni, T., Ikegawa, S., and Komi, P.V. 2001. Concentric force enhancement during human movement. *Acta Physiologica Scandinavica* 173: 369-377.

Fleck, S.J. 1983. Bridging the gap: Interval training physiological basis. *NSCA Journal* 5: 40: 57-62.

Fleck, S.J. 1988. Cardiovascular adaptations to resistance training. *Medicine and Science in Sports and Exercise* 20: S146-S151.

Fleck, S.J. 1998. *Successful long-term weight training*. Chicago: NTP/Contemporary Publishing Group, Inc.

Fleck, S.J. 1999. Periodized strength training: A critical review. *Journal of Strength and Conditioning Research* 13: 82-89.

Fleck, S.J. 2002. Cardiovascular responses to strength training. In *Strength & power in sport*, edited by P.V. Komi, 387-406. Oxford: Blackwell Science.

Fleck, S.J., Bartels, R., Fox, E.L., and Kraemer, W. 1982. Isokinetic total work increases and peak force training cut-off points. *National Strength and Conditioning Association Journal* 4 (2): 20-21.

Fleck, S.J., Bennett, J.B. III, Kraemer, W.J., and Baechle, T.R. 1989. Left ventricular hypertrophy in highly strength trained males. *Sports Cardiology 2nd International Conference Volume Two*, pp. 303-311.

Fleck, S.J., Case, S., Puhl, J., and Van Handle, P. 1985. Physical and physiological characteristics of elite women volleyball players. *Canadian Journal of Applied Sport Science* 10: 122-126.

Fleck, S.J., and Dean, L.S. 1987. Previous resistance-training experience and the pressor response during resistance exercise. *Journal of Applied Physiology* 63: 116-120.

Fleck, S.J., Henke, C., and Wilson, W. 1989. Cardiac MRI of elite junior Olympic weight lifters. *International Journal of Sports Medicine* 10: 329-333.

Fleck, S.J., and Kontor, K. 1986. Complex training. *National Strength and Conditioning Association Journal* 8: 66-69.

Fleck, S.J., and Schutt, R.C. 1985. Types of strength training. *Clinics in Sports Medicine* 4:159-169.

Florini, J.R. 1987. Hormonal control of muscle growth. *Muscle and Nerve* 10: 577-598.

Florini, J.R., Ewton, D.Z., and Coolican, S.A. 1996. Growth hormone and the insulin-like growth factor system in myogenesis. *Endocrine Reviews* 17: 481-517.

Florini, J.R., Samuel, D.S., Ewton, D.Z., Kirk, C., and Sklar, R.M. 1996. Stimulation of myogenic differentiation by a neuregulin, glial growth factor 2: Are neuregulins the long-sought muscle trophic factors secreted by nerves? *The Journal of Biological Chemistry* 271: 12699-12702.

Fogelholm, M., Kaprio, J., and Sarna, S. 1994. Healthy lifestyles of former Finnish world class athletes. *Medicine and Science in Sports and Exercise* 26: 224-229.

Ford, H.T., Puckett, J.R., Drummond, J.P., Sawyer, K., Gantt, K., and Fussell, C. 1983. Effects of three combinations of plyometric and weight training programs on selected physical fitness test items. *Perceptual and Motor Skills* 56: 919-922.

Fowles, J.R., MacDougall, J.D., Tarnopolsky, M.A., Sale, D.G., Roy, B.D., and Yarasheski, K.E. 2000. The effects of acute passive stretch on muscle protein synthesis in humans. *Canadian Journal of Applied Physiology* 25: 165-180.

Fox, E.L. 1979. *Sports physiology*. Philadelphia: Saunders.

Fox, E.L., and Mathews, D.K. 1981. *The physiological basis of physical education and athletics*. Philadelphia: Saunders.

Freedson, P.S., Micheuic, P.M., Loucks, A.B., and Birandola, R.M. 1983. Physique, body composition, and psychological characteristics of competitive female body builders. *Physician and Sportsmedicine* 11: 85-93.

Friden, J., Sjostrom, M., and Ekblom, B. 1983. Myofibrillar damage following intense eccentric exercise in man. *International Journal of Sports Medicine* 4: 170-176.

Frisch, R.E., and McArthur, J.W. 1974. Menstrual cycles: Fatness as a determinant of minimum weight and height necessary for their onset. *Science* 185: 949-951.

Froelicher, V.F. 1983. *Exercise testing and training*. New York: LeJacq.

Frontera, W.R., Hughes, V.A., Lutz, K.J., and Evans, W.J. 1991. A cross-sectional study of muscle strength and mass in 45- to 78-year-old men and women. *Journal of Applied Physiology* 71: 644-650.

Frontera, W.R., Meredith, C.N., O'Reilly, K.P., Knuttgen, H.G., and Evans, W.J. 1988. Strength conditioning in older men: Skeletal muscle hypertrophy and improved function. *Journal of Applied Physiology* 64: 1038-1044.

Frontera, W.R., Suh, D., Krivickas, L.S., Hughes, V.A., Goldstein, R., and Roubenoff, R. 2000. Skeletal muscle fiber quality in older men and women. *American Journal Physiology Cell Physiology* 279: C611-C618.

Frost, R.A., and Lang, C.H. 1999. Differential effects of insulin-like growth factor I (IGF-I) and IGF-binding protein-1 on protein metabolism in human skeletal muscle cells. *Endocrinology* 140: 3962-3970.

Fry, A.C., Allemeier, C.A., and Staron, R.S. 1994. Correlation between percentage of fiber type area and myosin heavy chain content in human skeletal muscle. *European Journal of Applied Physiology and Occupational Physiology* 68: 246-251.

Fry, A.C., and Kraemer, W.J. 1991. Physical performance characteristics of American collegiate football players. *Journal of Applied Sport Science Research* 5: 126-138.

Fry, A.C., and Kraemer, W.J. 1997. Resistance exercise overtraining and overreaching. Neuroendocrine responses. *Sports Medicine* 23: 106-129.

Fry, A.C., Kraemer, W.J., and Ramsey, L.T. 1998. Pituitary-adrenal-gonadal responses to high-intensity resistance exercise overtraining. *Journal of Applied Physiology* 85: 2352-2359.

Fry, A.C., Kraemer, W.J., Stone, M.H., Warren, B.J., Fleck, S.J., Kearney, J.T., and Gordon, S.E. 1994. Endocrine responses to overreaching before and after 1 year of weightlifting. *Canadian Journal of Applied Physiology* 19: 400-410.

Fry, A.C., Kraemer, W.J., Stone, M.J., Fleck, S.J., Kearney, J.T., Triplett, N.T., and Gordon, S.E. 1995. Acute endocrine responses with long-term weightlifting in a 51-year old male weightlifter. *Journal of Strength and Conditioning Research* 9: 193 (abstract).

Fry, A.C., Kraemer, W.J., van Borselen, F., Lynch, J.M., Marsit, J.L, Roy, E.P., Triplett, N.T., and Knuttgen, H.G. 1994. Performance decrements with high-intensity resistance exercise overtraining. *Medicine and Science in Sports and Exercise* 26: 1165-1173.

Fry, A.C., Stone, M.H., Thrush, J.T., and Fleck, S.J. 1995. Precompetition training sessions enhance competitive performance of high anxiety junior weightlifters. *Journal of Strength and Conditioning Research* 9: 37-42.

Fryburg, D.A. 1994. Insulin-like growth factor I exerts growth hormone- and insulin-like actions on human muscle protein metabolism. *American Journal of Physiology* 267: E331-E336.

Fryburg, D.A. 1996. NG-monomethyl-L-arginine inhibits the blood flow but not the insulin-like response of forearm muscle to IGF-I: Possible role of nitric oxide in muscle protein synthesis. *Journal of Clinical Investigation* 97: 1319-1328.

Fryburg, D.A., and Barrett, E.J. 1995. Insulin, growth hormone and IGF-I regulation of protein metabolism. *Diabetes Reviews* 3: 93-112.

Fryburg, D.A., Jahn, L.A., Hill, S.A., Oliveras, D.M., and Barrett, E.J. 1995. Insulin and insulin-like growth factor-I enhance human skeletal muscle protein anabolism during hyperaminoacidemia by different mechanisms. *Journal of Clinical Investigation* 96: 722-729.

Fukunaga, T., Funato, K., and Ikegawa, S. 1992. The effects of resistance training on muscle area and strength in prepubescent age. *Annals of Physiology and Anthropology* 11: 357-364.

Gaja, B. 1965. The new revolutionary phase or sequence system of training. *Iron Man* 26: 14-17.

Gardner, G. 1963. Specificity of strength changes of the exercised and nonexercised limb following isometric training. *Research Quarterly* 34: 98-101.

Garfinkel, S., and Cafarelli, E. 1992. Relative changes in maximal force, emg, and muscle cross-sectional area after isometric training. *Medicine and Science in Sports and Exercise* 24: 1220-1227.

Garhammer, J. 1989. Weight lifting and training. In *Biomechanics of sport*, edited by C.L. Vaughan, 169-211. Boca Raton, FL: CRC Press.

Garhammer, J., and Takano, B. 1992. Training for weightlifting. *Strength and Power in Sports* 5: 357-381.

Gasser, G.A.,and Brooks, G.A. 1979. Metabolism and lactate after prolonged exercise to exhaustion. *Medicine and Science in Sports* 10: 47.

Gehri, D.J., Ricard, M.D., Kleiner, D.M., and Kirkendall, D.T. 1998. A comparison of plyometric training techniques for improving vertical jump ability and energy production. *Journal of Strength and Conditioning Research* 12: 85-89.

George, K.P., Wolfe, L.A., Burggraf, G.W., and Norman, R. 1995. Electrocardiographic and echocardiographic characteristics of female athletes. *Medicine and Science in Sports and Exercise* 27: 1362-1370.

Gettman, L.R., and Ayers, J.J. 1978. Aerobic changes through 10 weeks of slow and fast speed isokinetic training. *Medicine and Science in Sports* 10: 47.

Gettman, L.R., Ayers, J.J., Pollock, M.L., Durstine, J.C., and Grantham, W. 1979. Physiological effects on adult men of circuit strength training and jogging. *Archives of Physical Medicine and Rehabilitation* 60: 115-120.

Gettman, L.R., Ayres, J.J., Pollock, M.L., and Jackson, A. 1978. The effect of circuit weight training on strength, cardiorespiratory function and body composition of adult men. *Medicine and Science in Sports* 10: 171-176.

Gettman, L.R., Culter, L.A., and Strathman, T. 1980. Physiological changes after 20 weeks of isotonic vs isokinetic circuit training. *Journal of Sports Medicine and Physical Fitness* 20: 265-274.

Gettman, L.R., and Pollock, M.L. 1981. Circuit weight training: A critical review of its physiological benefits. *The Physician and Sportsmedicine* 9: 44-60.

Gibala, M.J., Interisano, S.A., Tarnopolsky, M.A., Roy, B.D., MacDonald, J.R., Yarasheski, K.E., and MacDougall, J.D. 2000. Myofibrillar disruption following acute concentric and eccentric resistance exercise in strength-trained men. *Canadian Journal of Physiology and Pharmacology* 78: 656-661.

Gillam, G.M. 1981. Effects of frequency of weight training on muscle strength enhancement. *Journal of Sports Medicine* 21: 432-436.

Giorgi, A., Wilson, G.J., Weatherby, R.P., and Murphy, A. 1998. Functional isometric weight training: Its effects on the development of muscular function and the endocrine system over an 8-week training period. *Journal of Strength and Conditioning Research* 12: 18-25.

Giustina, A., and Veldhuis, J.D. 1998. Pathophysiology of the neuroregulation of growth hormone secretion in experimental animals and the human. *Endocrine Reviews* 19: 717-797.

Gladden, L.B., and Colacino, D. 1978. Characteristics of volleyball players and success in a national tournament. *Journal of Sports Medicine and Physical Fitness* 18: 57-64.

Godard, M.P., Wygand, J.W., Carpinelli, R.N., Catalano, S., and Otto, R.M. 1998. Effects of accentuated eccentric resistance training on concentric knee extensor strength. *Journal of Strength and Conditioning Research* 12: 26-29.

Goldberg, A.P. 1989. Aerobic and resistance exercise modify risk factors for coronary heart disease. *Medicine and Science in Sports and Exercise* 21: 669-674.

Goldberg, L., Elliot, D.L., and Kuehl, K.S. 1988. Cardiovascular changes at rest and during mixed static and dynamic exercise after weight training. *Journal of Applied Sport Science Research* 2: 42-45.

Goldberg, L., Elliot, D.L., and Kuehl, K.S. 1994. A comparison of the cardiovascular effects of running and weight training. *Journal of Strength and Conditioning Research* 8: 219-224.

Golden, C.L., and Dudley, G.A. 1992. Strength after bouts of eccentric or concentric actions. *Medicine and Science in Sports and Exercise* 24: 926-933.

Goldspink, G. 1992. Cellular and molecular aspects of adaptation in skeletal muscle. In *Strength and power in sport*, edited by P.V. Komi, 211-229. Oxford: Blackwell Scientific.

Goldspink, G. 1998. Cellular and molecular aspects of muscle growth, adaptation and aging. *Gerontology* 15: 35-43.

Goldspink, G. 1999. Changes in muscle mass and phenotype and the expression of autocrine and systemic growth factors by muscle in response to stretch and overload. *Journal of Anatomy* 194: 323-334.

Goldspink, G., and Yang, S.Y. 2001. Effects of activity on growth factor expression. *International Journal of Sport Nutrition and Exercise Metabolism* 11: S21-S27.

Gollhofer, A. 1987. Innervation characteristics of m. gastrocnemius during landing on different surfaces. In *Biomechanics XB*, edited by B. Johnson, 701-706. Champaign, IL: Human Kinetics.

Gollnick, P.D., Timson, B.F., Moore, R.L., and Riedy, M. 1981. Muscular enlargement and number of fibers in skeletal muscles of rats. *Journal of Applied Physiology: Respiratory, Environmental and Exercise Physiology* 50: 936-943.

Gonyea, W.J. 1980. Role of exercise in inducing increases in skeletal muscle fiber number. *Journal of Applied Physiology: Respiratory, Environmental and Exercise Physiology* 48: 421-426.

Gonyea, W.J., and Sale, D. 1982. Physiology of weight-lifting exercise. *Archives of Physical Medicine and Rehabilitation* 63: 235-237.

Gonyea, W.J., Sale, D., Gonyea, F., and Mikesky, A. 1986. Exercise induced increases in muscle fiber number. *European Journal of Applied Physiology* 55: 137-141.

Gonzalez-Camarena, R., Carrasco-Sosa, S., Roman-Ramos, R., Gaitan-Gonzalez, M.J., Medina-Banuelos, V., and Azpiroz-Leehan, J. 2000. Effect of static and dynamic exercise on heart rate and blood pressure variabilities. *Medicine and Science in Sports and Exercise* 32: 1719-1728.

Gordon, S.E., Davis, B.S., Carlson, C.J., and Booth, F.W. 2001. ANG II is required for optimal overload-induced skeletal muscle hypertrophy. *American Journal of Physiology* 280: E150-E159.

Gordon, S.E., Kraemer, W.J., and Pedro, J.G. 1991. Increased acid-base buffering capacity via dietary supplementation: Anaerobic exercise implications. *Journal of Applied Nutrition* 43: 40-48.

Gordon, S.E., Kraemer, W.J., Vos, N.H., Lynch, J.M., and Knuttgen, H.G. 1994. Effect of acid base balance on the growth hormone response to acute, high-intensity cycle exercise. *Journal of Applied Physiology* 76: 821-829.

Gotshalk, L.A., Loebel, C.C., Nindl, B.C., Putukian, M., Sebastianelli, W.J., Newton, R.U., Häkkinen, K., and Kraemer, W.J. 1997. Hormonal responses to multiset versus single-set heavy-resistance exercise protocols. *Canadian Journal of Applied Physiology* 22: 244-255.

Gotshall, R.W., Gootman, J., Byrnes, W.C., Fleck, S.J., and Volovich, T.C. 1999. Noninvasive characterization of the blood pressure response to the double-leg press exercise. *Journal of Exercise Physiology online* 2, www.css.edu/users/tboone2.

Grassi, B., Cerretelli, P., Narici, M.V., and Marconi, C. 1991. Peak anaerobic power in master athletes. *European Journal of Applied Physiology* 62: 394-399.

Graves, J.E., and James, R.J. 1990. Concurrent augmented feedback and isometric force generation during familiar and unfamiliar muscle movements. *Research Quarterly for Exercise and Sport* 61: 75-79.

Graves, J.E., Pollock, M.L., Foster, D.N., Leggett, S.H., Carpenter, D.M., Vuoso, R., and Jones, A. 1990. Effects of training frequency and specificity on isometric lumbar extension strength. *Spine* 15: 504-509.

Graves, J.E., Pollock, M.L., Jones, A.E., Colvin, A.B., and Leggett, S.H. 1989. Specificity of limited range of motion variable resistance training. *Medicine and Science in Sports and Exercise* 21: 84-89.

Graves, J.E., Pollock, M.L., Leggett, S.H., Braith, R.W., Carpenter, D.M., and Bishop, L.E. 1988. Effect of reduced frequency on muscular strength. *International Journal of Sports Medicine* 9: 316-319.

Graves, J.E., Pollock, M.I., Leggett, S.H., Carpenter, D.M., Fix, C.R., and Fulton, M.N. 1992. Limited range-of-motion lumbar extension strength training. *Medicine and Science in Sports and Exercise* 24: 128-133.

Gray, D.P., and Dale, E. 1984. Variables associated with secondary amenorrhea in women runners. *Journal of Sports Sciences* 1: 55-67.

Green, H., Dahly, A., Shoemaker, K., Goreham, C., Bombardier, E., and Ball-Burnett, M. 1999. Serial effects of high-resistance and prolonged endurance training on Na⁺-K⁺ pump concentration and enzymatic activities in human vastus lateralis. *Acta Physiologica Scandinavica* 165: 177-184.

Green, H., Goreham, C., Ouyang, J., Ball-Burnett, M., and Ranney, D. 1998. Regulation of fiber size, oxidative potential, and capillarization in human muscle by resistance exercise. *American Journal of Physiology* 276: R591-R596.

Green, H., Grange, F., Chin, C., Goreham, C., and Ranney, D. 1998. Exercise-induced decreases in sarcoplasmic reticulum Ca²⁺-ATPase activity attenuated by high-resistance training. *Acta Physiologica Scandinavica* 164: 141-146.

Green, H.J. 1986. Muscle power: Fiber type recruitment, metabolism and fatigue. In *Human muscle power,* edited by N.L. Jones, N. McCartney, and A.J. McComas, 65-79. Champaign, IL: Human Kinetics.

Greenspan, F.S. 1994. The thyroid gland. In *Basic and clinical endocrinology,* edited by F.S. Greenspan, and J.D. Baxter, 4th ed., 160-226. Norwalk, CT: Appleton and Lange.

Griffin, J., Tooms, R., Vander Zwaag, R., Bertorini, T., and O'Toole, M. 1993. Eccentric muscle performance of elbow and knee muscle groups and untrained men and women. *Medicine and Science in Sports and Exercise* 25: 936-944.

Grimby, G., Bjorntorp, P., Fahlen, M., Hoskins, T.A., Hook, O., Oxhof, H., and Saltin, B. 1973. Metabolic effects of isometric training. *Scandinavian Journal of Chemical Laboratory Investigation* 31: 301-305.

Grimby, G., and Hannerz, J. 1977. Firing rate and recruitment order of toe extensor motor units in different modes of voluntary contraction. *Journal of Physiology (London)* 264: 867-879.

Grimby, G., Hannerz, J., and Hedman, B. 1981. The fatigue and voluntary discharge properties of single motor units in man. *Journal of Physiology* 36: 545-554.

Grumbs, V.L., Seagal, D., Halligan, J.B., and Lower, G. 1982. Bilateral radius and ulnar fractures in adolescent weight lifters. *American Journal Sports Medicine* 10: 375-379.

Guezennec, Y., Leger. L., Lhoste, F., Aymonod, M., and Pesquies, P.C. 1986. Hormone and metabolite response to weight-training sessions. *International Journal of Sports Medicine* 7:100-105.

Guyton, A.C. 1991. *Textbook of medical physiology.* 8th ed. Philadelphia: W.B. Saunders.

Haennel, R., Teo, K.K., Quinney, A., and Kappagoda, T. 1989. Effects of hydraulic circuit training on cardiovascular function. *Medicine and Science in Sports and Exercise* 21: 605-612.

Hagberg, J.M., Ehsoni, A.A., Goldring, D., Hernandez, A., Sincore, D.R., and Holloszy, J.O. 1984. Effect of weight training on blood pressure and hemodynamics in hypertensive adolescents. *Journal of Pediatrics* 104: 147-151.

Haggmark, T., Jansson, E., and Eriksson, E. 1982. Fiber type area and metabolic potential of the thigh muscle in man after knee surgery and immobilization. *International Journal of Sports Medicine* 2: 12-17.

Haggmark, T., Jansson, E., and Svane, B. 1978. Cross-sectional area of the thigh muscle in man measured by computed tomography. *Scandinavian Journal of Clinical and Laboratory Investigation* 38: 354-360.

Häkkinen, K. 1985. Factors influencing trainability of muscular strength during short term and prolonged training. *National Strength and Conditioning Association Journal* 7: 32-37.

Häkkinen, K. 1987. Force production characteristics of leg extensor, trunk flexor and extensor muscles in male and female basketball players. *Journal of Sports Medicine and Physical Fitness* 31: 325-331.

Häkkinen, K. 1989. Neuromuscular and hormonal adaptations during strength and power training. *Journal of Sports Medicine* 29: 9-26.

Häkkinen, K. 1992. Neuromuscular responses in male and female athletes to two successive strength training sessions in one day. *Journal of Sports Medicine and Physical Fitness* 32: 234-242.

Häkkinen, K. 1993. Changes in physical fitness profile in female basketball players during the competitive season including explosive strength training. *Journal of Sports Medicine and Physical Fitness* 33: 19-26.

Häkkinen K., Alen, M., Kallinen, M., Newton, R.U., and Kraemer, W.J. 2002. Neuromuscular adaptation during prolonged strength training, detraining and re-strength training in middle aged and elderly people. *European Journal of Applied Physiology* 83: 51-62.

Häkkinen, K., Alen, M., and Komi, P.V. 1985. Changes in isometric force- and relaxation-time, electromyographic and muscle fibre characteristics of human skeletal muscle during strength training and detraining. *Acta Physiologica Scandinavica* 125: 573-585.

Häkkinen, K., and Häkkinen, A. 1991. Muscle cross-sectional area, force production and relaxation characteristics in women at different ages. *European Journal of Applied Physiology* 62: 410-414.

Häkkinen, K., and Kallinen, M. 1994. Distribution of strength training volume into one or two daily sessions on muscular adaptations in female athletes. *Electromyography and Clinical Neurophysiology* 34: 117-124.

Häkkinen, K., Kallinen, M., and Komi, P.V. 1994. Neuromuscular adaptations in strength athletes during strength training distributed into one or two daily sessions. *European Journal of Applied Physiology* 68: 269-270.

Häkkinen, K., and Komi, P. 1981. Effect of different combined concentric and eccentric muscle work on maximal strength development. *Journal of Human Movement Studies* 7: 33-44.

Häkkinen, K., and Komi, P.V. 1983. Changes in neuromuscular performance in voluntary and reflex contraction during strength training in man. *International Journal of Sports Medicine* 4: 282-288.

Häkkinen, K., and Komi, P.V. 1985a. Changes in electrical and mechanical behavior of leg extensor muscles during heavy resistance strength training. *Scandinavian Journal of Sports Science* 7: 55-64.

Häkkinen, K., and Komi, P.V. 1985b. Effect of explosive type strength training on electromyographic and force production characteristics of leg extensor muscles during concentric and various stretch-shortening cycle exercises. *Scandinavian Journal of Sports Science* 7: 65-76.

Häkkinen, K., and Komi, P.V. 1985c. Changes in electrical and mechanical behavior of leg extensor muscles during heavy resistance strength training. *Scandinavian Journal of Sports Science* 7: 55-64.

Häkkinen, K., and Komi, P.V. 1986. Effects of fatigue and recovery on electromyographic and isometric force- and relaxation-time characteristics of human skeletal muscle. *European Journal of Applied Physiology* 55: 588-596.

Häkkinen, K., Komi, P.V., and Alen, M. 1985. Effect of explosive type strength training on isometric force- and relaxation-time, electromyographic and muscle fibre characteristics of leg extensor muscles. *Acta Physiologica Scandinavica* 125: 587-600.

Häkkinen, K., Komi, P.V., Alen, M., and Kauhanen, H. 1987. EMG, muscle fibre and force production characteristics during a 1 year training period in elite weightlifters. *European Journal of Applied Physiology* 56: 419-427.

Häkkinen, K., Komi, P.V., and Tesch, P.A. 1981. Effect of combined concentric and eccentric strength training and detraining on force-time, muscle fiber and metabolic characteristics of leg extensor muscles. *Scandinavian Journal of Sports Science* 3: 50-58.

Häkkinen, K., Kraemer, W.J., and Newton, R. 1997. Muscle activation and force production during bilateral and unilateral concentric and isometric contractions of the knee extensors in men and women at different ages. *Electromyography Clinical Neurophysiology* 37: 131-142.

Häkkinen, K., Kraemer, W.J., Newton, R.U., and Alen, M. 2001. Changes in electromyographic activity, muscle fibre and force production characteristics during heavy resistance/power strength training in middle-aged and older men and women. *Acta Physiologica Scandinavica* 141: 51-62.

Häkkinen, K., Newton, R.U., Gordon, S.E., McCormick, M., Volek, J.S., Nindl, B.C., Gotshalk, L.A., Campbell, W.W., Evans, W.J., Häkkinen, A., Humphries, B., and Kraemer, W.J. 1998. Changes in muscle morphology, electromyographic activity, and force production characteristics during progressive strength training in young and older men. *Journal of Gerontology: Biological Medical Sciences* 53: 415-423.

Häkkinen, K., and Pakarinen, A. 1991. Serum hormones in male strength athletes during intensive short term strength training. *European Journal of Applied Physiology* 63: 194-199.

Häkkinen, K., and Pakarinen, A. 1993. Muscle strength and serum testosterone, cortisol and SHBG concentrations in middle-aged and elderly men and women. *Acta Physiologica Scandinavica* 148:199-207.

Häkkinen, K., and Pakarinen, A. 1995. Acute hormonal responses to heavy resistance exercise in men and women at different ages. *International Journal of Sports Medicine* 16: 507-513.

Häkkinen, K., Pakarinen, A., Alen, M., Kauhanen, H., and Komi, P.V. 1987. Relationships between training volume, physical performance capacity, and serum hormone concentration during prolonged training in elite weight lifters. *International Journal of Sports Medicine* 8: 61-65.

Häkkinen, K., Pakarinen, A., Alen, M., Kauhanen, H., and Komi, P.V. 1988a. Neuromuscular and hormonal responses in elite athletes to two successive strength training sessions in one day. *European Journal of Applied Physiology* 57: 133-139.

Häkkinen, K., Pakarinen, A., Alen, M., Kauhanen, H., and Komi, P.V. 1988b. Daily hormonal and neuromuscular responses to intensive strength training in 1 week. *International Journal of Sports Medicine* 9: 422-428.

Häkkinen, K., Pakarinen, A., Alen, M., Kauhanen, H., and Komi, P.V. 1988c. Neuromuscular and hormonal adaptations in athletes to strength training in two years. *Journal of Applied Physiology* 65: 2406-2412.

Häkkinen, K., Pakarinen, A., Alen, M., and Komi, P.V. 1985. Serum hormones during prolonged training of neuromuscular performance. *European Journal of Applied Physiology* 53: 287-293.

Häkkinen, K., Pakarinen, A, and Kallinen, M. 1992. Neuromuscular adaptations and serum hormones in women during short-term intensive strength training. *European Journal of Applied Physiology* 64: 106-111.

Häkkinen, K., Pakarinen, A., Komi, P.V., Ryushi, T., and Kauhanen, H. 1989. Neuromuscular adaptations and hormone balance in strength athletes, physically active males, and females during intensive strength training. In *Proceedings of the XII International Congress of Biomechanics*, no.8, edited by R.J. Gregor, R.F. Zernicke, and W.C. Whiting, 889-894. Champaign, IL: Human Kinetics.

Häkkinen, K., Pakarinen, A., Kraemer, W.J., Häkkinen, A., Valkeinen, H., and Alen, M. 2001. Selective muscle hypertrophy, changes in EMG and force, and serum hormones during strength training in older women. *Journal of Applied Physiology* 91: 569-580.

Häkkinen, K., Pakarinen, A., Kraemer, W.J., Newton, R.U., and Alen, M. 2000. Basal concentrations and acute responses of serum hormones and strength development during heavy resistance training in middle-aged and elderly men and women. *Journal of Gerontology: Biological Sciences, Medical Sciences* 55: B95-B105.

Häkkinen, K., Pakarinen, A., Kyrolainen, H., Cheng, S., Kim, D.H., and Komi, P.V. 1990. Neuromuscular adaptations and serum hormones in females during prolonged power training. *International Journal of Sports Medicine* 11: 91-98.

Häkkinen, K., Pakarinen, A., Newton, R.U., and Kraemer, W.J. 1998. Acute hormone responses to heavy resistance lower and upper extremity exercise in young versus old men. *European Journal of Applied Physiology* 77: 312-319.

Hall, Z.W., and Ralston, E. 1989. Nuclear domains in muscle cells. *Cell* 59: 771-772.

Hamada, T., Sale, D.G., MacDougall, J.D., and Tarnopolsky, M.A. 2000. Postactivation potentiation, fiber type, and twitch contraction time in human knee extensor muscles. *Journal of Applied Physiology* 88: 2131-2137.

Hamil, B.P. 1994. Relative safety of weightlifting and weight training. *Journal of Strength and Conditioning Research* 8: 53-57.

Hamilton, W.F., Woodbury, R.A., and Harper, H.T. 1943. Arterial, cerebrospinal, and venous pressures in man during cough and strain. *American Journal of Physiology* 141: 42-50.

Hamlin, M.J., and Quigley, B.M. 2001. Quadriceps concentric and eccentric exercise 2: Differences in muscle strength, fatigue and EMG activity in eccentrically-exercised sore and non-sore muscles. *Journal of Science and Medicine in Sport* 4: 104-115.

Hammond, G.L., Kontturi, M.,Vihko, P., and Vihko, R. 1974. Serum steroids in normal males and patients with prostatic diseases. *Clinical Endocrinology* 9: 113-121.

Harder, D. 2000. *Strength and speed,* 6th ed. Castro Valley, CA: Education Plus.

Harman, E. 1983. Resistive torque analysis of 5 Nautilus exercise machines. *Medicine and Science in Sports and Exercise* 15: 113.

Harman, E.A., Rosenstein, R., Frykman, P., and Nigro, G. 1989. Effects of a belt on intra-abdominal pressure during weight lifting. *Medicine and Science in Sports and Exercise* 21: 186-190.

Harries, U.J., and Bassey, E.J. 1990. Torque-velocity relationships for the knee extensors in women in their 3rd and 7th decades. *European Journal of Applied Physiology* 60: 87-190.

Harris, K.A., and Holly, R.G. 1987. Physiological responses to circuit weight training in borderline hypertensive subjects. *Medicine and Science in Sports and Exercise* 19: 246-252.

Harr Romey, B.M., Denier Van Der Gon, J.J., and Gielen, C.C. 1982. Changes in recruitment order of motor units in the human biceps muscle. *Experimental Neurology* 78: 360-368.

Hass, C.J., Feigenbaum, M.S., and Franklin, B.A. 2001. Prescription of resistance training for healthy populations. *Sports Medicine* 31: 953-964.

Hass, C.J., Garzarella, L., de Hoyos, D., and Pollock, M.L. 2000. Single versus multiple sets in long-term recreational weightlifters. *Medicine and Science in Sports and Exercise* 32: 235-242.

Hatfield, F.C. 1981. *Powerlifting: A scientific approach.* Chicago: Contemporary Books.

Hatfield, F.C. 1989. *Power: A scientific approach.* Chicago: Contemporary Books.

Hatfield, F.C., and Krotee, M.L. 1978. *Personalized weight training for fitness and athletics from theory and practice.* Dubuque, IA: Kendall/Hunt.

Hather, B.M., Mason, C.E., and Dudley, G.A. 1991. Histochemical demonstration of skeletal muscle fiber types and capillaries on the same transverse section. *Clinical Physiology* (Oxford) 11: 127-134.

Hather, B.M., Tesch, P.A., Buchanan, P., and Dudley, G.A. 1992. Influence of eccentric actions on skeletal muscle adaptations to resistance training. *Acta Physiologica Scandinavica* 143: 177-185.

Hatta, H., Atomi, Y., Yamamoto, Y., Shinohara, S., and Yamada, S. 1989. Incorporation of blood lactate and glucose into tissues in rats after short-duration strenuous exercise. *International Journal of Sports Medicine* 10: 272-278.

Hawke, T.J., and Garry, D.J. 2001. Myogenic satellite cells: Physiology to molecular biology. *Journal of Applied Physiology* 91: 534-551.

Hawkins, S.A., Schroeder, E.T., Wiswell, R.A., Jaque, S.V., Marcell, T.J., and Costa, K. 1999. Eccentric muscle action increases site-specific osteogenic response. *Medicine and Science in Sports and Exercise* 31: 1287-1292.

Haykowsky, M.J., Quinney, H.A., Gillis, R., and Thompson, C.R. 2000. Left ventricular morphology in junior and master resistance trained athletes. *Medicine and Science in Sports and Exercise* 32: 349-352.

Hayward, V.H., Johannes Ellis, S.M., and Romer, J.F. 1986. Gender differences in strength. *Research Quarterly for Exercise and Sport* 57: 154-159.

Heinonen, A., Sievanen, H., Kannus, P., Oja, P., and Vuori, I. 1996. Effects of unilateral strength training and detraining on bone mineral mass and estimated mechanical characteristics of upper limb bones in young women. *Journal of Bone Mineral Research* 11: 490-501.

Heitkamp, H.C., Horstmann, T., Mayer, F., Weller, J., and Dickhuth, H.H. 2001. Gains in strength and muscular balance after balance training. *International Journal of Sports Medicine* 22: 285-290.

Hejna, W.F., Rosenberg, A., Buturusis, D.J., and Krieger, A. 1982. The prevention of sports injuries in high school students through strength training. *National Strength and Conditioning Association Journal* 4: 28-31.

Henneman, E., Somjen, G., and Carpenter, D.O. 1985. Functional significance of cell size in spinal motorneurons. *Journal of Neurophysiology* 28: 560-580.

Hennessy, L., and Kilty, J. 2001. Relationship of the stretch-shortening cycle to sprint performance and trained female athletes. *Journal of Strength and Conditioning Research* 15: 326-331.

Hennessy, L.C., and Watson, A.W.S. 1994. The interference effects of training for strength and endurance simultaneously. *Journal of Strength and Conditioning Research* 8: 12-19.

Henriksson-Larsen, K. 1985. Distribution, number, and size of different types of fibers in whole cross-sections of female m. tibialis anterior. An enzyme histochemical study. *Acta Physiologica Scandinavica* 123: 229-235.

Hermansen, L., Machlum, S., Pruett, E.R., Vaage, O., Waldrum, H., and Wessel-Aas, T. 1976. Lactate removal at rest and during exercise. In *Metabolic adaptation to prolonged physical exercise*, edited by H. Howard and J.R. Pootsmans, 101-105. Basel: Birhauser Verlag.

Herrick, A.B., and Stone, W.J. 1996. The effects of periodization versus progressive resistance exercise on upper and lower body strength in women. *Journal of Strength and Conditioning Research* 10: 72-76.

Hetherington, M.R. 1976. Effect of isometric training on the elbow flexion force torque of grade five boys. *Research Quarterly for Exercise and Sport* 47: 41-47.

Hettinger, R. 1961. *Physiology of strength.* Springfield, IL: Charles C. Thomas.

Hettinger, R., and Muller, E. 1953. Muskelleistung und muskeltraining. *Arbeits Physiology* 15: 111-126.

Hewett, T.E. 2000. Neuromuscular and hormonal factors associated with knee injuries in female athletes' strategies for intervention. *Sports Medicine* 29: 313-327.

Hewett, T.E., Lindenfeld, T.N., Riccobene, J.V., and Noyes, F.R. 1999. The effect of neuromuscular training on the incidence of knee injury in female athletes: A prospective study. *American Journal of Sports Medicine* 27:699-706.

Hickson, R.C. 1980. Interference of strength development by simultaneously training for strength and endurance. *European Journal of Applied Physiology* 45: 255-269.

Hickson, R.C., Dvorak, B.A., Gorostiaga, E.M., Kurowski, T.T., and Foster, C. 1988. Potential for strength and endurance training to amplify endurance performance. *Journal of Applied Physiology* 65: 2285-2290.

Hickson, R.C., Hidaka, K. and Foster, C. 1994. Skeletal muscle fiber type, resistance training, and strength-related performance. *Medicine and Science in Sports and Exercise* 26: 593-598.

Hickson, R.C., Hidaka, K., Foster, C., Falduto, M.T., and Chatterton, R.T. 1994. Successive time courses of strength development and steroid hormone responses to heavy-resistance training. *Journal of Applied Physiology* 76: 663-670.

Hickson, R.C., and Marone, J.R. 1993. Exercise and inhibition of glucocorticoid-induced muscle atrophy. *Exercise and Sports Sciences Reviews* 21: 135-167.

Hickson, R.C., Rosenkoetter, M.A., and Brown, M.M. 1980. Strength training effects on aerobic power and short-term endurance. *Medicine and Science in Sports and Exercise* 12: 336-339.

Hikida, R.S., Staron, R.S., Hagerman, F.C., Walsh, S., Kaiser, E., Shell, S., and Hervey, S. 2000. Effects of high-intensity resistance training on untrained older men. II. Muscle fiber characteristics and nucleo-cytoplasmic relationships. *Journal of Gerontology: A Biological Sciences Medical Sciences* 55: B347-B354.

Hikida, R.S., Van Nostran, S., Murray, J.D., Staron, R.S., Gordon, S.E., and Kraemer, W.J. 1997. Myonuclear loss in atrophied soleus muscle fibers. *Anatomical Record* 247: 350-354.

Hildebrandt, W., Schutze, H., and Stegemann, J. 1992. Cardiovascular limitations of active recovery from strenuous exercise. *European Journal of Applied Physiology and Occupational Physiology* 64: 250-257.

Hill, D.W., and Butler, S.D. 1991. Hemodynamic responses to weightlifting exercise. *Sports Medicine* 12: 1-7.

Ho, K.W., Roy, R.R., Tweedle, C.D., Heusner, W.W., Van Huss, W.D., and Carrow, R. 1980. Skeletal muscle fiber splitting with weight-lifting exercise in rats. *American Journal of Anatomy* 157: 433-440.

Hoeger, W.W.K., Barette, S.L., Hale, D.F., and Hopkins, D.R. 1987. Relationship between repetitions and selected percentages of one repetition maximum. *Journal of Applied Sport Science Research* 1: 11-13.

Hoeger, W.W.K., Hopkins, D.R., Barette, S.L. and Hale, D.F. 1990. Relationship between repetitions and selected percentages of one repetition maximum: A comparison between untrained and trained males and females. *Journal of Applied Sport Science Research* 4: 47-54.

Hoffman, J.R., Fry, A.C., Howard, R., Maresh, C.M., and Kraemer, W.J. 1991. Strength, speed and endurance changes during the course of a division I basketball season. *Journal of Applied Sport Science Research* 3: 144-149.

Hoffman, J.R., and Kalfeld, S. 1998. The effect of resistance training on injury rate and performance in a self-defense instructors course for women. *Journal of Strength and Conditioning Research* 12: 52-56.

Hoffman, J.R., Kraemer, W.J., Fry, A.C., Deschenes, M., Kemp, M. 1990. The effects of self-selection for frequency of training in a winter conditioning program for football. *Journal of Applied Sport Science Research* 4: 76-82.

Hoffman, T., Stauffer, R.W., and Jackson, A.S. 1979. Sex difference in strength. *American Journal of Sports Medicine* 7: 265-267.

Hogan, M.C., Gladden, L.B., Kurdak, S.S., and Poole, D.C. 1995. Increased (lactate) in working dog muscle reduces tension development independent of pH. *Medicine and Science in Sports and Exercise* 27: 371-377.

Holmdahl, D.C., and Ingelmark, R.E. 1948. Der bau des Gelenknorpels unterverschiedenen funktionellen Verhaltnissen. *Acta Anatomica* 6: 113-116.

Hortobagyi, T., Devita, P., Money, J., and Barrier, J. 2001. Effects of standard and eccentric overload strength training in young women. *Medicine and Science in Sports and Exercise* 33: 1206-1212.

Hortobagyi, T., Hill, J.P., Houmard, J.A., Fraser, D.D., Lambert, N.J., and Israel, R.G. 1996. Adaptive responses to muscle lengthening and shortening in humans. *Journal of Applied Physiology* 80: 765-772.

Hortobagyi, T., Houmard, J.A., Stevenson, J.R., Fraser, D.D., Johns, R.A., Israel, R.G. 1993. The effects of detraining on power athletes. *Medicine and Science in Sports and Exercise* 25: 929-935.

Hortobagyi, T., Katch, F.I., and LaChance, P.F. 1991. Effects of simultaneous training for strength and endurance on upper and lower body strength and running performance. *Journal of Sports Medicine and Physical Fitness* 31: 20-30.

Horvath, B. 1959. What's new in muscles? *Muscle Sculpture* 2: 39-44.

Hostler, D., Crill, M.T., Hagerman, F.C., and Staron, R.S. 2001. The effectiveness of 0.5-lb. increments in progressive resistance exercise. *Journal of Strength and Conditioning Research* 15: 86-91.

Hostler, D., Schwirian, C.I., Campos, G., Toma, K., Crill, M.T., Hagerman, G.R., Hagerman, F.C., and Staron, R.S. 2001. Skeletal muscle adaptations in elastic resistance-trained young men and women. *European Journal of Applied Physiology* 86: 112-118.

Housh, D.J., Housh, T.J., Johnson, G.O., and Chu, W.K. 1992. Hypertrophic response to unilateral concentric isokinetic training. *Journal of Applied Physiology* 73: 65-70.

Housh, D.J., Housh, T.J., Weir, J.P., Weir, L.L., Evetovich, T.K., and Dolin, P.E. 1998. Effects of unilateral eccentric-only dynamic constant external resistance training on quadriceps femoris cross-sectional area. *Journal of Strength and Conditioning Research* 12: 192-198.

Housh, T.J., Housh, D.J., Weir, J.P., and Weir, L.L. 1996. Effects of eccentric-only resistance training and detraining. *International Journal of Sports Medicine* 17: 145-148.

Houston, M.E., Froese, E.A., Valeriote, S.P., Green, H.J., and Ramey, D.A. 1983. Muscle performance, morphology and metabolic capacity during strength training and detraining: A one leg model. *European Journal of Applied Physiology and Occupational Physiology* 51: 25-135.

Houston, M.E., Norman, R.W., and Froese, E.A. 1988. Mechanical measures during maximal velocity knee extension exercise and their relation to fiber composition of the human vastus lateralis muscle. *European Journal of Applied Physiology* 58: 1-7.

Howald, H. 1982. Training-induced morphological and functional changes in skeletal muscle. *International Journal of Sports Medicine* 3: 1-12.

Howell, J.N., Fuglevand, A.J., Walsh, M.L., and Bigland-Ritche, B. 1995. Motor unit activity during isometric and concentric-eccentric contractions of the human first dorsal interosseous muscle. *Journal of Neurophysiology* 74: 901-904.

Hughes, V.A., Frontera, W.R., Dallal, G.E., Lutz, K.J., Fisher, E.C., and Evans, W.J. 1995. Muscle strength and body composition: Associations with bone density in older subjects. *Medicine and Science in Sports and Exercise* 27: 967-974.

Hughes, V.A., Frontera, W.R., Weed, M., Evans, W.J., Dallal, G.E., Roubenoff, R., and Fiatarone, M.A. 2001. Longitudinal muscle strength changes in older adults: Influence of muscle mass, physical activity, and health. *Journal of Gerontology: Biological Sciences, Medical Sciences* 56: B209-B217.

Hultman, E., Bergstrom, J., and Anderson, N.M. 1967. Breakdown and resynthesis of phosphorylcreatine and adenosine triphosphate in connection with muscular work in man. *Scandinavian Journal of Clinical Investigation* 19: 56-66.

Humphries, B., Newton, R.U., Bronks, R., Marshall, S., McBride, J., Triplett-McBride, T., Häkkinen, K., Kraemer, W.J., and Humphries, N. 2000. Effect of exercise intensity on bone density, strength, and calcium turnover in older women. *Medicine and Science in Sports and Exercise* 32: 1043-1050.

Hunter, G.R., Demment, R., and Miller, D. 1987. Development of strength and maximum oxygen uptake during simultaneous training for strength and endurance. *Journal of Sports Medicine and Physical Fitness* 27:269-275.

Hunter, G.R., McGuirk, J., Mitrano, N., Pearman, P., Thomas, B., and Arrington, R. 1989. The effects of a weight training belt on blood pressure during exercise. *Journal of Applied Strength and Conditioning Research* 3:13-18.

Hunter, G.R., Wetzstein, C.J., Fields, D.A., Brown, A., Bamman, M.M. 2000. Resistance training increases total energy expenditure and free-living physical activity in older adults. *Journal of Applied Physiology* 89: 977-984.

Hunter, G.R. 1985. Changes in body composition, body build and performance associated with different weight training frequencies in males and females. *National Strength and Conditioning Association Journal* 7: 26-28.

Hunter, G.R., and Culpepper, M.I. 1995. Joint angle specificity of fixed mass versus hydraulic resistance knee flexion training. *Journal of Strength and Conditioning Research* 9: 13-16.

Hunter, G.R., and Treuth, M.S. 1995. Relative training intensity and increases in strength in older women. *Journal of Strength and Conditioning Research* 9: 188-191.

Hunter, G.R., Wetzstein, C.J., McLafferty, C.L. Jr., Zuckerman, P.A., Landers, K.A., Bamman, M.M. 2001. High-resistance versus variable-resistance training in older adults. *Medicine and Science in Sports and Exercise* 33: 1759-1764.

Hunter, J.P., and Marshall, R.N. 2002. Effects of power and flexibility training on vertical jump technique. *Medicine and Science in Sports and Exercise* 34: 470-486.

Hunter, S.K., Thompson, M.W., Ruell, P.A., Harmer, A.R., Thom, J.M., Gwinn, T.H., and Adams, R.D. 1999. Human skeletal sarcoplasmic reticulum Ca2+ uptake and muscle function with aging and strength training. *Journal of Applied Physiology* 86: 1858-1865.

Hurley, B. 1995. Strength training in the elderly to enhance health status. *Medicine Exercise Nutrition and Health* 4: 217-229.

Hurley, B.F. 1989. Effects of resistance training on lipoprotein-lipid profiles: A comparison to aerobic exercise training. *Medicine and Science in Sports and Exercise* 21: 689-693.

Hurley, B.F., Hagberg, J.M., Goldberg, A.P., Seals, D.R., Ehsani, A.A., Brennan, R.E., and Holloszy, J.O. 1988. Resistive training can reduce coronary risk factors without altering VO$_2$ max or percent body fat. *Medicine and Science in Sports and Exercise* 20: 150-154.

Hurley, B.F., Hagberg, J.M., Seals, D.R., Ehsani, A.A., Goldberg, A.P., and Holloszy, J.O. 1987. Glucose tolerance and lipid-lipoprotein levels in middle-age powerlifters. *Clinical Physiology* 7: 11-19.

Hurley, B.F., Seals, D.R., Ehsani, A.A., Cartier, L.J., Dalsky, G.P., Hagberg, J.M., and Holloszy, J.O. 1984. Effects of high-intensity strength training on cardiovascular function. *Medicine and Science in Sports and Exercise* 16: 483-488.

Hurley, B.F., Seals, D.R., Hagberg, J.M., Goldberg, A.C., Ostrove, S.M., Holloszy, J.O., Wiest, W.G., and Goldberg, A.P. 1984. High-density-lipoprotein cholesterol in bodybuilders vs. powerlifters. *Journal of the American Medical Association* 252: 507-513.

Huston, L.J., and Wojtys, E.M. 1996. Neuromuscular performance characteristics in elite female athletes. *American Journal of Sports Medicine* 24: 427-436.

Hutton, R.S., and Atwater, S.W. 1992. Acute and chronic adaptations of muscle proprioceptors in response to increased use. *Sports Medicine* 14: 406-421.

Huxley A.F. 2000. Cross-bridge action: Present views, prospects, and unknowns. *Journal of Biomechanics* 33: 1189-1195.

Huxley, A.F., and Niedergerke, R. 1954. Structural changes in muscle during contraction. *Nature* 173: 971-972.

Huxley, H.E., and Hanson, E.J. 1954. Changes in cross-striations of muscle during contraction and stretch and their structural interpretation. *Nature* 173: 973-976.

Hyatt, J.-P.K., and Clarkson, P.M. 1998. Creatine kinase release and clearance using mm variants following repeated bouts of eccentric exercise. *Medicine and Science in Sports and Exercise* 30: 1059-1065.

Hymer, W.C., Kirshnan, K., Kraemer, W.J., Welsch, J., and Lanham, W. 2000. Mammalian pituitary growth hormone: Applications of free flow electrophoresis. *Electrophoresis* 21: 311-317.

Hymer, W.C., Kraemer, W.J., Nindl, B.C., Marx, J.O., Benson, D.E., Welsch, J.R., Mazzetti, S.A., Volek, J.S., and Deaver, D.R. 2001. Characteristics of circulating growth hormone in women following acute heavy resistance exercise. *American Journal of Physiology: Endocrinology and Metabolism* 281: E878-E887.

Ichinose, Y., Kanehisa, H., Ito, M., Kawakami, Y., and Fukunaga, T. 1998. Relationship between muscle fiber pennation and force capability in Olympic athletes. *International Journal of Sports Medicine* 19: 541-546.

Iellamo, F., Legramante, J.M., Raimondi, G., Castrucci, F., Damiani, C., Foti, C., Peruzzi, G., and Caruso, I. 1997. Effects of isokinetic, isotonic and isometric submaximal exercise on heart rate and blood pressure. *European Journal of Applied Physiology* 75: 89-96.

Ikai, M., and Fukunaga, T. 1970. A study on training effect on strength per unit cross-sectional area of muscle by means of ultrasonic measurement. *European Journal of Applied Physiology* 28: 173-180.

Ikai, M., and Steinhaus, A.H. 1961. Some factors modifying the expression of human strength. *Journal of Applied Physiology* 16: 157-163.

Imamura, K., Ashida, H., Ishikawa, T., and Fujii, M. 1983. Human major psoas muscle and sacrospinalis muscle in relation to age: A study by computed tomography. *Journal of Gerontology* 38: 678-681.

Ingelmark, B.E., and Elsholm, R. 1948. A study on variations in the thickness of the articular cartilage in association with rest and periodical load. *Uppsala Lakaretorenings Foxhandlinger* 53: 61-64.

Ingjer, F. 1969. Effects of endurance training on muscle fiber ATP-ase activity, capillary supply and mitochondrial content in man. *Journal of Physiology* 294: 419-432.

Ishida, K., Moritani, T., and Itoh, K. 1990. Changes in voluntary and electrically induced contractions during strength training and detraining. *European Journal of Applied Physiology* 60: 244-248.

Ivey, F.M., Tracy, B.L., Lemmer, J.T., NessAiver, M., Metter, E.J., Fozard, J.L., and Hurley, B.F. 2000. Effects of strength training and detraining on muscle quality: Age and gender comparisons. *Journal of Gerontology Aging Biological Science Medicine Science* 55: B152-B157.

Izquierdo, M., Häkkinen, K., Ibanez, J., Garrues, M., Anton, A., Zuniga, A., Larrion, J.L., and Gorostiaga, E.M. 2001. Effects of strength training on muscle power and serum hormones in middle aged and older men. *Journal of Applied Physiology* 90: 1497-1507.

Jackson, A., Jackson, T., Hnatek, J., and West, J. 1985. Strength development: Using functional isometric in isotonic strength training program. *Research Quarterly for Exercise and Sport* 56: 324-337.

Jacobson, B.H. 1986. A comparison of two progressive weight training techniques on knee extensor strength. *Athletic Training* 21: 315-318, 390.

Jacobson, P.C., Bever, W., Brubb, S.A., Taft, T.N., and Talmage, R.V. 1984. Bone density in female: College athletes and older athletic female. *Journal of Orthopaedic Research* 2: 328-332.

Jakobi, J.M., and Chilibeck, P.D. 2001. Bilateral and unilateral contractions: Possible differences in maximal voluntary force. *Canadian Journal of Applied Physiology* 26: 12-33.

Janssen, I., Heymsfield, S.B., Wang, Z., and Ross, R. 2000. Skeletal muscle mass and distribution in 468 men and women aged 18-80 yr. *Journal of Applied Physiology* 89: 81-88.

Jefferson, L.S., and Kimball, S.R. 2001. Translational control of protein synthesis: Implications for understanding changes in skeletal muscle mass. *International Journal of Sport Nutrition and Exercise Metabolism* 11: S143-S149.

Jenkins, N., and Mintowt-Czyz, W. 1986. Bilateral fracture separations of the distal radial epiphysis during weightlifting. *British Journal of Sports Medicine* 20: 72-73.

Jenkins, W.L., Thackaberry, M., and Killian, C. 1984. Speed-specific isokinetic training. *Journal of Orthopaedic and Sports Physical Therapy* 6: 181-183.

Jensen, C., and Fisher, G. 1979. *Scientific basis of athletic conditioning.* Philadelphia: Lea and Febiger.

Johansson, P.H., Linstrom, L., Sundelin, G., and Lindstrom, B. 1999. The effects of preexercise stretching on muscular soreness, tenderness and force loss following heavy eccentric exercise. *Scandinavian Journal of Medicine Science Sports* 9: 219-225.

Johnson, B.L., Adamczy, K.J.W., Tennoe, K.O., and Stromme, S.B. 1976. A comparison of concentric and eccentric muscle training. *Medicine and Science in Sports* 8: 35-38.

Johnson, C.C., Stone, M.H., Lopez, S.A., Hebert, J.A., Kilgore, L.T., and Byrd, R.J. 1982. Diet and exercise in middle-age men. *Journal of the American Dietetic Association* 81: 695-701.

Johnson, J.H., Colodny, S., and Jackson, D. 1990. Human torque capability versus machine resistive torque for four eagle resistance machines. *Journal of Applied Sport Science Research* 4: 83-87.

Jones, A. 1973. The best kind of exercise. *Ironman* 32: 36-38.

Jones, D.A., and Rutherford, O.M. 1987. Human muscle strength training: The effects of three different regimes and the nature of the resultant changes. *Journal of Physiology* 391: 1-11.

Jones, K., Hunter, G., Fleisig, G., Escamilla, R., and Lemak, L. 1999. The effects of compensatory acceleration on upper-body strength and power in collegiate football players. *Journal of Strength and Conditioning Research* 13: 99-105.

Jozsi, A.C., Campbell, W.W., Joseph, L., Davey, S.L., and Evans, W.J. 1999. Changes in power with resistance training in older and younger men and women. *Journal of Gerontology: Biological Sciences* 54: M591-M596.

Jubrias, S.A., Esselman, P.C., Price, L.B., Cress, M.E., and Conley, K.E. 2001. Large energetic adaptations of elderly muscle to resistance and endurance training. *Journal of Applied Physiology* 90: 1663-1670.

Kadi F., Bonnerud, P., Eriksson, A., and Thornell, L.E. 2000. The expression of androgen receptors in human neck and limb muscles: Effects of training and self-administration of androgenic-anabolic steroids. *Histochemistry and Cell Biology* 113: 25-29.

Kadi, F. Eriksson, A., Holmner, S., Butler-Browne, G.S., and Thornell, L.E. 1999. Cellular adaptation of the trapezius muscle in strength-trained athletes. *Histochemistry and Cell Biology* 111: 189-195.

Kadi, F., and Thornell, L.E. 2000. Concomitant increases in myonuclear and satellite cell content in female trapezius muscle following strength training. *Histochemistry and Cell Biology* 113: 99-103.

Kahn, J.F., Kapitaniak, B., and Monod, H. 1985. Comparisons of two modalities when exerting isometric contractions. *European Journal of Applied Physiology* 54: 331-335.

Kalra, P.S., Sahu, A., and Kalra, S.P. 1990. Interleukin-1 inhibits the ovarian steroid-induced luteinizing hormone surge and release of hypothalamic luteinizing hormone-releasing hormone in rats. *Endocrinology* 126: 2145-2152.

Kamen, G., Kroll, W., and Ziagon, S.T. 1984. Exercise effects upon reflex time components in weight lifters and distance runners. *Medicine and Science in Sports and Exercise* 13: 198-204.

Kamen, G., and Roy A. 2000. Motor unit synchronization in young and elderly adults. *European Journal of Applied Physiology* 81: 403-410.

Kanakis, C., and Hickson, C. 1980. Left ventricular responses to a program of lower-limb strength training. *Chest* 78: 618-621.

Kanehisa, H., Ikegawa, S., Tsunoda, N., and Fukunaga, T. 1994. Strength and cross-sectional area of knee extension muscles in children. *European Journal of Applied Physiology* 68: 402-405.

Kanehisa, H., Ikegawa, S., and Fukunaga, T. 1998. Body composition and cross-sectional areas of limb lean tissues in Olympic weight lifters. *Scandinavian Journal of Medicine and Science in Sports* 8: 271-278.

Kanehisa, H., and Miyashita, M. 1983a. Effect of isometric and isokinetic muscle training on static strength and dynamic power. *European Journal of Applied Physiology* 50: 365-371.

Kanehisa, H., and Miyashita, M. 1983b. Specificity of velocity in strength training. *European Journal of Applied Physiology* 52: 104-106.

Kanehisa, H., Nagareda, H., Kawakami, Y., Akima, H., Masani, K., Kouzaki, M., and Fukanaga, T. 2002. Effects of equivolume isometric training programs comprising medium or high resistance on muscle size and strength. *European Journal of Applied Physiology* 87: 112-119.

Kanehisa, H., Okuyama, H., Ikegawa, S., and Fukunga, T. 1996. Sex difference in force generation capacity during repeated maximal knee extensions. *European Journal of Applied Physiology* 73: 557-562.

Kaneko, M., Fuchimoto, T., Toji, H., and Suei, K. 1983. Training effect of different loads on the force-velocity relationship and mechanical power output in human muscle. *Scandinavian Journal of Sports Science* 5: 50-55.

Karlsson, J., Bonde-Petersen, F., Henriksson, J., and Knuttgen, H.G. 1975. Effects of previous exercise with arms or legs on metabolism and performance in exhaustive exercise. *Journal of Applied Physiology* 38: 208-211.

Katch, U.L., Katch, F.I., Moffatt, R., and Gittleson, M. 1980. Muscular development and lean body weight in body builders and weight lifters. *Medicine and Science in Sports and Exercise* 12: 340-344.

Katz, B. 1939. The relationship between force and speed in muscular contraction. *Journal of Physiology* 96: 45-64.

Kauhanen, H., and Häkkinen, K. 1989. Short term effects of voluminous heavy resistance training and recovery on the snatch technique in weightlifting. In *Proceedings of the XII International Congress of Biomechanics,* edited by R.J. Gregor, R.F. Zernicke, and W.C. Whitting. Abstract, 31.

Kawakami, Y., Abe T., and Fukunaga T. 1993. Muscle-fiber pennation angles are greater in hypertrophied than in normal muscles. *Journal of Applied Physiology* 74: 2740-2744.

Kawakami, Y., Abe, T., Kuno, S., and Fukunaga, T. 1995. Training induced changes in muscle architecture and specific tension. *European Journal of Applied Physiology* 72: 37-43.

Kearns, C.F., Abe, T., and Brechue, W.F. 2000. Muscle enlargement in sumo wrestlers includes increased muscle fascicle length. *European Journal of Applied Physiology* 83: 289-296.

Keeler, L.K., Finkelstein, L.H., Miller, W., and Fernhall, B. 2001. Early-phase adaptations of traditional speed vs. superslow resistance training on strength and aerobic capacity in sedentary individuals. *Journal of Strength and Conditioning Research* 15: 309-314.

Kell, R.T., Bell, G., and Quinney, A. 2001. Musculoskeletal fitness, health and quality of life. *Sports Medicine* 31: 863-873.

Kelley, G.A., Kelley, K.S., and Tran, Z.V. 2000. Exercise and bone mineral density in men: A meta-analysis. *Journal of Applied Physiology* 88: 1730-1736.

Kelley G.A., Kelley, K.S., and Tran, Z.V. 2001. Resistance training and bone mineral density in women: A meta-analysis of controlled trials. *American Journal of Physical Medicine and Rehabilitation* 80: 65-77.

Kellis, E., and Baltzopoulos, V. 1995. Isokinetic eccentric exercise. *Sports Medicine* 19: 202-222.

Kent-Braun, J.A., Ng, A.V., and Young, K. 2000. Skeletal muscle contractile and noncontractile components in young and older women and men. *Journal of Applied Physiology* 88: 662-668.

Keogh, J.W.L., Wilson, G.J., and Weatherby, R.P. 1999. A cross-sectional comparison of different resistance training techniques in the bench press. *Journal of Strength and Conditioning Research* 13: 247-258.

Kerr, D. Ackland, T., Maslen, B., Morton, A., and Prince, R. 2001. Resistance training over 2 years increases bone mass in postmenopausal women. *Journal of Bone and Mineral Research* 16: 175-181.

Kesperek, S.J., Conway, G.R., Krayeski, D.S., and Lohne, J.J. 1992. A reexamination of the effect of exercise on rate of muscle protein degradation. *American Journal of Physiology* 263: E1144-E1150.

Keul, J., Haralambei, G., Bruder, M., and Gottstein, H.J. 1978. The effect of weight lifting exercise on heart rate and metabolism in experienced lifters. *Medicine and Science in Sports and Exercise* 10: 13-15.

Khan, K., McKay, H.A., Haapassalo, H., Bennell, K.L., Forwood, M.R., Kannus, P., and Wark, J.D. 2000. Does childhood and adolescence provide a unique opportunity for exercise to strengthen the skeleton? *Journal of Science and Medicine in Sport* 3: 150-164.

King, D.S., Sharp, R.L., Vukovich, M.D., Brown, G.A., Reifenrath, T.A., Uhl, N., and Parsons, K.A. 1999. Effect of oral androstenedione on serum testosterone and adaptations to resistance training in young men: A randomized controlled trial. *Journal of the American Medical Association* 281: 2020-2028.

Kitai, T.A., and Sale, D.G. 1989. Specificity of joint angle in isometric training. *European Journal of Applied Physiology* 58: 744-748.

Kjaer, M., and Secher, N.H. 1992. Neural influences on cardiovascular and endocrine responses to static exercise in humans. *Sports Medicine* 13: 303-319.

Kleiner, D.M., Blessing, D.L., Davis, W.R., and Mitchell, J.W. 1996. Acute cardiovascular responses to various forms of resistance exercise. *Journal of Strength and Conditioning Research* 10: 56-61.

Kleiner, D.M., Blessing, D.L., Mitchell, J.W., and Davis, W.R. 1999. A description of the acute cardiovascular responses to isokinetic resistance at three different speeds. *Journal of Strength and Conditioning Research* 13: 360-366.

Kleiner, S.M., Bazzarre, T.L., and Ainsworth, B.E. 1994. Nutritional status of nationally ranked elite bodybuilders. *International Journal of Sports Medicine* 4: 54-69.

Klitgaard, H., Ausoni, S., and Damiani, E. 1989. Sarcoplasmic reticulum of human skeletal muscle: Age-related changes and effect of training. *Acta Physiologica Scandinavica* 137: 23-31.

Klitgaard, H., Mantoni, M., Schiaffino, S., Ausoni, S., Gorza, L., Laurent-Winter, C., Schnohr, P., and Saltin, B. 1990. Function, morphology and protein expression of ageing skeletal muscle: A cross-sectional study of elderly men with different training backgrounds. *Acta Physiologica Scandinavica* 140: 41-54.

Knapik, J.J., Mawdsley, R.H., and Ramos, M.U. 1983. Angular specificity and test mode specificity of isometric and isokinetic strength training. *Journal of Orthopedic Sports Physical Therapy* 5: 58-65.

Knapik, J.J., Wright, J.E., Kowal, D.M., and Vogel, J.A. 1980. The influence of U.S. Army basic initial entry training on the muscular strength of men and women. *Aviation, Space and Environmental Medicine* 51: 1086-1090.

Knuttgen, H.G., and Kraemer, W.J. 1987. Terminology and measurement in exercise performance. *Journal of Applied Sport Science Research* 1: 1-10.

Knuttgen, H.G., and Saltin, B. 1972. Muscle metabolites and oxygen uptake in short-term submaximal exercise in man. *Journal of Applied Physiology* 32: 690-694.

Kokkonen, J., Bangerter, B., Roundy, E., and Nelson, A. 1988. Improved performance through digit strength gains. *Research Quarterly for Exercise and Sport* 59: 57-63.

Komi, P.V. 1979. Neuromuscular performance: Factors influencing force and speed production. *Scandinavian Journal of Sports Sciences* 1:2-15.

Komi, P.V., and Buskirk, E.R. 1972. Effect of eccentric and concentric muscle conditioning on tension and electrical activity of human muscle. *Ergonomics* 15: 417-434.

Komi, P.V., and Häkkinen, K. 1988. Strength and power. In *The Olympic book of sports medicine,* edited by A. Dirix, H.G. Knuttgen, and K. Tittel, 183. Boston: Blackwell Scientific.

Komi, P.V., Kaneko, M., and Aura, O. 1987. EMG activity of the leg extensor muscles with special reference to mechanical efficiency in concentric and eccentric exercise. *International Journal of Sports Medicine* 8: 22-29.

Komi, P.V., and Karlsson, J. 1978. Skeletal muscle fiber types, enzyme activities and physical performance in young males and females. *Acta Physiologica Scandinavica* 103: 210-218.

Komi, P.V., Linnamo, V., Ventoinen, P., and Sillanpaa, M. 2000. Force and EMG power spectrum during eccentric and concentric actions. *Medicine and Science in Sports and Exercise* 32: 1757-1762.

Komi, P.V., Suominen, H., Heikkinen, E., Karlsson, J., and Tesch, P. 1982. Effects of heavy resistance and explosive-type strength training methods on mechanical, functional, and metabolic aspects of performance. In *Exercise and sport biology,* edited by P.V. Komi, 90-102. Champaign, IL: Human Kinetics.

Koutedakis, Y., Boreham, C., Kabitsis, C., Sharp, N.C.C. 1992. Seasonal deterioration of selected physiological variables in elite male skiers. *International Journal of Sports Medicine* 13: 548-551.

Kovaleski, J.E., and Heitman, R.J. 1993a. Effects of isokinetic velocity spectrum exercise on torque production. *Sports Medicine, Training and Rehabilitation* 4: 67-71.

Kovaleski, J.E., and Heitman, R.J. 1993b. Interaction of velocity and progression order during isokinetic velocity spectrum exercise. *Isokinetics and Exercise Science* 3: 118-122.

Kovaleski, J.E., Heitman, R.J., Scaffidi, F.M., and Fondren, F.B. 1992. Effects of isokinetic velocity spectrum exercise on average power and total work. *Journal of Athletic Training* 27: 54-56.

Kovaleski, J.E., Heitman, R.H., Trundle, T.L., and Gilley, W.F. 1995. Isotonic preload versus isokinetic knee extension resistance training. *Medicine and Science in Sports and Exercise* 27: 895-899.

Kowalchuk, J.M., Heigenhauser, F.J.F., Lininger, MI., Obminski, G., Sutton, J.R., and Jones, N.L. 1988. Role of lungs and inactive muscle in acid-base control after maximal exercise. *Journal of Applied Physiology* 65: 2090-2096.

Koziris, L.P., Hickson, R.C., Chatterton, R.T., Groseth, R.T., Christie, J.M., Goldflies, D.G., and Unterman, T.G. 1999. Serum levels of total and free IGF-1 and IGFBP-3 are increased and maintained in long-term training. *Journal of Applied Physiology* 86: 1436-1442.

Koziris, L.P., Kraemer; W.J., Patton, J.F., Triplett, N.T., Fry, A.C., Gordon, S.E., and Knuttgen, H.G. 1996. Relationship of aerobic power to anaerobic performance indices. *Journal of Strength and Conditioning Research* 10: 35-39.

Kraemer, W.J. 1983a. Detraining the "bulked-up" athlete: Prospects for lifetime health and fitness. *National Strength and Conditioning Association Journal* 5: 10-12.

Kraemer, W.J. 1983b. Exercise prescription in weight training: A needs analysis. *National Strength and Conditioning Association Journal* 5: 64-65.

Kraemer, W.J. 1983c. Exercise prescription in weight training: Manipulating program variables. *National Strength and Conditioning Association Journal* 5: 58-59.

Kraemer, W.J. 1988. Endocrine responses to resistance exercise. *Medicine and Science in Sports and Exercise* 20 (Suppl.): S152-S157.

Kraemer, W.J. 1992a. Endocrine responses and adaptations to strength training. In *Strength and power in sports,* edited by P.V. Komi, 291-304. Boston: Blackwell Scientific.

Kraemer, W.J. 1992b. Hormonal mechanisms related to the expression of muscular strength and power. In *Strength and power in sports,* edited by P.V. Komi, 64-76. Boston: Blackwell Scientific.

Kraemer, W.J. 1994. Neuroendocrine responses to resistance exercise. In *Essentials of strength and conditioning,* edited by T.R. Baechle, 86-107. Champaign, IL: Human Kinetics.

Kraemer, W.J. 1997. A series of studies: The physiological basis for strength training in American football: Fact over philosophy. *Journal of Strength and Conditioning Research* 11: 131-142.

Kraemer, W.J., Aguilera, B.A., Terada, M., Newton, R.U., Lynch, J.M., Rosendaal, G., McBride, J.M., Gordon, S.E., and Häkkinen, K. 1995. Responses of IGF-I to endogenous increases in growth hormone after heavy-resistance exercise. *Journal of Applied Physiology* 77: 206-211.

Kraemer, W.J., Clemson, A., Triplett, N.T., Bush, J.A., Newton, R.U., and Lynch, J.M. 1996. The effects of plasma cortisol evaluation on total and differential leukocyte counts in response to heavy-resistance exercise. *European Journal of Applied Physiology* 73(1-2): 93-97.

Kraemer, W.J., Deschenes, M.R., and Fleck, S.J. 1988. Physiological adaptations to resistance exercise implications for athletic conditioning. *Sports Medicine* 6: 246-256.

Kraemer, W.J., Dudley, G.A., Tesch, P.A., Gordon, S.E., Hather, B.M., Volek, J.S., and Ratamess, N.A. 2001. The influence of muscle action on the acute growth hormone response to resistance exercise and short-term detraining. *Growth Hormone and IGF Research* 11: 75-83.

Kraemer, W.J., Dziados, J.E., Marchitelli, L.J., Gordon, S.E., Harman, E.A., Mello, R., Fleck, S.J., Frykman, P.N., and Triplett, N.T. 1993. Effects of different heavy-resistance exercise protocols on plasma B-endorphin concentrations. *Journal of Applied Physiology* 74: 450-459.

Kraemer, W.J., and Fleck, S.J. 1993. *Strength training for young athletes.* Champaign IL: Human Kinetics.

Kraemer, W.J., Fleck, S.J., Dziados, J.E., Harman, E., Marchitelli, L.J., Gordon, S.E., Mello, R., Frykman, P.N., Koziris, L.P., and Triplett, N.T. 1993. Changes in hormonal concentrations following different heavy resistance exercise protocols in women. *Journal of Applied Physiology* 75: 594-604.

Kraemer, W.J., Fleck, S.J. and Evans, W.J. 1996. Strength and power training: Physiological mechanisms of adaptation. In *Exercise and sport sciences reviews,* edited by J.O. Holoszy, 363-398. Baltimore: Williams & Wilkins.

Kraemer, W.J., Fleck, S.J., Maresh, C.M., Ratamess, N.A., Gordon, S.E., Goetz, K.L., Harman, E.A., Frykman, P.N., Volek, J., Mazzetti, S.A., Fry, A.C., Marchitelli, L.J., and Patton, J.F. 1999. Acute hormonal responses to a single bout of heavy resistance exercise in trained power lifters and untrained men. *Canadian Journal of Applied Physiology* 24: 524-537.

Kraemer, W.J., and Fry, A.C. 1995. Strength testing: Development and evaluation of methodology. In *Physiological assessment of human fitness,* edited by P. Maud and C. Foster. Champaign, IL: Human Kinetics.

Kraemer, W.J., Fry, A.C., Rubin, M.R., Triplett-McBride, T., Gordon, S.E., Koziris, L.P., Lynch, J.M., Volek, J.S., Meuffels, D.E., Newton, R.U., and Fleck, S.J. 2001. Physiological and performance responses to tournament wrestling. *Medicine and Science in Sports and Exercise* 33: 1367-1378.

Kraemer, W.J., Fry, A.C., Warren, B.J., Stone, M.H., Fleck, S.J., Kearney, J.T., Conroy, B.P., Maresh, C.M., Weseman, C.A., Triplett, N.T., and Gordon, S.E. 1992. Acute hormonal responses of elite junior weightlifters. *International Journal of Sports Medicine* 12: 228-235.

Kraemer, W.J., Gordon, S.E., Fleck, S.J., Marchitelli, L.J., Mello, R., Dziados, J.E., Friedl, K., Harman, E., Maresh, C., and Fry, A.C. 1991. Endogenous anabolic hormonal and growth factor responses to heavy resistance exercise in males and females. *International Journal of Sports Medicine* 12: 228-235.

Kraemer, W.J., and Gotshalk, L.A. 2000. Physiology of American football. In *Exercise and sport science,* edited by W.E. Garrett and D.T. Kirkendall, 798-813. Philadelphia: Lippincott, Williams & Wilkins.

Kraemer, W.J., Häkkinen, K., Newton, R.U., McCormick, M., Nindl, B.C., Volek, J.S., Gotshalk, L.A., Fleck, S.J., Campbell, W.W., Gordon, S.E., Farrell, P.A., and Evans, W.J. 1998. Acute hormonal responses to heavy resistance exercise in younger and older men. *European Journal of Applied Physiology* 77: 206-211.

Kraemer, W.J., Häkkinen, K., Newton, R. U., Nindl, B.C., Volek, J.S., McCormick, M., Gotshalk, L.A., Gordon, S.E., Fleck, S.J., Campbell, W.W., Putukian, M., and Evans, W.J. 1999. Effects of heavy-resistance training on hormonal response patterns in younger vs. older men. *Journal of Applied Physiology* 87: 982-992.

Kraemer, W.J., Keuning, M., Ratamess, N.A., Volek, J.S., McCormick, M., Bush, J.A., Nindl, B.C., Gordon, S.E., Mazzetti, S.A., Newton, R.U., Gomez, A.L., Wickham, R.B., Rubin, M.R., and Häkkinen, K. 2001. Resistance training combined with bench-stepping enhances women's health profile. *Medicine and Science in Sports and Exercise* 33: 259-269.

Kraemer, W.J., and Koziris, L.P. 1992. Muscle strength training: Techniques and considerations. *Physical Therapy Practice* 2: 54-68.

Kraemer, W.J., and Koziris, L.P. 1994. Olympic weightlifting and power lifting. In *Physiology and nutrition for competitive sport,* edited by D.R. Lamb, H.G. Knuttgen, and R. Murray, 1-54. Carmel, IN: Cooper.

Kraemer, W.J., Koziris, L.P., Ratamess, N.A., Häkkinen, K., Triplett-McBride, N.T., Fry, A.C., Gordon, S.E., Volek, J.S., French, D.N., Rubin, M.R., Gomez, A.L., Sharman, M.J., Lynch, J.M., Izquierdo, M., and Fleck, S.J. 2002. Detraining produces minimal changes in physical performance and hormonal variables in recreationally strength-trained men. *Journal of Strength and Conditioning Research* 16: 373-382.

Kraemer, W.J., Loebel, C.C., Volek, J.S., Ratamess, N.A., Newton, R.U., Wickham, R.B., Gotshalk, L.A., Duncan, N.D., Mazzetti, S.A., Gomez, A.L., Rubin, M.R., Nindl, B.C., and Häkkinen, K. 2001. The effect of heavy resistance exercise on the circadian rhythm of salivary testosterone in men. *European Journal of Applied Physiology* 84: 13-18.

Kraemer, W.J., Marchitelli, L., McCurry, D., Mello, R., Dziados, J.E., Harman, E., Frykman, P., Gordon, S.E., and Fleck, S.J. 1990. Hormonal and growth factor responses to heavy resistance exercise. *Journal of Applied Physiology* 69: 1442-1450.

Kraemer, W.J., Mazzetti, S.A., Nindl, B.C., Gotshalk, L.A., Volek, J.S., Bush, J.A., Marx, J.O., Dohi, K., Gomez, A.L., Miles, M., Fleck, S.J., Newton, R.U., and Häkkinen, K. 2001. Effect of resistance training on women's strength/power and occupational performances. *Medicine and Science in Sports and Exercise* 33: 1011-1025.

Kraemer, W.J., and Newton, R.U. 2000. Training for muscular power. *Physical and Medical Rehabilitation Clinics of North America* 11: 341-368.

Kraemer, W.J., Noble, B.J., Culver, B.W., and Clark, M.J. 1987. Physiologic responses to heavy-resistance exercise with very short rest periods. *International Journal of Sports Medicine* 8: 247-252.

Kraemer, W.J., Patton, J., Gordon, S.E., Harman, E.A., Deschenes, M.R., Reynolds, K., Newton, R.U., Triplett, N.T., and Dziados, J.E. 1995. Compatibility of high intensity strength and endurance training on hormonal and skeletal muscle adaptations. *Journal of Applied Physiology* 78: 976-989.

Kraemer, W.J., Patton, J.F., Knuttgen, H.G., Marchitelli, L.J., Cruthirds, C., Damokosh, A., Harman, E., Frykman, P., and Dziados, J.E. 1989. Hypothalamic pituitary-adrenal responses to short duration high-intensity cycle exercise. *Journal of Applied Physiology* 66: 161-166.

Kraemer, W.J., and Ratamess, N.A. 2000. Physiology of resistance training: Current issues. In *Orthopaedic Physical Therapy Clinics of North America: Exercise Technologies* 9: 4, pp. 467-513. Philadelphia: W.B. Saunders.

Kraemer, W.J., Ratamess, N., Fry, A.C., Triplett-McBride, T., Koziris, L.P., Bauer, J.A., Lynch, J.M., and Fleck, S.J. 2000. Influence of resistance training volume and periodization on physiological and performance adaptations in collegiate women tennis players. *The American Journal of Sports Medicine* 28: 626-633.

Kraemer, W.J., Staron, R.S., Hagerman, F.C., Hikida, R.S., Fry, A.C., Gordon, S.E., Nindl, B.C., Gotshalk, L.A., Volek, J.S., Marx, J.O., Newton, R.U., and Häkkinen, K. 1998. The effects of short-term resistance training on endocrine function in men and women. *European Journal of Applied Physiology* 78: 69-76.

Kraemer, W.J., Vogel, J.A., Patton, J.F., Dziados, J.E., and Reynolds, K.L. 1987. The effects of various physical training programs on short duration high intensity load bearing performance and the Army physical fitness test. *USARIEM Technical Report,* 30/87 August.

Kraemer, W.J., Volek, J.S., Bush, J.A., Putukian, M., and Sebastianelli, W.J. 1998. Hormonal responses to consecutive days of heavy-resistance exercise with or without nutritional supplementation. *Journal of Applied Physiology* 85: 1544-1555.

Kramer, J.B., Stone, M.H., O'Bryant, H.S., Conley, M.S., Johnson, R.L., Nieman, D.C., Honeycutt, D.R., and Hoke, T.P. 1997. Effects of single vs. multiple sets of weight training: Impact of volume, intensity, and variation. *Journal of Strength and Conditioning Research* 11: 143-147.

Kubo, K., Kanehisa, H., Ito, M., and Fukunaga, T. 2001. Effects of isometric training on the elasticity of human tendon structures in vivo. *Journal of Applied Physiology* 91: 26-32.

Kubo, K., Kanehisa, H., and Fukunaga, T. 2002. Effects of resistance and stretching training programmes on the viscoelastic properties of human tendon structures *in vivo. Journal of Physiology* 538: 219-226.

Kujala, U.M., Sarna, S., Kaprio, J., Tikkanen, H.O., and Koskenvuo, M. 2000. Natural selection to sports, later physical activity habits, and coronary heart disease. *British Journal of Sports Medicine* 34: 445-449.

Kumagai, K., Abe, T., Brechue, W.F., Ryushi, T., Takano, S., and Mizuno, M. 2000. Sprint performance is related to muscle fascicle length in male 100-m sprinters. *Journal of Applied Physiology* 88: 811-816.

Kusintz, I., and Kenney, C. 1958. Effects of progressive weight training on health and physical fitness of adolescent boys. *Research Quarterly* 29: 295-301.

Lacerte, M., deLateur, B.J., Alquist, A.D., and Questad, K.A. 1992. Concentric versus combined concentric-eccentric isokinetic training programs: Effect on peak torque of human quadriceps femoris muscle. *Archives of Physical Medicine and Rehabilitation* 73: 1059-1062.

LaChance, P.F. and Hortobagyi, T. 1994. Influence of cadence on muscular performance during push-up and pull-up exercises. *Journal of Strength and Conditioning Research* 8: 76-79.

Laidlaw, D.H., Kornatz, K.W., Keen, D.A., Suzuki, S., and Enoka, R.M. 1999. Strength training improves the steadiness of slow lengthening contractions performed by old adults. *Journal of Applied Physiology* 87: 1786-1795.

Lamb, D.R. 1978. *Physiology of exercise: Response and adaptations.* New York: Macmillan.

Lander, J.E., Bates, B.T., Sawhill, J.A., and Hamill, J.A. 1985. Comparison between free-weight and isokinetic bench pressing. *Medicine and Science in Sports and Exercise* 17: 344-353.

Lander, J.E., Hundley, J.R., and Simonton, R.L. 1992. The effectiveness of weight-belts during multiple repetitions of the squat exercise. *Medicine and Science in Sports and Exercise* 24: 603-609.

Lander, J.E., Simonton, R., and Giacobbe, J. 1990. The effectiveness of weight-belts during the squat exercise. *Medicine and Science in Sports and Exercise* 22: 117-126.

Landers, K.A., Hunter, G.R., Wetzstein, C.J., Bamman, M.M., and Weisier, R.L. 2001. The interrelationship among muscle mass, strength, and the ability to perform physical tasks of daily living in younger and older women. *Journal of Gerontology: Biological Sciences, Medical Sciences* 56: B443-B448.

Larsson, L. 1978. Morphological and functional characteristics of the aging skeletal muscle in man. *Acta Physiological Scandinavica* 457 (Suppl.): 1-36.

Larsson, L. 1982. Physical training effects on muscle morphology in sedentary males at different ages. *Medicine, Science, and Sports Exercise* 14: 203-206.

Larsson, L. 1983. Histochemical characteristics of human skeletal muscle during aging. *Acta Physiologica Scandinavica* 117: 469-471.

Lathinghouse, L.H., and Trimble, M.H. 2000. Effects of isometric quadriceps activation on the q-angle in women before and after quadriceps exercise. *Journal of Orthopaedic and Sports Physical Therapy* 30:211-216.

Laubach, L.L. 1976. Comparative muscular strength of men and women: A review of the literature. *Aviation, Space and Environmental Medicine* 47: 534-542.

Laurent, D., Reutenauer, H., Payen, J.F., Favre-Javin, A., Eterradossi, J., Lekas, J.F., and Rossi, A. 1992. Muscle bioenergetics in skiers: Studies using NMR. *International Journal of Sports Medicine* 13 (Suppl. 1): S150-S152.

Laurent, G.J., Sparrow, M.P., Bates, P.C., and Millward, D.J. 1978. Collagen content and turnover in cardiac and skeletal muscles of the adult fowl and the changes during stretch induced growth. *Biochemistry Journal* 176: 419-427.

Laursen, P.B., and Jenkins, D.G. 2002. The scientific basis for high-intensity interval training: Optimizing training programs and maximizing performance in highly trained endurance athletes. *Sports Medicine* 32: 53-73.

Laycoe, R.R., and Marteniuk, R.G. 1971. Leaning and tension as factors in strength gains produced by static and eccentric training. *Research Quarterly* 42: 299-305.

Layne, J.E., and Nelson, M.E. 1999. The effects of progress of resistance training on bone density: A review. *Medicine and Science in Sports and Exercise* 3: 25-30.

Lebenstedt, M., Platte, P., and Pirke, K.M. 1999. Reduced resting metabolic rate in athletes with menstrual disorders. *Medicine and Science in Sports and Exercise* 31: 1250-1256.

Lebrun, C.M. 1994. The effect of the phase of the menstrual cycle and the birth control pill on athletic performance. *Clinics in Sports Medicine* 13: 419-441.

Lee, A., Craig, B.W., Lucas, J., Pohlman, R., and Stelling, H. 1990. The effect of endurance training, weight training and a combination of endurance and weight training on blood lipid profile of young males subjects. *Journal of Applied Sport Science Research* 4: 68-75.

Legwold, G. 1982. Does lifting weights harm a prepubescent athlete? *Physician and Sportsmedicine* 10: 141-144.

Leiger, A.B., and Milner, T.E. 2001. Muscle function at the wrist after eccentric exercise. *Medicine and Science in Sports and Exercise* 33: 612-620.

Leighton, J. 1955. Instrument and technique for measurement of range of joint motion. *Archives of Physical Medicine and Rehabilitation* 38: 24-28.

Leighton, J. 1957. Flexibility characteristics of three specialized skill groups of champion athletes. *Archives of Physical Medicine and Rehabilitation* 38: 580-583.

Leighton, J.R., Holmes, D., Benson, J., Wooten, B., and Schmerer, R. 1967. A study of the effectiveness of ten different methods of progressive resistance exercise on the development of strength, flexibility, girth and body weight. *Journal of the Association of Physical and Mental Rehabilitation* 21: 78-81.

Lemmer, J.T., Hurlbut, D.E., Martel, G.F., Tracy, B.L., Ivey, F.M., Metter, E.J., Fozard, J.L., Fleg, J.L., and Hurley, B.F. 2000. Age and gender responses to strength training and detraining. *Medicine and Science in Sports and Exercise* 32: 1505-1512.

Lemmer, J.T., Ivey, F.M., Ryan, A.S., Martel, G.F., Hurlbut, D.E., Metter, J.E., Fozard, J.L., Fleg, J.L., and Hurley, B.F. 2001. Effect of strength training on resting metabolic rate and physical activity: Age and gender comparisons. *Medicine and Science in Sports and Exercise* 33: 532-541.

Lemon, P.W., and Mullin, J.P. 1980. Effect of initial muscle glycogen levels on protein catabolism during exercise. *Journal of Applied Physiology: Respiratory, Environmental and Exercise Physiology* 48: 624-629.

LeMura, L.M., Von Duvillard, S.P., Andreacci, J.A., Klebez, J.M., Chelland, S.A., and Russo, J. 2000. Lipid and lipoprotein profiles, cardiovascular fitness, body composition, and diet during and after resistance, aerobic and combination training in young women. *European Journal of Applied Physiology* 82: 451-458.

Lesmes, G.R., Costill, D.L., Coyle, E.F., and Fink, W.J. 1978. Muscle strength and power changes during maximal isokinetic training. *Medicine and Science in Sports* 4: 266-269.

Lewis, A.J., Wester, T.J., Burrin, D.G., and Dauncey, M.J. 2000. Exogenous growth hormone induces somatotrophic gene expression in neonatal liver and skeletal muscle. *American Journal of Physiology* 278: R838-R844.

Lewis, S., Nygaard, E., Sanchez, J., Egelbald, H., and Saltin, B. 1984. Static contraction of the quadriceps muscle in man: Cardiovascular control and responses to one-legged strength training. *Acta Physiologica Scandinavica* 122: 341-353.

Lexell, J., Hendriksson-Larsen, K., Winblad, B., and Sjostrom, M. 1983. Distribution of different fiber types in human skeletal muscles: Effects of aging studied in whole muscle cross section. *Muscle Nerve* 6: 588-595.

Lexell, J., Taylor, C.C., and Sjostrom, M. 1988. What is the cause of the ageing strophy? Total number, size and proportion of different fiber types studied in whole vastus lateralis muscle from 15- to 83-year-old men. *Journal of Neurological Sciences* 84: 275-294.

Liederman, E. 1925. *Secrets of strength*. New York: Earle Liederman.

Lind, A.R., and Petrofsky, J.S. 1978. Isometric tension from rotary stimulation of fast and slow cat muscles. *Muscle and Nerve* 1: 213-218.

Lindh, M. 1979. Increase of muscle strength from isometric quadriceps exercises at different knee angles. *Scandinavian Journal of Rehabilitation Medicine* 11: 33-36.

Linsenbardt, S.T., Thomas, T.R., and Madsen, R.W. 1992. Effect of breathing technique on blood pressure response to resistance exercise. *British Journal of Sports Medicine* 26: 97-100.

Lithinghouse, L.H., and Trimble, M.H. 2000. Effects of isometric quadriceps activation on the q-angle in women before and after quadriceps exercise. *Journal of Orthopedic and Sports Physical Therapy* 20:211-230.

Liu, H., Liu, P., and Qin, X. 1987. *Investigation of menstrual cycle and female weightlifters*. Beijing: Department of Exercise Physiology, National Institue of Sports Science.

Lloyd, T., Buchanan, J.R., Bitzer, S., Waldman, C.J., Myers, C., and Ford, B.G. 1987. Interrelationship of diet, athletic activity, menstrual status and bone density in collegiate women. *Amerian Journal of Clinical Nutrition* 46: 681-684.

Lombardi, V.P., and Troxel, R.K. 1999. Weight training injuries & deaths in the U.S. *Medicine and Science in Sports and Exercise* 31: S93.

Longcope, C. 1996. Dehydroepiandrosterone metabolism. *Journal of Endocrinology* 150 (Suppl.): S125-S127.

Loucks, A.B., and Horvath, S.M. 1985. Athletic amenorrhea: A review. *Medicine and Science in Sports and Exercise* 17: 56-72.

Loughna, P.T., Mason, P., and Bates, P.C. 1992. Regulation of insulin-like growth factor I gene expression in skeletal muscle. *Symposium of the Society for Experimental Biology* 46: 319-330.

Ludbrook, J., Faris, I.B., Iannos, J., Jamieson, G.G., and Russel, W.J. 1978. Lack of effect of isometric handgrip exercise on the responses of the carotid sinus baroreceptor reflex in man. *Clinical Science and Molecular Medicine* 55: 189-194.

Lund, H., Vestergaard-Poulsen, P., Kanstrup, I.-L., and Sejrsen, P. 1998. The effect of passive stretching on delayed onset muscle soreness, and other detrimental effects following eccentric exercise. *Scandinavian Journal of Medicine and Science in Sports* 8: 216-221.

Lusiani, L., Ronsisvalle, G., Bonanome, A., Castellani, V., Macchia, C., and Pagan, A. 1986. Echocardiographic evaluation of the dimensions and systolic properties of the left ventricle in freshman athletes during physical training. *European Heart Journal* 7: 196-203.

Luthi, J.M., Howald, H., Claassen, H., Rosler, K., Vock, P., and Hoppler, H. 1986. Structural changes in skeletal muscle tissue with heavy-resistance exercise. *International Journal of Sports Medicine* 7: 123-127.

Lyle, N., and Rutherford, O.M. 1998. A comparison of voluntary versus stimulated strength training of the human abductor pollicis muscle. *Journal Sports Sciences* 16: 267-270.

Lyman, S., Fleisig, G.S., Waterbor, J.W., Funkhouser, E.M., Pulley, L., Andrews, J.R., Osiniki, E.D., and Roseman, J.M. 2001. Longitudinal study of elbow and shoulder pain in youth baseball pitchers. *Medicine and Science in Sports and Exercise* 33: 1803-1810.

Lynch, N.A., Metter, E.J., Lindle, R.S., Fozard, J.L., Tobin, J.D., Roy, T.A., Fleg, J.L., and Hurley, B.F. 1999. Muscle quality. I. use associated differences between arm and leg muscle groups. *Journal of Applied Physiology* 86: 188-194.

Macaluso, A., De Vitto, G., Felici, F., and Nimmo, M.A. 2000. Electromyogram changes during sustained contraction after resistance training in women in their 3rd and 8th decades. *European Journal of Applied Physiology* 82: 418-424.

MacDougall, J.D. 1986. Adaptability of muscle to strength training—A cellular approach. In *Biochemistry of exercise VI*, 501-513. Champaign, IL: Human Kinetics.

MacDougall, J.D. 1992. Hypertrophy or hyperplasia. In *Strength and power in sport*, edited by P.V. Komi, 230-238. Oxford: Blackwell Scientific.

MacDougall, J.D., Gibala, M.J., Tarnopolsky, M.A., MacDonald, J.R., Interisano, S.A., and Yarasheski, K.E. 1995. The time course for elevated muscle protein synthesis following heavy resistance exercise. *Canadian Journal of Applied Physiology* 20: 480-486.

MacDougall, J.D., Hicks, A.L., MacDonald, J.R., McKelvie, R.S., Green, H.J., and Smith, K.M. 1998. Muscle performance and enzymatic adaptations to sprint interval training. *Journal of Applied Physiology* 84: 2138-2142.

MacDougall, J.D., Sale, D.G., Alway, S.E., and Sutton, J.R. 1984. Muscle fiber number in biceps brachii in bodybuilders and control subjects. *Journal of Applied Physiology* 57: 1399-1403.

MacDougall, J.D., Sale, D.G., Elder, G.C.B., and Sutton, J.R. 1982. Muscle ultrastructural characteristics of elite powerlifters and bodybuilders. *European Journal of Applied Physiology* 48: 117-126.

MacDougall, J.D., Sale, D.G., Moroz, J.R., Elder, G.C.B., Sutton, J.R., Howald, H. 1979. Mitochondrial volume density in human skeletal muscle following heavy resistance training. *Medicine and Science in Sports* 11: 164-166.

MacDougall, J.D., Tarnopolsky, M.A., Chesley, A., and Atkinson, S.A. 1992. Changes in muscle protein synthesis following heavy resistance exercise in humans: A pilot study. *Acta Physiologica Scandinavica* 146: 403-404.

MacDougall, J.D., Tuxen, D., Sale, D.G., Moroz, J.R., and Sutton, J.R. 1985. Arterial blood pressure response to heavy resistance exercise. *Journal of Applied Physiology* 58: 785-790.

MacDougall, J.D., Ward, G.R., Sale, D.G., and Sutton, J.R. 1977. Biochemical adaptations of human skeletal muscle to heavy resistance training and immobilization. *Journal of Applied Physiology* 43: 700-703.

Maddalozzo, G.F., and Snow, C.M. 2000. High intensity resistance training: Effects on bone in older men and women. *Calcification Tissue International* 66: 399-404.

Madsen, N., and McLaughlin, T. 1984. Kinematic factors influencing performance and injury risk in the bench press exercise. *Medicine and Science in Sports and Exercise* 16: 429-437.

Maffiuletti, N.A., and Martin, A. 2001. Progressive versus rapid rate of contraction during 7 wk of isometric resistance training. *Medicine and Science in Sports and Exercise* 33: 1220-1227.

Magnusson, S.P. 1998. Passive properties of human skeletal muscle during stretch maneuvers: A review. *Scandinavian Journal of Medicine, Science and Sports* 8: 65-77.

Magnusson, S.P., Aagaard, P., and Nielson, J. J. 2000. Passive energy return after repeated stretches on the hamstring muscle-tendon unit. *Medicine and Science in Sports and Exercise* 32: 1160-1164.

Mair, J., Mayr, M., Muller, E., Koller, A., Haid, C., Artner-Dworzak, E., Calzolari, C., Larue, C., and Pushchendorf, B. 1995. Rapid adaptation to eccentric exercise-induced muscle damage. *International Journal of Sports Medicine* 16: 352-356.

Manning, R.J., Graves, J.E., Carpenter, D.M., Leggett, S.H., and Pollock, M.L. 1990. Constant vs. variable resistance knee extension training. *Medicine and Science in Sports and Exercise* 22: 397-401.

Mannion, A.F., Jakeman, P.M., and Willan, P.L.T. 1992. Effect of isokinetic training of the knee extensors on isokinetic strength and peak power output during cycling. *European Journal of Applied Physiology* 65: 370-375.

Manore, M.M., Thompson, J., and Russo, M. 1993. Diet and exercise strategies of a world-class bodybuilder. *International Journal of Sports Medicine* 3: 76-86.

Marcinik, E.J., Potts, J., Schlabach, G., Will, S., Dawson, P., and Hurley, B.F. 1991. Effects of strength training on lactate threshold and endurance performance. *Medicine and Science in Sports and Exercise* 23: 739-743.

Maresh, C.M., Abraham, A., DeSouza, M.J., Deschenes, M.R., Kraemer, W.J., Armstrong, L.E., Maguire, M.S., Gabaree, C.L., and Hoffman, J.R. 1992. Oxygen consumption following exercise of moderate intensity and duration. *European Journal of Applied Physiology* 65: 421-424.

Maresh, C.M., Allison, T.G., Noble, B.J., Drash, A., and Kraemer, W.J. 1989. Substrate and endocrine responses to race-intensity exercise following a marathon run. *International Journal of Sports Medicine* 10: 101-106.

Markiewitz, A.D., and Andrish, J.T. 1992. Hand and wrist injuries in the preadolescent athlete. *Clinics in Sports Medicine* 11: 203-225.

Markov, G., Spengler, C.M., Knopfli-Lenzin, C., Stuessi, C., and Boutellier, U. 2001. Respiratory muscle training increases cycling endurance without affecting cardiovascular responses to exercise. *European Journal of Applied Physiology* 85: 223-239.

Martin, A., Martin, I., and Morlon, B. 1995. Changes induced by eccentric training on force-velocity relationships of the elbow flexor muscles. *European Journal of Applied Physiology* 72: 183-185.

Marx, J.O., Ratamess, N.A., Nindl, B.C., Gotshalk, L.A., Volek, J.S., Dohi, K., Bush, J.A., Gomez, A.L., Mazzetti, S.A., Fleck, S.J., Häkkinen, K., Newton, R.U., and Kraemer, W.J. 2001. Low-volume circuit versus high-volume periodized resistance training in women. *Medicine and Science in Sports and Exercise* 33: 635-643.

Massey, B.H., and Chaudet, N.L. 1956. Effects of heavy resistance exercise on range of joint movement in young male adults. *Research Quarterly* 27: 41-51.

Masterson, G. 1999. The impact of menstrual phases on anaerobic power performance in collegiate women. *Journal of Strength and Conditioning Research* 13: 325-329.

Masterson, G.L., and Brown, S.P. 1993. Effects of weighted rope jump training on power performance tests in collegians. *Journal of Strength and Conditioning Research* 7: 108-114.

Matavulj, D., Kukolj, M., Ugarkovic, D., Tihanyi, J., and Jaric, S. 2001. Effects of plyometric training on jumping performance in junior basketball players. *Journal of Sports Medicine and Physical Fitness* 41: 159-164.

Matheson, J.W., Kernozek, T.W., Fater, D.C., and Davies, G.J. 2001. Electromyographic activity and applied load during seated quadriceps exercises. *Medicine and Science in Sports and Exercise* 33: 1713-1725.

Maud, R.J., and Shultz, B.B. 1986. Gender comparisons and anaerobic power and anaerobic capacity tests. *British Journal of Sports Medicine* 20: 51-54.

Maughan, R.J., Harmon, M., Leiper, J.B., Sale, D., and Delman, A. 1986. Endurance capacity of untrained males and females in isometric and dynamic muscular contractions. *European Journal of the Applied Physiology* 55: 395-400.

Mayhew, J.L., Ball, T.E., and Bowen, J.C. 1992. Prediction of bench press ability from submaximal repetitions before and after training. *Sports Medicine Training and Rehabilitation* 3: 195-201.

Mayhew, J.L., and Gross, P.M. 1974. Body composition changes in young women with high intensity weight training. *Research Quarterly* 45: 433-440.

Mayhew, J.L., and Salm, P.C. 1990. Gender differences and anaerobic power tests. *European Journal of Applied Physiology* 60: 133-138.

Mazzetti, S.A., Kraemer, W.J., Volek, J.S., Duncan, N.D., Ratamess, N.A., Gómez, A.L., Newton, R.U., Häkkinen, K., and Fleck, S.J. 2000. The influence of direct supervision of resistance training on strength performance. *Medicine and Science in Sports and Exercise* 32: 1043-1050.

Mazzetti, S.A., Ratamess, N.A., and Kraemer, W.J. 2000. Pumping down: After years of bulking up, when they graduate, strength-trained athletes must be shown how to safely detrain. *Training and Conditioning* 10: 10-13.

McBride, J.M., Triplett-McBride, T., Davie, A., and Newton, R.U. 1999. A comparison of strength and power characteristics between power lifters, Olympic lifters, and sprinters. *Journal of Strength and Conditioning Research* 13: 58-66.

McCall, G.E., Byrnes, W.C., Dickinson, A., Pattany, P.M., and Fleck, S.J. 1996. Muscle fiber hypertrophy, hyperplasia, and capillary density in college men after resistance training. *Journal of Applied Physiology* 81: 2004-2012.

McCall, G.E., Byrnes, W.C., Fleck, S.J., Dickinson, A., and Kraemer, W.J. 1999. Acute and chronic hormonal responses to resistance training designed to promote muscle hypertrophy. *Canadian Journal of Applied Physiology* 24: 96-107.

McCall, G.E., Grindeland, R.E., Roy, R.R., and Edgerton, V.R. 2000. Muscle afferent activity modulates bioassayable growth hormone in human plasma. *Journal of Applied Physiology* 89: 1137-1141.

McCarrick, M.J., and Kemp, J.G. 2000. The effect of strength training and reduced training on rotator cuff musculature. *Clinical Biomechanics* 15 (Suppl. 1): S42-S45.

McCarthy, J.P., Agre, J.C., Graf, B.K., Poziniak, M.A., and Vailas, A.C. 1995. Compatibility of adaptive responses with combining strength and endurance training. *Medicine and Science in Sports and Exercise* 27: 429-436.

McCartney, N., McKelvie, R.S., Martin, J., Sale, D.G., and MacDougall, J.D. 1993. Weight-training induced attenuation of the circulatory response of older males to weight lifting. *Journal of Applied Physiology* 74: 1056-1060.

McDonagh, M.J.N., and Davies, C.T.M. 1984. Adaptive response of mammalian skeletal muscle to exercise with high loads. *European Journal of Applied Physiology* 52: 139-155.

McDonagh, M.J.N., Hayward, C.M., and Davies, C.T.M. 1983. Isometric training in human elbow flexor muscles. *Journal of Bone and Joint Surgery* 65: 355-358.

McGee, D., Jessee, T.C., Stone, M.H., and Blessing, D. 1992. Leg and hip endurance adaptations to three weight-training programs. *Journal of Applied Sports Science Research* 6: 92-95.

McHugh, M.P., Tyler, T.F., Greenberg, S.C., and Gleim, G. 2002. Differences and activation patterns between eccentric and concentric quadriceps contractions. *Journal of Sports Sciences* 20: 83-91.

McKenna, M.J., Harmer, A.R., Fraser, S.F., and Li, J.L. 1996. Effects of training on potassium, calcium and hydrogen ion regulation in skeletal muscle and blood during exercise. *Acta Physiologica Scandinavica* 156: 335-346.

McKenna, M.J., Heigenhauser, G.J., McKelvie, R.S., Obminski, G., MacDougall, J.D., and Jones, N.L. 1997. Enhanced pulmonary and active skeletal muscle gas exchange during intense exercise after spring training in men. *Journal of Physiology* 501: 703-716.

McLaughlin, T.M., Dillman, C.J., and Lardner, T.J. 1977. A kinematic model of performance of the parallel squat. *Medicine and Science in Sports* 9: 128-133.

McLester, J.R., Bishop, P., and Guilliams, M.E. 2000. Comparison of 1 day and 3 day per week of equal volume resistance training in experienced subjects. *Journal of Strength and Conditioning Research* 14: 273-281.

McLoughlin, P., McCaffrey, N., and Moynihan, J.B. 1991. Gentle exercise with previously inactive muscle group hastens the decline of blood lactate concentration after strenuous exercise. *European Journal of Applied Physiology* 62: 274-278.

McMorris, R.O., and Elkins, E.C. 1954. A study of production and evaluation of muscular hypertrophy. *Archives of Physical Medicine and Revocation* 35: 420-426.

McNair, P.J., Dombroski, E.W., Hewson, D.J., and Stanley, S.N. 2001. Stretching at the ankle joint: Viscoelastic response to holds and continuous passive motion. *Medicine and Science in Sports and Exercise* 33: 354-358.

Meltzer, D.E. 1994. Age dependence of Olympic weightlifting ability. *Medicine and Science in Sports and Exercise* 26: 1053-1067.

Meredith, C.N., Frontera, W.R., O'Reilly, K.P., and Evans, W.J. 1992. Body composition in elderly men: Effect of dietary modification during strength training. *Journal of American Geriatric Society* 40: 155-162.

Mero, A. 1988. Blood lactate production and recovery from anaerobic exercise in trained and untrained boys. *European Journal of Applied Physiology* 57: 660-666.

Mero, A., Luthtanen, P., Vitasalo, J.T., and Komi, P.V. 1981. Relationship between maximal running velocity, muscle fiber characteristics, force production and force relaxation of sprinters. *Scandinavian Journal of Sport Science* 3: 16-22.

Messier, S.P., and Dill, M.E. 1985. Alterations in strength and maximal oxygen uptake consequent to Nautilus circuit weight training. *Research Quarterly in Exercise and Sport* 56: 345-351.

Meyer, R.A., and Terjung, R.L. 1979. Differences in ammonia and adenylate metabolism in contracting fast and slow muscle. *American Journal of Physiology* 237: C11-C18.

Meyers, C.R. 1967. Effect of two isometric routines on strength, size and endurance in exercised and non-exercised arms. *Research Quarterly* 38: 430-440.

Micheli, L.J. 1983. Overuse injuries and children's sports: The growth factor. *Orthopedic Clinics of North America* 14: 337-360.

Micheli, L.J., and Wood, R. 1995. Back pain in young athletes: Significant differences from adults in causes and patterns. *Archives of Pediatric and Adolescent Medicine* 149: 15-18.

Miles, D.S., Owens, J.J., Golden, J.C., and Gotshall, R.W. 1987. Central and peripheral hemodynamics during maximal leg extension exercise. *European Journal of Applied Physiology* 56: 12-17.

Miller, A.E.J., MacDougall, J.D., Tarnopolsky, M.A., and Sale, D.G. 1992. Gender differences in strength and muscle fiber characteristics. *European Journal of Applied Physiology* 66: 254-262.

Miller, B.P. 1982. The effects of plyometric training on the vertical jump performance of adult female subjects. *British Journal of Sports Medicine* 16: 113-115.

Miller, W.J., Sherman, W.M., and Ivy, J.L. 1984. Effect of strength training on glucose tolerance and post-glucose insulin response. *Medicine and Science in Sports and Exercise* 16: 539-543.

Milner-Brown, H.S., Stein, R.B., and Yemin, R. 1973. The orderly recruitment of human motor units during voluntary contractions. *Journal of Physiology* 230: 359-370.

Misner, S.E., Broileau, R.A., Massey, B.H., and Mayhew, J. 1974. Alterations in the body composition of adult men during selected physical training. *Journal of the American Geriatrics Society* 22: 33-38.

Moffatt, R.J., Wallace, M.B., and Sady, S.P. 1990. Effect of anabolic steroids on lipoprotein profiles of female weight lifters. *Physician and Sportsmedicine* 18: 106-115.

Moffroid, M.T., and Whipple, R.H. 1970. Specificity of speed of exercise. *Physical Therapy* 50: 1693-1699.

Moffroid, M.T., Whipple, R.H., Hofkosh, J., Lowman, E., and Thistle, H. 1969. A study of isokinetic exercise. *Physical Therapy* 49: 735-747.

Mohr, K.J., Pink, N.M., Elsner, C., Kvitne, R.S. 1998. Electromyographic investigation of stretching: The effect of warm-up. *Clinical Journal of Sports Medicine* 8: 215-220.

Moldoveanu, A.I., Shephard, R.J., and Shek, P.N. 2001. The cytokine response to physical activity and training. *Sports Medicine* 31: 115-144.

Mont, M.A., Cohen, D.B., Campbell, K.R., Gravare, K., and Mathur, S.K. 1994. Isokinetic concentric versus eccentric training of shoulder rotators with functional evaluation of performance enhancement in elite tennis players. *American Journal of Sports Medicine* 22: 513-517.

Mookerjee, S., and Ratamess, N.A. 1999. Comparison of strength differences and joint action durations between full and partial range-of-motion bench press exercise. *Journal of Strength Conditioning Research* 13: 76-81.

Moore, M.A., and Hutton, R.S. 1980. Electromyographic investigation of muscle stretching techniques. *Medicine and Science in Sports and Exercise* 12: 322-329.

Morales, J., and Sobonya, S. 1996. Use of submaximal repetition tests for predicting 1-rm strength in class athletes. *Journal of Strength and Conditioning Research* 10: 186-189.

Morehouse, C. 1967. Development and maintenance of isometric strength of subjects with diverse initial strengths. *Research Quarterly* 38: 449-456.

Morgan, D.W., Cruise, R.J., Girardin, B.W., Lutz-Schneider, V., Morgan, D.H., and Qi, W.M. 1986. HDL-C concentrations in weight-trained, endurance trained, and sedentary females. *Physician and Sportsmedicine* 14: 166-181.

Morganti, C.M., Nelson, M.E., Fiatarone, M.A., Dallal, G.E., Economos, C.D., Crawford, B.M., and Evans, W.J. 1995. Strength improvements with 1 yr of progressive resistance training in older women. *Medicine and Science in Sports and Exercise* 27: 906-912.

Moritani, T. 1992. Time course of adaptations during strength and power training. In *Strength and power in sport,* edited by P.V. Komi, 226-278. Oxford: Blackwell.

Moritani, T., and DeVries, H.A. 1979. Neural factors versus hypertrophy in the time course of muscle strength gain. *American Journal of Physical Medicine* 82: 521-524.

Moritani, T., and DeVries, H.A. 1980. Potential for gross hypertrophy in older men. *Journal of Gerontology* 35: 672-682.

Morrey, M.A., and Hensrud, D.D. 1999. Risk of medical events in a supervised health and fitness facility. *Medicine and Science in Sports and Exercise* 31: 1233-1236.

Morrissey, M.C., Harman, E.A., Frykman, P.N., and Han, K.H. 1998. Early phase differential effects of slow and fast barbell squat training. *American Journal of Sports Medicine* 26: 221-230.

Morris, C.J., Tolfroy, K., and Coppack, R.J. 2001. Effects of short-term isokinetic training on standing long-jump performance in untrained men. *Journal of Strength and Conditioning Research* 15: 498-502.

Morrow, J.R., Jackson, A.S., Hosler, W.W., and Kachurick, J.K. 1979. The importance of strength, speed and body size for team success in women's intercollegiate volleyball. *Research Quarterly* 50: 429-437.

Morrow, T., and Hostler, W.W. 1981. Strength comparisons and untrained men and trained women athletes. *Medicine and Science in Sports and Exercise* 13: 194-198.

Mosher, P.E., Underwood, S.A., Ferguson, M.A., and Arnold, R.O. 1994. Effects of 12 weeks of aerobic circuit weight training on anaerobic capacity, muscular strength, and body composition in college-age women. *Journal of Strength and Conditioning Research* 8: 144-140.

Moskwa, C.A., and Nicholas, J.A. 1989. Musculoskeletal risk factors in the young athlete. *Physician and Sportsmedicine* 17: 45-59.

Moss, B.M., Refsnes, P.E., Abildgaard, A., Nicolaysen, K., and Jensen, J. 1997. Effects of maximal effort strength training with different loads on dynamic strength, cross-sectional area, load-power, and load-velocity relationships. *European Journal of Applied Physiology* 75: 193-199.

Mujika, I., and Padilla, S. 2001. Muscular characteristics of detraining in humans. *Medicine and Science in Sports and Exercise* 33: 1297-1303.

Mulligan, S.E., Fleck, S.J., Gordon, S.E., Koziris, L.P., Triplett-McBride, N.T., and Kraemer, W.J. 1996. Influence of resistance exercise volume on serum growth hormone and cortisol concentrations in women. *Journal of Strength and Conditioning Research* 10: 256-262.

Murphy, A.J., Wilson, G.J., Pryor, J.F., and Newton, R.U. 1995. Isometric assessment of muscular function: The effect of joint angle. *Journal of Applied Biomechanics* 11: 205-215.

Murray, M.P., Duthie, E.H., Gambert, S.T., Sepic, S.B., and Mollinger, L.A. 1985. Age-related differences in knee muscle strength in normal women. *Journal of Gerontology* 40: 275-280.

Nagaya, N., and Herrera, A.A. 1995. Effects of testosterone on synaptic efficacy at neuromuscular junctions in asexually dimorphic muscle of male frogs. *Journal of Physiology* 483: 141-153.

Nakamaru, Y., and Schwartz, A. 1972. The influence of hydrogen ion concentration on calcium binding and release by skeletal muscle sarcoplasmic reticulum. *Journal of General Physiology* 59: 22-32.

Nakoao, M., Inoue, Y., and Murakami, H. 1995. Longitudinal study of the effect of high-intensity weight training on aerobic capacity. *European Journal of Applied Physiology* 70: 20-25.

Nardone, A., Romano, C., and Schieppati, M. 1989. Selective recruitment of high-threshold human motor units during voluntary isometric lengthening of active muscles. *Journal of Physiology (London)* 409: 451-471.

Narici, M.V., Roi, G.S., Landoni, L., Minetti, A.E., and Cerretelli, P. 1989. Changes in force, cross-sectional area and neural activation during strength training and detraining of the human quadriceps. *European Journal of Applied Physiology* 59: 310-319.

National Strength and Conditioning Association. 1996. Youth resistance training: Position statement paper and literature review. Colorado Springs: NSCA.

Nattiv, A., Agonstini, R., Drinkwater, B., and Yeager, K.K. 1994. The female athlete triad: The inter-relatedness of disorder eating, amenorrhea, and osteoporosis. *Clinics in Sports Medicine* 13: 405-418.

Naughton, G., Farpour-Lambert, N.J., Carlson, J., Bradney, M., and Van Praagh, E. 2000. Physiological issues surrounding the performance of adolescent athletes. *Sports Medicine* 30: 309-325.

Neder, J.A., Luiz, E.N., Shinzato, G.T., Andrade, M.S., Peres, C., and Silva, A.C. 1999. Reference values for concentric knee isokinetic strength and power in nonathletic men and women from both 20 to 80 years old. *Journal of Orthopedic and Sports Physical Therapy* 29: 116-126.

Nelson, A.G., Allen, J.D., Cornwell, C., and Kookonen, J. 2001. Inhibition of maximal voluntary isometric torque production by acute stretching is joint-angle specific. *Research Quarterly Exercise and Sport* 72: 68-70.

Nelson, A.G. Guillory, I.K., Cornwell, C., and Kookonen, J. 2001. Inhibition of maximal voluntary isokinetic torque production following stretching is velocity specific. *Journal of Strength and Conditioning Research* 15: 241-246.

Nelson, A.G., and Kokkonen, J. 2001. Acute ballistic muscle stretching inhibits maximal strength performance. *Research Quarterly Exercise and Sport* 72: 415-419.

Nelson, G.A., Arnall, D.A., Loy, S.F., Silvester, L.J., and Conlee, R.K. 1990. Consequences of combining strength and endurance training regimens. *Physical Therapy* 70: 287-294.

Nelson, M.E., Fiatarone, M.A., Morganti, C.M., Trice, I., Greenberg, R.A., and Evans, W.J. 1994. Effects of high-intensity strength training on multiple risk factors for osteoporotic fractures. *Journal of the American Medical Association* 272: 1909-1914.

Nelson, R.M., Soderberg, G.L., and Urbscheit, N.L. 1984. Alteration of motor-unit discharge characteristics in aged humans. *Physical Therapy* 64: 29-34.

Nemoto, E.M., Hoff, J.T., and Sereringhaus, W.J. 1974. Lactate uptake and metabolism by brain during hyperlactacidemia and hypoglycemia. *Stroke* 5: 353-359.

Newton, R.U., Häkkinen, K., Kraemer, W.J., McCormick, M., Volek, J., Gordon, S.E., Campbell, W.W., and Evans. W.J. 1995. Resistance training and the development of muscle strength and power in young versus older men. In *XV Congress of the International Society of Biomechanics*, University of Jyväskylä, Finland, pp. 672-673.

Newton, R.U. and Kraemer, W.J. 1994. Developing explosive muscular power: Implications for a mixed methods training strategy. *Journal of Strength and Conditioning* 16: 20-31.

Newton, R.U., Kraemer, W.J., and Häkkinen, K. 1999. Effects of ballistic training on preseason preparation of elite volleyball players. *Medicine and Science in Sports and Exercise* 31: 323-330.

Newton, R.U., Kraemer, W.J., Häkkinen, K., Humphries, B.J., and Murphy, A.J. 1996. Kinematics, kinetics, and muscle activation during explosive upper body movements: Implications for power development. *Journal of Applied Biomechanics* 12: 31-43.

Newton, R.U., and Wilson, G.J. 1993a. The kinetics and kinematics of powerful upper body movements: The effects of load. Abstracts of the International Society of Biomechanics XIVth Congress, Paris, 4-8 July, p. 1510.

Newton, R.U., and Wilson, G.J. 1993b. Reducing the risk of injury during plyometric training: The effect of dampeners. *Sports Medicine, Training and Rehabilitation* 4: 1-7.

Nichols, D.L., Sanborn, C.F., Bonnick, S.L., Gench, B., and DiMarco, N. 1995. Relationship of regional body composition to bone mineral density in college females. *Medicine and Science in Sports and Exercise* 27: 178-182.

Nichols, D.L., Sanborn, C.F., and Love, A.M. 2001. Resistance training and bone mineral density in adolescent females. *Journal of Pediatrics* 139: 494-499.

Nichols, J.F., Hitzelberger, L.M., Sherman, J.G., and Patterson, P. 1995. Effects of resistance training on muscular strength and functional abilities of community-dwelling older adults. *Journal of Aging and Physical Activity* 3: 238-250.

Nielsen, B., Nielsen, K., Behrendt-Hansen, M., and Asmussen, E. 1980. Training of "a functional muscular strength" in girls 7-19 years old. In *Children and exercise IX*, eds. K. Berg and B. Eriksson, 69-77. Baltimore, MD: Diversity Park Press.

Nindl, B.C., Harman, E.A., Marx, J.O., Gotshalk, L.A., Frykman, P.N., Lammi, E., Palmer, C., and Kraemer, W.J. 2000. Regional body composition changes in women after 6 months periodized physical training. *Journal of Applied Physiology* 88: 2251-2259.

Nindl, B.C., Hymer, W.C., Deaver, D.R., and Kraemer, W.J. 2001. Growth hormone pulsability profile characteristics following acute heavy resistance exercise. *Journal of Applied Physiology,* 91: 163-172.

Nindl, B.C., Kraemer, W.J., Gotshalk, L.A., Marx, J.O., Volek, J.S., Bush, J.A., Häkkinen, K., Newton, R.U., and Fleck, S.J. 2001. Testosterone responses after acute resistance exercise in women: Effects of regional fat distribution. *International Journal of Sports Nutrition and Metabolism* 11: 451-465.

Nindl, B.C., Kraemer, W.J., Marx, J.O., Arciero, P.J., Dohi, K., Kellogg, M.D., and Loomis, G.A. 2001. Overnight responses of the circulating IGF-1 system after acute heavy-resistance exercise. *Journal of Applied Physiology* 90: 1319-1326.

Norris, D.O. 1980. *Vertebrate endocrinology.* Philadelphia: Lea and Febiger.

Nosaka, K., and Clarkson, P.M. 1995. Muscle damage following repeated bouts of high force eccentric exercise. *Medicine and Science in Sports and Exercise* 27: 1263-1269.

Nosaka, K., Clarkson, P.M., McGuiggin, M.E., and Byrne, J.M. 1991. Time course of muscle damage after high force eccentric exercise. *European Journal of Applied Physiology* 63: 70-76.

Nosaka, K., and Newton, M. 2002. Difference in the magnitude of muscle damage between maximal and submaximal eccentric loading. *Journal of Strength and Conditioning Research* 16: 202-208.

Nyburgh, K.H., Bachrach, L.K., Lewis, B., Kent, K., and Marcus, R. 1993. Low bone mineral density at axial and appendicular sites in amenorrheic athletes. *Medicine and Science in Sports and Exercise* 25: 1197-1202.

O'Bryant, H.S., Byrd, R., and Stone, M.H. 1988. Cycle ergometer performance and maximum leg and hip strength adaptations to two different methods of weight training. *Journal of Applied Sport Science Research* 2: 27-30.

O'Hagan, F.T., Sale, D.G., MacDougall, J.D., and Garner, S.H. 1995a. Comparative effectiveness of accommodating and weight resistance training modes. *Medicine and Science in Sports and Exercise* 27: 1210-1219.

O'Hagen, F.T., Sale, D.G., MacDougal, J.D., and Garner, S.H. 1995b. Response to resistance training in young women and men. *International Journal of Sports Medicine* 16: 314-321.

Ohtsuki, T. 1981. Decrease in grip strength induced by simultaneous bilateral exertion with reference to finger strength. *Ergonomics* 24: 37-48.

O'Shea, K.L., and O'Shea, J.P. 1989. Functional isometric weight training: Its effects on dynamic and static strength. *Journal of Applied Sport Science Research* 3: 30-33.

O'Shea, P. 1966. Effects of selected weight training programs on the development of strength and muscle hypertrophy. *Research Quarterly* 37: 95-102.

Osternig, L.R., Robertson, R.N., Troxel, R.K., and Hansen, P. 1990. Differential responses to proprioceptive neuromuscular facilitation (PNF) stretch techniques. *Medicine and Science in Sports and Exercise* 22: 106-111.

Ostrowski, K., Wilson, G.J., Weatherby, R., Murphy, P.W., and Lyttle, A.D. 1997. The effect of weight training volume on hormonal output and muscular size and function. *Journal of Strength and Conditioning Research* 11: 148-154.

Oteghen, S.L. 1975. Two speeds of isokinetic exercise as related to the vertical jump performance of women. *Research Quarterly* 46: 78-84.

Ozmun, J.C., Mikesky, A.E., and Surburg, P.R. 1994. Neuromuscular adaptations following prepubescent strength training. *Medicine and Science in Sports and Exercise* 26: 510-514.

Paasuke, M., Ereline, J., Gapeyeva, H., Sirkel, S., and Sander, P. 2000. Age-related differences in twitch contractile properties of plantarflexor muscles in women. *Acta Physiologica Scandinavica* 170: 51-57.

Paavolainen, L., Häkkinen, K., Hamalainen, I., Nummela, A., Rusko, H. 1999. Explosive-strength training improves 5-km running time by improving running economy and muscle power. *Journal of Applied Physiology* 86: 1527-1533.

Pacak, K., Palkovits, M., Yadid, G., Kvetnansky, R., Kopin, I.J., and Goldstein, D.S. 1998. Heterogeneous neurochemical responses to different stressors: A test of Selye's doctrine of nonspecificity. *American Journal of Physiology* 275: R1247-R1255.

Paddon-Jones, D., and Abernathy, P.J. 2001. Acute adaptation to low-volume eccentric exercise. *Medicine and Science in Sports and Exercise* 33: 1213-1219.

Paffenbarger, R.S., Hyde, R.T., Wing, A.L., Steinmetz, C.H. 1984. A natural history of athleticism and cardiovascular health. *Journal of the American Medical Association* 252: 491-495.

Page, B. 1966. Latest muscle building technique. *Muscle Builder* 14: 20-21.

Parkhouse, W.S., Coupland, D.C., Li, C., and Vanderhoek, K.J. 2000. IGF-1 bioavailability is increased by resistance training in older women with low bone mineral density. *Mechanisms of Aging Development* 113: 75-83.

Path, G., Bornstein, S.R., Ehrhart-Bornstein, M., and Scherbaum, W.A. 1997. Interleukin-6 and the interleukin-6 receptor in the human adrenal gland: expression and effects on steroidogenesis. *Journal of Clinical Endocrinology and Metabolism* 82: 2343-2349.

Pavlath, G.K., Rich, K., Webster, S.G., and Blau, H.M. 1989. Localization of muscle gene products in nuclear domains. *Nature* 337: 570-573.

Payne, V.G., Morrow, J.R. Jr., Johnson, L., and Dalton, S.N. 1997. Resistance training in children and youth: A meta-analysis. *Research Quarterly for Exercise and Sport* 68: 80-88.

Pearson, A.C., Schiff, M., Mrosek, D., Labovitz, A.J., and Williams, G.A. 1986. Left ventricular diastolic function in weight lifters. *American Journal of Cardiology* 58: 1254-1259.

Pearson, D.R., and Costill, D.L. 1988. The effects of constant external resistance exercise and isokinetic exercise training on work-induced hypertrophy. *Journal of Applied Sport Science Research* 3: 39-41.

Pecci, M.A., and Lombardo, J.A. 2000. Performance-enhancing supplements. *Physical Medicine Rehabilitation Clinics of North America* 11: 949-960.

Perrault, H., and Turcotte, R.A. 1994. Exercise-induced cardiac hypertrophy fact or fallacy? *Sports Medicine* 17: 288-308.

Perrone, C.E., Fenwick-Smith, D., and Vandenburgh, H.H. 1995. Collagen and stretch modulate autocrine secretion of insulin-like growth factor-1 and insulin-like growth factor binding proteins from differentiated skeletal muscle cells. *The Journal of Biological Chemistry* 270: 2099-2106.

Petersen, S., Wessel, J., Bagnall, K., Wilkens, H., Quinney, A., and Wenger, H. 1990. Influence of concentric resistance training on concentric and eccentric strength. *Archives of Physical Medicine and Rehabilitation* 71: 101-105.

Petersen, S.R., Miller, G.D., Quinney, H.A., and Wenger, H.A. 1987. The effectiveness of a mini-cycle on velocity-specific strength acquisition. *Journal of Orthopaedic and Sports Physical Therapy* 9: 156-159.

Peterson, J.A. 1975. Total conditioning: A case study. *Athletic Journal* 56: 40-55.

Petit, M.A., Prior, J.C., and Barr, S.L. 1999. Running and ovulation positively change cancellous bone in premenopausal women. *Medicine and Science in Sports and Exercise* 31: 780-787.

Pette, D., and Staron, R.S. 1990. Cellular and molecular diversities of mammalian skeletal muscle fibers. *Review of Physiology, Biochemistry and Pharmacology* 116: 2-75.

Pette, D., and Staron, R.S. 2001. Transitions of muscle fiber phenotypic profiles. *Histochemistry and Cell Biology* 115: 359-372.

Pfeiffer, R., and Francis, R. 1986. Effects of strength training on muscle development in prepubescent, pubescent and postpubescent males. *Physician and Sportsmedicine* 14: 134-143.

Phillips, S.K., Bruce, S.A., Newton, D., and Woledge, R.C. 1992. The weakness of old age is not due to failure of muscle activation. *Journal of Gerontology: Medical Sciences* 47: 45-49.

Phillips, S.M. 2000. Short-term training: When do repeated bouts of resistance exercise become training? *Canadian Journal of Applied Physiology* 25: 185-193.

Phillips, S.M., Tipton, K.D., Aarsland, A., Wolf, S.E., and Wolfe, R.R. 1997. Mixed muscle protein synthesis and breakdown after resistance exercise in humans. *American Journal of Physiology* 273: E99-E107.

Phillips, S.M., Tipton, K.D., Ferrando, A.A., and Wolfe, R.R. 1999. Resistance training reduces the acute exercise-induced increase in muscle protein turnover. *American Journal of Physiology* 276: E118-E124.

Pichon, C.E., Hunter, G.R., Morris, M., Bond, R.L., and Metz, J. 1996. Blood pressure and heart rate response and metabolic cost of circuit versus traditional weight training. *Journal of Strength and Conditioning Research* 10: 153-156.

Pierce, K., Rozenek, R., and Stone, M.H. 1993. Effects of high volume weight training on lactate, heart rate, and perceived exertion. *Journal of Strength and Conditioning Research* 7: 211-215.

Piers, L.S., Soares, M.J., McCormack, L.M., and O'Dea, K. 1998. Is there evidence for an age-related reduction in metabolic rate? *Journal of Applied Physiology* 85: 2196-2204.

Pincivero, D.M., Gear, W.S., Sterner, R.L., and Karunakara, R.G. 2000. Gender differences in the relationship between quadriceps work and fatigue during high-intensity exercise. *Journal of Strength and Conditioning Research* 14: 202-206.

Pincivero, D.M., Lephart, S.M., and Karunakara, R.G. 1997. Effects of rest interval on isokinetic strength and functional performance after short term high intensity training. *British Journal of Sports Medicine* 31: 229-234.

Pipes, T.V. 1978. Variable resistance versus constant resistance strength training in adult males. *European Journal of Applied Physiology* 39: 27-35.

Pipes, T.V. 1979. Physiological characteristics of elite body builders. *Physician and Sportsmedicine* 7: 116-126.

Pizzimenti, M.A. 1992. Mechanical analysis of the Nautilus leg curl machine. *Canadian Journal of Sport Science* 17: 41-48.

Ploutz, L.L., Tesch, P.A., Biro, R.L., and Dudley, G.A. 1994. Effect of resistance training on muscle use during exercise. *Journal of Applied Physiology* 76: 1675-1681.

Ploutz-Snyder, L.L., and Giamis, E.L. 2001. Orientation and familiarization to 1 RM strength testing in old and young women. *Journal of Strength and Conditioning Research* 15: 519-523.

Ploutz-Snyder, L.L., Giamis, E.L., and Rosenbaum, A.E. 2001. Resistance training reduces susceptibility to eccentric exercise-induced muscle dysfunction in older women. *Journal of Gerontology: Biological Sciences, Medical Sciences* 56: B384-B390.

Polhemus, R., Burkhart, E., Osina, M., and Patterson, M. 1981. The effects of plyometric training with ankle and vest weights on conventional weight training programs for men and women. *National Strength Coaches Association Journal* 2: 13-15.

Pollock, M.H., Graves, J.E., Bamman, M.M., Leggett, S.H., Carpenter, D.M., Carr, C., Cirulli, J., Makozich, J., and Fulton, M. 1993. Frequency and volume of resistance training: Effect on cervical extension strength. *Archives of Physical Medicine and Rehabilitation* 74: 1080-1086.

Poole, H. 1964. Multi-poundage sets. *Muscle Builder* 14: 20-21.

Pope, R.P., Herbert, R.D., Kirwan, J.D., and Graham, B.J. 2000. A randomized trial of preexercise stretching for prevention of lower-limb injury. *Medicine and Science in Sports and Exercise* 32: 271-277.

Potteiger, J.A., Lockwood, R.H., Haub, M.D., Dolezal, B.A., Almuzaini, K.S., Schroeder, J.M., and Zebras, C.J. 1999. Muscle power and fiber characteristics following 8 weeks of plyometric training. *Journal of Strength and Conditioning Research* 13: 275-279.

Powers, W.E., Browning, F.M., and Groves, B.R. 1978. The super overload: The new method for improving muscular strength. *Journal of Physical Education* (March/April): 10-12.

Prevost, M.C., Nelson, A.G.E., and Maraj, B.K.V. 1999. The effect of two days of velocity specific isokinetic training on torque production. *Journal of Strength and Conditioning Research* 13: 35-39.

Prior, J.C., Vigna, Y.M., and McKay, D.W. 1992. Reproduction for the athletic female: New understandings of physiology and management. *Sports Medicine* 14: 190-199.

Pruit, L.A., Jackson, R.D., Bartels, R.L., and Lehnard, H.J. 1992. Weight-training effects on bone mineral density in early post-menopausal women. *Journal of Bone Mineral Research* 7: 179-185.

Puhl, J., Case, S., Fleck, S., and Van Handel, P. 1982. Physical and physiological characteristics of elite volleyball players. *Research Quarterly for Exercise and Sport* 53: 257-262.

Pyka, G., Wiswell, R.A., and Marcus, R. 1992. Age-dependent effect of resistance exercise on growth hormone secretion in people. *Journal of Clinical Endocrinology and Metabolism* 75: 404-407.

Quaedackers, M.E., Van Den Brink, C.E., Wissink, S., Schreurs, R.H., Gustafsson, J.K., Van Der, J.A., Saag, P.T., and Van Der Burg, B.B. 2001. 4-hydroxytamoxifen transrepresses nuclear factor-kappa B activity in human osteoblastic U2-OS cells through estrogen receptor (ER) alpha, not through ER beta. *Endocrinology* 142: 1156-1166.

Raastad, T., Bjoro, T., and Hallen, J. 2000. Hormonal responses to high- and moderate-intensity strength exercise. *European Journal of Applied Physiology* 82: 121-128.

Rack, D.M.H., and Westbury, D.R. 1969. The effects of length and stimulus rate on isometric tension in the cat soleus. *Journal of Physiology* 204: 443-460.

Rains, C.B., Weltman, A.W., Cahil, B.R., Janney, C.A., Tippett, S.R., and Katch, F.I. 1987. Strength training for prepubescent males: Is it safe? *American Journal Sports Medicine* 15: 483-489.

Ramos, E., Frontera, W.R., Llopart, A., and Feliciano, D. 1998. Muscle strength and hormonal levels and adolescents: gender related differences. *International Journal of Sports Medicine* 19: 526-531.

Ramsay, J.A., Blimkie, C.J.R., Smith, K., Garner, S., MacDougall, J.D., and Sale, D.G. 1990. Strength training effects and prepubescent boys. *Medicine and Science in Sports and Exercise* 22: 605-614.

Rarick, G.L., and Larson, G.L. 1958. Observations on frequency and intensity of isometric muscular effort in developing static muscular strength in post-pubescent males. *Research Quarterly* 29: 333-341.

Rasch, P. 1971. Isometric exercise and gains of muscular strength. In *Frontiers of fitness*, edited by R. Shepard, 98-111. Springfield: Thomas.

Rasch, P., and Morehouse, L. 1957. Effect of static and dynamic exercises on muscular strength and hypertrophy. *Journal of Applied Physiology* 11: 29-34.

Rasch, P.J., and Pierson, W.R. 1964. One position versus multiple positions in isometric exercise. *American Journal of Physical Medicine* 43: 10-12.

Rasch, P.J., Preston, W.R., and Logan, G.A. 1961. The effect of isometric exercise upon the strength of antagonistic muscles. *Internationale Zeitschrift fur Angewandte Physiologie Einschliesslich Arbitsphysiologie* 19: 18-22.

Read, M.M., and Cisar, C. 2001. The influence of varied rest interval lengths on depth jump performance. *Journal of Strength and Conditioning Research* 15: 279-283.

Reis, E., Frick, U., and Schmidbleicher, D. 1995. Frequency variations of strength training sessions triggered by the phases of the menstrual cycle. *International Journal of Sportsmedicine* 16: 545-550.

Rhea, M.R., Alvar, B.A., Burkett, L.N., and Ball, S.D. 2003. A meta-analysis to determine the dose response for strength development. *Medicine and Science in Sports and Exercise* 35: 456-464.

Rhea, M.R., Ball, S.D., Phillips, W.T., and Burkett, L.N. 2002. A comparison of linear and daily undulating periodized programs with equated volume and intensity for strength. *Journal of Strength and Conditioning Research* 16: 250-255.

Richford, C. 1966. *Principles of successful body building.* Alliance, NE: Iron Man Industries.

Rico, H., Gonzalez-Riola, J., Revilla, L.F., Gomez-Castresana, F., and Escribano, J. 1994. Cortical versus trabecular bone mass: Influence of activity on both bone components. *Calcified Tissue International* 37: 325-330.

Rimmer, E., and Sleivert, G. 2000. Effects of a plyometrics intervention program on sprint performance. *Journal of Strength and Conditioning Research* 14: 295-301.

Roberts, J.M., and Wilson, K. 1999. Effect of stretching duration on active and passive range of motion in the lower extremity. *British Journal of Sports Medicine* 33: 259-263.

Robinson, J.M., Stone, M.H., Johnson, R.L., Penland, C.M., Warren, B.J., and Lewis, R.D. 1995. Effects of different weight training exercise/rest intervals on strength, power, and high intensity exercise endurance. *Journal of Strength and Conditioning Research* 9: 216-221.

Rogers, M.A., and Evans, W.J. 1993. Changes in skeletal muscle with aging: Effects of exercise training. In *Exercise and sport sciences reviews*, Volume 21, edited by J.O. Holloszy. Baltimore, MD: Williams & Wilkins.

Rooney, K.J., Herbert, R.D., and Balwave, R.J. 1994. Fatigue contributes to the strength training stimulus. *Medicine and Science in Sports and Exercise* 26: 1160-1164.

Rooyackers, O.E., and Nair, K.S. 1997. Hormonal regulation of human muscle protein metabolism. *Annual Reviews in Nutrition* 17: 457-485.

Ross, A., Leveritt, M., and Riek, S. 2001. Neural influences on sprint running: Training adaptations and acute responses. *Sports Medicine* 31: 409-425.

Roth, D.A., Stanley, W.C., and Brooks, G.A. 1988. Induced lactacidemia does not affect postexercise O_2 consumption. *Journal of Applied Physiology* 65: 1045-1049.

Roth, S.M., Martel, G.F., Ivey, F.M., Lemmer, J.T., Tracy, B.L., Hurlbut, D.E., Metter, E.J., Hurley, B.F., and Rogers, M.A. 1999. Ultrastructural muscle damage in young vs. older men after high-volume, heavy resistance strength training. *Journal of Applied Physiology* 86: 1833-1840.

Roth, S.M., Martel, G.F., Ivey, F.M., Lemmer, J.T., Tracy, B.L., Hurlbut, D.E., Metter, E.J., Hurley, B.F., and Rogers, M.A. 2000. High-volume, heavy-resistance strength training and muscle damage in young and older women. *Journal of Applied Physiology* 86: 1112-1118.

Roth, S.M., Martel G.F., Ivey, F.M., Lemmer, J.T., Tracy, B.L., Metter, E.J., Hurley, B.F., and Rogers, M.A. 2001. Skeletal muscle satellite cell characteristics in young and older men and women after heavy resistance strength training. *Journal of Gerontology: A Biological Sciences Medical Sciences* 56: B240-B247.

Roubenoff, R. 2001. Origins and clinical relevance of sarcopenia. *Canadian Journal of Applied Physiology* 26: 78-89.

Rowe, T.A. 1979. Cartilage fracture due to weight lifting. *British Journal of Sports Medicine* 13: 130-131.

Rowell, L.B., Kranning, K.K., Evans, T.O., Kennedy, J.W., Blackman, J.R., and Kusumi, F. 1966. Splanchnic removal of lactate and pyruvate during prolonged exercise in man. *Journal of Applied Physiology* 21: 1773-1783.

Rowlinson, S.W., Waters, M.J., Lewis, U.J., and Barnard, R. 1996. Human growth hormone fragments 1-43 and 44-191: In vitro somatogenic activity and receptor binding characteristics in human and nonprimate systems. *Endocrinology* 137: 90-95.

Roy, B.D., Tarnopolsky, M.A., MacDougall, J.D., Fowles, J., and Yarasheski, K.E. 1997. Effect of glucose supplement timing on protein metabolism after resistance training. *Journal of Applied Physiology* 82: 1882-1888.

Rubin, M.R., Kraemer, W.J., Nindl, B.C., Marx, J.O., Gotshalk, L.A., Welch, J.R., and Hymer, W.C. 2000. Periodized resistance training potentiates in vivo bioactivity of human growth hormone. *Medicine and Science in Sports and Exercise* 32: S186

Rudman, D., Feller, A.G., Nagraj, H.S., Gergans, G.A., Lalitha, P.Y., Goldberg, A.F., Schlenker, R.A., Cohn, L., Rudman, I.W., and Mattson, D.E. 1990. Effects of human growth hormone in men over 60 years old. *The New England Journal of Medicine* 323: 1-6.

Russell-Jones, D.L., Umpleby, A., Hennessey, T., Bowes, S., Shojaee-Moradies, F., Hopkins, K., Jackson, N., Kelly, J., Jones, R., and Sonksen, P. 1994. Use of leucine clamp to demonstrate that IGF-I actively stimulates protein synthesis in normal humans. *American Journal of Physiology* 267: E591-598.

Ryan, J.R., and Salciccioli, G.G. 1976. Fractures of the distal radial epiphysis in adolescent weight lifters. *Sports Medicine* 4: 26-27.

Ryschon, T.W., Fowler, M.D., Wysong, R.E., Anthony, A.R., and Balaban, R.S. 1997. Efficiency of human skeletal muscle in vivo: Comparison of isometric, concentric, and eccentric muscle action. *Journal of Applied Physiology* 83: 867-874.

Ryushi, T., Häkkinen, K., Kauhanen, H., and Komi, P.V. 1988. Muscle fiber characteristics, muscle cross-sectional area and force production in strength athletes, physically active males and females. *Scandinavian Journal of Sports Science* 10: 7-15.

Sadamoto, T., Bonde-Peterson, F., and Suzuki, Y. 1983. Skeletal muscle tension, flow pressure and EMG during sustained isometric contractions in humans. *European Journal of Applied Physiology* 51: 395-408.

Sahlin, K., and Ren, J.M. 1989. Relationship of contraction capacity to metabolic changes during recovery from a fatiguing contraction. *Journal of Applied Physiology* 67: 648-654.

Sailors, M., and Berg, K. 1987. Comparison of responses to weight training in pubescent boys and men. *Journal of Sports Medicine* 27: 30-37.

Sale, D.G. 1992. Neural adaptations to strength training. In *Strength and power in sport,* edited by P.V. Komi, 249-265. Boston: Blackwell Scientific.

Sale, D.G., MacDougall, J.D., Alway, S.E., and Sutton, J.R. 1987. Voluntary strength and muscle characteristics in untrained men and women and male bodybuilders. *Journal of Applied Physiology* 62: 1786-1793.

Sale, D.G., MacDougall, J.D., Jacobs, I., and Garner, S. 1990. Interaction between concurrent strength and endurance training. *Journal of Applied Physiology* 68: 260-270.

Sale, D.G., MacDougall, J.D., Upton, A.R.M., and McComas, A.J. 1983. Effect of strength training upon motoneuron excitability in man. *Medicine and Science in Sports and Exercise* 15: 57-62.

Sale, D.G., Moroz, D.E., McKelvie, R.S., MacDougall, J.D., and McCartney, N. 1993. Comparison of blood pressure response to isokinetic and weight-lifting exercise. *European Journal of Applied Physiology* 67: 115-120.

Sale, D.G., Moroz, D.E., McKelvie, R.S., MacDougall, J.D., and McCartney, N. 1994. Effect of training on the blood pressure response to weight lifting. *Canadian Journal of Applied Physiology* 19: 60-74.

Saltin, B., and Astrand, P.O. 1967. Maximal oxygen uptake in athletes. *Journal of Applied Physiology* 23: 353-358.

Sanborn, K., Boros, R., Hruby, J., Schilling, B., O'Bryant, H., Johnson, R., Hoke, T., Stone, M., and Stone, M.H. 2000. Performance effects of weight training with multiple sets not to failure versus a single set to failure in women. *Journal of Strength and Conditioning Research* 14: 328-331.

Santana, J.C. 2000. *Functional training: Breaking the bonds of traditionalism.* Boca Raton, FL: Optimum Performance Systems.

Sapolsky, R.M., Romero, L.M., and Munck, A.U. 2000. How do glucocorticoids influence stress responses? Integrating permissive, suppressive, stimulatory, and preparative actions. *Endocrine Reviews* 21: 55-89.

Saxton, J.M., Clarkson, P.M., James, R., Miles, M., Westerfer, M., Clark, S., and Donnelly, A.E. 1995. Neuromuscular dysfunction following eccentric exercise. *Medicine and Science in Sports and Exercise* 27: 1185-1193.

Saxton, J.M., and Donnelly, A.E. 1995. Light concentric exercise during recovery from exercise-induced muscle damage. *International Journal of Sports Medicine* 16: 347-351.

Sayers, S.P., and Clarkson, P.M. 2001. Force recovery after eccentric exercise in males and females. *European Journal of Applied Physiology* 84: 122-126.

Sayers, S.P., Clarkson, P.M., Rouzier, P.A., and Kamen, G. 1999. Adverse events associated with eccentric exercise protocols: Six case studies. *Medicine and Science in Sports and Exercise* 31: 1697-1702.

Sayers, S.P., Harackiewicz, D.V., Harman, E.A., Frykman, P.N., and Rosensyein, M.T. 1999. Cross-validation of three jump power equations. *Medicine and Science in Sports and Exercise* 31: 572-577.

Scala, D., McMillian, J., Blessing, D., Rozenek, R., and Stone, M. 1987. Metabolic cost of a preparatory phase of training in weightlifting: A practical observation. *Journal of Applied Sports Science Research* 1: 48-52.

Schantz, P. 1982. Capillary supply in hypertrophied human skeletal muscle. *Acta Physiologica Scandinavica* 114: 635-637.

Schantz, P., Randall-Fox, E., Hutchinson, W., Tyden, A., and Astrand, P.O. 1983. Muscle fibre type distribution, muscle cross-sectional area and maximal voluntary strength in humans. *Acta Physiologica Scandinavica* 117: 219-226.

Schantz, P., Randall-Fox, E., Norgen, P., and Tyden, A. 1981. The relationship between the mean muscle fibre area and the muscle cross-sectional area of the thigh in subjects with large differences in thigh girth. *Physiologica Scandinavica* 113: 537-539.

Scharf, H.-P., Eckhardt, R., Maurus, M., and Puhl, W. 1994. Metabolic and hemodynamic changes during isokinetic muscle training. *International Journal of Sports Medicine* 15: S56-S59.

Schiotz, M.K., Potteiger, J.A., Huntsinger, P.G., and Denmark, D.C. 1998. The short-term effects of periodized and constant-intensity training on body composition, strength, and performance. *Journal of Strength and Conditioning Research* 12: 173-178.

Schlumberger, A., Stec, J., and Schmidtbleicher, D. 2001. Single- vs. multiple-set strength training in women. *Journal of Strength and Conditioning Research* 15: 284-289.

Schmidtbleicher, D. 1994. Training for power events. In *Strength and power and sport,* edited by P. V. Komi. 381-395. London: Blackwell Scientific.

Schmidtbleicher, D., and Gollhofer, A. 1982.Neuromuskulare Untersuchungen zur Bestimmung individueller Belatungsgrossen fur ein Tiefsprungtraining. *Leistungssport* 12: 298-307.

Schmidtbleicher, D., Gollhofer, A., and Frick, U. 1988. Effects of stretch-shortening type training on the performance capability and innervation characteristics of leg extensor muscles. In *Biomechanics XI-A*, edited by G. deGroot, A. Hollander, P. Huijing, and G. van Ingen Schenau, vol. 7-A, 185-189. Amsterdam: Free University Press.

Schneider, V., Arnold, B., Martin, K., Bell, D., and Crocker, P. 1998. Detraining effects in college football players during the competitive season. *Journal of Strength and Conditioning Research* 12: 42-45.

Schnoebelen-Combes, S., Louveau, I., Postel-Vinay, M.C., and Bonneau, M. 1996. Ontogeny of GH receptor and GH-binding protein in the pig. *Journal of Endocrinology* 148: 249-255.

Schott, J., McCully, K., and Rutherford, O.M. 1995. The role of metabolites in strength training II. Short versus long isometric contractions. *European Journal of Applied Physiology* 71: 337-341.

Schultz, R.W. 1967. Effect of direct practice and repetitive sprinting and weight training on selected motor performance tasks. *Research Quarterly* 38: 108-118.

Schwab, R., Johnson, G.O., Housh, T.J., Kinder, J.E., and Weir, J.P. 1993. Acute effects of different intensities of weight lifting on serum testosterone. *Medicine and Science in Sports and Exercise* 25: 1381-1385.

Scoles, G. 1978. Depth jumping! Does it really work? *Athletic Journal* 58: 48-75.

Seaborne, D., and Taylor, A.W. 1984. The effect of speed of isokinetic exercise on training transfer to isometric strength in the quadriceps. *Journal of Sports Medicine* 24: 183-188.

Seals, D.R. 1993. Influence of active muscle size on sympathetic nerve discharge during isometric contractions in humans. *Journal of Applied Physiology* 75: 1426-1431.

Secher, N.H. 1975. Isometric rowing strength of experienced and inexperienced oarsmen. *Medicine and Science in Sports and Exercise* 7: 280-283.

Secher, N.H., Rorsgaard, S., and Secher, O. 1978. Contralateral influence on recruitment of curarized muscle fibers during maximal voluntary extension of the legs. *Acta Physiologica Scandinavica* 130: 455-462.

Seger, J.Y., Arvidsson, B., and Thorstensson, A. 1998. Specific effects of eccentric and concentric training on muscle strength and morphology in humans. *European Journal of Applied Physiology* 79: 49-57.

Selye, H. 1936. A syndrome produced by diverse nocuous agents. *Nature* 138: 32.

Serresse, O., Lortie, G., Bouchard, C., and Boulay, M.R. 1988. Estimation of the contribution of the various energy systems during maximal work of short duration. *International Journal of Sports Medicine* 9: 456-460.

Sewall, L., and Micheli, L. 1986. Strength training for children. *Journal of Pediatric Orthopedics* 6: 143-146.

Sforzo, G.A., and Touey, P.R. 1996. Manipulating exercise order affects muscular performance during a resistance exercise training session. *Journal of Strength and Conditioning Research* 10: 20-24.

Sharman, M.J., Newton, R.U., Triplett-McBride, T., McGuigan, M.R., McBride, J.M., Häkkinen, A., Häkkinen, K., and Kraemer, W.J. 2001. Changes in myosin heavy chain composition with heavy resistance training in 60- to 70-year-old men and women. *European Journal of Applied Physiology* 84 (1-2): 127-132.

Sharp, M.A. 1994. Physical fitness and occupational performance of women in the U.S. Army. *Work* 2: 80-92.

Shaw, C.E., McCully, K.K., and Posner, J.D. 1995. Injuries during the one repetition maximum assessment in the elderly. *Journal of Cardiopulmonary Rehabilitation* 15: 283-287.

Shellock, F.G., and Prentice, W.E. 1985. Warming-up and stretching for improved physical performance and prevention of sports related injuries. *Sports Medicine* 2: 267-278.

Shephard, R.J. 2000a. Exercise and training in women, part I: Influence of gender on exercise and training responses. *Canadian Journal of Applied Physiology* 25:19-34.

Shephard, R.J. 2000b. Exercise and training in women, part II: Influence of menstrual cycle and pregnancy on exercise responses. *Canadian Journal of Applied Physiology* 25: 35-54.

Shinohara, M., Kouzaki, M., Yoshihisa, T., and Fukunaga, T. 1998. Efficacy of tourniquet ischemia for strength training with low resistance. *European Journal of Applied Physiology* 77: 189-191.

Siegal, J., Camaione, D., and Manfredi, T. 1989. The effects of upper body resistance training in prepubescent children. *Pediatrics Exercise Science* 1: 145-154.

Silvester, L.J., Stiggins, C., McGown, C., and Bryce, G. 1984. The effect of variable resistance and free-weight training programs on strength and vertical jump. *National Strength and Conditioning Association Journal* 5: 30-33.

Singh, M.A., Ding, W., Manfredi, T.J., Solares, G.S., O'Neill, E.F., Clements, K.M., Ryan, N.D., Kehayias, J.J., Fielding, R.A., and Evans, W.J. 1999. Insulin-like growth factor I in skeletal muscle after weight-lifting exercise in frail elders. *American Journal of Physiology* 277: E135-E143.

Sinnett, A.M., Berg, K., Latin, R.W., and Noble, J.M. 2001. The relationship between field tests of anaerobic power and 10-km run performance. *Journal of Strength and Conditioning Research* 15: 405-412.

Sinning, W.E. 1974. Body composition assessment of college wrestlers. *Medicine and Science in Sports* 6: 139-145.

Skutek, M., van Griensven, M., Zeichen, J., Brawer, N., and Bosch, U. 2001. Cyclic mechanical stretching modulates secretion pattern of growth factors in human tendon fibroblasts. *European Journal of Applied Physiology* 86: 48-52.

Slawinski, J., Demarle, A., Koralsztein, J.P., and Billat, V. 2001 Effect of supra-lactate threshold training on the relationship between mechanical stride descriptors and aerobic energy cost in trained runners. *Archives of Physiology and Biochemistry* 109: 110-116.

Smith, L.L. 2000. Cytokine hypothesis of overtraining: A physiological adaptation to excessive stress? *Medicine and Science in Sports and Exercise* 32: 317-331.

Smith, L.L., Bruentz, M.H., Cheier, T.C., McCammon, M.R., Houmard, J.A., Franklin, M.E., and Israel, R.G. 1993. The effects of static and ballistic stretching on delayed onset muscle soreness and creatine kinase. *Research Quarterly Exercise and Sport* 64: 103-107.

Smith, M.J., and Melton, P. 1981. Isokinetic versus isotonic variable resistance training. *American Journal of Sports Medicine* 9: 275-279.

Smith, M.L., and Raven, B.P. 1986. Cardiovascular responses to lower body negative pressure in endurance and static exercise trained men. *Medicine and Science in Sports and Exercise* 18: 545-550.

Smith, R.C., and Rutherford, O.M. 1995. The role of metabolites in strength training I. A comparison of eccentric and concentric contractions. *European Journal of Applied Physiology* 71: 332-236.

Snoecky, L.H.E.H., Abeling, H.F.M., Lambrets, J.A.C., Schmitz, J.J.F., Verstappen, F.T.J., and Reneman, R.S. 1982. Echocardiographic dimensions in athletes in relation to their training programs. *Medicine and Science in Sports and Exercise* 14: 42-54.

Snow, C.M., Rosen, C.J., and Robinson, T.L. 2000. Serum IGF-I is higher in gymnasts than runners and predicts bone and lean mass. *Medicine and Science in Sports and Exercise* 32: 1902-1907.

Sorichter, S., Mair, J., Koller, A., Secnik, P., Parrak, V., Haid, C., Muller, E., and Puschendorf, B. 1997. Muscular adaptation and strength during the early phase of eccentric training: Influence of the training frequency. *Medicine and Science in Sports and Exercise* 29: 1646-1652.

Spataro, A., Pellicca, A., Proschan, M.A., Granata, M., Spataro, A., Bellone, P., Caselli, G., Biffi, A., Vecchio, C., and Maron, B.J. 1994. Morphology of the "athlete's heart" assessed by echocardiography in 947 elite athletes representing 27 sports. *American Journal of Cardiology* 74: 802-806.

Spence, D.W., Disch, J.G., Fred, H.C., and Coleman, A.E. 1980. Descriptive profiles of highly skilled women volleyball players. *Medicine and Science in Sports and Exercise* 12: 299-302.

Speroff, L., and Redwine, D.B. 1980. Exercise and menstrual function. *Physician and Sportsmedicine* 8: 42-48.

Spitzer, J.J. 1974. Effect of lactate infusion on canine myocardial free fatty acid metabolism in vivo. *American Journal of Physiology* 22: 213-217.

Sprynarova, S., and Parizkova, J. 1971. Functional capacity and body composition in top weight lifters, swimmers, runners, and skiers. *International fur Angewandte Physiolgie* 29: 184-194.

Stadler, M.A., Noble, B.J., and Wilkerson, J.G. 1990. The effects of supplemental weight training for ballet dancers. *Journal of Applied Sport Science Research* 4: 94-102.

Staff, P.H. 1982. The effect of physical activity on joints, cartilage, tendons and ligaments. *Scandinavian Journal of Social Medicine* 290 (Suppl.): 59-63.

Stanforth, P.R., Painter, T.L., and Wilmore, J.H. 1992. Alteration in concentric strength consequent to powercise and universal gym circuit training. *Journal of Applied Sport Science Research* 6: 152-157.

Stanley, W.C. 1991. Myocardial lactate metabolism during exercise. *Medicine and Science in Sports and Exercise* 23: 920-924.

Starkey, D.B., Pollock, M.L., Ishida, Y., Welsch, M.A., Brechue, W.F., Graves, J.E., and Feigenbaum, M.S. 1996. Effect of resistance training volume on strength and muscle thickness. *Medicine and Science in Sports and Exercise* 28: 1311-1320.

Staron, R.S., Hagerman, F.C., and Hikida, R.S. 1981. The effects of detraining on an elite power lifter. *Journal of Neurological Sciences* 51: 247-257.

Staron, R.S., Hagerman, F.C., Hikida, R.S., Murray, T.F., Hosteler, D.P., Crill, M.T., Ragg, K.E., and Toma, K. 2001. Fiber type composition of the vastus lateralis muscle of young men and women. *Journal of Histochemistry and Cytochemistry* 48: 623-630.

Staron, R.S., and Hikida, R.S. 2001. Muscular responses to exercise and training. In *Exercise and Sport Science*, edited by W. E. Garrett Jr. and D.T. Kirkendall. Philadelphia: Lippincott Williams & Wilkins.

Staron, R.S., Hikida, R.S., and Hagerman, F.C. 1983. Reevaluation of human muscle fast-twitch subtypes: Evidence for a continuum. *Histochemistry* 78: 33-39.

Staron, R.S., and Johnson, P. 1993. Myosin polymorphism and differential expression in adult human skeletal muscle. *Comparative Biochemical Physiology* 106B: 463-475.

Staron, R.S., Karapondo, D.L., Kraemer, W.J., Fry, A.C., Gordon, S.E., Falkel, J.E., Hagerman, F.C., and Hikida, R.S. 1994. Skeletal muscle adaptations during the early phase of heavy-resistance training in men and women. *Journal of Applied Physiology* 76: 1247-1255.

Staron, R.S., Leonardi, M.J., Karapondo, D.L., Malicky, E.S., Falkel, J.E., Hagerman, F.C., and Hikida, R.S. 1991. Strength and skeletal muscle adaptations in heavy-resistance-trained women after detraining and retraining. *Journal of Applied Physiology* 70: 631-640.

Staron, R.S., Malicky, E.S., Leonardi, M.J., Falkel, J.E., Hagerman, F.C., and Dudley, G.A. 1989. Muscle hypertrophy and fast fiber type conversions in heavy resistance-trained women. *European Journal of Applied Physiology* 60: 71-79.

Staron, R.S., Murray, T.F., Gilders, R.M., Hagerman, R.C., Hikida, R.S., and Ragg, K.E. 2000. Influence of resistance training on serum lipid and lipoprotein concentrations in young men and women. *Journal of Strength and Conditioning Research* 14: 37-44.

Stauber, W.T., Clarkson, P.M., Fritz, V.K., and Evans, W.J. 1990. Extracellular matrix disruption and pain after eccentric muscle action. *Journal of Applied Physiology* 69: 868-874.

Steben, R.E., and Steben, A.H. 1981. The validity of the stretch-shortening cycle in selected jumping events. *Journal of Sports Medicine* 21: 28-37.

Steinhaus, A.H. 1954. Some selected facts from physiology and the physiology of exercise applicable to physical rehabilitation. Paper presented to the study group on body mechanics, Washington, DC.

Stoessel, L., Stone, M.H., Keith, R., Marple, D., and Johnson, R. 1991. Selected physiological, psychological and performance characteristics of national-caliber United States women weightlifters. *Journal of Strength and Conditioning Research* 5: 87-95.

Stone, M.H. 1992. Connective tissue and bone response to strength training. In *Strength and power training in sport*, edited by P.V. Komi, 279-290. Oxford: Blackwell Scientific.

Stone, M.H., Fleck, S.J., Triplett, N.R., and Kraemer, W.J. 1991. Physiological adaptations to resistance training exercise. *Sports Medicine* 11: 210-231.

Stone, M.H., Johnson, R.C., and Carter, D.R. 1979. A short term comparison of two different methods of resistance training on leg strength and power. *Athletic Training* 14: 158-160.

Stone, M.H., Nelson, J.K., Nader, S., and Carter, D. 1983. Short-term weight training effects on resting and recovery heart rates. *Athletic Training* Spring: 69-71.

Stone, M.H., O'Bryant, H., and Garhammer, J.G. 1981. A hypothetical model for strength training. *Journal of Sports Medicine and Physical Fitness* 21: 342-351.

Stone, M.H., Plisk, S.S., Stone, M.E., Schilling, B.K., O'Bryant, H.S., and Pierce, K.C. 1998. Athletic performance development: Volume load—1 set vs. multiple sets, training velocity and training variation. *Strength and Conditioning* 20: 22-31.

Stone, M.H., Potteiger, J.A., Pierce, K.C., Proulx, C.M., O'Bryant, H.S., Johnson, R.L., and Stone, M.E. 2000. Comparison of the effects of three different weight-training programs on the one repetition maximum squat. *Journal of Strength and Conditioning Research* 14: 332-337.

Stone, M.H., Wilson, G.D., Blessing, D., and Rozenek, R. 1983. Cardiovascular responses to short-term Olympic style weight-training in young men. *Canadian Journal of Applied Sport Science* 8: 134-139.

Stone, W.J., and Coulter, S.P. 1994. Strength/endurance effects from three resistance training protocols with women. *Journal of Strength and Conditioning Research* 8: 231-234.

Stowers, T., McMillian, J., Scala, D., Davis, V., Wilson, D., and Stone, M. 1983. The short-term effects of three different strength-power training methods. *National Strength and Conditioning Association Journal* 5: 24-27.

Strasburger, C.J., Wu, Z., Pfaulm, C., and Dressendorfer, R.A. 1996. Immunofunctional assay of human growth hormone (hGH) in serum: A possible consensus of quantitative hGH measurement. *Journal of Clinical Endocrinology and Metabolism* 81: 2613-2620.

Straub, W.F. 1968. Effect of overload training procedures upon velocity and accuracy of the overarm throw. *Research Quarterly* 39: 370-379.

Sugiura, T., Matoba, H., Miyata, H., Kawai, Y,, and Murakami, N. 1992. Myosin heavy chain isoform transition in aging fast and slow muscles of the rat. *Acta Physiological Scandinavica* 144: 419-423.

Sullivan, M.K., Dejulia, J.J., and Worrell, T.W. 1992. Effect of pelvic position and stretching method on hamstring muscle flexibility. *Medicine and Science in Sports and Exercise* 24: 1383-1389.

Swanson, S.C., and Caldwell, G.E. 2000. An integrated biomechanical analysis of high speed incline and level treadmill running. *Medicine and Science in Sports and Exercise* 32: 1146-1155.

Syrovy, I., and Gutmann, E. 1970. Changes in speed of contraction and ATPase activity in striated muscle during old age. *Experimental Gerontology* 5: 31-35.

Szanberg, E., Jefferson, L.S., Lundholm, K., and Kimball, S.R. 1997. Postprandial stimulation of muscle protein synthesis is independent of changes in insulin. *American Journal of Physiology* 272: E841-847.

Szczypaczewska, M., Nazar, K., and Kaciuba-Uscilko, H. 1989. Glucose tolerance and insulin response to glucose load in body builders. *International Journal of Sports Medicine* 10: 34-37.

Taaffe, D.R., and Marcus, R. 1997. Dynamic muscle strength alterations to detraining and retraining in elderly men. *Clinical Physiology* 17: 311-324.

Taaffe, D.R., Pruitt, L., Reim, J., Hintz, R.L., Butterfield, G., Hoffman, A.R., and Marcus, R. 1994. Effect of recombinant human growth hormone on the muscle strength response to resistance exercise in elderly men. *Journal of Clinical Endocrinology and Metabolism* 79: 1361-1366.

Takarada, Y., and Ishii, N. 2002. Effects of low-intensity resistance exercise with short interest rest period on muscular function in middle-aged women. *Journal of Strength and Conditioning Research* 16: 123-128.

Takarada, Y., Takazawa, H., Sato, Y., Takebayashi, S., Tanaka, Y., and Ishii, Y. 2000. Effects of resistance exercise combined with moderate vascular occlusion on muscular function in humans. *Journal of Applied Physiology* 88: 2097-2106.

Talag, T.S. 1973. Residual muscular soreness as influenced by concentric, eccentric, and static contractions. *Research Quarterly* 44:458-461.

Tanner, J.M. 1964. *The physique of the Olympic athlete*. London: Allen and Unwin.

Tarnopolsky, M.A., Atkinson, S.A., MacDougall, J.D., Senor, B.B., Lemon, P.W., and Schwarcz, H. 1991. Whole body leucine metabolism during and after resistance exercise in fed humans. *Medicine and Science in Sports and Exercise* 23: 326-333.

Tarnopolsky, M.A., MacDougall, J.D., and Atkinson, S.A. 1988. Influence of protein intake and training status on nitrogen balance and lean body mass. *Journal of Applied Physiology* 64:187-193.

Tatro, D.L., Dudley, G.A., and Convertino, V.A. 1992. Carotidcardiac baroreflex response and LBNP tolerance following resistance training. *Medicine and Science in Sports and Exercise* 24: 789-796.

Taylor, J.M., Thompson, H.S., Clarkson, P.M., Miles, M.P., and DeSouza, M.J. 2000. Growth hormone response to an acute bout of resistance exercise in weight-trained and non-weight-trained women. *Journal of Strength and Conditioning Research* 14: 220-227.

Tesch, P.A. 1987. Acute and long-term metabolic changes consequent to heavy-resistance exercise. *Medicine and Science in Sports and Exercise* 26: 67-89.

Tesch, P.A. 1992. Short- and long-term histochemical and biochemical adaptations in muscle. In *Strength and power in sport*, edited by P.V. Komi, 239-248. Oxford: Blackwell Scientific.

Tesch, P.A., and Dudley, G.A. 1994. *Muscle meets magnet.* Published by P.A. Tesch, Stockholm, Sweden. Distributed by BookMaster, Inc, Mansfield, OH.

Tesch, P.A., Dudley, G.A., Duvoisin, M.R., Hather, B.M., and Harris, R.T. 1990. Force and EMG signal patterns during repeated bouts of concentric or eccentric muscle actions. *Acta Physiologica Scandinavica* 138: 263-271.

Tesch, P.A., Hjort, H., and Balldin, U.I. 1983. Effects of strength training on G tolerance. *Aviation, Space, and Environmental Medicine* 54: 691-695.

Tesch, P.A., Komi, P.V., and Häkkinen, K. 1987. Enzymatic adaptations consequent to long-term strength training. *International Journal of Sports Medicine* 8 (Suppl.): 66-69.

Tesch P.A., and Larsson L. 1982. Muscle hypertrophy in bodybuilders. *European Journal of Applied Physiology* 49: 301-306.

Tesch, P.A., Thorsson, A., and Colliander, E.B. 1990. Effects of eccentric and concentric resistance training on skeletal muscle substrates, enzyme activities and capillary supply. *Acta Physiologica Scandinavica* 140: 575-580.

Tesch, P.A., Thorsson, A., and Essen-Gustavsson, B. 1989. Enzyme activities of FT and ST muscle fibers in heavy-resistance trained athletes. *Journal of Applied Physiology* 67: 83-87.

Tesch, P.A., Thorsson, A., and Kaiser, P. 1984. Muscle capillary supply and fiber type characteristics in weight and power lifters. *Journal of Applied Physiology* 56: 35-38.

Tesch, P.A., Wright, J.E., Vogel, J.A., Daniels, W.L., Sharp, D.S., and Sjodin, B. 1985. The influence of muscle metabolic characteristics on physical performance. *European Journal of Applied Physiology* 54: 237-243.

Tharion, W.J., Rausch, T.M., Harman, E.A., and Kraemer, W.J. 1991. Effects of different resistance exercise protocols on mood states. *Journal of Applied Sport Science Research* 5: 60-65.

Thepaut-Mathieu, C., Van Hoecke, J., and Martin, B. 1988. Myoelectrical and mechanical changes linked to length specificity during isometric training. *Journal of Applied Physiology* 64: 1500-1505.

Thissen, J.P., Ketelslegers, J.M., and Underwood, L.E. 1994. Nutritional regulation of the insulin-like growth factors. *Endocrine Reviews* 15: 80-101.

Thistle, H.G., Hislop, H.J., Moffroid, M., and Lowman, E.W. 1967. Isokinetic contraction: A new concept in resistive exercise. *Archives of Physical Medicine and Rehabilitation* 48: 279-282.

Thompson, C.W., and Martin, E.T. 1965. Weight training and baseball throwing speed. *Journal of the Association of Physical and Mental Rehabilitation* 19: 194-196.

Thompson, D.B., and Chapman, A.E. 1988. The mechanical response of active human muscle during and after stretch. *European Journal of Applied Physiology* 57: 691-697.

Thompson, P.D., Sadanian, A., Cullinane, E.M., Bodziony, K.S., Catlin, D.H., Torek-Both, G., and Douglas, P.S. 1992. Left ventricular function is not impaired in weight-lifters who use anabolic steroids. *Journal of the American College of Cardiology* 19: 278-282.

Thorstensson, A. 1977. Observations on strength training and detraining. *Acta Physiologica Scandinavica* 100: 491-493.

Thorstensson, A., Hulten, B., von Dolben, W., and Karlsson, J. 1976. Effect of strength training on enzyme activities and fibre characteristics in human skeletal muscles. *Acta Physiologica Scandinavica* 96: 392-398.

Thorstensson, A., Karlsson, J., Viitasalo, J., Luhtanen, P., and Komi, P. 1976. Effect of strength training on EMG of human skeletal muscle. *Acta Physiologica Scandinavica* 98: 232-236.

Thrash, K., and Kelly, B. 1987. Flexibility and strength training. *Journal of Applied Sports Science Research* 1: 74-75.

Tikkanen, H.O., Naveri, H., and Harkonen, M. 1996. Skeletal muscle fiber distribution influences serum high-density lipoprotein cholesterol level. *Atherosclerosis* 120: 1-5.

Timonen, S., and Procope, B.J. 1971. Premenstrual syndrome and physical exercise. *Acta Obstetrica et Gynaecologica Scandinavica* 50: 331-337.

Timson, B.F., Bowlin, B.K., Dudenhoeffer, G.A., and George, J.B. 1985. Fiber number, area, and composition of mouse soleus muscle following enlargement. *Journal of Applied Physiology: Respiratory, Environmental and Exercise Physiology* 58: 619-624.

Tipton, C.M., Matthes, R.D., Maynard, J.A., and Carey, R.A. 1975. The influence of physical activity on ligaments and tendons. *Medicine and Science in Sports* 7: 34-41.

Tipton, K.D., Rasmussen, B.B., Miller, S.L., Wolf, S.E., Owens-Stovall, S.K., Petrini, B.E., and Wolfe, R.R. 2001. Timing of amino acid-carbohydrate ingestion alters anabolic response of muscle to resistance exercise. *American Journal of Physiology* 281: E197-206.

Tipton, K.D., and Wolfe, R.R. 1998. Exercise-induced changes in protein metabolism. *Acta Physiologica Scandinavica* 162: 377-387.

Todd, T. 1985. Historical perspective: The myth of the muscle-bound lifter. *National Strength and Conditioning Association Journal* 7: 37-41.

Tomberline, J.P., Basford, J.R., Schwen, E.E., Orte, P.A., Scott, S.C., Laughman, R.K., and Ilstrud, D.M. 1991. Comparative study of isokinetic eccentric and concentric quadriceps training. *The Journal of Orthopaedic and Sports Physical Therapy* 14: 31-36.

Tomlin, D.L., and Wenger, H.A. 2001. The relationship between aerobic fitness and recovery from high intensity intermittent exercise. *Sports Medicine* 31: 1-11.

Tomten, S.E., Falch, J.A., Birkenland, K.I., Hemmersbach, P., and Hostmark, A.T. 1998. Bone mineral density and menstrual irregularities. A comparative study on cortical and trabecular bone structures in runners with alleged normal eating behavior. *International Journal of Sportsmedicine* 19: 92-97.

Too, D., Wakatama, E.J., Locati, L.L., and Landwer, G.E. 1998. Effect of precompetition bodybuilding diet and training regime on body composition and blood chemistry. *Journal of Sports Medicine and Physical Fitness* 238: 45-52.

Trivedi, B., and Dansforth, W.H. 1966. Effect of pH on the kinetics of frog muscle phosphofructokinase. *Journal of Biology Chemistry* 241: 4110-4112.

Tsolakis, C., Messinis, D., Stergiolas, A., and Dessypris, A. 2000. Hormonal responses after strength training and detraining in prepubertal and pubertal boys. *Journal of Strength and Conditioning Research* 14: 399-404.

Tsuzuku, S., Ikegami, Y., and Yabe, K. 1998. Effects of high-intensity resistance training on bone mineral density in young male powerlifters. *Calcification Tissue International* 63: 283-286.

Tsuzuku, S., Shimokata, H., Ikegami, Y., Yabe, K., and Wasnich, R.D. 2001. Effects of high versus low-intensity resistance training on bone mineral density in young males. *Calcification Tissue International* 68: 342-347.

Tucci, J.T., Carpenter, D.M., Pollock, M.L., Graves, J.E., and Leggett, S.H. 1992. Effect of reduced frequency of training and detraining on lumbar extension strength. *Spine* 17: 1497-1501.

Turner, J.D., Rotwein, P., Novakofski, J., and Bechtel, P.J. 1988. Induction of messenger RNA for IGF-I and –II during growth hormone-stimulated muscle hypertrophy. *American Journal of Physiology* 255: E513-517.

Turto, H., Lindy, S., and Halme, J. 1974. Protocollagen proline hydroxylase activity in work-induced hypertrophy of rat muscle. *American Journal of Physiology* 226: 63-65.

Twisk. J.W.R. 2001. Physical activity guidelines for children and adolescents a critical review. *Sports Medicine* 31: 617-627.

Twisk, J.W.R., Kemper, H.C.G., and van Mechelen, W. 2000. Tracking of activity and fitness and the relationship with cardiovascular disease risk factors. *Medicine and Science in Sports and Exercise* 32: 1455-1461.

Urhausen, A., and Kindermann, W. 1992. Echocardiographic findings in strength- and endurance-trained athletes. *Sports Medicine* 13: 270-284.

Van der Ploeg, G.E., Brooks, A.G., Withers, R.T., Dollman, J., Leaney, F., and Chatterton, B.E. 2001. Body composition changes in female bodybuilders during preparation for competition. *European Journal of Clinical Nutrition* 55: 268-277.

Vandervoot, A.A., Sale, D.G., and Moroz, J. 1984. Comparison of motor unit activation during unilateral and bilateral leg extensions. *Journal of Applied Physiology: Respiratory, Environmental and Exercise Physiology* 56: 46-51.

Vandervoot, A.A., and Symons, T.B. 2001. Functional and metabolic consequences of sarcopenia. *Canadian Journal of Applied Physiology* 26: 90-101.

Vanhelder, W.P., Radomski, M.W., and Goode, R.C. 1984. Growth hormone responses during intermittent weight lifting exercise in men. *European Journal of Applied Physiology and Occupational Physiology* 53: 31-34.

Verhoshanski, V. 1967. Are depth jumps useful? *Track and Field* 12: 9.

Vermeulen, A., Rubens, R., and Verdonck, L. 1972. Testosterone secretion and metabolism in male senescence. *Journal of Clinical Endocrinology* 34: 730-735.

Viitassalo, J.T., Komi, P.V., and Karovonen, M.J. 1979. Muscle strength and body composition as determinants of blood pressure in young men. *European Journal of Applied Physiology* 42: 165-173.

Vitcenda, M., Hanson, P., Folts, J., and Besozzi, M. 1990. Impairment of left ventricular function during maximal isometric dead lifting. *Journal of Applied Physiology* 691: 2062-2066.

Volek, J.S., Duncan, N.D., Mazzetti, S.A., Staron, R.S., Putukian, M.P., Gomez, A.L., Pearson, D.R., Fink, W.J., and Kraemer, W.J. 1999. Performance and muscle fiber adaptations to creatine supplementation and heavy resistance training. *Medicine and Science in Sports and Exercise* 31: 1147-1156.

Volek, J.S., and Kraemer, W.J. 1996. Creatine supplementation: its effect on human muscular performance and body composition. *Journal of Strength and Conditioning Research* 10: 200-210.

Volek, J.S., Kraemer, W.J., Bush, J.A., Incledon, T., and Boetes, M. 1997. Testosterone and cortisol in relationship to dietary nutrients and resistance exercise. *Journal of Applied Physiology* 82: 49-54.

Volpe, S.L., Walberg-Rankin, J., Rodman, K.W., and Sebolt, D.R. 1993. The effect of endurance running on training adaptations in women participating in a weight lifting program. *Journal of Strength and Conditioning Research* 7: 101-107.

Vorobyev, A.N. 1988. Part 12: Musculo-skeletal and circulatory effects of weightlifting. *Soviet Sports Review* 23: 144-148.

Vossen, J.E., Kramer, J.E., Burke, D.G., and Vossen, D.P. 2000. Comparison of dynamic push-up training and plyometric push-up training on upper-body power and strength. *Journal of Strength and Conditioning Research* 14: 248-253.

Vrijens, J. 1978. Muscle strength development in the pre- and post-pubescent age. *Medicine and Sports* (Basel) 11: 152-158.

Wagner, D.R., and Kocak, M.S. 1997. A multivariate approach to assessing anaerobic power following a plyometric training program. *Journal of Strength and Conditioning Research* 11: 251-255.

Walberg, J.L., and Johnston, C.S. 1991. Menstrual function and eating behavior in female recreational weight lifters and competitive body builders. *Medicine and Science in Sports and Exercise* 23: 30-36.

Walberg-Rankin, J., Edmonds, C.E., and Gwazdauskas, F.C. 1993. Diet and weight changes of female bodybuilders before and after competition. *International Journal of Sports Medicine* 3: 87-102.

Walberg-Rankin, J., Franke, W.D., and Gwazdauskas, F.C. 1992. Response of beta-endorphin and estradiol to resistance exercise in females during energy balance and energy restriction. *International Journal of Sports Medicine*, 13: 542-547.

Waldeger, S., Busch, G.L., Kaba, N.K., Zempel, G., Ling, H., Heidland, A., Haussinger, D., and Lang, F. 1997. Effect of cellular hydration on protein metabolism. *Mineral and Electrolyte Metabolism* 23: 201-205.

Waldman, R., and Stull, G. 1969. Effects of various periods of inactivity on retention of newly acquired levels of muscular endurance. *Research Quarterly* 40: 393-401.

Walker, P.M., Brunotte, F., Rouhier-Marcer, I., Cottin, Y., Casillas, J.M., Gras, P., and Didier, J.P. 1998. Nuclear magnetic resonance evidence of different muscular adaptations after resistance training. *Archives of Physical Medicine and Rehabilitation* 79: 1391-1398.

Wallace, J.D., Cuneo, R.C., Bidlingmaier, M., Lundberg, P.A., Carlsson, L., Luiz, C., Boguszewski, C.L., Hay, J., Healy, M.L., Napoli, R., Dall, R., Rosén, T., and Strasburger, C.J. 2001. The response of molecular isoforms of growth hormone to acute exercise in trained adult males. *Journal of Clinical Endocrinology and Metabolism* 86: 200-206.

Wallace, M.B., Lim, J., Cutler, A., and Bucci, L. 1999. Effects of dehydroepiandrosterone vs. androstenedione supplementation in men. *Medicine and Science in Sports and Exercise* 31: 1788-1792.

Wallace, M.B., Moffatt, R.J., Haymes, E.M., and Green, N.R. 1991. Acute effects of resistance exercise on parameters of lipoprotein metabolism. *Medicine and Science in Sports and Exercise* 23: 199-204.

Wang, N., Hikida, R.S., Staron, R.S., and Simoneau, J.-A. 1993. Muscle fiber types of women after resistance training-quantitative ultrastructure and enzyme activity. *Pflugers Archives* 424: 494-502.

Ward, J., and Fisk, G.H. 1964. The difference in response of the quadriceps and biceps brachii muscles to isometric and isotonic exercise. *Archives of Physical Medicine and Rehabilitation* 45: 612-620.

Ware, J.S., Clemens, C.T., Mayhew, J.L., and Johnston, T.J. 1995. Muscular endurance repetitions to predict bench press and squat strength in college football players. *Journal of Strength and Conditioning Research* 9: 99-103.

Warren, B.J., Stone, M.H., Kearney, J.T., Fleck S.J., Johnson, R.L., Wilson, G.D., and Kraemer, W.J. 1992. Performance measures, blood lactate and plasma ammonia as indicators of overwork in elite junior weightlifters. *International Journal of Sports Medicine* 13: 372-376.

Warren, G.L., Hermann, K.M., Ingallis, C.P., Masselli, M.A., and Armstrong, R.B. 2000. Decreased EMG median frequency during a second bout of eccentric contractions. *Medicine and Science in Sports and Exercise* 32: 820-829.

Wasserman, D.H., Connely, C.C., and Pagliassotti, M.J. 1991. Regulation of hepatic lactate balance during exercise. *Medicine and Science in Sports and Exercise* 23: 912-919.

Weaver, C.M., Teegarden, D., Lyle, R.M., McCabe, G.P., McCabe, L.D., Proullx, W., Kern, M., Sedlock, D., Anderson, D.D., Hillberry, B.M., Peacock, M., and Johnston, c.C. 2001. Impact of exercise on bone health and contraindication of oral contraceptive use in young women. *Medicine and Science in Sports and Exercise,* 33:873-880.

Weider, J. 1954. Cheating exercises build the biggest muscles. *Muscle Builder* 3: 60-61.

Weir, J.P., Housh, D.J., Housh, T.J., and Weir, L.L. 1997. The effect of unilateral concentric weight training and detraining on joint angle specificity, cross-training, and the bilateral deficit. *Journal of Orthopedic Sports Physical Therapy* 25: 264-270.

Weir, J.P., Housh, T.J., and Weir, L.L. 1994. Electromyographic evaluation of joint angle specificity and cross-training after isometric training. *Journal of Applied Physiology* 77: 197-201.

Weir, J.P., Housh, T.J., Weir, L.L., and Johnson, G.O. 1995. Effects of unilateral isometric strength training and joint angle specificity and cross training. *European Journal of Applied Physiology* 70: 337-343.

Weiss, L.W., Coney, H.D., and Clark, F.C. 1999. Differential functional adaptations to short-term low-, moderate-, and high-repetition weight training. *Journal of Strength and Conditioning Research* 13: 236-241.

Weiss, L.W., Cureton, K.J., and Thompson, F.N. 1983. Comparison of serum testosterone and androstenedione responses to weight lifting in men and women. *European Journal of Applied Physiology* 50: 413-419.

Wells, J.B., Jokl, E., and Bohanen, J. 1973. The effects of intense physical training upon body composition of adolescent girls. *Journal of the Association for Physical and Mental Rehabilitation* 17: 63-72.

Weltman, A., Janney, C., Rians, C., Strand, K., Berg, B., Tippit, S., Wise, J., Cahill, B., and Katch, F. 1986. The effects of hydraulic resistance strength training in pre-pubertal males. *Medicine and Science in Sports and Exercise* 18: 629-638.

Westcott, W. 1994. High-intensity training. *Nautilus* 4 (1): 5-8.

Westcott, W. 1995. High intensity strength training. *IDEA Personal Trainer* 6: 9.

Westcott, W.L., Winett, R.A., Anderson, E.S., Wojcik, J.R., Loud, R.L.R., Cleggett, E., and Glover, S. 2001. Effects of regular and slow speed resistance training on muscle strength. *Journal of Sports Medicine and Physical Fitness* 41: 154-158.

Wickiewicz, T.L., Roy, R.R., Powell, P.L., Perrine, J.J., and Edgerton, B.R. 1984. Muscle architecture and force-velocity relationships in humans. *Journal of Applied Physiology: Respiratory, Environmental and Exercise Physiology* 57: 435-443.

Widholm, O. 1979. Dysmenorrhea during adolescence. *Act Obstetrica et Gynaecologica Scandinavic* 87:61-66.

Wiemann, K., and Hahn, K. 1997. Influences of strength, stretching, and circulatory exercises on flexibility parameters of the human hamstrings. *International Journal of Sports Medicine* 18: 340-346.

Willett, G.M., Hyde, J.E., Uhrlaub, M.B., Wendl, C.L., and Karst, G.M. 2001. Relative activity of abdominal muscles during commonly prescribed strengthening exercises. *Journal of Strength and Conditioning Research* 15: 480-485.

Williams, A.G., Ismail, A.N., Sharma, A., and Jones, D.A. 2002. Effects of resistance exercise volume and nutritional supplementation on anabolic and catabolic hormones. *European Journal of Applied Physiology* 86(4): 315-321.

Williams, M., and Stutzman, L. 1959. Strength variation throughout the range of joint motion. *Physical Therapy Review* 39: 145-152.

Williams, N.I., Bullen, B.A., McArthur, J.W., Skrinar, G.S., and Turnbull, B.A. 1999. Effects of short-term strenuous endurance exercise upon corpus luteum function. *Medicine and Science in Sports and Exercise* 31: 949-958.

Williams, N.I., Young, J.C., McArthur, J.W., Bullen, B., Skrinar, G.S., and Turnbull, B. 1995. Strenuous exercise with caloric restriction: Effect on luteinizing hormone secretion. *Medicine and Science in Sports and Exercise* 27: 1390-1398.

Williams, P.T., Stefanick, M.L., Vranizan, K.M., and Wood, P.D. 1994. The effects of weight loss of exercise or by dieting on plasma high-density lipoprotein (HDL) levels in man with low, intermediate, and normal-to-high HDL at baseline. *Metabolism* 43: 917-924.

Willoughby, D.S. 1992. A comparison of three selected weight training programs on the upper and lower body strength of trained males. *Annual Journal Applied Research in Coaching Athletics* March: 124-146.

Willoughby, D.S. 1993. The effects of meso-cycle-length weight training programs involving periodization and partially equated volumes on upper and lower body strength. *Journal of Strength and Conditioning Research* 7: 2-8.

Willoughby, D.S., Chilek, D.R., Schiller, D.A., and Coast, J.R. 1991. The metabolic effects of three different free weight parallel squatting intensities. *Journal of Human Movement Studies* 21: 53-67.

Willy, R.M., Kyle, B.A., Moore, S.A., and Chileboun, G.S. 2001 Effect of cessation and resumption of static hamstring muscle stretching on joint range of motion. *Journal of Orthopedic Sports Physical Therapy* 31: 138-144.

Wilmore, J.H. 1974. Alterations in strength, body composition, and anthropometric measurements consequent to a 10-week weight training program. *Medicine and Science in Sports* 6: 133-138.

Wilmore, J.H., and Costill DL. 1994. *Physiology of sport and exercise*. Champaign, IL: Human Kinetics.

Wilmore, J.H., Parr, R.B., Girandola, R.N., Ward, P., Vodak, P.A., Barstow, T.J., Pipes, T.V., Romero, G.T., and Leslie, P. 1978. Physiological alterations consequent to circuit weight training. *Medicine and Science in Sports* 10: 79-84.

Wilson, G.J. 1994. Strength and power in sport. In *Applied anatomy and biomechanics in sport*, edited by J. Bloomfield, T.R. Aukland, and B.C., Elliott, 110-208. Boston: Blackwell Scientific.

Wilson, G.J., and Murphy, A.J. 1996. The use of isometric tests of muscular function in athletic assessment. *Sports Medicine* 22: 19-37.

Wilson, G.J., Newton, R.U., Murphy, A.J., and Humphries, B.J. 1993. The optimal training load for the development of dynamic athletic performance. *Medicine and Science in Sports and Exercise* 25: 1279-1286.

Wilt, F. 1968. Training for competitive running. In *Exercise physiology*, edited by H.B. Falls, 395-414. New York: Academic Press.

Winters, K.M., and Snow, C.M. 2000. Detraining reverses positive effects of exercise on the musculoskeletal system in premenopausal women. *Journal of Bone and Mineral Research* 15: 2495-2503.

Wiswell, R.A., Hawkins, S.A., Jaque, S.V., Hyslop, D., Constantino, N., Tarpenning, K., Marcell, T., Schroeder, E.T. 2001. Relationship between physiological loss, performance decrement, and age in master athletes. *Journal of Gerontology: Biological Sciences, Medical Sciences* 56: M618-M626.

Withers, R.T. 1970. Effect of varied weight-training loads on the strength of university freshmen. *Research Quarterly* 41: 110-114.

Withers, R.T., Noell, C.J., Whittingham, N.O., Chatterton, B.E., Schultz, C.G., and Keeves, J.P. 1997. Body composition changes in elite male bodybuilders during preparation for competition. *Australian Journal of Science and Medicine in Sport* 29: 11-16.

Wolfe, L.A., Cunningham, D.A., and Boughner, D.R. 1986. Physical conditioning effects on cardiac dimensions: A review of echocardiographic studies. *Canadian Journal of Applied Sport Science* 11: 66-79.

Wolfe, R.R. 2000. Effects of insulin on muscle tissue. *Current Opinion in Clinical Nutrition and Metabolic Care* 3: 67-71.

Wolinsky, F.D., and Fitzgerald, J.F. 1994. Subsequent hip fracture among older adults. *American Journal of Public Health* 84: 1316-1318.

Wright, J.E. 1980. Anabolic steroids and athletics. In *Exercise and sport sciences reviews*, edited by R.S. Hutton and D.I. Miller, 149-202. The Franklin Institute.

Wright, J.R., McCloskey, D.I., and Fitzpatrick, R.C. 2000. Effects of systemic arterial blood pressure on the contractile force of a human hand muscle. *Journal of Applied Physiology* 88: 1390-1396.

Yao, W., Fuglevand, R.J., and Enoka, R.M. 2000. Motor-unit synchronization increases EMG amplitude and decreases force steadiness of simulated contractions. *Journal of Neurophysiology* 83: 441-452.

Yaresheski, K.E. 1994. Growth hormone effects on metabolism, body composition, muscle mass and strength. *Exercise and Sport Sciences Reviews* 22: 288-312.

Yaresheski, K.E., Campbell, J.A., Smith, K., Rennie, M.J., Holloszy, J.O., and Bier, D.M. 1992. Effect of growth hormone and resistance exercise on muscle growth in young men. *American Journal of Applied Physiology* 262: E261-E267.

Yaresheski, K.E., Zachwieja, J.J., and Bier, D.M. 1993. Acute effects of resistance exercise on muscle protein synthesis rate in young and elderly men and women. *American Journal of Applied Physiology* 265: 210-214.

Yaresheski, K.E., Zachwieja, J.J., Campbell, J.A., and Bier, D.M. 1995. Effect of growth hormone and resistance exercise on muscle growth and strength in older men. *American Journal of Physiology* 268: E268-E276.

Yates, J.W., and Kamon, E. 1983. A comparison of peak and constant angle torque-velocity curves in fast and slow twitch populations. *European Journal of Applied Physiology* 51: 67-74.

Young, A., and Skelton, D.A. 1994. Applied physiology of strength and power in old age. *International Journal of Sports Medicine* 15: 149-151.

Young, A., Stokes, M., and Crowe, M. 1984. Size and strength of the quadriceps muscles of old and young women. *European Journal of Clinical Investigation* 14: 282-287.

Young, N., Formica, C., Szmukler, G., and Seeman, E. 1994. Bone density at weight-bearing and non-weight-bearing sites in ballet dancers: The effects of exercise, hypogonadism, and body weight. *Journal of Endocrinology Metabolism* 78: 449-454.

Young W., and Elliott, S. 2001. Acute effects of static stretching, proprioceptive neuromuscular facilitation stretching, and maximum voluntary contractions on explosive force production and jumping performance. *Research Quarterly Exercise and Sport* 72: 273-279.

Young, W.B. 1993. Training for speed/strength: Heavy versus light loads. *National Strength and Conditioning Association Journal* 15: 34-42.

Young, W.B., and Bilby, G.E. 1993. The effect of voluntary effort to influence speed of contraction on strength, muscular power and hypertrophy development. *Journal of Strength and Conditioning Research* 7: 172-178.

Young W.B., McDowell, M.H., and Scarlett, B.J. 2001. Specificity of sprint and agility training methods. *Journal of Strength and Conditioning Research* 15: 315-319.

Yudkin, J., and Cohen, R.D. 1974. The contribution of the kidney to the removal of a lactic acid load under normal and acidotic conditions in the conscious rat. *Clinical Science and Molecular Medicine* 46: 9.

Zapf, J. 1997. Total and free IGF serum levels. *European Journal of Endocrinology* 136: 146-147.

Zatsiorsky, V. 1995. *Science and practice of strength training*. Champaign, IL: Human Kinetics.

Zemper, E.D. 1990. Four year study of weight room injuries in national sample of college football teams. *National Strength and Conditioning Association Journal* 12: 32-34.

Zernicke, R.F., and Loitz, B.J. 1992. Exercise related adaptations in connective tissue. In *Strength and power in sport*, edited by P.V. Komi, 77-95. Oxford: Blackwell Scientific.

Zinovieff, A. 1951. Heavy resistance exercise: The Oxford technique. *British Journal of Physical Medicine* 14: 129-132.

Zrubak, A. 1972. Body composition and muscle strength of body builders. *Acta Facultatis Rerum Naturalium Universitatis Comenianae Anthropologia* 11: 135-144.

Index

About the Authors

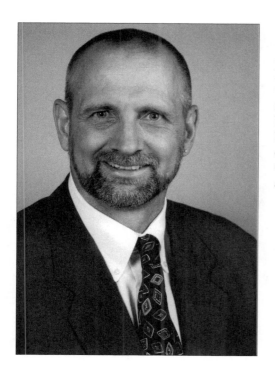

Steven J. Fleck is chair of the sport science department at Colorado College in Colorado Springs. He earned a PhD in exercise physiology from The Ohio State University in 1978. He has headed the physical conditioning program of the U.S. Olympic Committee, served as strength coach for the German Volleyball Association, and coached high school track, basketball, and football. Dr. Fleck is a past vice president of basic and applied research for the National Strength and Conditioning Association (NSCA) and is a fellow of the American College of Sports Medicine (ACSM). He was honored in 1991 as the NSCA Sport Scientist of the Year.

William J. Kraemer is a professor in the department of kinesiology working in the Human Performance Laboratory at the University of Connecticut at Storrs. He also is a professor in the department of physiology and neurobiology and a professor of medicine at the University of Connecticut Health Center School of Medicine. He earned a PhD in physiology and biochemistry from the University of Wyoming in 1984. Dr. Kraemer is a past president of the National Strength and Conditioning Association (NSCA) and a fellow in the American College of Sports Medicine (ACSM). He was awarded the NSCA's Lifetime Achievement , Outstanding Award (1994) and the Education of the Year Award (2002). He is also editor-in-chief of the *Journal of Strength and Conditioning Research*.

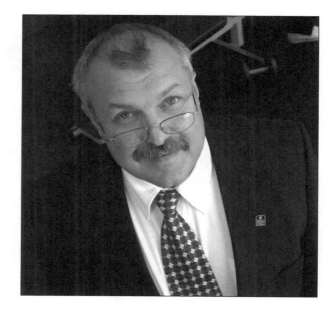

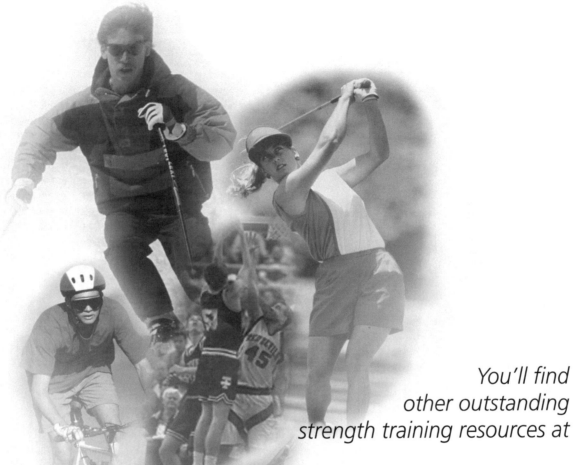